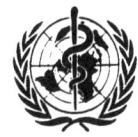

WORLD HEALTH ORGANIZATION

INTERNATIONAL AGENCY FOR RESEARCH ON CANCER

# IARC MONOGRAPHS
## ON THE
# EVALUATION OF CARCINOGENIC
# RISKS TO HUMANS

Diesel and Gasoline Engine Exhausts
and Some Nitroarenes

VOLUME 46

This publication represents the views and expert opinions
of an IARC Working Group on the
Evaluation of Carcinogenic Risks to Humans,
which met in Lyon,

14–21 June 1988

1989

# IARC MONOGRAPHS

In 1969, the International Agency for Research on Cancer (IARC) initiated a programme on the evaluation of the carcinogenic risk of chemicals to humans involving the production of critically evaluated monographs on individual chemicals. In 1980, the programme was expanded to include the evaluation of the carcinogenic risk associated with exposures to complex mixtures.

The objective of the programme is to elaborate and publish in the form of monographs critical reviews of data on carcinogenicity for chemicals and complex mixtures to which humans are known to be exposed, and on specific exposures, to evaluate these data in terms of human risk with the help of international working groups of experts in chemical carcinogenesis and related fields, and to indicate where additional research efforts are needed.

This project is supported by PHS Grant No. 5-UO1 CA33193-06 awarded by the US National Cancer Institute, Department of Health and Human Services. Additional support has been provided by the Commission of the European Communities since 1986.

©International Agency for Research on Cancer 1989

ISBN 92 832 1246 0

ISSN 0250-9555

All rights reserved. Application for rights of reproduction or translation, in part or *in toto*, should be made to the International Agency for Research on Cancer.

Distributed for the International Agency for Research on Cancer
by the Secretariat of the World Health Organization

PRINTED IN THE UK

# CONTENTS

NOTE TO THE READER .................................................... 5

LIST OF PARTICIPANTS .................................................. 7

PREAMBLE ............................................................. 11
    Background ....................................................... 13
    Objective and Scope .............................................. 13
    Selection of Topics for Monographs ............................... 14
    Data for Monographs .............................................. 15
    The Working Group ................................................ 15
    Working Procedures ............................................... 15
    Exposure Data .................................................... 16
    Biological Data Relevant to the Evaluation of Carcinogenicity to Humans .... 17
    Evidence for Carcinogenicity in Experimental Animals ............. 18
    Other Relevant Data in Experimental Systems and Humans ........... 20
    Evidence for Carcinogenicity in Humans ........................... 21
    Summary of Data Reported ......................................... 24
    Evaluation ....................................................... 25
    References ....................................................... 28

GENERAL REMARKS ON THE AGENTS CONSIDERED ............................. 31

THE MONOGRAPHS

    Diesel and gasoline engine exhausts .............................. 41
        Composition of engine exhausts ............................... 41
            Introduction ............................................. 41
            Diesel engine exhaust .................................... 47
            Gasoline engine exhaust .................................. 53
            Comparison of emissions from different engines ........... 57
        Occurrence and analysis ...................................... 58
            Occupational exposure .................................... 58
                Workers whose predominant exhaust exposure is that from diesel
                engines ................................................ 59
                Workers whose predominant exhaust exposure is that from gasoline
                engines ................................................ 69
            Environmental exposure ................................... 74
            Analysis ................................................. 80

## CONTENTS

Biological data relevant to the evaluation of carcinogenic risk to humans ... 88
  Carcinogenicity studies in animals ... 88
    Diesel engine exhaust ... 88
    Gasoline engine exhaust ... 98
  Other relevant data ... 105
    Experimental systems ... 105
    Humans ... 128
  Epidemiological studies of carcinogenicity to humans ... 132
    Introduction ... 132
    Mortality and morbidity statistics ... 133
    Cohort studies ... 133
    Case-control studies ... 138
    Childhood cancer ... 145
  Summary of data reported and evaluation ... 148
  References ... 155

Some nitroarenes
  3,7-Dinitrofluoranthene ... 189
  3,9-Dinitrofluoranthene ... 195
  1,3-Dinitropyrene ... 201
  1,6-Dinitropyrene ... 215
  1,8-Dinitropyrene ... 231
  7-Nitrobenz[a]anthracene ... 247
  6-Nitrobenzo[a]pyrene ... 255
  6-Nitrochrysene ... 267
  2-Nitrofluorene ... 277
  1-Nitronaphthalene ... 291
  2-Nitronaphthalene ... 303
  3-Nitroperylene ... 313
  1-Nitropyrene ... 321
  2-Nitropyrene ... 359
  4-Nitropyrene ... 367

SUMMARY OF FINAL EVALUATIONS ... 375

APPENDIX 1. ACTIVITY PROFILES FOR GENETIC AND RELATED TESTS ... 377

SUPPLEMENTARY CORRIGENDA TO VOLUMES 1–45 ... 419

CUMULATIVE INDEX TO THE *MONOGRAPHS* SERIES ... 421

# NOTE TO THE READER

The term 'carcinogenic risk' in the *IARC Monographs* series is taken to mean the probability that exposure to an agent will lead to cancer in humans.

Inclusion of an agent in the *Monographs* does not imply that it is a carcinogen, only that the published data have been examined. Equally, the fact that an agent has not yet been evaluated in a monograph does not mean that it is not carcinogenic.

The evaluations of carcinogenic risk are made by international working groups of independent scientists and are qualitative in nature. No recommendation is given for regulation or legislation.

Anyone who is aware of published data that may alter the evaluation of the carcinogenic risk of an agent to humans is encouraged to make this information available to the Unit of Carcinogen Identification and Evaluation, International Agency for Research on Cancer, 150 cours Albert Thomas, 69372 Lyon Cedex 08, France, in order that the agent may be considered for re-evaluation by a future working group.

Although every effort is made to prepare the monographs as accurately as possible, mistakes may occur. Readers are requested to communicate any errors to the Unit of Carcinogen Identification and Evaluation, so that corrections can be reported in future volumes.

# IARC WORKING GROUP ON THE EVALUATION OF CARCINOGENIC RISKS TO HUMANS: DIESEL AND GASOLINE ENGINE EXHAUSTS AND SOME NITROARENES

## Lyon, 14–21 June 1988

**Members**

F.A. Beland, Division of Biochemical Toxicology HFT-110, National Center for Toxicological Research, Jefferson, AR 72079, USA

A. Brøgger, Department of Genetics, Institute for Cancer Research, The Norwegian Radium Hospital, Montebello, 0310 Oslo 3, Norway (*Chairman*)

R.A. Cartwright, Leukaemia Research Fund for Clinical Epidemiology at the University of Leeds, Department of Pathology, 17 Springfield Mount, Leeds LS2 9NG, UK

U. Heinrich, Fraunhofer Institute for Toxicology and Aerosol Research, Nikolai Fuchs Strasse 1, 3000 Hannover 61, Federal Republic of Germany

B. Holmberg, Department of Toxicology, National Institute of Occupational Health, 17184 Solna, Sweden

J. Jacob, Biochemical Institute of Environmental Carcinogens, Lurup 4, 2070 Grosshansdorf, Federal Republic of Germany

M. Jacobsen, Institute of Occupational Medicine, Roxburgh Place, Edinburgh EH8 9SU, UK

V.A. Koblyakov, Laboratory of Chemical Carcinogenesis, Institute of Carcinogenesis, Cancer Research Center, Kashirskoye shosse 24, 115478 Moscow, USSR

J. Lewtas, Genetic Bioassay Branch (MD 68), Health Effects Research Laboratory, Environmental Protection Agency, Research Triangle Park, NC 27711, USA (*Vice-chairman*)

J. McCammon, Division of Standards Development and Technology Transfer, National Institute for Occupational Safety and Health, 4676 Columbia Parkway, Cincinnati, OH 45226, USA

R.O. McClellan, Lovelace Inhalation Toxicology Research Institute, PO Box 5890, Albuquerque, NM 87185, USA

O. Pelkonen, Department of Pharmacology and Toxicology, University of Oulu, Kajaanintie 52 D, 90220 Oulu, Finland

J.M. Peters, Division of Occupational Health, Department of Preventive Medicine, University of Southern California School of Medicine, Parkview Medical Building B-306, Los Angeles, CA 90033, USA

F. Pott, Medical Institute of Environmental Hygiene of the University of Düsseldorf, Postfach 5634, 4000 Düsseldorf 1, Federal Republic of Germany

J.N. Pritchard, Environmental Medical Sciences Division, Harwell Laboratory, Building 551, Harwell, Oxfordshire OX11 0RA, UK

H.S. Rosenkranz, Department of Environmental Health Sciences, Case Western Reserve University School of Medicine, Cleveland, OH 44106, USA

T. Sanner, Laboratory for Environmental and Occupational Cancer, Institute for Cancer Research, The Norwegian Radium Hospital, Montebello, 0310 Oslo 3, Norway

D. Schuetzle, Analytical Sciences Department, Ford Motor Co. Scientific Research Laboratory, Room S-3083, 20 000 Rotunda Drive, Dearborn, MI 48121, USA

F.E. Speizer, Channing Laboratory, Harvard Medical School, 180 Longwood Avenue, Boston, MA 02115, USA

A. Tossavainen, Institute for Occupational Health, Topeliuksenkatu 41 a A, 00250 Helsinki, Finland

H. Tsuda, Department of Pathology, Nagoya City University Medical School, 1 Kawasumi, Muzuho-cho, Mizuho-ku, Nagoya 467, Japan

P. Vineis, Department of Biomedical Science and Human Oncology, Chair of Tumour Epidemiology, University of Turin, via Santena 7, 10126 Turin, Italy

**Representatives/Observers**

*Representative of the National Cancer Institute*

D. Silverman[1], Division of Cancer Etiology, National Cancer Institute, Landow Building, Room 3B04, Bethesda, MD 20892, USA

*Representative of the Commission of the European Communities*

E. Krug, Commission of the European Communities, Health and Safety Directorate, Bâtiment Jean Monnet, Plateau du Kirchberg, BP 1907, 2920 Luxembourg, Grand Duchy of Luxembourg

---

[1]Unable to attend

*Representative of Tracor Technology Resources, Inc.*

S. Olin, Tracor Technology Resources, Inc., 1601 Research Boulevard, Rockville, MD 20850, USA

*Committee of Common Market Automobile Constructors*

H. Klingenberg, Department of Research—Measurement Techniques, Volkswagen AG, Postfach, 3180 Wolfsburg, Federal Republic of Germany

*Health Effects Institute*

R. Shaikh, Health Effects Institute, 215 First Street, Cambridge, MA 02142, USA

*International Organization of Motor Vehicle Manufacturers*

W. Stoeber, Fraunhofer Institute for Toxicology and Aerosol Research, Nikolai Fuchs Strasse 1, 3000 Hannover 61, Federal Republic of Germany

**Secretariat**

A. Aitio, Unit of Carcinogen Identification and Evaluation (*Officer in Charge of the Programme*)
H. Bartsch, Unit of Enviromental Carcinogens and Host Factors
J.R.P. Cabral, Unit of Mechanisms of Carcinogenesis
E. Cardis, Unit of Biostatistics Research and Informatics
M. Coleman, Unit of Descriptive Epidemiology
M. Friesen, Unit of Environmental Carcinogens and Host Factors
M.-J. Ghess, Unit of Carcinogen Identification and Evaluation
M. Gilbert, International Programme on Chemical Safety, World Health Organization, Geneva, Switzerland
E. Heseltine, Lajarthe, Montignac, France
T. Kauppinen, Unit of Carcinogen Identification and Evaluation (*Co-secretary*)
D. Mietton, Unit of Carcinogen Identification and Evaluation
R. Montesano, Unit of Mechanisms of Carcinogenesis
I. O'Neill, Unit of Environmental Carcinogens
C. Partensky, Unit of Carcinogen Identification and Evaluation
I. Peterschmitt, Unit of Carcinogen Identification and Evaluation, Geneva, Switzerland
R. Saracci, Unit of Analytical Epidemiology
D. Shuker, Unit of Environmental Carcinogens and Host Factors
L. Shuker, Unit of Carcinogen Identification and Evaluation (*Co-secretary*)
L. Simonato, Unit of Analytical Epidemiology
L. Tomatis, Director

V. Turusov, Director's Office
J.D. Wilbourn, Unit of Carcinogen Identification and Evaluation
H. Yamasaki, Unit of Mechanisms of Carcinogenesis

*Secretarial assistance*
- J. Cazeaux
- M. Lézère
- S. Reynaud

# PREAMBLE

# IARC MONOGRAPHS PROGRAMME ON THE EVALUATION OF CARCINOGENIC RISKS TO HUMANS[1]

## PREAMBLE

### 1. BACKGROUND

In 1969, the International Agency for Research on Cancer (IARC) initiated a programme to evaluate the carcinogenic risk of chemicals to humans and to produce monographs on individual chemicals. The *Monographs* programme has since been expanded to include consideration of exposures to complex mixtures of chemicals (which occur, for example, in some occupations and as a result of human habits) and of exposures to other agents, such as radiation and viruses. With Supplement 6(1), the title of the series was modified from *IARC Monographs on the Evaluation of the Carcinogenic Risk of Chemicals to Humans* to *IARC Monographs on the Evaluation of Carcinogenic Risks to Humans*, in order to reflect the widened scope of the programme.

The criteria established in 1971 to evaluate carcinogenic risk to humans were adopted by the working groups whose deliberations resulted in the first 16 volumes of the *IARC Monographs* series. Those criteria were subsequently re-evaluated by working groups which met in 1977(2), 1978(3), 1979(4), 1982(5) and 1983(6). The present preamble was prepared by two working groups which met in September 1986 and January 1987, prior to the preparation of Supplement 7(7) to the *Monographs* and was modified by a working group which met in November 1988(8).

### 2. OBJECTIVE AND SCOPE

The objective of the programme is to prepare, with the help of international working groups of experts, and to publish in the form of monographs, critical reviews and evaluations of evidence on the carcinogenicity of a wide range of agents to which humans are or may be exposed. The *Monographs* may also indicate where additional research efforts are needed.

---

[1]This project is supported by PHS Grant No. 5 UO1 CA33193-06 awarded by the US National Cancer Institute, Department of Health and Human Services, and with a subcontract to Tracor Technology Resources, Inc. Since 1986, this programme has also been supported by the Commission of the European Communities.

The *Monographs* represent the first step in carcinogenic risk assessment, which involves examination of all relevant information in order to assess the strength of the available evidence that, under certain conditions of exposure, an agent could alter the incidence of cancer in humans. The second step is quantitative risk estimation, which is not usually attempted in the *Monographs*. Detailed, quantitative evaluations of epidemiological data may be made in the *Monographs*, but without extrapolation beyond the range of the data available. Quantitative extrapolation from experimental data to the human situation is not undertaken.

These monographs may assist national and international authorities in making risk assessments and in formulating decisions concerning any necessary preventive measures. **The evaluations of IARC working groups are scientific, qualitative judgements about the degree of evidence for carcinogenicity provided by the available data on an agent. These evaluations represent only one part of the body of information on which regulatory measures may be based. Other components of regulatory decisions may vary from one situation to another and from country to country, responding to different socioeconomic and national priorities. Therefore, no recommendation is given with regard to regulation or legislation, which are the responsibility of individual governments and/or other international organizations.**

The *IARC Monographs* are recognized as an authoritative source of information on the carcinogenicity of chemicals and complex exposures. A users' survey, made in 1984, indicated that the *Monographs* are consulted by various agencies in 45 countries. Each volume is generally printed in 4000 copies for distribution to governments, regulatory bodies and interested scientists. The *Monographs* are also available *via* the Distribution and Sales Service of the World Health Organization.

## 3. SELECTION OF TOPICS FOR MONOGRAPHS

Topics are selected on the basis of two main criteria: (i) that they concern agents for which there is evidence of human exposure, and (ii) that there is some evidence or suspicion of carcinogenicity. The term 'agent' is used to include individual chemical compounds, groups of chemical compounds, physical agents (such as radiation) and biological factors (such as viruses) and mixtures of agents such as occur in occupational exposures and as a result of personal and cultural habits (like smoking and dietary practices). Chemical analogues and compounds with biological or physical characteristics similar to those of suspected carcinogens may also be considered, even in the absence of data on carcinogenicity.

The scientific literature is surveyed for published data relevant to an assessment of carcinogenicity; the IARC surveys of chemicals being tested for carcinogenicity(8) and directories of on-going research in cancer epidemiology(9) often indicate those agents that may be scheduled for future meetings. An ad-hoc working group convened by IARC in 1984 gave recommendations as to which chemicals and exposures to complex mixtures should be evaluated in the *IARC Monographs* series(10).

As significant new data on subjects on which monographs have already been prepared become available, re-evaluations are made at subsequent meetings, and revised monographs are published.

## 4. DATA FOR MONOGRAPHS

The *Monographs* do not necessarily cite all the literature concerning the subject of an evaluation. Only those data considered by the Working Group to be relevant to making the evaluation are included.

With regard to biological and epidemiological data, only reports that have been published or accepted for publication in the openly available scientific literature are reviewed by the working groups. In certain instances, government agency reports that have undergone peer review and are widely available are considered. Exceptions may be made on an ad-hoc basis to include unpublished reports that are in their final form and publicly available, if their inclusion is considered pertinent to making a final evaluation (see pp. 25 *et seq*.). In the sections on chemical and physical properties and on production, use, occurrence and analysis, unpublished sources of information may be used.

## 5. THE WORKING GROUP

Reviews and evaluations are formulated by a working group of experts. The tasks of this group are five-fold: (i) to ascertain that all appropriate data have been collected; (ii) to select the data relevant for the evaluation on the basis of scientific merit; (iii) to prepare accurate summaries of the data to enable the reader to follow the reasoning of the Working Group; (iv) to evaluate the results of experimental and epidemiological studies; and (v) to make an overall evaluation of the carcinogenicity of the agent to humans.

Working Group participants who contributed to the consideration and evaluation of the agents within a particular volume are listed, with their addresses, at the beginning of each publication. Each participant who is a member of a working group serves as an individual scientist and not as a representative of any organization, government or industry. In addition, representatives from national and international agencies and industrial associations are invited as observers.

## 6. WORKING PROCEDURES

Approximately one year in advance of a meeting of a working group, the topics of the monographs are announced and participants are selected by IARC staff in consultation with other experts. Subsequently, relevant biological and epidemiological data are collected by IARC from recognized sources of information on carcinogenesis, including data storage and retrieval systems such as CANCERLINE, MEDLINE and TOXLINE. Bibliographical sources for data on genetic and related effects and on teratogenicity include EMIC, ETIC and TOXLINE.

The major collection of data and the preparation of first drafts of the sections on chemical and physical properties, on production and use, on occurrence, and on analysis are carried out under a separate contract funded by the US National Cancer Institute. Efforts are made to supplement this information with data from other national and international sources. Representatives from industrial associations may assist in the preparation of sections on production and use.

Production and trade data are obtained from governmental and trade publications and, in some cases, by direct contact with industries. Separate production data on some agents may not be available because their publication could disclose confidential information. Information on uses is usually obtained from published sources but is often complemented by direct contact with manufacturers.

Six months before the meeting, reference material is sent to experts, or is used by IARC staff, to prepare sections for the first drafts of monographs. The complete first drafts are compiled by IARC staff and sent, prior to the meeting, to all participants of the Working Group for review.

The Working Group meets in Lyon for seven to eight days to discuss and finalize the texts of the monographs and to formulate the evaluations. After the meeting, the master copy of each monograph is verified by consulting the original literature, edited and prepared for publication. The aim is to publish monographs within nine months of the Working Group meeting.

## 7. EXPOSURE DATA

Sections that indicate the extent of past and present human exposure, the sources of exposure, the persons most likely to be exposed and the factors that contribute to exposure to the agent under study are included at the beginning of the monograph.

Most monographs on individual chemicals or complex mixtures include sections on chemical and physical data, and production, use, occurrence and analysis. In other monographs, for example on physical agents, biological factors, occupational exposures and cultural habits, other sections may be included, such as: historical perspectives, description of an industry or habit, exposures in the work place or chemistry of the complex mixture.

The Chemical Abstracts Services Registry Number, the latest Chemical Abstracts Primary Name and the IUPAC Systematic Name are recorded. Other synonyms and trade names are given, but the list is not necessarily comprehensive. Some of the trade names may be those of mixtures in which the agent being evaluated is only one of the ingredients.

Information on chemical and physical properties and, in particular, data relevant to identification, occurrence and biological activity are included. A separate description of technical products gives relevant specifications and includes available information on composition and impurities.

The dates of first synthesis and of first commercial production of an agent are provided; for agents which do not occur naturally, this information may allow a reasonable estimate to be made of the date before which no human exposure to the agent could have occurred. The dates of first reported occurrence of an exposure are also provided. In addition, methods of synthesis used in past and present commercial production and different methods of production which may give rise to different impurities are described.

Data on production, foreign trade and uses are obtained for representative regions, which usually include Europe, Japan and the USA. It should not, however, be inferred that those areas or nations are necessarily the sole or major sources or users of the agent being evaluated.

Some identified uses may not be current or major applications, and the coverage is not necessarily comprehensive. In the case of drugs, mention of their therapeutic uses does not necessarily represent current practice nor does it imply judgement as to their clinical efficacy.

Information on the occurrence of an agent in the environment is obtained from data derived from the monitoring and surveillance of levels in occupational environments, air, water, soil, foods and animal and human tissues. When available, data on the generation, persistence and bioaccumulation of the agent are also included.

Statements concerning regulations and guidelines (e.g., pesticide registrations, maximal levels permitted in foods, occupational exposure limits) are included for some countries as indications of potential exposures, but they may not reflect the most recent situation, since such limits are continuously reviewed and modified. The absence of information on regulatory status for a country should not be taken to imply that that country does not have regulations with regard to the subject under consideration.

The purpose of the section on analysis is to give the reader an overview of current methods cited in the literature, with emphasis on those widely used for regulatory purposes. No critical evaluation or recommendation of any of the methods is meant or implied. Methods for monitoring human exposure are also given, when available. The IARC publishes a series of volumes, *Environmental Carcinogens: Selected Methods of Analysis*(11), that describe validated methods for analysing a wide variety of agents.

## 8. BIOLOGICAL DATA RELEVANT TO THE EVALUATION OF CARCINOGENICITY TO HUMANS

The term 'carcinogen' is used in these monographs to denote an agent that is capable of increasing the incidence of malignant neoplasms; the induction of benign neoplasms may in some circumstances (see p. 19) contribute to the judgement that an agent is carcinogenic. The terms 'neoplasm' and 'tumour' are used interchangeably.

Some epidemiological and experimental studies indicate that different agents may act at different stages in the carcinogenic process, probably by fundamentally different mechanisms. In the present state of knowledge, the aim of the *Monographs* is to evaluate evidence of carcinogenicity at any stage in the carcinogenic process independently of the underlying mechanism involved. There is as yet insufficient information to implement classification according to mechanisms of action(6).

Definitive evidence of carcinogenicity in humans can only be provided by epidemiological studies. Evidence relevant to human carcinogenicity may also be provided by experimental studies of carcinogenicity in animals and by other biological data, particularly those relating to humans.

The available studies are summarized by the working groups, with particular regard to the qualitative aspects discussed below. In general, numerical findings are indicated as they appear in the original report; units are converted when necessary for easier comparison. The Working Group may conduct additional analyses of the published data and use them in their assessment of the evidence and may include them in their summary of a study; the results of such supplementary analyses are given in square brackets. Any comments are also made in square brackets; however, these are kept to a minimum, being restricted to those instances in which it is felt that an important aspect of a study, directly impinging on its interpretation, should be brought to the attention of the reader.

## 9. EVIDENCE FOR CARCINOGENICITY IN EXPERIMENTAL ANIMALS

For several agents (e.g., 4-aminobiphenyl, bis(chloromethyl)ether, diethylstilboestrol, melphalan, 8-methoxypsoralen (methoxsalen) plus UVR, mustard gas and vinyl chloride), evidence of carcinogenicity in experimental animals preceded evidence obtained from epidemiological studies or case reports. Information compiled from the first 41 volumes of the *IARC Monographs*(12) shows that, of the 44 agents for which there is *sufficient* or *limited evidence* of carcinogenicity to humans (see p. 25), all 37 that have been tested adequately experimentally produce cancer in at least one animal species. Although this association cannot establish that all agents that cause cancer in experimental animals also cause cancer in humans, nevertheless, **in the absence of adequate data in humans, it is biologically plausible and prudent to regard agents for which there is** *sufficient evidence* **(see p. 26) of carcinogenicity in experimental animals as if they presented a carcinogenic risk to humans.**

The monographs are not intended to summarize all published studies. Those that are inadequate (e.g., too short a duration, too few animals, poor survival; see below) or are judged irrelevant to the evaluation are generally omitted. They may be mentioned briefly, particularly when the information is considered to be a useful supplement to that of other reports or when they provide the only data available. Their inclusion does not, however, imply acceptance of the adequacy of the experimental design or of the analysis and interpretation of their results. Guidelines for conducting adequate long-term carcinogenicity experiments have been outlined (e.g., ref. 13).

The nature and extent of impurities or contaminants present in the agent being evaluated are given when available. Mention is made of all routes of exposure by which the agent has been adequately studied and of all species in which relevant experiments have been performed. Animal strain, sex, numbers per group, age at start of treatment and survival are reported.

Experiments in which the agent was administered in conjunction with known carcinogens or factors that modify carcinogenic effects are also reported. Experiments on the carcinogenicity of known metabolites and derivatives may be included.

*(a) Qualitative aspects*

The overall assessment of the carcinogenicity of an agent involves several considerations of qualitative importance, including (i) the experimental conditions under which the test was performed, including route and schedule of exposure, species, strain, sex, age, duration of follow-up; (ii) the consistency with which the agent has been shown to be carcinogenic, e.g., in how many species and at which target organ(s); (iii) the spectrum of neoplastic response, from benign tumours to malignant neoplasms; and (iv) the possible role of modifying factors.

Considerations of importance to the Working Group in the interpretation and evaluation of a particular study include: (i) how clearly the agent was defined; (ii) whether the dose was adequately monitored, particularly in inhalation experiments; (iii) whether the doses used were appropriate and whether the survival of treated animals was similar to that of controls; (iv) whether there were adequate numbers of animals per group; (v) whether animals of both sexes were used; (vi) whether animals were allocated randomly to groups; (vii) whether the duration of observation was adequate; and (viii) whether the data were adequately reported. If available, recent data on the incidence of specific tumours in historical controls, as well as in concurrent controls, should be taken into account in the evaluation of tumour response.

When benign tumours occur together with and originate from the same cell type in an organ or tissue as malignant tumours in a particular study and appear to represent a stage in the progression to malignancy, it may be valid to combine them in assessing tumour incidence. The occurrence of lesions presumed to be preneoplastic may in certain instances aid in assessing the biological plausibility of any neoplastic response observed.

Among the many agents that have been studied extensively, there are few instances in which the only neoplasms induced were benign. Benign tumours in experimental animals frequently represent a stage in the evolution of a malignant neoplasm, but they may be 'endpoints' that do not readily undergo transition to malignancy. However, if an agent is found to induce only benign neoplasms, it should be suspected of being a carcinogen and it requires further investigation.

*(b) Quantitative aspects*

The probability that tumours will occur may depend on the species and strain, the dose of the carcinogen and the route and period of exposure. Evidence of an increased incidence of neoplasms with increased exposure strengthens the inference of a causal association between the exposure to the agent and the development of neoplasms.

The form of the dose-response relationship can vary widely, depending on the particular agent under study and the target organ. Since many chemicals require metabolic activation before being converted into their reactive intermediates, both metabolic and pharmacokinetic aspects are important in determining the dose-response pattern. Saturation of steps such as absorption, activation, inactivation and elimination of the carcinogen may produce nonlinearity in the dose-response relationship, as could saturation of processes such as DNA repair(14,15).

*(c) Statistical analysis of long-term experiments in animals*

Factors considered by the Working Group include the adequacy of the information given for each treatment group: (i) the number of animals studied and the number examined histologically, (ii) the number of animals with a given tumour type and (iii) length of survival. The statistical methods used should be clearly stated and should be the generally accepted techniques refined for this purpose(15,16). When there is no difference in survival between control and treatment groups, the Working Group usually compares the proportions of animals developing each tumour type in each of the groups. Otherwise, consideration is given as to whether or not appropriate adjustments have been made for differences in survival. These adjustments can include: comparisons of the proportions of tumour-bearing animals among the 'effective number' of animals alive at the time the first tumour is discovered, in the case where most differences in survival occur before tumours appear; life-table methods, when tumours are visible or when they may be considered 'fatal' because mortality rapidly follows tumour development; and the Mantel-Haenszel test or logistic regression, when occult tumours do not affect the animals' risk of dying but are 'incidental' findings at autopsy.

In practice, classifying tumours as fatal or incidental may be difficult. Several survival-adjusted methods have been developed that do not require this distinction(15), although they have not been fully evaluated.

## 10. OTHER RELEVANT DATA IN EXPERIMENTAL SYSTEMS AND HUMANS

*(a) Structure-activity considerations*

This section describes structure-activity correlations that are relevant to an evaluation of the carcinogenicity of an agent.

*(b) Absorption, distribution, excretion and metabolism*

Concise information is given on absorption, distribution (including placental transfer) and excretion. Kinetic factors that may affect the dose-reponse relationship, such as saturation of uptake, protein binding, metabolic activation, detoxification and DNA-repair processes, are mentioned. Studies that indicate the metabolic fate of the agent in experimental animals and humans are summarized briefly, and comparisons of data from animals and humans are made when possible. Comparative information on the relationship between exposure and the dose that reaches the target site may be of particular importance for extrapolation between species.

*(c) Toxicity*

Data are given on acute and chronic toxic effects (other than cancer), such as organ toxicity, immunotoxicity, endocrine effects and preneoplastic lesions. Effects on reproduction, teratogenicity, feto- and embryotoxicity are also summarized briefly.

*(d) Genetic and related effects*

Tests of genetic and related effects may indicate possible carcinogenic activity. They can also be used in detecting active metabolites of known carcinogens in human or animal body fluids, in detecting active components in complex mixtures and in the elucidation of possible mechanisms of carcinogenesis.

The available data are interpreted critically by phylogenetic group according to the endpoints detected, which may include DNA damage, gene mutation, sister chromatid exchange, micronuclei, chromosomal aberrations, aneuploidy and cell transformation. The concentrations (doses) employed are given and mention is made of whether an exogenous metabolic system was required. When appropriate, these data may be represented by bar graphs (activity profiles), with corresponding summary tables and listings of test systems, data and references. Detailed information on the preparation of these profiles is given in an appendix to those volumes in which they are used.

Positive results in tests using prokaryotes, lower eukaryotes, plants, insects and cultured mammalian cells suggest that genetic and related effects (and therefore possibly carcinogenic effects) could occur in mammals. Results from such tests may also give information about the types of genetic effect produced by an agent and about the involvement of metabolic activation. Some endpoints described are clearly genetic in nature (e.g., gene mutations and chromosomal aberrations), others are to a greater or lesser degree associated with genetic effects (e.g., unscheduled DNA synthesis). In-vitro tests for tumour-promoting activity and for cell transformation may detect changes that are not necessarily the result of genetic alterations but that may have specific relevance to the process of carcinogenesis. A critical appraisal of these tests has been published(13).

Genetic or other activity detected in the systems mentioned above is not always manifest in whole mammals. Positive indications of genetic effects in experimental mammals and in humans are regarded as being of greater relevance than those in other organisms. The demonstration that an agent can induce gene and chromosomal mutations in whole mammals indicates that it may have the potential for carcinogenic activity, although this activity may not be detectably expressed in any or all species tested. The relative potency of agents in tests for mutagenicity and related effects is not a reliable indicator of carcinogenic potency. Negative results in tests for mutagenicity in selected tissues from animals treated *in vivo* provide less weight, partly because they do not exclude the possibility of an effect in tissues other than those examined. Moreover, negative results in short-term tests with genetic endpoints cannot be considered to provide evidence to rule out carcinogenicity of agents that act through other mechanisms. Factors may arise in many tests that could give misleading results; these have been discussed in detail elsewhere(13).

The adequacy of epidemiological studies of reproductive outcomes and genetic and related effects in humans is evaluated by the same criteria as are applied to epidemiological studies of cancer.

## 11. EVIDENCE FOR CARCINOGENICITY IN HUMANS

### (a) Types of studies considered

Three types of epidemiological studies of cancer contribute data to the assessment of carcinogenicity in humans — cohort studies, case-control studies and correlation studies. Rarely, results from randomized trials may be available. Case reports of cancer in humans exposed to particular agents are also reviewed.

Cohort and case-control studies relate individual exposures to the agent under study to the occurrence of cancer in individuals, and provide an estimate of relative risk (ratio of incidence in those exposed to incidence in those not exposed) as the main measure of association.

In correlation studies, the units of investigation are usually whole populations (e.g., in particular geographical areas or at particular times), and cancer incidence is related to a summary measure of the exposure of the population to the agent under study. Because individual exposure is not documented, however, a causal relationship is less easy to infer from correlation studies than from cohort and case-control studies.

Case reports generally arise from a suspicion, based on clinical experience, that the concurrence of two events — that is, exposure to a particular agent and occurrence of a cancer — has happened rather more frequently than would be expected by chance. Case reports usually lack complete ascertainment of cases in any population, definition or enumeration of the population at risk and estimation of the expected number of cases in the absence of exposure.

The uncertainties surrounding interpretation of case reports and correlation studies make them inadequate, except in rare instances, to form the sole basis for inferring a causal relationship. When taken together with case-control and cohort studies, however, relevant case reports or correlation studies may add materially to the judgement that a causal relationship is present.

Epidemiological studies of benign neoplasms and presumed preneoplastic lesions are also reviewed by working groups. They may, in some instances, strengthen inferences drawn from studies of cancer itself.

*(b) Quality of studies considered*

It is necessary to take into account the possible roles of bias, confounding and chance in the interpretation of epidemiological studies. By 'bias' is meant the operation of factors in study design or execution that lead erroneously to a stronger or weaker association between an agent and disease than in fact exists. By 'confounding' is meant a situation in which the relationship between an agent and a disease is made to appear stronger or to appear weaker than it truly is as a result of an association between the agent and another agent that is associated with either an increase or decrease in the incidence of the disease. In evaluating the extent to which these factors have been minimized in an individual study, working groups consider a number of aspects of design and analysis as described in the report of the study. Most of these considerations apply equally to case-control, cohort and correlation studies. Lack of clarity of any of these aspects in the reporting of a study can decrease its credibility and its consequent weighting in the final evaluation of the exposure.

Firstly, the study population, disease (or diseases) and exposure should have been well defined by the authors. Cases in the study population should have been identified in a way that was independent of the exposure of interest, and exposure should have been assessed in a way that was not related to disease status.

Secondly, the authors should have taken account in the study design and analysis of other variables that can influence the risk of disease and may have been related to the exposure of interest. Potential confounding by such variables should have been dealt with either in the design of the study, such as by matching, or in the analysis, by statistical adjustment. In cohort studies, comparisons with local rates of disease may be more appropriate than those with national rates. Internal comparisons of disease frequency among individuals at different levels of exposure should also have been made in the study.

Thirdly, the authors should have reported the basic data on which the conclusions are founded, even if sophisticated statistical analyses were employed. At the very least, they should have given the numbers of exposed and unexposed cases and controls in a case-control study and the numbers of cases observed and expected in a cohort study. Further tabulations by time since exposure began and other temporal factors are also important. In a cohort study, data on all cancer sites and all causes of death should have been given, to avoid the possibility of reporting bias. In a case-control study, the effects of investigated factors other than the agent of interest should have been reported.

Finally, the statistical methods used to obtain estimates of relative risk, absolute cancer rates, confidence intervals and significance tests, and to adjust for confounding should have been clearly stated by the authors. The methods used should preferably have been the generally accepted techniques that have been refined since the mid-1970s. These methods have been reviewed for case-control studies(17) and for cohort studies(18).

(c) *Quantitative considerations*

Detailed analyses of both relative and absolute risks in relation to age at first exposure and to temporal variables, such as time since first exposure, duration of exposure and time since exposure ceased, are reviewed and summarized when available. The analysis of temporal relationships can provide a useful guide in formulating models of carcinogenesis. In particular, such analyses may suggest whether a carcinogen acts early or late in the process of carcinogenesis(6), although such speculative inferences cannot be used to draw firm conclusions concerning the mechanism of action of the agent and hence the shape (linear or otherwise) of the dose-response relationship below the range of observation.

(d) *Criteria for causality*

After the quality of individual epidemiological studies has been summarized and assessed, a judgement is made concerning the strength of evidence that the agent in question is carcinogenic for humans. In making its judgement, the Working Group considers several criteria for causality. A strong association (i.e., a large relative risk) is more likely to indicate causality than a weak association, although it is recognized that relative risks of small magnitude do not imply lack of causality and may be important if the disease is common. Associations that are replicated in several studies of the same design or using different epidemiological approaches or under different circumstances of exposure are more likely to represent a causal relationship than isolated observations from single studies. If there are inconsistent results among investigations, possible reasons are sought (such as differences in amount of exposure), and results of studies judged to be of high quality are given more weight than those from studies judged to be methodologically less sound. When suspicion of carcinogenicity arises largely from a single study, these data are not combined with those from later studies in any subsequent reassessment of the strength of the evidence.

If the risk of the disease in question increases with the amount of exposure, this is considered to be a strong indication of causality, although absence of a graded response is not necessarily evidence against a causal relationship. Demonstration of a decline in risk after cessation of or reduction in exposure in individuals or in whole populations also supports a causal interpretation of the findings.

Although the same carcinogenic agent may act upon more than one target, the specificity of an association (i.e., an increased occurrence of cancer at one anatomical site or of one morphological type) adds plausibility to a causal relationship, particularly when excess cancer occurrence is limited to one morphological type within the same organ.

Although rarely available, results from randomized trials showing different rates among exposed and unexposed individuals provide particularly strong evidence for causality.

When several epidemiological studies show little or no indication of an association between an exposure and cancer, the judgement may be made that, in the aggregate, they show evidence of lack of carcinogenicity. Such a judgement requires first of all that the studies giving rise to it meet, to a sufficient degree, the standards of design and analysis described above. Specifically, the possibility that bias, confounding or misclassification of exposure or outcome could explain the observed results should be considered and excluded with reasonable certainty. In addition, all studies that are judged to be methodologically sound should be consistent with a relative risk of unity for any observed level of exposure to the agent and, when considered together, should provide a pooled estimate of relative risk which is at or near unity and has a narrow confidence interval, due to sufficient population size. Moreover, no individual study nor the pooled results of all the studies should show any consistent tendency for relative risk of cancer to increase with increasing level of exposure to the agent. It is important to note that evidence of lack of carcinogenicity obtained in this way from several epidemiological studies can apply only to the type(s) of cancer studied and to dose levels of the agent and intervals between first exposure to it and observation of disease that are the same as or less than those observed in all the studies. Experience with human cancer indicates that, for some agents, the period from first exposure to the development of clinical cancer is seldom less than 20 years; latent periods substantially shorter than 30 years cannot provide evidence for lack of carcinogenicity.

## 12. SUMMARY OF DATA REPORTED

In this section, the relevant experimental and epidemiological data are summarized. Only reports, other than in abstract form, that meet the criteria outlined on p. 15 are considered for evaluating carcinogenicity. Inadequate studies are generally not summarized: such studies are usually identified by a square-bracketed comment in the text.

*(a) Exposures*

Human exposure is summarized on the basis of elements such as production, use, occurrence in the environment and determinations in human tissues and body fluids. Quantitative data are given when available.

## (b) Experimental carcinogenicity data

Data relevant to the evaluation of the carcinogenicity of the agent in animals are summarized. For each animal species and route of administration, it is stated whether an increased incidence of neoplasms was observed, and the tumour sites are indicated. If the agent produced tumours after prenatal exposure or in single-dose experiments, this is also indicated. Dose-response and other quantitative data may be given when available. Negative findings are also summarized.

## (c) Human carcinogenicity data

Results of epidemiological studies that are considered to be pertinent to an assessment of human carcinogenicity are summarized. When relevant, case reports and correlation studies are also considered.

## (d) Other relevant data

Structure-activity correlations are mentioned when relevant.

Toxicological information and data on kinetics and metabolism in experimental animals are given when considered relevant. The results of tests for genetic and related effects are summarized for whole mammals, cultured mammalian cells and nonmammalian systems.

Data on other biological effects in humans of particular relevance are summarized. These may include kinetic and metabolic considerations and evidence of DNA binding, persistence of DNA lesions or genetic damage in humans exposed to the agent.

When available, comparisons of such data for humans and for animals, and particularly animals that have developed cancer, are described.

## 13. EVALUATION

Evaluations of the strength of the evidence for carcinogenicity arising from human and experimental animal data are made, using standard terms.

It is recognized that the criteria for these evaluations, described below, cannot encompass all of the factors that may be relevant to an evaluation of the carcinogenicity of an agent. In considering all of the relevant data, the Working Group may assign the agent to a higher or lower category than a strict interpretation of these criteria would indicate.

### (a) Degrees of evidence for carcinogenicity in humans and in experimental animals and supporting evidence

It should be noted that these categories refer only to the strength of the evidence that these agents are carcinogenic and not to the extent of their carcinogenic activity (potency) nor to the mechanism involved. A classification may change as new information becomes available.

#### (i) Human carcinogenicity data

The evidence relevant to carcinogenicity from studies in humans is classified into one of the following categories:

*Sufficient evidence of carcinogenicity*: The Working Group considers that a causal relationship has been established between exposure to the agent and human cancer. That is, a positive relationship has been observed between the exposure to the agent and cancer in studies in which chance, bias and confounding could be ruled out with reasonable confidence.

*Limited evidence of carcinogenicity*: A positive association has been observed between exposure to the agent and cancer for which a causal interpretation is considered by the Working Group to be credible, but chance, bias or confounding could not be ruled out with reasonable confidence.

*Inadequate evidence of carcinogenicity*: The available studies are of insufficient quality, consistency or statistical power to permit a conclusion regarding the presence or absence of a causal association.

*Evidence suggesting lack of carcinogenicity*: There are several adequate studies covering the full range of doses to which human beings are known to be exposed, which are mutually consistent in not showing a positive association between exposure to the agent and any studied cancer at any observed level of exposure. A conclusion of 'evidence suggesting lack of carcinogenicity' is inevitably limited to the cancer sites, circumstances and doses of exposure and length of observation covered by the available studies. In addition, the possibility of a very small risk at the levels of exposure studied can never be excluded.

In some instances, the above categories may be used to classify the degree of evidence for the carcinogenicity of the agent for specific organs or tissues.

(ii) *Experimental carcinogenicity data*

The evidence relevant to carcinogenicity in experimental animals is classified into one of the following categories:

*Sufficient evidence of carcinogenicity*: The Working Group considers that a causal relationship has been established between the agent and an increased incidence of malignant neoplasms or of an appropriate combination of benign and malignant neoplasms (as described on p. 19) in (a) two or more species of animals or (b) two or more independent studies in one species carried out at different times or in different laboratories or under different protocols.

Exceptionally, a single study in one species might be considered to provide sufficient evidence of carcinogenicity when malignant neoplasms occur to an unusual degree with regard to incidence, site, type of tumour or age at onset.

In the absence of adequate data on humans, it is biologically plausible and prudent to regard agents for which there is *sufficient evidence* of carcinogenicity in experimental animals as if they presented a carcinogenic risk to humans.

*Limited evidence of carcinogenicity*: The data suggest a carcinogenic effect but are limited for making a definitive evaluation because, e.g., (a) the evidence of carcinogenicity is restricted to a single experiment; or (b) there are unresolved questions regarding the adequacy of the design, conduct or interpretation of the study; or (c) the agent increases the incidence only of benign neoplasms or lesions of uncertain neoplastic potential, or of certain neoplasms which may occur spontaneously in high incidences in certain strains.

*Inadequate evidence of carcinogenicity*: The studies cannot be interpreted as showing either the presence or absence of a carcinogenic effect because of major qualitative or quantitative limitations.

*Evidence suggesting lack of carcinogenicity*: Adequate studies involving at least two species are available which show that, within the limits of the tests used, the agent is not carcinogenic. A conclusion of evidence suggesting lack of carcinogenicity is inevitably limited to the species, tumour sites and doses of exposure studied.

(iii) *Supporting evidence of carcinogenicity*

The other relevant data judged of sufficient importance as to affect the making of the overall evaluation are indicated.

(b) *Overall evaluation*

Finally, the total body of evidence is taken into account; the agent is described according to the wording of one of the following categories, and the designated group is given. The categorization of an agent is a matter of scientific judgement, reflecting the strength of the evidence derived from studies in human and in experimental animals and from other relevant data.

*Group 1 — The agent is carcinogenic to humans.*

This category is used only when there is *sufficient evidence* of carcinogenicity in humans.

*Group 2*

This category includes agents for which, at one extreme, the degree of evidence of carcinogenicity in humans is almost sufficient, as well as those for which, at the other extreme, there are no human data but for which there is experimental evidence of carcinogenicity. Agents are assigned to either 2A (probably carcinogenic) or 2B (possibly carcinogenic) on the basis of epidemiological, experimental and other relevant data.

*Group 2A — The agent is probably carcinogenic to humans.*

This category is used when there is *limited evidence* of carcinogenicity in humans and *sufficient evidence* of carcinogenicity in experimental animals. Exceptionally, an agent may be classified into this category solely on the basis of *limited evidence* of carcinogenicity in humans or of *sufficient evidence* of carcinogenicity in experimental animals strengthened by supporting evidence from other relevant data.

*Group 2B — The agent is possibly carcinogenic to humans.*

This category is generally used for agents for which there is *limited evidence* in humans in the absence of *sufficient evidence* in experimental animals. It may also be used when there is *inadequate evidence* of carcinogenicity in humans or when human data are nonexistent but there is *sufficient evidence* of carcinogenicity in experimental animals. In some instances, an agent for which there is *inadequate evidence* or no data in humans but *limited evidence* of carcinogenicity in experimental animals together with supporting evidence from other relevant data may be placed in this group.

*Group 3 — The agent is not classifiable as to its carcinogenicity to humans.*

Agents are placed in this category when they do not fall into any other group.

*Group 4 — The agent is probably not carcinogenic to humans.*

This category is used for agents for which there is *evidence suggesting lack of carcinogenicity* in humans together with *evidence suggesting lack of carcinogenicity* in experimental animals. In some circumstances, agents for which there is *inadequate evidence* of or no data on carcinogenicity in humans but *evidence suggesting lack of carcinogenicity* in experimental animals, consistently and strongly supported by a broad range of other relevant data, may be classified in this group.

### References

1. IARC (1987) *IARC Monographs on the Evaluation of Carcinogenic Risks to Humans*, Supplement 6, *Genetic and Related Effects: An Updating of Selected* IARC Monographs *from Volumes 1 to 42*, Lyon
2. IARC (1977) *IARC Monographs Programme on the Evaluation of the Carcinogenic Risk of Chemicals to Humans. Preamble (IARC intern. tech. Rep. No. 77/002)*, Lyon
3. IARC (1978) *Chemicals with* Sufficient Evidence *of Carcinogenicity in Experimental Animals* — IARC Monographs *Volumes 1–17 (IARC intern. tech. Rep. No. 78/003)*, Lyon
4. IARC (1979) *Criteria to Select Chemicals for* IARC Monographs *(IARC intern. tech. Rep. No. 79/003)*, Lyon
5. IARC (1982) *IARC Monographs on the Evaluation of the Carcinogenic Risk of Chemicals to Humans*, Supplement 4, *Chemicals, Industrial Processes and Industries Associated with Cancer in Humans (IARC Monographs, Volumes 1 to 29)*, Lyon
6. IARC (1983) *Approaches to Classifying Chemical Carcinogens According to Mechanism of Action (IARC intern. tech. Rep. No. 83/001)*, Lyon
7. IARC (1987) *IARC Monographs on the Evaluation of Carcinogenic Risks to Humans*, Supplement 7, *Overall Evaluations of Carcinogenicity: An Updating of* IARC Monographs *Volumes 1 to 42*, Lyon
8. IARC (1973-1988) *Information Bulletin on the Survey of Chemicals Being Tested for Carcinogenicity*, Numbers 1–13, Lyon

   Number  1 (1973)  52 pages
   Number  2 (1973)  77 pages
   Number  3 (1974)  67 pages
   Number  4 (1974)  97 pages
   Number  5 (1975)  88 pages
   Number  6 (1976) 360 pages
   Number  7 (1978) 460 pages
   Number  8 (1979) 604 pages
   Number  9 (1981) 294 pages
   Number 10 (1983) 326 pages
   Number 11 (1984) 370 pages
   Number 12 (1986) 385 pages
   Number 13 (1988) 404 pages

9. Muir, C. & Wagner, G., eds (1977–88) *Directory of On-going Studies in Cancer Epidemiology 1977–88 (IARC Scientific Publications)*, Lyon, International Agency for Research on Cancer

10. IARC (1984) *Chemicals and Exposures to Complex Mixtures Recommended for Evaluation in IARC Monographs and Chemicals and Complex Mixtures Recommended for Long-term Carcinogenicity Testing (IARC intern. tech. Rep. No. 84/002)*, Lyon

11. *Environmental Carcinogens. Selected Methods of Analysis:*

    Vol. 1. *Analysis of Volatile Nitrosamines in Food (IARC Scientific Publications No. 18)*. Edited by R. Preussmann, M. Castegnaro, E.A. Walker & A.E. Wasserman (1978)

    Vol. 2. *Methods for the Measurement of Vinyl Chloride in Poly(vinyl chloride), Air, Water and Foodstuffs (IARC Scientific Publications No. 22)*. Edited by D.C.M. Squirrell & W. Thain (1978)

    Vol. 3. *Analysis of Polycyclic Aromatic Hydrocarbons in Environmental Samples (IARC Scientific Publications No. 29)*. Edited by M. Castegnaro, P. Bogovski, H. Kunte & E.A. Walker (1979)

    Vol. 4. *Some Aromatic Amines and Azo Dyes in the General and Industrial Environment (IARC Scientific Publications No. 40)*. Edited by L. Fishbein, M. Castegnaro, I.K. O'Neill & H. Bartsch (1981)

    Vol. 5. *Some Mycotoxins (IARC Scientific Publications No. 44)*. Edited by L. Stoloff, M. Castegnaro, P. Scott, I.K. O'Neill & H. Bartsch (1983)

    Vol. 6. *N-Nitroso Compounds (IARC Scientific Publications No. 45)*. Edited by R. Preussmann, I.K. O'Neill, G. Eisenbrand, B. Spiegelhalder & H. Bartsch (1983)

    Vol. 7. *Some Volatile Halogenated Hydrocarbons (IARC Scientific Publications No. 68)*. Edited by L. Fishbein & I.K. O'Neill (1985)

    Vol. 8. *Some Metals: As, Be, Cd, Cr, Ni, Pb, Se, Zn (IARC Scientific Publications No. 71)*. Edited by I.K. O'Neill, P. Schuller & L. Fishbein (1986)

    Vol. 9. *Passive Smoking (IARC Scientific Publications No. 81)*. Edited by I.K. O'Neill, K.D. Brunnemann, B. Dodet & D. Hoffmann (1987)

12. Wilbourn, J., Haroun, L., Heseltine, E., Kaldor, J., Partensky, C. & Vainio, H. (1986) Response of experimental animals to human carcinogens: an analysis based upon the IARC Monographs Programme. *Carcinogenesis, 7*, 1853–1863

13. Montesano, R., Bartsch, H., Vainio, H., Wilbourn, J. & Yamasaki, H., eds (1986) *Long-term and Short-term Assays for Carcinogenesis — A Critical Appraisal (IARC Scientific Publications No. 83)*, Lyon, International Agency for Research on Cancer

14. Hoel, D.G., Kaplan, N.L. & Anderson, M.W. (1983) Implication of nonlinear kinetics on risk estimation in carcinogenesis. *Science, 219*, 1032–1037

15. Gart, J.J., Krewski, D., Lee, P.N., Tarone, R.E. & Wahrendorf, J. (1986) *Statistical Methods in Cancer Research, Vol. 3, The Design and Analysis of Long-term Animal Experiments (IARC Scientific Publications No. 79)*, Lyon, International Agency for Research on Cancer

16. Peto, R., Pike, M.C., Day, N.E., Gray, R.G., Lee, P.N., Parish, S., Peto, J., Richards, S. & Wahrendorf, J. (1980) *Guidelines for simple, sensitive significance tests for carcinogenic effects in long-term animal experiments*. In: *IARC Monographs on the Evaluation of the Carcinogenic Risk of Chemicals to Humans, Supplement 2, Long-term and Short-term Screening Assays for Carcinogens: A Critical Appraisal*, Lyon, pp. 311–426

17. Breslow, N.E. & Day, N.E. (1980) *Statistical Methods in Cancer Research*, Vol. 1, *The Analysis of Case-control Studies* (*IARC Scientific Publications No. 32*), Lyon, International Agency for Research on Cancer

18. Breslow, N.E. & Day, N.E. (1987) *Statistical Methods in Cancer Research*, Vol. 2, *The Design and Analysis of Cohort Studies* (*IARC Scientific Publications No. 82*), Lyon, International Agency for Research on Cancer

# GENERAL REMARKS ON THE AGENTS CONSIDERED

This forty-sixth volume of *IARC Monographs* covers diesel and gasoline engine exhausts and 15 nitroarenes. It is related to Volume 45 (IARC, 1989), which dealt with occupational exposures in petroleum refining and with crude oil and the major petroleum fuels, since the engine exhausts considered in the present volume originate from the use of two major petroleum fuels — gasoline and diesel fuel — primarily in vehicles. This volume also complements Volume 35 (IARC, 1985), in which the relevant data on soots formed during the domestic or institutional combustion of heating fuels are summarized and evaluated. Diesel and gasoline engine exhaust emissions all contain soot, which is defined as carbon-containing material produced as a by-product of incomplete combustion or pyrolysis. The genetic activity and tumorigenicity of soot extracts (tars) from diesel and gasoline engine exhausts have been compared with those of soot extracts from coal, wood and fuel oil (Lewtas, 1985).

*Engine exhausts*

The main sources of engine exhausts are vehicles: automobiles, buses, trucks, trains, ships, boats, heavy construction equipment, fork-lift trucks, tractors and jet aircraft, although diesel- and gasoline-fuelled engines are also used as stationary power sources. Jet engine exhausts were not considered in this volume, since no study relevant to an evaluation of their carcinogenicity was available. The Working Group was aware of some data on the analysis of the chemical composition of jet engine exhaust (Black *et al.*, 1977; McCammon & Crandall, 1980; McCartney *et al.*, 1986) and on pollutant concentrations in airports (Judd, 1971; Bastress, 1973). One study showed, however, that emissions from diesel- and gasoline-driven tank trucks and other vehicles at airports may cause heavier exposure than emissions from jet airplanes (McCammon *et al.*, 1981). Particle extracts from jet airplanes have been shown to be mutagenic (McCartney *et al.*, 1986). One epidemiological study addressed exposure to jet fuel exhaust (Siemiatycki *et al.*, 1988); due to the small number of exposed subjects, however, risk estimates were difficult to evaluate.

Engine exhausts are complex mixtures containing thousands of chemical compounds in the particulate and gaseous phases. Many components of engine exhausts have also been found in tobacco smoke and other combustion products. Table 1 lists agents that have been identified in engine exhausts and that have been evaluated by the IARC. The monograph on diesel and gasoline engine exhausts is not a review of data on these or other specific substances in engine exhausts but covers only experimental studies in which the whole exhaust or a major fraction of it has been tested. The few studies of exhaust irradiated with ultraviolet light are also discussed.

**Table 1. Agents identified in engine exhausts that have been evaluated in *IARC Monographs* volumes**

| Agent | Evidence of carcinogenicity[a] | | |
|---|---|---|---|
| | Humans | Animals | Group |
| Acetaldehyde | I | S | 2B |
| Acridines | | | |
|   Benz[c]acridine | ND | L | 3 |
|   Dibenz[a,h]acridine | ND | S | 2B |
|   Dibenz[a,j]acridine | ND | S | 2B |
| Acrolein | I | I | 3 |
| Benzene | S | S | 1 |
| 1,3-Butadiene | I | S | 2B |
| 1,2-Dibromoethane (ethylene dibromide) | I | S | 2A |
| 1,2-Dichloroethane | ND | S | 2B |
| Ethylene | ND | ND | 3 |
| Formaldehyde | L | S | 2A |
| Lead and lead compounds | | | |
|   Inorganic | I | S | 2B |
|   Organolead | I | I | 3 |
| Methylbromide | I | L | 3 |
| Nitroarenes | | | |
|   3,7-Dinitrofluoranthene[b] | ND | L | 3 |
|   3,9-Dinitrofluoranthene[b] | ND | L | 3 |
|   1,3-Dinitropyrene[b] | ND | L | 3 |
|   1,6-Dinitropyrene[b] | ND | S | 2B |
|   1,8-Dinitropyrene[b] | ND | S | 2B |
|   9-Nitroanthracene | ND | ND | 3 |
|   6-Nitrobenzo[a]pyrene[b] | ND | L | 3 |
|   3-Nitrofluoranthene | ND | I | 3 |
|   2-Nitrofluorene[b] | ND | S | 2B |
|   1-Nitronaphthalene[b] | ND | I | 3 |
|   2-Nitronaphthalene[b] | ND | I | 3 |
|   1-Nitropyrene[b] | ND | S | 2B |
| Polycyclic aromatic compounds | | | |
|   Anthanthrene | ND | L | 3 |
|   Anthracene | ND | I | 3 |
|   Benz[a]anthracene | ND | S | 2A |
|   Benzo[b]fluoranthene | ND | S | 2B |
|   Benzo[j]fluoranthene | ND | S | 2B |
|   Benzo[k]fluoranthene | ND | S | 2B |
|   Benzo[ghi]fluoranthene | ND | I | 3 |
|   Benzo[a]fluorene | ND | I | 3 |
|   Benzo[b]fluorene | ND | I | 3 |
|   Benzo[ghi]perylene | ND | I | 3 |
|   Benzo[c]phenanthrene | ND | I | 3 |
|   Benzo[a]pyrene | ND | S | 2A |
|   Benzo[e]pyrene | ND | I | 3 |
|   Chrysene | ND | L | 3 |

**Table 1 (contd)**

| Agent | Evidence of carcinogenicity[a] | | |
|---|---|---|---|
| | Humans | Animals | Group |
| Coronene | ND | I | 3 |
| Cyclopenta[*cd*]pyrene | ND | L | 3 |
| Dibenz[*a,h*]anthracene | ND | S | 2A |
| Dibenzo[*a,e*]pyrene | ND | S | 2B |
| Dibenzo[*a,h*]pyrene | ND | S | 2B |
| 1,4-Dimethylphenanthrene | ND | I | 3 |
| Fluoranthene | ND | I | 3 |
| Fluorene | ND | I | 3 |
| Indeno[1,2,3-*cd*]pyrene | ND | S | 2B |
| 2-Methylchrysene | ND | L | 3 |
| 3-Methylchrysene | ND | L | 3 |
| 4-methylchrysene | ND | L | 3 |
| 5-Methylchrysene | ND | S | 2B |
| 6-Methylchrysene | ND | L | 3 |
| 1-Methylphenanthrene | ND | I | 3 |
| Perylene | ND | I | 3 |
| Phenanthrene | ND | I | 3 |
| Pyrene | ND | I | 3 |
| Triphenylene | ND | I | 3 |
| Propylene | ND | ND | 3 |

[a]From Supplement 7 (IARC, 1987), unless otherwise indicated; I, inadequate evidence; L, limited evidence; ND, no adequate data; S, sufficient evidence; 1, Group 1 — the agent is carcinogenic to humans; 2A, Group 2A — the agent is probably carcinogenic to humans; 2B, Group 2B — the agent is possibly carcinogenic to humans; 3, Group 3 — the agent is not classifiable as to its carcinogenicity to humans

[b]In this volume

In 1980, there were approximately 320 million passenger cars in the world, and approximately 75 million trucks and 20 million buses. The major increase in the world vehicle fleet occurred during 1950–70, with a substantial tapering off of this increase in subsequent years (Swedish Ministry of Agriculture, 1983). Diesel cars have virtually disappeared from the US market but currently account for 18% of new registrations in the countries of the European Community (Henssler & Gospage, 1987).

Intensive research was begun in the 1970s to develop internal combustion engines capable of meeting the emission control standards adopted in various parts of the world. This has resulted in the development of control techniques common to gasoline and diesel engines, including improved engine design and the use of exhaust gas recirculation and oxidation catalysts. Gasoline engines have been adapted for use of double and three-way catalysts, primarily intended to reduce emission of nitrogen oxides (Swedish Ministry of Agriculture, 1983). Air pollution standards which became effective in 1975 in the USA (US Environmental Protection Agency, 1972, 1974) necessitated the use of catalytic converters on passenger cars sold in that country, which entailed the simultaneous introduction of unleaded gasoline to avoid poisoning the active catalyst within the converter. Unleaded gasoline was introduced in Japan in 1972 (Swedish Ministry of Agriculture, 1979). The introduction of unleaded gasoline in the European Community was proposed in 1984 (Commission of the European Communities, 1984; Henssler & Gospage, 1987); with effect from 1 October 1989, new vehicles with engine capacities greater than 2 l must have a catalytic converter (Commission of the European Communities, 1985). Leaded regular gasoline has been banned in the Federal Republic of Germany since 1 February 1988 (Bundesministerium für Umwelt, Naturschutz und Reaktorsicherheit, 1987; CONCAWE, 1988). The sale of leaded regular gasoline was prohibited in Switzerland from 1 July 1986 (Conseil Fédéral Suisse, 1985), and, since 1 October 1987, all cars have had to be equipped with a catalytic converter; the same regulation has applied to light motorcycles since 1 October 1988 (Département Fédéral de l'Intérieur de Suisse, 1986).

Diesel engines have become the predominant source of industrial power, due in part to their ruggedness and power efficiency. Diesel locomotives were introduced on railroads in Canada and the USA in 1928 and in Germany in 1932. The 'dieselization' of railroads occurred rapidly in the USA: 5% of the locomotives used in 1943 had diesel engines (Anon., 1966), but 95% conversion had taken place by 1959 (Garshick *et al.*, 1987). The introduction of diesel engines into underground coal mines began in Germany in 1927, in Belgium and France soon after, and in the UK in 1939 (Harrington & East, 1947). In the USA, diesel engines were first used in a Pennsylvania limestone mine in 1939 and in underground coal mines in 1946; their use in coal mines in the USA was not common as recently as 1977, but since that time there has been a five-fold increase. The worldwide use of diesel engines in mining applications has advanced steadily since their introduction (Daniel, 1984).

A substantial effort throughout the world during the late 1970s and 1980s resulted in improved characterization of emissions from light-duty diesel engines. Unfortunately, much less information is available with regard to heavy-duty diesel engines. It would be particularly important to characterize exhaust emissions from diesel railroad locomotives, which might be of value in interpreting the results of epidemiological studies of railroad workers.

Because of the differences in the characteristics of exhausts from different types of motors — diesel/gasoline, light duty/heavy duty, catalytic/noncatalytic — every attempt was made to identify the exhaust tested in the studies considered. With respect to experimental studies, therefore, a number of early studies in which the type of engine exhaust was not specified were not considered by the Working Group, except in the absence of comparable data on specific exhaust types.

In interpreting the results of studies of complex mixtures, such as those in which animals are exposed to vehicle exhausts, it is important that the atmospheres to which the animals were exposed be characterized in as much detail as possible. The relevance of characterizing the various components, such as specific gases (e.g., nitrogen dioxide) and particulate material (e.g., diesel soot and associated organic compounds), is apparent when it is recognized that each may play a role in producing disease. For example, nitrogen dioxide and carbonaceous particles may irritate respiratory tract epithelium, and organic compounds may interact with DNA.

In rats exposed to high levels of whole diesel exhaust, long-term clearance of soot particles from the lungs is impaired and there is a build-up of the lung burden of soot that is in excess of the levels predicted from observations at low levels of exposure. At high levels of exposure, chronic active inflammation accompanies the focal accumulation of 'sequestered' soot in alveolar macrophages. In these areas, epithelial cell hyperplasia, progressive fibrosis and squamous metaplasia have been observed. Similar changes have been noted in studies with other materials in which increased incidences of lung tumours have been observed. The potential role of the lung 'overload' phenomenon and the associated pathology in the pathogenesis of lung tumours due to inhaled particles is not yet clear, and further research is needed in view of the prominent role of lung carcinogenicity in rats exposed to diesel engine exhaust.

The relevance to the human situation of impaired clearance in animals also awaits clarification. There is a severe lack of information on the effects on humans of engine exhausts. In particular, there are no data on the deposition and clearance of inhaled diesel exhaust particles. However, it should be noted that impairment of the pulmonary clearance of insoluble particles has been observed in cigarette smokers (Bohning *et al.*, 1982; Freedman *et al.*, 1984), who deposit gram quantities of tar per week (Pritchard, 1987). On the basis of a 320-day half-time for the pulmonary clearance of insoluble particles (Bailey *et al.*, 1982), life-time occupational exposure to, for example, 0.3 mg/m$^3$ (Gamble *et al.*, 1987) would result in a lung burden of approximately 50 mg. Scaling down to rats on the basis of relative lung weights by a factor of 250 (human:rat; Xu & Yu, 1987) would bring this burden to within an order of magnitude of that which impairs pulmonary clearance in rats.

Although it is clear that exposure of animals to engine exhausts results in the induction of lung tumours, it should be noted that complete necropsies were performed in only a few studies (e.g., Heinrich *et al.*, 1986; Mauderly *et al.*, 1987), and the presence or absence of tumours at sites other than the lung was not reported. Such data would be of interest in view of the epidemiological evidence of bladder cancer. It is to be hoped that site-specific tumour incidences will be reported in future studies. In considering data on bladder tumours, it should be noted that there are species differences in their induction by certain classes of chemicals.

*Nitroarenes*

Nitroarenes are found mainly in engine exhausts, and diesel engines, especially, produce considerable amounts. Monographs on some nitroarenes are included in this volume on the basis of the availability of data on carcinogenic activity in experimental animals; no epidemiological data were available on individual nitroarenes. It should be noted that 6-nitrochrysene, 7-nitrobenz[*a*]anthracene, 3-nitroperylene, 2-nitropyrene and 4-nitropyrene have not been found in engine exhausts, although three of these (6-nitrochrysene, 2-nitropyrene and 4-nitropyrene) have been found in extracts of environmental airborne particles.

The nitroarenes found in engine exhausts are listed in Table 1. Some were evaluated previously (IARC, 1984), and only those for which additional data on carcinogenicity have become available since the earlier evaluation have been re-evaluated in this volume. It was originally planned to include 3,4-dinitrofluoranthene in this volume, but no data on its carcinogenicity were available. It induced DNA damage (Nakagawa *et al.*, 1987) and mutation in bacteria (Tokiwa *et al.*, 1986; Nakagawa *et al.*, 1987).

It should be noted that most of the biological data on the nitroarenes considered in this volume relate to the compounds alone; however, in the environment, nitroarenes occur predominantly in association with carbonaceous particles. As demonstrated in the monograph on 1-nitropyrene, association with particles substantially prolongs residence time. In the evaluation and testing of polycyclic aromatic compounds for carcinogenicity, detailed knowledge of impurities is important, and identification of possibly carcinogenic impurities is essential if lack of carcinogenicity is to be established and if a compound is carcinogenic only when administered at high doses. Thus, the levels of impurities present in a substance and the limit of detection of the analytical method used are stated as precisely as possible.

Genetic activity profiles were prepared for the individual nitroarenes but not for diesel or gasoline engine exhaust materials, since it would not be appropriate to plot data on complex mixtures on the basis of dissimilar samples. The most extensive data base exists for particle extracts of engine exhausts, for which the units (e.g., $\mu g/ml$ for *in-vitro* tests and $mg/kg$ for *in-vivo* tests) would be suitable for use in profiles.

Mindful of the procedures adopted in the preparation of earlier volumes in this series of *Monographs* (see Preamble, p. 15, section 4), the Working Group reviewed and referred to reports other than those published as part of the general scientific literature only when this was considered to be pertinent to making a final evaluation of carcinogenicity and provided that the reports were readily available. The Working Group wishes to draw attention to a series of peer-reviewed reports available from the Health Effects Institute (Cambridge, MA, USA) that include information on the health effects of automobile emissions and of some of the nitroarenes described in this volume.

## References

Anon. (1966) *Encyclopaedia Britannica*, Vol. 18, Chicago, IL, W. Benton, p. 1119

Bailey, M.R., Fry, F.A. & James, A.C. (1982) The long-term clearance kinetics of insoluble particles from the human lung. *Ann. occup. Hyg.*, 26, 273–290

Bastress, E.K. (1973) Impact of aircraft exhaust emissions at airports. *Environ. Sci. Technol.*, 7, 811–816

Black, M.S., Rehg, W.R., Sievers, R.E. & Brooks, J.J. (1977) Gas chromatographic technique for compound class analysis of jet engine exhaust. *J. Chromatogr.*, 142, 809–822

Bohning, D.E., Atkins, H.L. & Cohn, S.H. (1982) Long-term particle clearance in man: normal and impaired. *Ann. occup. Hyg.*, 26, 259–271

Bundesministerium für Umwelt, Naturschutz und Reatorsicherheit (Federal Ministry for Environmental Affairs) (1987) Decree on change in decree on lead content of gasoline (Ger.). *Bundesgesetzblatt*, 1, 2810

Commission of the European Communities (1984) Proposal for a Council amending Directive 70/220/EEC on the approximation of the laws of the Member States relating to measures to be taken against air pollution by gases from engines of motor vehicles. *Off. J. Eur. Communities*, *C178*, 9–12

Commission of the European Communities (1985) Council Directive of 20 March 1985 concerning the comparison of legislations of Member States relative to the lead content of gasoline. *Off. J. Eur. Communities*, *L96*, 25–29

CONCAWE (1988) *Current Status and Trends in Unleaded Gasoline Demand. Western Europe, January 1988*, The Hague

Conseil Fédéral Suisse (Federal Council of Switzerland) (1985) *Ordinance on Air Protection* (Fr.), Bern, p. 60

Daniel, J.H., Jr (1984) *Diesels in Underground Mining: A Review and an Evaluation of an Air Quality Monitoring Methodology* (*Bureau of Mines Report of Investigations (RI) 8884*), Washington DC, US Department of the Interior, Bureau of Mines

Département Fédéral de l'Intérieur Suisse (Swiss Federal Department of the Interior) (1986) *Prescriptions for Exhaust Gases from Light and Heavy Cars and from Light and Heavy Motorcycles* (Fr.), Bern

Freedman, A.P., Street, M.C. & Camplone, D. (1984) Effect of cigarette smoking on alveolar particulate clearance. *J. Aerosol Sci.*, *15*, 237–240

Gamble, J., Jones, W. & Minshall, S. (1987) Epidemiological-environmental study of diesel bus garage workers: acute effects of $NO_2$ and respirable particulate on the respiratory system. *Environ. Res.*, *42*, 201–214

Garshick, E., Schenker, M.B., Muñoz, A., Segal, M., Smith, T.J., Woskie, S.R., Hammond, S.K. & Speizer, F.E. (1987) A case-control study of lung cancer and diesel exhaust exposure in railroad workers. *Am. Rev. respir. Dis.*, *135*, 1242–1248

Harrington, D. & East, J.H., Jr (1947) *Diesel Equipment in Underground Mining* (*Bureau of Mines Information Circular (IC) 7406*), Washington DC, US Department of the Interior, Bureau of Mines

Heinrich, U., Peters, L., Mohr, U., Bellmann, B., Fuhst, R., Ketkar, M.B., König, J., König, H. & Pott, F. (1986) *Investigation of Subacute and Chronic Effects of Gasoline Engine Exhaust on Rodents* (Ger.) (*FAT Series No. 55*), Frankfurt/Maine, Forschungvereinigung Automobiltechnik e.V.

Henssler, H. & Gospage, S. (1987) *The Exhaust Emission Standards of the European Community, SP-718, Motor Vehicle Pollution Control — A Global Perspective* (*SAE Technical Paper Series*), Warrendale, PA, The Engineering Society for Advancing Mobility

IARC (1984) *IARC Monographs on the Evaluation of the Carcinogenic Risk of Chemicals to Humans*, Vol. 33, *Polynuclear Aromatic Compounds, Part 2, Carbon Blacks, Mineral Oils and Some Nitroarenes*, Lyon, pp. 171–222

IARC (1985) *IARC Monographs on the Evaluation of the Carcinogenic Risk of Chemicals to Humans*, Vol. 35, *Polynuclear Aromatic Compounds, Part 4, Bitumens, Coal-tars and Derived Products, Shale-oils and Soots*, Lyon

IARC (1987) *IARC Monographs on the Evaluation of Carcinogenic Risks to Humans*, Supplement 7, *Overall Evaluations of Carcinogenicity: An Updating of* IARC Monographs *Volumes 1 to 42*, Lyon

IARC (1989) *IARC Monographs on the Evaluation of Carcinogenic Risks to Humans*, Vol. 45, *Occupational Exposures in Petroleum Refining; Crude Oil and Major Petroleum Fuels*, Lyon

Judd, H.J. (1971) Levels of carbon monoxide recorded on aircraft flight decks. *Aerosp. Med.*, 42, 344–348

Lewtas, J. (1985) *Combustion emissions: characterization and comparison of their mutagenic and carcinogenic activity*. In: Stich, H.F., ed., *Carcinogens and Mutagens in the Environment*, Vol. V, *The Workplace: Sources of Carcinogens*, Boca Raton, FL, CRC Press, pp. 59–74

Mauderly, J.L., Jones, R.K., Griffith, W.C., Henderson, R.F. & McClellan, R.O. (1987) Diesel exhaust is a pulmonary carcinogen in rats exposed chronically by inhalation. *Fundam. appl. Toxicol.*, 9, 208–221

McCammon, C.S. & Crandall, M.S. (1980) *Industrial Hygiene In-depth Survey Report of Exposure of Fuelmen at Allied New York Services, Inc., JFK International Airport (US NTIS PB82-183625)*, Cincinnati, OH, National Institute for Occupational Safety and Health

McCammon, C.S., Halperin, W.F. & Lemen, R.A. (1981) Carbon monoxide exposure from aircraft fueling vehicles. *Arch. environ. Health*, 36, 136–138

McCartney, M.A., Chatterjee, B.F., McCoy, E.C., Mortimer, E.A., Jr & Rosenkranz, H.S. (1986) Airplane emissions: a source of mutagenic nitrated polycyclic aromatic hydrocarbons. *Mutat. Res.*, 171, 99–104

Nakagawa, R., Horikawa, K., Sera, N., Kodera, Y. & Tokiwa, H. (1987) Dinitrofluoranthene: induction, identification and gene mutation. *Mutat. Res.*, 191, 85–91

Pritchard, J.N. (1987) *Respiratory Deposition of Tar Aerosols in Cigarette Smokers*, PhD Thesis, University of Essex, Department of Chemistry

Siemiatycki, J., Gérin, M., Stewart, P., Nadon, L., Dewar, R. & Richardson, L. (1988) Associations between several sites of cancer and ten types of exhaust and combustion products. Results from a case-referent study in Montreal. *Scand. J. Work Environ. Health*, 14, 79–90

Swedish Ministry of Agriculture (1979) *Motor Vehicles and Air Pollution. Statement of Problems, Programme of Investigation. A Status Report from the Swedish Government Committee on Automotive Air Pollution*, Stockholm, p. 45

Swedish Ministry of Agriculture (1983) *Motor Vehicles and Cleaner Air. Report of the Swedish Government Committee on Automotive Air Pollution*, Stockholm, pp. 169, 176

Tokiwa, H., Otofuji, T., Nakagawa, R., Horikawa, K., Maeda, T., Sano, N., Izumi, E. & Otsuka, H. (1986) Dinitro derivatives of pyrene and fluoranthene in diesel emission particulates and their tumorigenicity in mice and rats. In: Ishinishi, N., Koizumi, A., McClellan, R.O. & Stöber, W., eds, *Carcinogenic and Mutagenic Effects of Diesel Engine Exhaust*, Amsterdam, Elsevier, pp. 253–270

US Environmental Protection Agency (1972) New motor vehicles and new motor vehicle engines. Title 40. Protection of environment. Part 85. Control of air pollution from new motor vehicles and new motor vehicle engines. *Fed. Reg.*, 37, 24250–24320

US Environmental Protection Agency (1974) Title 40. Protection of environment. Part 85. Control of air pollution from new motor vehicles and new motor vehicle engines. Miscellaneous amendments. *Fed. Reg.*, 39, 18074–18088

Xu, G.B. & Yu, C.P. (1987) Deposition of diesel exhaust particles in mammalian lungs. A comparison between rodents and man. *Aerosol Sci. Technol.*, 7, 117–123

# THE MONOGRAPHS

# DIESEL AND GASOLINE ENGINE EXHAUSTS

## 1. Composition of Engine Exhausts

### 1.1 Introduction

Diesel and gasoline engines are the major power train sources used in vehicles. They are both internal, intermittent combustion engines. In diesel engines, the fuel is self-ignited as it is injected into air that has been heated by compression. In gasoline engines, the fuel is ignited by sparking-plugs. The fuels used in diesel and gasoline engines also differ, with diesel fuel consisting of higher boiling range petroleum fractions (see IARC, 1989). Primarily because of its higher density, a litre of diesel fuel contains approximately 13% more energy than a litre of gasoline.

There are two categories of diesel engine: open-chamber or direct-injection engines are preferred for heavy-duty applications because they offer the best fuel economy; divided-chamber or indirect-injection engines have been preferred for light-duty applications because they are less sensitive to differences in fuels, have a wider range of speeds (and therefore greater power:weight ratio), run more quietly and emit fewer pollutants (National Research Council, 1982).

The major products of the complete combustion of petroleum-based fuels in an internal combustion engine are carbon dioxide (13%) and water (13%), with nitrogen from air comprising most (73%) of the remaining exhaust. A very small portion of the nitrogen is converted to nitrogen oxides and some nitrated hydrocarbons. Some excess oxygen may be emitted, depending on the operating conditions of the engine. Gasoline engines are designed to operate at a nearly stoichiometric ratio (air:fuel ratio, ≃14.6:1); diesel engines operate with excess air (air:fuel ratio, ≃25–30:1; Lassiter & Milby, 1978).

Incomplete combustion results in the emission of carbon monoxide, unburnt fuel and lubricating oil (Yamaki *et al.*, 1986) and of oxidation and nitration products of the fuel and lubricating oil. These incomplete combustion products comprise thousands of chemical components present in the gas and particulate phases (Zaebst *et al.*, 1988); some specific chemical species and classes found in engine exhausts are listed in Table 1. The concentration of a chemical species in vehicle exhaust is a function of several factors, including engine type, engine operating conditions, fuel and lubricating oil composition and emission control system (Johnson, 1988).

**Table 1. Some compounds and classes of compounds in vehicle engine exhaust**[a]

Gas phase
- Acrolein
- Ammonia
- Benzene
- 1,3-Butadiene
- Formaldehyde
- Formic acid
- Heterocyclics and derivatives[b]
- Hydrocarbons ($C_1$–$C_{18}$) and derivatives[b]
- Hydrogen cyanide
- Hydrogen sulfide
- Methane
- Methanol
- Nitric acid
- Nitrous acid
- Oxides of nitrogen
- Polycyclic aromatic hydrocarbons and derivatives[b]
- Sulfur dioxide
- Toluene

Particulate phase
- Heterocyclics and derivatives[b]
- Hydrocarbons ($C_{14}$–$C_{35}$) and derivatives[b]
- Inorganic sulfates and nitrates
- Metals (e.g., lead and platinum)
- Polycyclic aromatic hydrocarbons and derivatives[b]

[a]From National Research Council (1983); Lies *et al.* (1986); Schuetzle & Frazier (1986); Carey (1987); Johnson (1988); Zaebst *et al.* (1988)

[b]Derivatives include acids, alcohols, aldehydes, anhydrides, esters, ketones, nitriles, quinones, sulfonates and halogenated and nitrated compounds, and multifunctional derivatives

Reports of measurements of polycyclic aromatic hydrocarbons (PAHs) emitted from spark-ignition gasoline engines first appeared in the literature in the 1950s (Kotin *et al.*, 1954) and early 1960s (Begeman & Colucci, 1962; Hoffmann & Wynder, 1962a). More recently, nitrated PAHs (nitroarenes) were detected in vehicle engine emissions. Some nitroarenes that have been identified in exhaust are listed in Table 2. Research has also been undertaken to determine if these compounds are formed as a result of the combustion process or subsequently in the exhaust. It has been shown in many studies that PAHs may undergo further reaction during sampling, but that these reactions can be minimized by using proper sampling apparatus and procedures (see section 2.3; Schuetzle, 1983; Schuetzle & Perez, 1983; Lies *et al.*, 1986).

## Table 2. Some nitroarenes identified in vehicle exhaust[a]

1,3-Dihydroxynitropyrene
2,5-Dinitrofluorene
2,7-Dinitrofluorene
2,7-Dinitro-9-fluorenone
1,3-Dinitropyrene
1,6-Dinitropyrene
1,8-Dinitropyrene
9-Methylcarbazole
1-Nitro-3-acetoxypyrene
9-Nitroanthracene
2-Nitroanthracene or -phenanthrene
x-Nitroanthracene or -phenanthrene (two isomers)[b]
6-Nitrobenzo[a]pyrene
x-Nitrobenzoquinoline[b]
2-Nitrobiphenyl
3-Nitrobiphenyl
4-Nitrobiphenyl
1-Nitrochrysene
x-Nitrodibenzothiophene (two isomers)[b]
x-Nitro-y,z-dimethylanthracene or -phenanthrene (five isomers)[b]
1-Nitrofluoranthene
3-Nitrofluoranthene
7-Nitrofluoranthene
8-Nitrofluoranthene
2-Nitrofluorene
3-Nitro-9-fluorenone
10-Nitro-1-methylanthracene or -phenanthrene
10-Nitro-9-methylanthracene or -phenanthrene
x-Nitro-y-methylanthracene or -phenanthrene[b]
1-Nitro-2-methylnaphthalene
3-Nitro-1-methylpyrene
6-Nitro-1-methylpyrene
8-Nitro-1-methylpyrene
1-Nitronaphthalene
2-Nitronaphthalene
2-Nitrophenanthrene
1-Nitropyrene
5-Nitroquinoline
8-Nitroquinoline
x-Nitroterphenyl[b]
x-Nitro-y,z,z'-trimethylanthracene or -phenanthrene (six isomers)[b]
x-Nitrotrimethylnaphthalene (three isomers)[b]

[a]From Nishioka et al. (1983); Manabe et al. (1985); Schuetzle & Jensen (1985); White (1985); Draper (1986)

[b]x, y, z, and z' imply position is unknown

Considerable effort has been made to identify mutagenic and carcinogenic chemicals in vehicle exhausts, primarily from diesel engines. Most effective has been the use of protocols combining short-term bioassays for genetic and related effects or for tumorigenicity with chemical analysis (Brune et al., 1978; Schuetzle et al., 1982; Grimmer et al., 1983a, 1984, 1987).

The use of the *Salmonella typhimurium* mutagenesis assay to study factors which may alter the emission of mutagens from diesel and gasoline engines has been reviewed (Claxton, 1983). Effects of engine design, fuel composition and operation on mutagenicity in *S. typhimurium* have been reported (Huisingh et al., 1978; Clark et al., 1981; Huisingh et al., 1981; Clark et al., 1982a,b,c; Ohnishi et al., 1982; Zweidinger, 1982; Clark et al., 1984; Schuetzle & Frazier, 1986). The effect of sampling methodology, environment (laboratory, tunnels and ambient urban air) and atmospheric transformation in the *S. typhimurium* mutagenesis assay have also been reported (Ohnishi et al., 1980; Claxton & Barnes, 1981; Pierson et al., 1983; Brooks et al., 1984). Typical factors that affect emissions are shown in Tables 3 and 4. The data on mutagenicity are included for comparative purposes to indicate the quantity of total genotoxic components. The reader is referred to section 3.2 (p. 119) for summaries of studies of the genetic effects of diesel and gasoline engine exhausts.

Table 3. Levels of emissions from various diesel and gasoline engines (1980–85; US Environmental Protection Agency Federal Test Procedure (FTP) cycle only) and their mutagenicity

|  | Heavy-duty diesel vehicle | Light-duty diesel vehicle | Light-duty gasoline vehicle | |
|---|---|---|---|---|
|  |  |  | Without catalytic converter | With catalytic converter |
| *Gas phase in mg/mile (mg/km)* | | | | |
| Benzene | – | $24^a$ (15) | $162^a$ (101) | $13^a$ (8) |
| Carbon monoxide | $10\,000^a$ (6250) | $1270^b$ (794) | $28\,500^b$ (17 813) | $12\,200^b$ (7625) |
| Formaldehyde | – | $20^a$ (13) | $56^a$ (35) | $4^a$ (3) |
| Nitrogen oxides | $28\,000^a$ (17 500) | $1270^b$ (794) | $3520^b$ (2200) | $2350^b$ (1469) |
| Propylene | – | – | $230^a$ (144) | $18^a$ (11) |
| Toluene | $11^a$ (7) | – | $215^a$ (134) | $32^a$ (20) |
| *Gas-phase PAHs and PAH derivatives in µg/mile (µg/km)$^a$* | | | | |
| Anthracene | 8960 (5600) | 2100 (1313) | 3200 (2000) | 60 (38) |
| Fluoranthene | 1240 (775) | 300 (188) | 450 (281) | 7 (4) |
|  | – | 910 (569) | 300 (188) | – |
| 2-Nitrofluorene | – | 90 (56) | – | – |
| Pyrene | 1580 (988) | 380 (238) | 580 (363) | 9 (6) |
|  | 1580 (988) | 1130 (706) | 200 (125) | – |
| *Particulate-phase PAHs and PAH derivatives in µg/mile (µg/km)* | | | | |
| Anthracene | $439^a$ (274) | $105^a$ (66) | $160^a$ (100) | $3^a$ (2) |
| Benzo[*a*]pyrene | $54^a$ (34) | $13^a$ (8) | $20^a$ (13) | $0.4^a$ (0.3) |
|  | – | $1^{a,c}$ (0.6) | $(1-10)^d$ | $(0.1-1)^d$ |

## Table 3 (contd)

| | Heavy-duty diesel vehicle | Light-duty diesel vehicle | Light-duty gasoline vehicle | |
|---|---|---|---|---|
| | | | Without catalytic converter | With catalytic converter |
| Benzo[a]pyrene (contd) | – | – | $3^e$ (2) | $0.1^e$ (0.06) |
| | – | – | $15^f$ (9) | $3^f$ (2) |
| | $142^a$ (89) | $34^a$ (21) | $15^b$ (9) | $2^b$ (1) |
| Benzo[e]pyrene | $64^a$ (40) | $15^a$ (9) | $23^a$ (14) | $0.4^a$ (0.3) |
| Fluoranthene | $933^a$ (538) | $224^a$ (140) | $340^a$ (213) | $5^a$ (3) |
| | – | $683^a$ (427) | $225^a$ (141) | – |
| | – | $933^a$ (583) | $224^a$ (140) | – |
| 2-Nitrofluorene | – | $97^a$ (61) | – | – |
| 1-Nitropyrene | $45^a$ (28) | $11^a$ (7) | $0.3^a$ (0.2) | $<0.1^a$ (<0.06) |
| | – | $4^c$ (3) | $0.2^f$ (0.1) | $0.2^f$ (0.1) |
| | – | $8^b$ (5) | $0.2^b$ (0.1) | $0.2^b$ (0.1) |
| Pyrene | $1182^a$ (739) | $284^a$ (178) | $431^a$ (269) | $7^a$ (4) |
| | – | $848^a$ (530) | $150^a$ (94) | – |
| | – | $284^f$ (178) | $19^f$ (12) | $10^f$ (6) |
| | – | $39^{a,c}$ (24) | $47^a$ (29) | $26^a$ (16) |
| Total PAH | | $200-1000^g$ (125–625) | | |
| *Other emissions* | | | | |
| Total particulate phase | | | | |
| in mg/km | $1036^h$ | $246^h$ | $62^h$ | $11^h$ |
| in mg/mile (mg/km) | – | – | $103^f$ (64) | $32^f$ (20) |
| Total extractable matter | | | | |
| in mg/km | $188^h$ | $124^h$ | $10^h$ | $6^h$ |
| in mg/mile (mg/kg) | – | – | $21^f$ (13) | $14^f$ (9) |
| *Mutagenicity* | | | | |
| TA98 (without activation) | | | | |
| rev/km | $226^h$ | $595\,000^h$ | $61\,000^h$ | $30\,000^h$ |
| rev/mile | – | $99\,000^{a,c}$ | $15\,000^a$ | $4000^a$ |
| rev/mile | – | $509\,000^b$ | $152\,000^b$ | $41\,000^b$ |
| TA98 (with activation) | | | | |
| rev/mile | | $590^{a,c}$ | $260^f$ | $80^f$ |
| rev/km | $40\,000-530\,000^i$ | $240\,000-320\,000$ | $180\,000^i$ | $30\,000^i$ |
| rev/mile | – | – | $258\,000^b$ | $71\,000^b$ |

[a]From Schuetzle & Frazier (1986); [b]from Zweidinger (1982); [c]see Table 4, 22% fuel aromaticity; [d]from Holmberg & Ahlborg (1983) [assumed to be FTP cycle]; [e]from Williams & Swarin (1979); [f]from Lang *et al.* (1981); [g]from Clark *et al.* (1982b); [h]from Schuetzle (1983); [i]from Lewtas & Williams (1986)

Table 4. Factors affecting rate of emission of polycyclic aromatic hydrocarbons in μg/mile (μg/km) from diesel engine exhausts and mutagenicity[a]

| | Vehicle[b] | | | | Fuel aromaticity[c] | | Engine conditions[d] | | |
|---|---|---|---|---|---|---|---|---|---|
| | A | B | C | D | 22% | 55% | Retarded timing | Standard timing | Advanced timing |
| Pyrene | 39 ± 16 (24 ± 10) | 62 ± 15 (39 ± 9) | 29 ± 15 (18 ± 9) | 24 ± 11 (15 ± 7) | 39 ± 18 (24 ± 11) | 125 ± 39 (78 ± 24) | 31 ± 20 (19 ± 13) | 39 ± 18 (24 ± 11) | 35 ± 22 (22 ± 14) |
| Benzo[a]pyrene | 1.3 ± 0.9 (0.8 ± 0.6) | 1.9 ± 0.1 (1.2 ± 0.06) | 1.6 ± 0.2 (1 ± 0.1) | 0.6 ± 0.1 (0.4 ± 0.06) | 1.3 ± 0.5 (0.8 ± 0.3) | 7.1 ± 3.6 (4.4 ± 2.3) | 1.7 ± 1.1 (1.1 ± 0.7) | 1.3 ± 0.5 (0.8 ± 0.3) | 1.5 ± 0.6 (0.9 ± 0.4) |
| Benzo[e]pyrene | 2.3 ± 1.2 (1.4 ± 0.8) | 5.1 ± 0.2 (3 ± 0.1) | 3.0 ± 0.4 (1.9 ± 0.3) | 1.3 ± 0.4 (0.8 ± 0.3) | 3.0 ± 1.1 (1.9 ± 0.7) | 10.3 ± 4.1 (6.4 ± 2.6) | 3.6 ± 2.1 (2.3 ± 1.3) | 3.0 ± 1.1 (1.9 ± 0.7) | 4.2 ± 0.5 (3 ± 0.3) |
| 1-Nitropyrene | 3.0 ± 1.0 (1.9 ± 0.6) | 7.8 ± 2.2 (4.9 ± 1.4) | 1.8 ± 0.9 (1.1 ± 0.6) | 3.8 ± 1.4 (2.4 ± 0.9) | 4.1 ± 1.9 (2.6 ± 1.2) | 3.7 ± 1.6 (2.3 ± 1) | 2.3 ± 0.5 (1.4 ± 0.3) | 4.1 ± 1.9 (2.6 ± 1.2) | 15.5 ± 7.7 (10 ± 5) |
| Nitrogen oxides in g/mile (g/km) | — | — | — | — | — | — | 0.9 ± 0.02 (0.6 ± 0.01) | 1.0 ± 0.01 (0.6 ± 0.006) | 1.3 ± 0.1 (0.8 ± 0.06) |
| Mutagenicity in 10⁶ rev/mile (10⁶ rev/km) | | | | | | | | | |
| TA98 (without activation) | 1.0 ± 0.4 (0.6 ± 0.2) | 1.3 ± 0.3 (0.8 ± 0.2) | 0.8 ± 0.3 (0.5 ± 0.2) | 0.8 ± 0.2 (0.5 ± 0.1) | 0.99 ± 0.35 (0.6 ± 0.2) | 2.9 ± 0.80 (1.8 ± 0.5) | 2.2 ± 1.6 (1.4 ± 1.0) | 3.4 ± 1.5 (2.1 ± 0.9) | 6.4 ± 2.7 (4.0 ± 1.7) |
| TA98 (with activation) | 0.5 ± 0.2 (0.3 ± 0.1) | 0.7 ± 0.2 (0.4 ± 0.1) | 0.6 ± 0.2 (0.4 ± 0.1) | 0.5 ± 0.1 (0.3 ± 0.06) | 0.61 ± 0.18 (0.4 ± 0.1) | 2.1 ± 0.49 (1.3 ± 0.3) | 1.0 ± 0.5 (0.6 ± 0.3) | 1.8 ± 0.7 (1.1 ± 0.4) | 2.5 ± 1.1 (1.6 ± 0.6) |

[a]From Schuetzle & Frazier (1986)
[b]Duplicate tests on each vehicle run on four different fuels of 22% aromatic composition
[c]Duplicate tests on four vehicles run at standard timing on four different fuels
[d]Duplicate tests on two vehicles

In the descriptions below of the chemical and physical characteristics of emissions from diesel and spark-ignition (gasoline) engines, primary emphasis is placed on the identification of PAHs in different engines, with different fuels and under various operating conditions.

## 1.2 Diesel engine exhaust

In reviewing the data, the reader should recognize that detailed chemical characterization of engine emissions, especially for nitroarenes, was performed mostly in the late 1970s and 1980s. During that period, substantial changes occurred in engine and emission control technologies, and additional changes are to be expected in the future. It is also reasonable to expect that the emissions characterized recently may not represent fully emissions in earlier times. The available data refer mainly to light-duty vehicles; quantitative data on emissions from heavy-duty diesel engines are relatively sparse. Because of these limitations, the data presented here should be considered only as illustrative of the emissions of internal combustion engines; they should not be interpreted as representative of either current emissions from the wide range of engines used at present or of those that may have occurred in the past.

Compounds emitted from diesel engines include all of the compounds and compound classes listed in Table 1. Diesel engines produce two to ten times more particulate emissions than gasoline engines (without catalytic converter) of comparable power output and two to 40 times more particulate emissions than gasoline engines equipped with a catalytic converter (Table 3). The particles consist primarily of elemental carbon (Ball, 1987; 60–80%, Zaebst *et al.*, 1988), sulfuric acid (2–7%; Pierson & Brachaczek, 1983) and some metallic species, e.g., iron from the engine and exhaust system (Lang *et al.*, 1981), barium from fuel (Hampton *et al.*, 1983) and zinc from lubricating oil (Hare & Baines, 1979), and adsorbed organic compounds (National Research Council, 1982).

*(a) Distribution in particulate and gas phases*

The distribution of emissions between the gas and particulate phases is determined by the vapour pressure, temperature and concentration of the individual species. The partitioning of constituents between the particulate and gas phases has been measured by several investigators (Hampton *et al.*, 1983; Schuetzle, 1983). On the basis of these data, an empirical relationship between the molecular weight and the particulate- to gas-phase partition coefficient (P:G) for several of these compounds was derived, as shown for the PAHs in Table 5 (Schuetzle & Frazier, 1986).

*(b) Gas-phase emissions*

Gas-phase emissions from diesel engines comprise $C_1$–$C_{18}$ hydrocarbons, two- to four-ring PAHs and nitrated and oxygenated derivatives of $C_1$–$C_{12}$ hydrocarbons and two- to three-ring PAHs. The $C_1$–$C_{10}$ hydrocarbons result almost entirely from the combustion process, which involves cracking of higher molecular weight materials (National Research Council, 1982). The quantities of some of these gas-phase species in diesel exhaust are given in Table 3.

Table 5. Particulate- to gas-phase partition coefficients for some polycyclic aromatic hydrocarbons in diesel exhaust[a]

| Compound | Molecular weight | Partition coefficient |
| --- | --- | --- |
| Phenanthrene | 178 | 0.05 |
| Anthracene | 178 | 0.05 |
| Pyrene | 202 | 0.75 |
| Fluoranthene | 202 | 0.75 |
| Benz[a]anthracene | 228 | 1.46 |
| Benzo[a]pyrene[b] | 252 | 21.00 |

[a]From Schuetzle & Frazier (1986), unless otherwise specified
[b]From Schuetzle (1983)

*(c) Particulate-phase emissions*

Diesel particles are aggregates of spherical primary particles of 0.1–0.5 μm (National Research Council, 1982). Those generated under laboratory conditions in dilution tunnels have mass or volume median diameters ranging from 0.15 to 0.50 μm, depending on the operating conditions (Cheng *et al.*, 1984). Smaller primary spheres, formed within the combustion cylinder, grow by agglomeration and by acting as nuclei for the condensation of organic compounds (Duleep & Dulla, 1980).

The elemental carbon core of the particles has a large surface area which greatly enhances adsorption of organic compounds. Larger particles (>0.2 μm) tend to be flaky in nature (Moore *et al.*, 1978). If an engine is running under low load, there may be incomplete combustion, leading to a relatively low particle concentration and a higher proportion of organic compounds associated with the core particles (Dutcher *et al.*, 1984).

A variety of solvents has been used to extract organic compounds from diesel particles (Bjørseth, 1983; see p. 80). The soluble organic fraction of diesel particles usually accounts for 15–45% of the total particulate mass. Figure 1 shows the distribution of mass for the various subfractions of a standard heavy-duty diesel particulate extract (Schuetzle *et al.*, 1985).

The nonpolar fractions contain hydrocarbons derived from unburnt fuel and lubricating oil. In addition, many PAHs in the molecular weight range of 178–320 have been identified. Some PAHs and thioarenes identified in diesel engine exhausts are listed in Table 6 (Tong & Karasek, 1984). The alkyl substituted derivatives of at least some PAHs are more abundant than the parent hydrocarbons. If the amount of dimethylanthracenes or dimethylphenanthrenes is taken as 1.00, the relative abundance of anthracene or phenanthrene is 0.27, that of the methyl derivatives, 0.54, and that of the trimethyl derivatives, 0.37 (Schuetzle *et al.*, 1981). Since moderately polar fractions have been found to contribute a significant proportion of the mutagenicity of the total soluble organic fraction, much effort has been expended to characterize them. The distribution of PAH derivatives in one light-duty diesel particulate extract is given in Table 7 (Schuetzle, 1983).

Fig. 1. Analytical scheme for fractionation of heavy-duty diesel particulates (National Bureau of Standards Standard Reference Material (NBS SRM)-1650)[a]

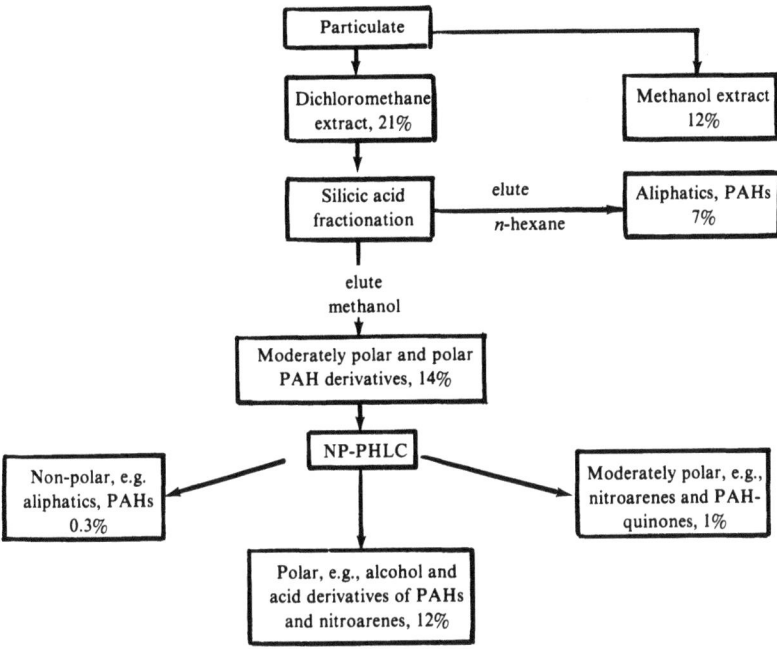

[a]From Schuetzle et al. (1985). Recoveries are given as weight percent of total particulate mass. NP-HPLC, normal phase-high-performance liquid chromatography

Table 6. Polycyclic aromatic comounds identified or tentatively identified in three light-duty diesel particulate extracts[a]

| Compound | Molecular weight | Concentration[b] ($\mu$g/g of extract) |
| --- | --- | --- |
| Acenaphthylene | 152 | 30 |
| Fluorene | 166 | 100–168 |
| Trimethylnaphthalene | 170 | 30–50 |
| Anthracene | 178 | 155–356 |
| Phenanthrene | 178 | 2186–4883 |
| Dimethylbiphenyl | 182 | 30–91 |
| Tetramethylnaphthalene | 184 | 50–152 |
| Dibenzothiophene | 184 | 129–246 |
| 4$H$-Cyclopenta[$def$]phenanthrene | 190 | 517–1033 |
| 2-Methylanthracene | 192 | 517–1522 |
| 2-Methylphenanthrene | 192 | 1099–1481 |
| 3-Methylphenanthrene | 192 | 929–1287 |
| Trimethylbiphenyl | 196 | 50 |

## Table 6 (contd)

| Compound | Molecular weight | Concentration[b] (μg/g of extract) |
|---|---|---|
| Methyldibenzothiophene | 198 | 101–323 |
| Benzacenaphthylene | 202 | 791–1643 |
| Fluoranthene | 202 | 3399–7321 |
| Pyrene | 202 | 3532–8002 |
| 2-Phenylnaphthalene | 204 | 650–1336 |
| Dimethylphenanthrene | 206 | 443–1046 |
| 2- or 9-Ethylphenanthrene | 206 | 388–464 |
| Dimethylphenanthrene or -anthracene | 206 | 86–585 |
| Benzo[def]dibenzothiophene | 208 | 254–333 |
| Ethyldibenzothiophene | 212 | 151–179 |
| Benzo[a]fluorene | 216 | 541–990 |
| Benzo[b]fluorene | 216 | 175–538 |
| Methylfluoranthene or -pyrene | 216 | 224–552 |
| 1-Methylpyrene | 216 | 144–443 |
| Ethylmethylphenanthrene or -anthracene | 220 | 286–432 |
| Benzo[ghi]fluoranthene | 226 | 217–418 |
| Cyclopenta[cd]pyrene | 226 | 869–1671 |
| Benz[a]anthracene | 228 | 463–1076 |
| Chrysene or triphenylene | 228 | 657–1529 |
| Benzonaphthothiophene | 234 | 30–126 |
| Benzo[b]naphtho[2,1-d]thiophene | 234 | 30–53 |
| Methylbenz[a]anthracene | 242 | 30–50 |
| 3-Methylchrysene | 242 | 50–192 |
| Benzo[b]fluoranthene | 252 | 421–1098 |
| Benzo[j]fluoranthene | 252 | 492–1367 |
| Benzo[k]fluoranthene | 252 | 91–289 |
| Benzo[e]pyrene | 252 | 487–946 |
| Benzo[a]pyrene | 252 | 208–558 |
| 1,2-Binaphthyl | 254 | 30–50 |
| 2,2-Binaphthyl | 254 | 89–283 |
| 1-Phenylphenanthrene | 254 | 89–163 |
| 9-Phenylphenanthrene | 254 | 30–94 |
| Phenylphenanthrene or -anthracene | 254 | 30–116 |
| Benzo[ghi]perylene | 276 | 443–1050 |
| Indeno[1,2,3-cd]pyrene | 276 | 30–93 |
| Dibenz[a,h]anthracene | 278 | 50–96 |
| Coronene | 300 | 301–521 |
| Dibenzopyrene or -[def,p]chrysene | 302 | 89–254 |

[a]From Tong & Karasek (1984)

[b]Concentrations of less than 50 μg/g extract were obtained by approximate calculation

Table 7. Distribution of polycyclic aromatic hydrocarbon (PAH) derivatives in the moderately polar fraction[a] of a light-duty diesel particulate extract[b]

| PAH derivative | Fraction (wt %) |
|---|---|
| PAH ketones | 24.7 |
| PAH carboxyaldehydes | 20.6 |
| PAH acid anhydrides | 9.1 |
| Hydroxy-PAH | 19.0 |
| PAH quinones | 12.0 |
| Nitro-PAH | 0.5 |
| Other oxygenated PAH | 14.1 |

[a]Comprising 9% of the particulate phase by weight
[b]Schuetzle (1983)

The types of nitroarenes identified in diesel vehicle particles are listed in Figure 2. More than 50 nitrated derivatives of PAHs have been identified tentatively and 23 have been identified positively. These compounds occur in very low concentrations in comparison with the other PAH derivatives (Schuetzle & Jensen, 1985). The concentrations of nitroarenes measured in a light-duty diesel particulate extract by a method with a 0.3-ppm ($\mu$g/g) limit of detection are given in Table 8. Overall, about 40% of the direct mutagenicity of diesel particulate extracts can be accounted for by 1-nitro-3-acetoxypyrenes, dinitropyrenes and 1-nitropyrene (Manabe et al., 1985). Studies in which biological and other methods were used to estimate the contribution of nitro-PAH to the genetic effects of diesel emissions are discussed in section 3.2.

Examples of compounds in the polar soluble organic fraction of diesel vehicle particulate extracts include phenols (1-naphthol, 2-naphthol, cresol), acids (benzoic, naphthoic, phthalic and phenathroic acid), bases (benzacridines, dibenzacridines, pyridine, aniline) and some polar nitroarenes (National Research Council, 1982).

*(d) Effect of engine source, fuel and operating conditions on emissions*

In this section, the influence of several factors on the emission of four compounds — pyrene, benzo[a]pyrene, benzo[e]pyrene and 1-nitropyrene — is summarized (Schuetzle & Frazier, 1986). Particulate samples were collected from four diesel vehicles produced by four major manufacturers, which run on a variety of diesel fuels under various operating conditions (see Table 4). Overall, the emission rates of these compounds varied by no more than a factor of three.

The emission of PAHs was increased by a factor of three to four when the aromaticity of the fuel (content of aromatic hydrocarbons) increased from 22 to 55%, resulting in 2–24 and 2–60 mg/l pyrene, respectively. Exhaust pipe emissions of pyrene were not related to the pyrene content of the fuel, indicating that the primary source of PAHs is their formation

Fig. 2. Types of nitro-polycyclic aromatic hydrocarbons (PAHs) and nitroheterocyclic compounds identified in diesel emission particulates[a]

| Compound type | Rings | Examples | Number reported | |
|---|---|---|---|---|
| | | | Tentative | Confirmed |
| NO$_2$-PAH | 2–5 | 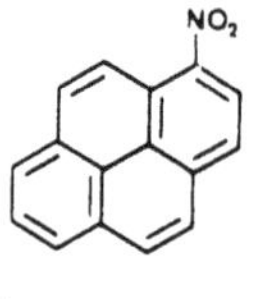 1-Nitropyrene | 10 | 9 |
| NO$_2$-alkyl-PAH | 2–4 | 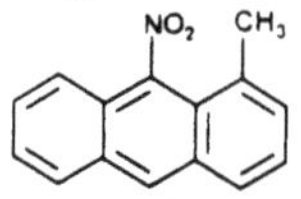 1-Methyl-9-nitroanthracene | 22 | 5 |
| NO$_2$-oxy-PAH | 3–4 | 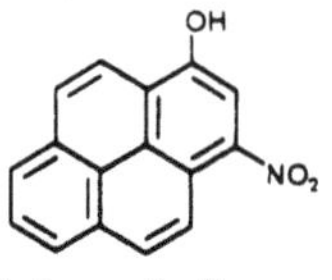 1-Hydroxy-3-nitropyrene | 10 | – |
| Di-NO$_2$-PAH | 2–4 | 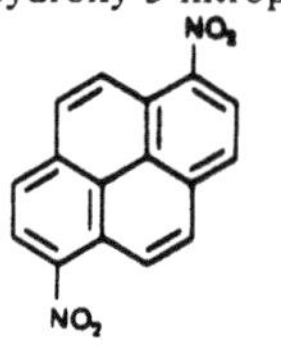 1,6-Dinitropyrene | 3 | 7 |
| NO$_2$-S-PAH | 2–3 | 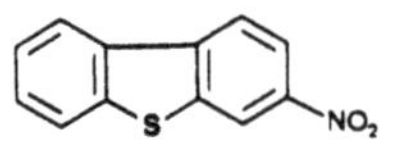 3-Nitrodibenzothiophene | 2 | – |
| NO$_2$-N-PAH | 2–3 | 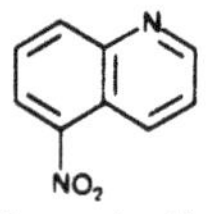 5-Nitroquinoline | 4 | 2 |

[a]From Schuetzle & Jensen (1985)

during the combustion process and not their presence in unburnt fuel in the exhaust. In contrast, fuel aromaticity had no effect on the emission of 1-nitropyrene, suggesting that nitrogen oxides, and not pyrene, are the limiting factor in the chemical formation of 1-nitropyrene (Schuetzle & Frazier, 1986).

Table 4 also presents data that demonstrate the effect of engine operating conditions on diesel emissions. Changes in engine timing have little effect on PAH emissions, but the 1-nitropyrene content increased by several fold, correlating with the increase in emissions of

Table 8. Concentrations of some nitroarenes ($\mu$g/g) in diesel particulate extracts

| Compound | Concentration | Reference |
|---|---|---|
| 1-Nitronaphthalene[a,b] | 0.95[c] | Paputa-Peck et al. (1983) |
| 2-Nitronaphthalene[a,b] | 0.35[c] | Paputa-Peck et al. (1983) |
| 2-Nitrofluorene[b] | 1.2[c] | Paputa-Peck et al. (1983) |
| 1-Nitropyrene[b] | 75 | Paputa-Peck et al. (1983) |
| 3-Nitrofluoranthene | 3.5[c] | Paputa-Peck et al. (1983) |
| 8-Nitrofluoranthene | 1.3[c] | Paputa-Peck et al. (1983) |
| 6-Nitrobenzo[a]pyrene[b] | 4.2[c] | Paputa-Peck et al. (1983) |
| 1,3-Dinitropyrene[b] | 0.30 | Paputa-Peck et al. (1983) |
| 1,6-Dinitropyrene[b] | 0.40 | Paputa-Peck et al. (1983) |
| 1,8-Dinitropyrene[b] | 0.53 | Paputa-Peck et al. (1983) |
| 2,7-Dinitrofluorene | 4.2, 6.0[d] | Schuetzle (1983) |
| 2,7-Dinitro-9-fluorenone | 3.0, 8.6[d] | Schuetzle (1983) |
| 1-Nitro-3-hydroxypyrene | 70 | Manabe et al. (1985) |
| 1-Nitro-3-acetoxypyrene | 6.3 | Manabe et al. (1985) |

[a]Tentative identification: confirmed by gas chromatographic retention times of authentic standards, but not by mass spectrometry

[b]Concentration estimated from chromatographic intensity by the Working Group within ± 50% error limits

[c]Considered in a monograph in this volume

[d]Two light-duty diesel particulate extracts

nitrogen oxides. Engine speed and load significantly affect the emission of nitroarenes in engine exhaust, as shown in Table 9. High load and high speed raise engine and exhaust temperatures, enhancing the partial oxidation of nitroarenes. Thus, the emission of nitroarenes, and possibly of other oxygenated PAH species, is highly dependent on source conditions (Schuetzle & Perez, 1983).

### 1.3 Gasoline engine exhaust

All research to date indicates that emissions from spark-ignition engines run on unleaded gasoline are qualitatively similar to the emissions from diesel engines (Alsberg et al., 1984; see Tables 3, 6 and 10). However, there are significant quantitative differences (see section 1.4). The data reported below relate to four-stroke engines, unless otherwise specified, although the emissions from two-stroke engines are qualitatively similar. Since several PAHs have been shown to be carcinogenic (IARC, 1983, 1987a), much research has been directed to the identification of individual compounds in these emissions (Table 10; Grimmer et al., 1977). As for diesel fuel, the emission of PAHs (measured as benzo[a]-pyrene) varies with the aromatic content of the gasoline (Schuetzle & Frazier, 1986).

Table 9. Effects of engine operating conditions on concentration of nitro-polycyclic aromatic hydrocarbons in heavy-duty diesel particles[a]

| Compound | Concentration in particles ($\mu g/g$)[b] | | |
|---|---|---|---|
| | HDD38, idle | HDD34, high speed, zero load | HDD4, high speed, full load |
| 2-Nitrofluorene | 84 (164) | 62 (134) | 1.9 (15) |
| 3-Nitro-9-fluorenone | 18 (35) | 7.9 (17) | 8 (63) |
| 2-Nitro-9-fluorenone | 10 (19) | 4.8 (10) | 3.7 (29) |
| 9-Nitroanthracene | 94 (184) | 16 (35) | 5.1 (40) |
| 9-Nitro-1-methylanthracene | 129 (252) | 13 (28) | 0.2 (1.6) |
| 3-Nitro-1,8-naphthalic acid anhydride | 23 (46) | 10 (22) | 22 (174) |
| 1-Nitropyrene | 14 (28) | 3 (6.5) | 0.13 (1) |
| 2,7-Dinitrofluorene | 15 (30) | 18 (39) | 3.9 (31) |
| 2,5-Dinitro-9-fluorenone | 5.5 (11) | 8 (17) | 2.1 (17) |
| 2,4,7-Trinitro-9-fluorenone | <1 (<2) | 0.4 (0.9) | NR[c] |
| 1,3-Dinitropyrene | <0.8 (<1.6) | 0.6 (1.3) | 0.4 (3.1) |
| 1,6-Dinitropyrene | <0.8 (<1.6) | 1.2 (2.6) | 0.8 (6.3) |
| 1,8-Dinitropyrene | <0.8 (<1.6) | 1.2 (2.6) | 0.8 (6.3) |
| 6-Nitrobenzo[a]pyrene | <3.2 (<6.5) | 1.6 (3.5) | 0.3 (2.4) |

[a]From Schuetzle & Perez (1983)

[b]Number in parentheses is concentration in extract in micrograms per gram; extraction of samples HDD38, HDD34 and HDD4 gave 51, 45.9 and 12.7% extractables, respectively.

[c]NR, not sufficiently resolved from several other components

Little detailed information is available on the occurrence of PAH derivatives (e.g., nitroarenes) in gasoline exhaust. Some acridines, including benz[c]acridine, dibenz[a,h]acridine and dibenz[a,j]acridine, have been identified in gasoline engine exhaust (Sawicki et al., 1965). 1,2-Dichloroethane (38–2900 $\mu g/m^3$) and 1,2-dibromoethane (22–1360 $\mu g/m^3$) have been measured in exhausts from engines run on leaded gasoline (Tsani-Bazaca et al., 1981). Methyl bromide has been found in the exhaust of cars using leaded (71–217 $\mu g/m^3$) and unleaded (<4–5 $\mu g/m^3$) gasoline (Harsch & Rasmussen, 1977).

The particles emitted from gasoline engines run on leaded fuel are physically different from particles emitted from diesel engines. Particles from gasoline engines are discrete, compact and dense. The mass median equivalent diameter of the particles, as measured along roads at steady speed ($\simeq$80 km/h) is 0.03–0.04 $\mu$m but increases to 0.2–0.4 $\mu$m when the vehicle is operated under cyclic conditions. Particulate mass comprises ammonium and lead sulfates, lead bromochloride and lead oxide, which are soluble in water. The proportion of organic solvent-extractable material is much smaller than that typically found in diesel particles (see Table 3). The remaining elemental carbon core of the particle has fewer sites available for adsorption of organic material, but quantitative comparisons with diesel particles are not available (Chamberlain et al., 1978).

Table 10. Polycyclic aromatic hydrocarbons identified in gasoline engine fuel and exhaust ($\mu$g/l of original or combusted fuel)[a]

| Compound | Molecular weight | Gasoline | Exhaust A[b] | Exhaust B[b] |
|---|---|---|---|---|
| Naphthalene | 128 | + | + | + |
| 1-Methylnaphthalene | 142 | + | + | + |
| 2-Methylnaphthalene | 142 | + | + | + |
| Acenaphthylene | 152 | + | + | + |
| Diphenylene | 152 | + | + | + |
| Acenaphthene | 154 | + | + | + |
| Diphenyl | 154 | + | + | + |
| 1,2-Dimethylnaphthalene | 156 | + | + | + |
| 1,3-Dimethylnaphthalene | 156 | + | + | + |
| 1,4-Dimethylnaphthalene | 156 | + | + | + |
| 1,5-Dimethylnaphthalene | 156 | + | + | + |
| 1,6-Dimethylnaphthalene | 156 | + | + | + |
| 1,7-Dimethylnaphthalene | 156 | + | + | + |
| 1,8-Dimethylnaphthalene | 156 | + | + | + |
| 2,3-Dimethylnaphthalene | 156 | + | + | + |
| 2,6-Dimethylnaphthalene | 156 | + | + | + |
| 2,7-Dimethylnaphthalene | 156 | + | + | + |
| 1-Ethylnaphthalene | 156 | + | + | + |
| 2-Ethylnaphthalene | 156 | + | + | + |
| Fluorene | 166 | + | + | + |
| Methylacenaphthylene* | 166 | + | + | + |
| Dibenzo[b,d]furan | 168 | − | + | + |
| Diphenylmethane | 168 | − | + | + |
| 2-Methyldiphenyl* | 168 | + | + | + |
| 3-Methyldiphenyl | 168 | + | + | + |
| 1,3,7-Trimethylnaphthalene | 170 | − | + | + |
| 1,6,7-Trimethylnaphthalene | 170 | + | + | + |
| 2,3,6-Trimethylnaphthalene | 170 | + | + | + |
| Anthracene | 178 | 1 555 | 534 | 642 |
| Phenanthrene | 178 | 15 700 | 2 930 | 2 356 |
| Methylfluorene* | 180 | + | + | + |
| 1-Methylfluorene | 180 | + | + | + |
| 2-Methylfluorene | 180 | + | + | + |
| 3,3'-Dimethyldiphenyl (m,m'-Ditolyl) | 182 | − | + | + |
| 4,4'-Dimethyldiphenyl (p,p'-Ditolyl) | 182 | + | + | + |
| 1,2-Diphenylethane | 182 | − | + | + |
| 4,5-Methylenephenanthrene | 190 |  | 473 | 762 |
| 3-Methylphenanthrene | 192 | 6 870 | 264 | 510 |
| 2-Methylphenanthrene | 192 | 7 730 | 269 | 578 |
| 2-Methylanthracene | 192 | 739 | 92 | 104 |
| 4- and 9-Methylphenanthrene | 192 | 1 243 | 190 | 330 |
| 1-Methylphenanthrene | 192 | 3 180 | 256 | 404 |
| Dimethylfluorene* | 194 | − to 372 | − to 161 | 184−192 |
| Dimethylfluorene* and 1-phenylnaphthalene | 194 / 204 | 143 | 37 | 108 |

**Table 10 (contd)**

| Compound | Molecular weight | Gasoline | Exhaust A[b] | Exhaust B[b] |
|---|---|---|---|---|
| Dimethyldiphenylenoxide* | 196 | + | + | + |
| Methyldiphenylethane* | 196 | + | + | + |
| Fluoranthene | 202 | 1 840 | 1 060 | 1 662 |
| Pyrene | 202 | 4 700 | 2 150 | 2 884 |
| 2-Phenylnaphthalene | 204 | 538 | 103 | 186 |
| Dimethylphenanthrene* | 206 | − to 1128 | − to 95 | − to 216 |
| Benzo[a]fluorene | 216 | 1 500 | 82 | 136 |
| Benzo[b]fluorene and benzo[c]fluorene | 216 | 1 420 | 65 | 112 |
| 1-Methylpyrene | 216 | + | + | + |
| 4-Methylpyrene | 216 | + | + | + |
| Cyclopento[cd]pyrene | 226 | − | 987 | 750 |
| Benzo[ghi]fluoranthene | 226 | 3 | 244 | 112 |
| Benz[a]anthracene | 228 | 39 | 83 | 50 |
| Benzo[c]phenanthrene | 228 | + | + | + |
| Chrysene | 228 | 52 | 123 | 85 |
| Triphenylene | 228 | 30 | 60 | 40 |
| 3-Methylchrysene | 242 | − | + | + |
| 2- and 5-Methylchrysene | 242 | 8 | 5 | 5 |
| 4- and 6-Methylchrysene | 242 | 8 | 5 | 5 |
| Benzo[b]fluoranthene | 252 | 159 | 48 | 19 |
| Benzo[k]fluoranthene | 252 | 9 | 17 | 7 |
| Benzo[j]fluoranthene | 252 | 9 | 27 | 11 |
| Benzo[e]pyrene | 252 | 307 | 59 | 37 |
| Benzo[a]pyrene | 252 | 133 | 81 | 50 |
| Perylene | 252 | 18 | 14 | 7 |
| 11H-Cyclopenta[qrs]benzo[e]pyrene (8,9-Methylenebenzo[e]pyrene) | 264 | 13 | 43 | 17 |
| 10H-Cyclopenta[mno]benzo[a]pyrene (10,11-Methylenebenzo[a]pyrene) | 264 | 5 | 18 | 8 |
| Anthanthrene | 276 | 20 | 17 | 26 |
| Benzo[ghi]perylene | 276 | 484 | 333 | 115 |
| Indeno[1,2,3-cd]fluoranthene | 276 | 16 | 32 | 12 |
| Indeno[1,2,3-cd]pyrene | 276 | 59 | 86 | 32 |
| Dibenz[a,h]anthracene | 278 | + | + | + |
| Dibenz[a,j]anthracene | 278 | + | + | + |
| Picene (Benzo[a]chrysene) | 278 | 1 | 1 | 1 |
| Benzo[ghi]cyclopenta[pqr]perylene (1,12-Methylenebenzo[ghi]perylene) | 288 | − | 41 | 19 |
| Coronene | 300 | 165 | 271 | 106 |
| Picene (Benzo[a]chrysene) (1,2,6,7-Dibenzopyrene) | 302 | 16 | − | − |

[a]From Grimmer et al. (1977); compounds that could not be identified are not included in the table.

[b]Exhaust A, vehicle with air-cooled four-cylinder engine (44 PS); Exhaust B, vehicle with water-cooled four-cylinder engine (68 PS)

+, characterized by mass spectrometry; concentrations given when available

−, not detected; limit of detection about 0.2 μg/l combusted fuel

*, isomer uncertain

## 1.4 Comparison of emissions from different engines

A number of studies have recently been undertaken to determine emissions from a wide variety of engines. Levels of selected gas and particulate species and of total particulate matter from light-duty diesel, heavy-duty diesel and gasoline engines (with and without catalytic converters) in 1980–85 are summarized in Table 3.

The levels of carbon monoxide and nitrogen oxides emitted are similar for light-duty diesel and for gasoline engines with catalytic converters. The particulate emission levels from light-duty and heavy-duty diesels are two to ten and eight to 40 times greater, respectively, than the emission levels from catalyst equipped light-duty gasoline engines (Table 3).

Fuel evaporation (e.g., from fuel lines and carburettors) has become relatively more important as a source of hydrocarbons since emissions from exhaust pipes have been reduced. Currently, fuel evaporation accounts for 30–60% of the total hydrocarbon emissions from passenger gasoline vehicles with catalytic converters. The vapour pressure of most current diesel fuels under ambient conditions is so low that emissions due to evaporation of diesel fuels are not significant (National Research Council, 1982).

The levels of PAHs in emissions from light-duty diesel engines and from gasoline engines without catalytic converters are comparable, although the diesel engines emit at least ten times more nitroarenes than the gasoline engines. Catalytic converters reduce the level of total PAHs by more than ten times (Table 3).

Nitric acid, which can react with PAHs to form nitroarenes, has been measured in diesel exhaust (Harris *et al.*, 1987), and Paputa-Peck *et al.* (1983) measured low-molecular-weight nitroarenes in diesel particles (Table 8). In view of the vapour pressure relationships, these nitroarenes would also be present in the gas phase (Hampton *et al.*, 1983). A value for 2-nitrofluorene is given in Table 3 (Schuetzle & Frazier, 1986). Liberti *et al.* (1984) found several gas-phase nitro-PAHs in diesel exhaust (Table 11).

Table 11. Gas-phase nitro-polycyclic aromatic hydrocarbons identified in diesel exhaust[a]

| Species | Relative concentration |
|---|---|
| x-Nitrofluorene[b] | 1.00 |
| 1-Nitronaphthalene | 0.10 |
| x-Methyl-1-nitronaphthalene[b] | 0.20 |
| 2-Nitronaphthalene | 0.30 |
| 2-Nitrofluorene | 0.75 |
| 9-Nitroanthracene | 0.50 |
| Dinitronaphthalene | 0.20 |

[a]From Liberti *et al.* (1984)

[b]x, position unknown

Aliphatic amines are present at very low concentrations in exhausts from cars equipped with catalytic converters. Total emissions were less than 2.2 mg/mile (1.4 mg/km), and average emission rates of monomethylamine and dimethylamine were no more than 0.3 and 0.1 mg/mile (0.2 and 0.06 mg/km), respectively (Cadle & Mulawa, 1980). Levels of 0.1−1.4 µg/m³ $N$-nitrosomorpholine and 0.5−17.2 µg/m³ $N$-nitrosodimethylamine were measured in crankcase gases of heavy-duty diesel engines (Goff et al., 1980). In one study in a vehicle tunnel, no $N$-nitrosodimethylamine was detected (detection limit, 0.1 µg/m³) in the air (Hampton et al., 1983).

## 2. Occurrence and Analysis

### 2.1 Occupational exposure

The occupational exposures to components of diesel engine exhaust of several groups of workers, including railroad workers, workers in mines with diesel-powered equipment, bus garage workers, truck drivers, fork-lift truck operators and fire-fighters, have been studied. The exposures of toll-booth attendants, border-station inspectors, traffic-control officers, professional drivers (truck, bus, taxi), car mechanics, car ferry workers, parking garage attendants and lumberjacks to components of gasoline engine exhaust have also been studied. Many workers are exposed to both diesel and gasoline engine exhausts. The extent of exposure to these specific exhausts in different occupational groups depends on many factors, such as country and time period considered; in addition, environmental exposure to exhausts (see section 2.2) influences the total exposure of workers.

A primary focus of this monograph is on human exposure to respirable particles emitted by diesel and gasoline engines. It is important in studying such exposures that the relative contributions from various types of engine exhaust be distinguished from each other and from those of other particulate sources. In source apportionment studies, chemical tracers are used which are unique to the combustion source, representative of the total particulate emissions, chemically stable, present in abundance, and easy to collect and analyse. Many compounds that may appear to be good tracers are not representative of the total sample, varying significantly with the fuel source, temperature of combustion and other factors.

Methods have been developed and used for apportioning the contribution of vehicle emissions from various sources. These are based upon the use of barium (a diesel fuel additive) and of lead for diesel and gasoline vehicles, respectively (Hampton et al., 1983; Johnson, 1988). The method may not be suitable for characterizing certain occupational exposures (e.g., mining, train and heavy-equipment operations) because barium is not typically used as a fuel additive in these applications.

Several new methods have been developed to apportion sources of occupational exposure to engine exhaust. For example, Currie and Klouda (1982) used measurements of $^{14}C/^{12}C$ to distinguish between carbon compounds in particles derived from combustion of old carbon sources (e.g., petroleum) and of contemporary carbon sources (e.g., wood, tobacco). Johnson et al. (1981) developed a thermal-optical analytical technique which has been used to apportion samples containing cigarette smoke and diesel exhaust particles (Zaebst et al., 1988). Cantrell et al. (1986) indicated that size selective sampling is a suitable method for distinguishing diesel particles from other particles in coal mines.

Unfortunately, for the studies of exposure reviewed in this section, the source apportionment techniques described above were not available. The data on components of engine exhausts, such as carbon monoxide, nitrogen oxides and sulfur dioxide, can be used to indicate the presence of engine exhaust but cannot be used to apportion exposures. Thus, information on single components reported in these studies cannot be used to rank relative exposures to total engine exhaust reliably, due to the variable relationships among the components resulting from factors such as engine speed, engine load and control techniques.

It should also be noted that occupational exposures to PAHs can be measured, but samples are typically not large enough to allow quantitative measurements to be made.

*(a) Workers whose predominant exhaust exposure is that from diesel engines*

(i) *Railroad workers*

Diesel locomotives were introduced on railroads in Canada and the USA in 1928 and in Germany in 1932. In the USA, the change-over to diesel engines was 95% complete by 1959 (Garshick et al., 1988).

Hobbs et al. (1977) reviewed the earlier literature on air contaminants in the environment of train crews. In addition, measurements of air contaminants in locomotives and cabooses were made during their passage through tunnels and during freighting and switch-yard operations. These authors estimated 8-h time-weighted averages (TWAs) for combined tunnel and freight operations, and Heino et al. (1978) evaluated levels of diesel exhaust components in locomotive cabs and round-houses in Finland (Table 12).

As part of a large epidemiological study on railroad workers, Hammond et al. (1984) presented data on components of diesel exhaust. The respirable particles collected had a dichloromethane extractable fraction of 46% (liquid chromatography fractionation), which was found to be composed of 45% aliphatic hydrocarbons, 33% olefinic and aromatic hydrocarbons and 23% polar compounds. The aromatic fraction included phenanthrene and alkylated phenanthrenes.

Woskie et al. (1988a) conducted an industrial hygiene survey of the US railroad industry as a part of epidemiological studies reported by Garshick et al. (1987, 1988). Personal exposure to respirable particles was measured and then corrected for the estimated contribution of cigarette smoke particulates. These data are presented in Table 13. Corrections for cigarette smoke were made by analysing composited respirable particulate samples for nicotine content; an adjusted respirable particulate concentration was then calculated for each job group, and the applicable average fraction of cigarette smoke was subtracted from the average respirable particulate concentration.

(ii) *Mine workers*

The first diesel engine-powered vehicles in underground mines were used in Germany in 1927 (Kaplan, 1959), and they are now used widely throughout the world (Daniel, 1984).

Table 12. Levels of air contaminants to which railroad workers are exposed

| Substance | Locomotive cabs | | | Freighting[b] (7.5-h TWA) | Switch-yard[b] (5-h TWA) | Caboose (8-h TWA in 1 tunnel trip)[b] | Roundhouses (mean; range)[a] |
|---|---|---|---|---|---|---|---|
| | Mean (range)[a] | Tunnels (8-h TWA)[b] | | | | | |
| | | 1 trip | 5 trips | | | | |
| Carbon monoxide (mg/m³) | — | 8.9 | 40.2 | 1.43 | 0.3 | 1.43 | — |
| Nitric oxide (mg/m³) | — | 5.7 | 27 | 0.2 | 0.09 | 2.4 | — |
| Nitrogen oxides (ppm) | 0.35 (ND–2.0) | | | | | | 2.55 (ND–10) |
| Nitrogen dioxide (mg/m³) | — | 0.04 | 0.06 | 0.04 | 0.06 | 0.02 | 0.26 (ND–0.4) |
| Total hydrocarbons (ppm) | — | 4.55 | 4.94 | 2.89 | 3.12 | 3.69 | — |
| Total aldehydes (as formaldehyde) | 0.01 (ND–0.1) mg/m³ | 0.07 ppm | 0.09 ppm | 0.05 ppm | 0.02 ppm | 0.14 ppm | 0.19 (ND–1.0) mg/m³ |
| Acrolein (mg/m³) | 0.02 (ND–0.2) | — | — | — | — | — | 0.07 (ND–0.5) |
| Total particulate matter (mg/m³) | 0.38 (0.1–0.8) | 0.05 | 0.07 | 0.16 | 0.01 | 0.27 | 1.99 (0.07–8.7) |

[a]From Heino et al. (1978)
[b]From Hobbs et al. (1977); TWA, time-weighted average (estimated)

ND, not detected

Table 13. Personal exposures to respirable particulate matter, and adjusted respirable particulate matter concentration[a], among railroad workers by job group[b]

| Exposure group | Job group | No. | Arithmetic mean (SD) of respirable particulate matter ($\mu g/m^3$) | Arithmetic mean (SD) of adjusted respirable particulate matter ($\mu g/m^3$) |
|---|---|---|---|---|
| Clerks | Clerk/station agent | 59 | 125 (75) | 42 (36) |
| Signal maintainers | Signal maintainer | 13 | 69 (39) | 58 (33) |
| Engineers/firers | Freight worker | 55 | 115 (67) | 94 (55) |
| | Yard worker | 50 | 108 (109) | 69 (70) |
| | Passenger | 23 | 75 (52) | 51 (35) |
| Brakers/conductors | Freight conductor | 62 | 126 (65) | 69 (52) |
| | Freight braker | 21 | 145 (80) | 102 (62) |
| | Passenger | 35 | 111 (62) | 104 (58) |
| | Yard worker | 32 | 180 (117) | 114 (76) |
| | Hostler | 8 | 231 (134) | 224 (130) |
| Shop workers | Electrician | 42 | 256 (332) | 192 (248) |
| | Machinist | 110 | 191 (146) | 147 (120) |
| | Supervisor, labourer and other shop workers | 24 | 244 (141) | 155 (83) |

[a]Cigarette smoke particulate matter subtracted from total respirable particulate matter (see text for explanation)
[b]From Woskie et al. (1988a); each sample was collected over a single work shift (7–12 h).

Other sources of exposure in mines include activities that produce large quantities of airborne particles, and blasting, which produces particles and gases such as methane and sulfur dioxide. In addition, these gases may be released spontaneously from the ore bed or from surrounding geological formations. Some exposures that may occur in mines, depending on the ores present, were evaluated by previous IARC working groups; these include radon (IARC, 1988), silica (IARC, 1987b), nickel (IARC, 1987a), chromium (IARC, 1987a) and asbestos (IARC, 1987a).

Lassiter and Milby (1978) gave examples of the levels of carbon monoxide and nitrogen dioxide that can be found at the diesel operator's position in an underground mine. On the basis of 2977 samples taken in 1963–72, the average concentration of carbon monoxide was 8.5 ppm (9.7 mg/m³), 5% of the samples containing >50 ppm (>57 mg/m³); 1504 samples contained an average concentration of 0.2 ppm (0.4 mg/m³) nitrogen dioxide, with 0.75% above 3 ppm (>6 mg/m³) and one sample >5 ppm (>10 mg/m³).

A study conducted for the US Bureau of Mines on levels of diesel exhaust components in 24 mines included two coal mines (Holland, 1978); the results are shown in Table 14. Anthracene and phenanthrene were found at measurable levels, but five other PAHs (benz[a]anthracene, benzo[a]pyrene, benzo[e]pyrene, chrysene and pyrene) were not.

**Table 14. Levels of diesel exhaust components (mg/m³) in 24 US mines**[a]

| Contaminant | Diesel exhaust source | | | Personal and area samples | | |
|---|---|---|---|---|---|---|
| | No. of samples | Mean | Range | No. of samples | Mean | Range |
| Carbon monoxide | 6 | 140 | 11.5–344 | 21 | 14.2 | 0–26.3 |
| Nitric oxide | 3 | 6.3 | <0.1–16.5 | 10 | 12.7 | 0.5–70 |
| Nitrogen dioxide | 5 | 16.8 | 1–40 | 29 | 1.6 | 0–11 |
| Sulfur dioxide | 5 | 0.3 | 0–<1 | 6 | 2.1 | 0–13 |
| Sulfuric acid | 4 | 12.8 | <0.2–46 | 9 | 0.3 | <0.004–2 |
| Formaldehyde | 10 | 7 | 0–42 | 23 | 0.8 | 0–8 |
| Acrolein | 7 | 2.1 | <0.1–3.2 | 16 | <0.4 | <0.02–<5 |
| Total particulate matter | 8 | 50.2 | 0.5–236 | 13 | 4.6 | 0.2–14 |
| Anthracene | 8 | 0.05 | 0.02–0.2 | 13 | 0.001 | 0.00005–0.004 |
| Phenanthrene | 8 | 0.001 | 0–0.008 | 13 | 0.01 | 0–0.17 |

[a]From Holland (1978)

Levels of air contaminants due to diesel emissions in other coal mines are summarized in Table 15.

The environment of six potash mines in New Mexico, USA, was investigated in 1976 (Attfield et al., 1982). The use of diesel equipment in these mines had begun between 1950 and 1966, and seven to 57 diesel-powered units were used. Environmental concentrations in production jobs and other areas in the six mines (based on 25–34 samples) were 6–10 mg/m³ carbon monoxide, 0.2–6.6 mg/m³ nitrogen dioxide and 0.1–4.0 ppm aldehydes.

Cornwell (1982) evaluated employee exposure to diesel emissions at a molybdenum mine in Colorado, USA. Diesel-powered equipment used in the mine included drills, five-yard load haul-dumps and two-yard load haul-dumps. Personal and area sampling was conducted for oxides of carbon, nitrogen and sulfur, formaldehyde, respirable particulate matter, PAHs and cyclohexane-soluble material (sum of particulate and gaseous samples). The results are shown in Table 16.

Daniel (1984) reported 0.2–1.3 ppm (0.4–2.6 mg/m³) nitrogen dioxide, 3.1–8.7 ppm (3.8–10.7 mg/m³) nitric oxide and 0.5–2.1 ppm (0.6–2.4 mg/m³) carbon monoxide in a South Dakota, USA, gold mine when samples were taken during the operation of a diesel mine vehicle. He found 0.3–0.6 ppm (0.8–1.6 mg/m³) sulfur dioxide, 0.1–0.3 mg/m³ sulfate, 0.4–1.7 mg/m³ respirable combustible dust and 1.1–4.4 mg/m³ total respirable dust.

(iii) *Bus garage and other bus workers*

Exposures of bus garage and other bus workers to diesel exhaust emissions are listed in Table 17. Few studies addressed other exposures that may occur in bus garages, such as to metal fumes from welding and similar operations and to asbestos during brake servicing.

Table 15. Levels of air contaminants (mg/m$^3$, unless otherwise specified) in coal mines

| Contaminant | Concentration | Sampling | Reference |
| --- | --- | --- | --- |
| Carbon monoxide | 8 (mean) | Personal | Lawter & Kendall (1977) |
| | 0–2.3 | Personal | Wheeler et al. (1981) |
| | 3.9–26.7 | Average of short-term area samples | Reger et al. (1982) |
| Nitrogen oxides | 0–5.2 ppm | Average of short-term area samples | Reger et al. (1982) |
| Nitrogen dioxide | 0.7 (mean) | Personal | Lawter & Kendall (1977) |
| | 0.06–0.5 | Personal | Wheeler et al. (1981) |
| | 0–1.1 | Average of short-term area samples | Reger et al. (1982) |
| | 0.06–1.5 | Range of full-shift area samples | Reger et al. (1982) |
| | 0.3–0.5 | Average of full-shift personal samples | Reger et al. (1982) |
| Nitric oxide | 3.7 (mean) | Personal | Lawter & Kendall (1977) |
| Aldehydes | 0.05 (mean) | Personal | Lawter & Kendall (1977) |
| | 0–0.01 | Personal | Wheeler et al. (1981) |
| Formaldehyde | 0.04 (mean) | Personal | Lawter & Kendall (1977) |
| 'Aromatics' | 0.7 (mean) | Personal | Lawter & Kendall (1977) |
| Cyclohexane-extractable hydrocarbons | 0.04–0.07 | Personal | Wheeler et al. (1981) |
| Total dust | 0–23.0 | Average of full-shift area samples | Reger et al. (1982) |
| Respirable dust | 0.6–1.7 | Personal | Wheeler et al. (1981) |
| | 0.9–2.7 | Average of full-shift personal samples | Reger et al. (1982) |
| | 0–16.1 | Range of full-shift area samples | Reger et al. (1982) |

Table 16. Air contaminant levels in a molybdenum mine[a]

| Contaminant | Concentration | Sampling |
| --- | --- | --- |
| Carbon monoxide | <1.1–6.1 mg/m$^3$ | 8-h TWA; area |
| Nitric oxide | ND–9.0 mg/m$^3$ | Area |
| Nitrogen dioxide | ND–6.4 | Area |
| | 0.08–0.78 mg/m$^3$ | 8-h TWA; area |
| | 0.06–4.32 mg/m$^3$ | 8-h TWA; personal |
| Sulfur dioxide | ND–0.05 mg/m$^3$ | Area |
| Formaldehyde | ND | Instantaneous area |
| Respirable particulate matter | 0.2–1.9 mg/m$^3$ | 8-h TWA; personal |
| Cyclohexane-soluble material | 0.02–0.93 mg/m$^3$ | 8-h TWA; personal |
| | 0.02–0.04 mg/m$^3$ | 8-h TWA; area |
| Benz[a]anthracene | 30–40 ng/m$^3$ | 8-h TWA; personal; in 2/15 samples |
| Benzo[a]pyrene | 40 ng/m$^3$ | 8-h TWA; personal; in 1/15 samples |
| Chrysene | 320 ng/m$^3$ | 8-h TWA; personal; in 1/15 samples |
| Fluoranthene | 60–340 ng/m$^3$ | 8-h TWA; personal; in 10/15 samples |
| | 70 ng/m$^3$ | 8-h TWA; area; in 1/4 samples |
| Pyrene | 80–480 ng/m$^3$ | 8-h TWA; personal; in 10/15 samples |
| | 140 ng/m$^3$ | 8-h TWA; area; in 1/4 samples |

[a]From Cornwell (1982); ND, not detected; TWA, time-weighted average

Table 17. Levels of air contaminants in bus garages (mg/m³, unless otherwise specified)

| Contaminant | Concentration | Sampling | Location | Time | Reference |
|---|---|---|---|---|---|
| Carbon monoxide | 2–18 | Diesel areas | Denver, CO, USA | March 1982 | Apol (1983) |
| | 7–11 | Terminal (background) | Denver, CO, USA | July–Sept. 1982 | Pryor (1983) |
| | 22–46 | Terminal (bus arrival/departure) | Denver, CO, USA | July–Sept. 1982 | Pryor (1983) |
| | 6–8 | Package receiving area | Denver, CO, USA | July–Sept. 1982 | Pryor (1983) |
| | 8–40 | Reservations room | Denver, CO, USA | July–Sept. 1982 | Pryor (1983) |
| | 8–401 | Air inlet | Denver, CO, USA | July–Sept. 1982 | Pryor (1983) |
| | <0.01–5.7 | Unspecified | Italy | – | del Piano et al. (1986) |
| | 1.7–24 | Personal, during periods of high activity | Sweden | – | Ulfvarson et al. (1987) |
| Nitric oxides as $NO_2$ | 0.8–1.4 | Air analysis | Egypt | 1965 | El Batawi & Noweir (1966) |
| | 2.6–2.8 | Close to exhaust | Egypt | 1965 | El Batawi & Noweir (1966) |
| Nitric oxide | 1.4–6.9 | Peak morning period | Denver, CO, USA | March 1982 | Apol (1983) |
| | 0.5–2.8 | Later morning period | Denver, CO, USA | March 1982 | Apol (1983) |
| Nitrous oxide | 0.3–1.0 | Personal, during periods of high activity | Sweden | – | Ulfvarson et al. (1987) |
| Nitrogen dioxide | 0.8–3.2 | Peak morning period | Denver, CO, USA | March 1982 | Apol (1983) |
| | 0.3–1.6 | Later morning period | Denver, CO, USA | March 1982 | Apol (1983) |
| | <0.07 | Package receiving area | Denver, CO, USA | June 1982 | Pryor (1983) |
| | 0.1–0.8 | Unspecified | Italy | – | del Piano et al. (1986) |
| | 0.3–1.1 | Personal, mean TWA | USA | – | Gamble et al. (1987) |
| | 0.2–1.1 | Personal, during periods of high activity | Sweden | – | Ulfvarson et al. (1987) |
| Sulfur dioxide | 0.14–0.86 | Air analysis | Egypt | 1965 | El Batawi & Noweir (1966) |
| | 1.8–2.1 | Close to exhaust | Egypt | 1965 | El Batawi & Noweir (1966) |
| | ≤0.13 | Morning period | Denver, CO, USA | March 1982 | Apol (1983) |
| | 0.03–0.18 | Personal, during periods of high activity | Denver, CO, USA | June 1982 | Pryor (1983) |
| | 0.03–1 | Unspecified | Italy | – | del Piano et al. (1986) |
| | <1.8 | Personal, during periods of high activity | Sweden | – | Ulfvarson et al. (1987) |
| Aldehydes | 0.7–1.8 | Air analysis | Egypt | 1965 | El Batawi & Noweir (1966) |
| | 42–52 | Close to exhaust | Egypt | 1965 | El Batawi & Noweir (1966) |
| Aldehydes[a] as formaldehyde | <0.3 ppm | Morning period | Denver, CO, USA | March 1982 | Apol (1983) |
| Formaldehyde | 0.04–0.8 | Personal, during periods of high activity | Sweden | – | Ulfvarson et al. (1987) |
| Acetaldehyde | 0.28–1.5 | Personal, during periods of high activity | Sweden | – | Ulfvarson et al. (1987) |
| | 2.3–9.5 ppm | Unspecified | Italy | – | del Piano et al. (1986) |

| Contaminant | Concentration | Sampling | Location | Time | Reference |
|---|---|---|---|---|---|
| PAH (ng/m$^3$) | | | | | |
| Anthanthrene | 0.05 | 1.00–5.00 h (no bus moving) | London, UK | June 1979 | Waller et al. (1985) |
| | 4.5 | 5.00–9.00 h (buses starting) | London, UK | June 1979 | Waller et al. (1985) |
| Benz[a]anthracene | <1–50 | Unspecified | Italy | – | del Piano et al. (1986) |
| Benzo[b]fluoranthene | <1–50 | Unspecified | Italy | – | del Piano et al. (1986) |
| Benzo[k]fluoranthene | <1–100 | Unspecified | Italy | – | del Piano et al. (1986) |
| Benzo[ghi]perylene | 1.1 | 1.00–5.00 h | London, UK | June 1979 | Waller et al. (1985) |
| | 27.2 | 5.00–9.00 h | London, UK | June 1979 | Waller et al. (1985) |
| | <1–30 | Unspecified | Italy | – | del Piano et al. (1986) |
| Benzo[a]pyrene | 0.6 | 1.00–5.00 h | London, UK | June 1979 | Waller et al. (1985) |
| | 13.0 | 5.00–9.00 h | London, UK | June 1979 | Waller et al. (1985) |
| | <1–20 | Unspecified | Italy | – | del Piano et al. (1986) |
| | <10 | Personal, during periods of high activity | Sweden | – | Ulfvarson et al. (1987) |
| Benzo[e]pyrene | 1.2 | 1.00–5.00 h | London, UK | June 1979 | Waller et al. (1985) |
| | 11.6 | 5.00–9.00 h | London, UK | June 1979 | Waller et al. (1985) |
| | <1–3 | Unspecified | Italy | – | del Piano et al. (1986) |
| Chrysene | <1–30 | Unspecified | Italy | – | del Piano et al. (1986) |
| Coronene | 0.8 | 1.00–5.00 h | London, UK | June 1979 | Waller et al. (1985) |
| | 13.6 | 5.00–9.00 h | London, UK | June 1979 | Waller et al. (1985) |
| Fluoranthene | 2–350 | Unspecified | Italy | – | del Piano et al. (1986) |
| Indeno[1,2,3-cd]pyrene | <1–330 | Unspecified | Italy | – | del Piano et al. (1986) |
| Pyrene | 2.5 | 1.00–5.00 h | London, UK | June 1979 | Waller et al. (1985) |
| | 17.5 | 5.00–9.00 h | London, UK | June 1979 | Waller et al. (1985) |
| | <1–460 | Unspecified | Italy | – | del Piano et al. (1986) |
| Hydrocarbons | | | | | |
| Benzene | ≤0.2 | Personal, during periods of high activity | Sweden | – | Ulfvarson et al. (1987) |
| Toluene | ≤0.2 | Personal, during periods of high activity | Sweden | – | Ulfvarson et al. (1987) |
| Total dust | <0.01–0.82 | Unspecified | Italy | – | del Piano et al. (1986) |
| | 0.46 | Personal, during periods of high activity | Sweden | – | Ulfvarson et al. (1987) |
| | 0.13–0.55 | TWA, including dust stirred up by buses | Denver, CO, USA | March 1982 | Apol (1983) |
| | 0.15–0.81 | Peak morning period | Denver, CO, USA | March 1982 | Apol (1983) |
| | 0.03–0.16 | Cyclohexane-soluble | Denver, CO, USA | March 1982 | Apol (1983) |
| | 0.01–0.09 | Unspecified | Denver, CO, USA | June 1982 | Pryor (1983) |
| | 0.17 | 1.00–5.00 h | London, UK | June 1979 | Waller et al. (1985) |
| | 0.58 | 5.00–9.00 h | London, UK | June 1979 | Waller et al. (1985) |

**Table 17 (contd)**

| Contaminant | Concentration | Sampling | Location | Time | Reference |
|---|---|---|---|---|---|
| Respirable dust | <0.01–0.73 | Unspecified | Italy | – | del Piano et al. (1986) |
|  | 0.12–0.61 | Personal, mean TWA | USA | – | Gamble et al. (1987a) |
| Metals ($\mu$g/m$^3$) |  |  |  |  |  |
| Cadmium | 0.3–0.5 | Unspecified | Italy | – | del Piano et al. (1986) |
| Chromium | <0.1–1.2 | Unspecified | Italy | – | del Piano et al. (1986) |
| Copper | <0.1–6.4 | Unspecified | Italy | – | del Piano et al. (1986) |
| Iron | 2.8–455 | Unspecified | Italy | – | del Piano et al. (1986) |
| Lead | <0.1–4.1 | Unspecified | Italy | – | del Piano et al. (1986) |
| Manganese | <0.1–4 | Unspecified | Italy | – | del Piano et al. (1986) |
| Nickel | <0.1–4.5 | Unspecified | Italy | – | del Piano et al. (1986) |
| Zinc | <0.1–15 | Unspecified | Italy | – | del Piano et al. (1986) |

[a]Including acetaldehyde, butyraldehyde, formaldehyde, propionaldehyde
PAH, polycyclic aromatic hydrocarbons; TWA, time-weighted average

The table includes the results of analyses of air during operations in two diesel bus garages in Egypt (El Batawi & Noweir, 1966) and measurements of airborne concentrations of diesel exhaust components in three bus repair facilities in Denver, CO, USA (Apol, 1983). In the latter study, sampling took place in March 1982 at several locations within each facility during peak dispatch and return times. A carbon monoxide level of 195 mg/m$^3$ was recorded in one garage early in the morning near buses with gasoline engines that were starting up. The author stated that exposure of drivers to this and higher levels for 10–15 min is possible. Pryor (1983) also conducted an industrial hygiene survey of diesel exhaust at the garage of a bus company in Denver, CO, in 1982, where buses with gasoline engines parked nearby. Area samples were taken to measure carbon monoxide, sulfur dioxide, nitrogen dioxide, total particulate matter and formaldehyde in the terminal and in package-receiving areas (Table 17). The high concentrations of carbon monoxide in the terminal dropped to the background concentration within a few minutes of bus arrival or departure. The higher levels of carbon monoxide in the reservation room and at the inlet corresponded to peak car traffic in the parking area, and dropped to a background level within 10–15 min of the end of the peak traffic.

Waller *et al.* (1985) measured pollutant levels in two diesel bus garages in London, UK, in 1979. Sampling took place close to the buses in an area of only limited worker exposure, so the data are said by the authors to present extreme upper limits only. Table 17 gives data on levels of PAHs near the door of one garage during two different periods. del Piano *et al.* (1986), reporting in an abstract, found concentrations of several air contaminants in Italian bus garages surveyed over two years, as shown in the table. Gamble *et al.* (1987a) studied 232 workers in four diesel bus garages in the USA. Mean TWA concentrations of respirable particles and nitrogen dioxide in personal samples, combined over three shifts and for all four garages, were reported (Table 17). Ulfvarson *et al.* (1987) measured personal exposures of workers in a bus garage with both large and small diesel-powered vehicles as well as gasoline-powered ones. Storage, engine warm-up, refuelling, washing and repairs were all performed at the garage. Elevated concentrations, especially of diesel exhaust, accumulated in garage bays in the morning, afternoon and evening when most of the buses were coming or going. Specific exposures in the garage as measured by personal sampling during these periods of high activity are detailed in Table 17.

(iv) *Truck drivers*

Ziskind *et al.* (1978) measured the concentrations of several gases in the cabins of heavy-duty diesel trucks under a variety of conditions. Concentrations of carbon monoxide, nitric oxide and nitrogen dioxide in the air and in the cabins were measured continuously. The maximal total concentrations in cabins measured during idling and road testing were as follows: carbon monoxide, 30 ppm (34 mg/m$^3$); nitric oxide, 2 ppm (2.5 mg/m$^3$); nitrogen dioxide, 3 ppm (6 mg/m$^3$). The maximal self-contamination concentrations (total cabin concentration minus ambient concentration) were: carbon monoxide, 10.5 ppm (12 mg/m$^3$); nitric oxide, 1.55 ppm (1.9 mg/m$^3$); nitrogen dioxide, 0.7 ppm (1.4 mg/m$^3$). The authors found a correlation between vehicle-induced concentrations of specific gases in cabins and several testing parameters, including condition of windows, type of cabin configuration and the presence of exhaust leaks and underside cabin openings.

The results of a study of truck drivers on roll-on roll-off ships by personal sampling over an entire work shift (Ulfvarson et al., 1987) are given in Table 18.

Table 18. Levels of airborne contaminants measured for truck drivers on Swedish roll-on roll-off ships $(mg/m^3)^a$

| Contaminant | Study I | Study II |
|---|---|---|
| Carbon monoxide | 1.4–2.7 | 1.1–5.1 |
| Nitrogen dioxide | 0.15–1.0 | 0.06–2.3 |
| Nitrous acid | 0.002–0.2 | Not reported |
| [Nitric oxide] | 0.1–0.8 | 0.2–0.7 |
| [Total hydrocarbons] | 12–14 | Not reported |
| Benzene | ⩽0.3 | Not reported |
| Toluene | <0.8 | Not reported |
| Formaldehyde | ⩽0.03 | 0.1–0.5 |
| Acetaldehyde | <1.6 | Not reported |
| Dust | 0.13–0.59 | 0.3–1.0 |

$^a$From Ulfvarson et al. (1987)

(v) *Fork-lift truck operators*

Breathing zone exposures were measured in an army ammunition depot in the USA in the winter of 1983 during the use of diesel-powered fork-lift trucks. PAHs, sulfur dioxide and carbon monoxide levels were below the detection limits [not given], while the concentration of particulate matter ranged from <0.01 to 1.3 mg/m$^3$, that of nitrogen dioxide from 0.1 to 3.2 ppm (<0.2–6.4 mg/m$^3$) and that of total sulfates from <10 to 32 μg/m$^3$. Area samples taken during the same test provided the following mean values: 1.1–2.6 ppm nitrogen oxides, 1.2–3.3 ppm (1.4–3.8 mg/m$^3$) carbon monoxide, 0.2–0.4 ppm (0.4–0.7 mg/m$^3$) sulfur dioxide and 7.4–8.5 ppm total hydrocarbons (Ungers, 1984). In a follow-up study in the summer of 1984 (Ungers, 1985), the level of PAHs was below the detection limit (3 ng/m$^3$), while breathing zone values during warehouse operations were in the following ranges: particles, 0.5–5.0 mg/m$^3$; sulfate, 0.02–0.6 mg/m$^3$; sulfite, <0.02–0.09 mg/m$^3$; nitric oxide, 1.6–13.6 mg/m$^3$; and nitrogen dioxide, 0.7–2.5 mg/m$^3$.

(vi) *Fire-fighters*

Fire-fighters are frequently and repeatedly exposed to diesel engine exhaust and other combustion products (Froines et al., 1987). Exposure to diesel exhaust occurs during response to an incident and in the fire station. When personal sampling was used to determine the exposures of fire-fighters in fire stations in three US cities — Boston, New York and Los Angeles — in 1985, total airborne particle levels (TWA) ranged from <0.1 to 0.48 mg/m$^3$. The authors predicted an average total particulate exposure of roughly 0.3 mg/m$^3$ on a typical day in Boston or New York. With an estimated 0.075 mg/m$^3$ contributed by background and smoking, exposure would be to approximately 0.225 mg/m$^3$ diesel exhaust particles and 0.054 mg/m$^3$ of dichloromethane extractable material. Sampling during simulated 'worst case' exposures in Los Angeles fire stations gave an upper bound concentration of 0.748 mg/m³ particles.

*(b) Workers whose predominant exhaust exposure is that from gasoline engines*

(i) *Toll-booth workers*

Ayres *et al.* (1973) evaluated exposure to engine exhaust for perions who worked in both a tunnel and in an adjacent toll plaza in New York City, USA (Table 19). The authors reported a close correlation among the concentrations of various pollutants, such that the level of carbon monoxide could be considered to be indicative of total automotive pollution levels. Following the installation of ventilation systems in toll booths, carbon monoxide levels dropped to 16—18 mg/m³.

Table 19. Levels of air contaminants (mg/m³, unless otherwise specified) to which toll-booth operators are exposed

| Contaminant | Concentration | Sampling | Reference |
|---|---|---|---|
| Carbon monoxide | 72 | 30-day average | Ayres *et al.* (1973) |
|  | 249 | Max hourly level | Ayres *et al.* (1973) |
|  | 26 ± 13 | Ambient 8-h TWA | Johnson *et al.* (1974) |
|  | 17.6—38.5 | Mean in booths | Burgess *et al.* (1977) |
|  | 150 | Max 8-h TWA (summer, tunnel booth) | Burgess *et al.* (1977) |
| Nitrogen oxides | 1.38 ppm | 30-day average | Ayres *et al.* (1973) |
|  | 6.13 ppm | Max hourly level | Ayres *et al.* (1973) |
| Nitrogen dioxide | 0.14 | 30-day average | Ayres *et al.* (1973) |
|  | 0.64 | Max hourly level | Ayres *et al.* (1973) |
|  | 0.08—0.20 | Mean in booths | Burgess *et al.* (1977) |
| Sulfur dioxide | 0.04—0.07 | Mean in booths | Burgess *et al.* (1977) |
| Aldehydes | 0.05 ppm | 30-day average | Ayres *et al.* (1973) |
|  | 0.16 ppm | Max hourly level | Ayres *et al.* (1973) |
| Acrolein | 0.007 | 30-day average | Ayres *et al.* (1973) |
|  | 0.03 | Max hourly level | Ayres *et al.* (1973) |
| Total hydrocarbons | 7.9 ppm | 30-day average | Ayres *et al.* (1973) |
|  | 29.6 ppm | Max hourly level | Ayres *et al.* (1973) |
|  | 5.7-19.8 ppm | Mean in booths | Burgess *et al.* (1977) |
| Lead | 30.9 µg/m³ | 30-day average | Ayres *et al.* (1973) |
|  | 98.0 µg/m³ | Max hourly level | Ayres *et al.* (1973) |
|  | 27.4 (5—87) µg/m³ | Ambient 8-h TWA | Johnson *et al.* (1974) |
|  | 7.7-16 µg/m³ | Mean respirable mass fraction | Burgess *et al.* (1977) |
| Manganese | <1 µg/m³ | Ambient 8-h TWA | Johnson *et al.* (1974) |
| Total suspended particulate matter | 0.04-0.75 |  | Burgess *et al.* (1977) |
|  | 0.2 (average) |  | Ayres *et al.* (1973) |
| Respirable mass fraction | 0.10 (average) |  | Burgess *et al.* (1977) |
| Respirable particles | 0.1 (average) |  | Ayres *et al.* (1973) |

A study of exposure to carbon monoxide of toll collectors on an interstate highway near Louisville, KY, USA, was reported by Johnson *et al.* (1974). Testing was conducted over a 12-day period in April 1973, and ambient concentrations of carbon monoxide, lead and manganese at three booths were determined as an overall mean 8-h TWA (Table 19). Carboxyhaemoglobin (COHb) levels in the workers were measured before and after shifts; typical pre-shift levels were 0.8–1.5%; the post-shift mean was 3.9%, with a range of 1.6–11.7%.

Burgess *et al.* (1977) evaluated the exposure of toll-booth collectors in the Boston area, at a tunnel and at two interchanges during 1972–74 (Table 19). Airborne lead levels in the work environment were roughly four times ambient urban levels; correlated increases were found in the hair and blood of the workers.

(ii) *Border-station inspectors*

Cohen *et al.* (1971) studied a group of such workers at the San Ysidro, CA, USA, station in 1969. Ambient and expired carbon monoxide levels were measured over roughly a 24-h period encompassing three shifts. Average hourly carbon monoxide levels were 15 mg/m$^3$ (8.00 to 16.00 h), 75 mg/m$^3$ (16.00 to 0.00 h) and 131 mg/m$^3$ (0.00 to 8.00 h); hourly levels ranged from 6 to 195 mg/m$^3$. Taking data from all shifts combined, nonsmoking individuals had significantly higher expired carbon monoxide levels at the end of the shift than before the shift, corresponding to COHb levels of 3.6% after the shift and 1.5% before the shift. For smokers, the estimated pre- and post-shift COHb levels, estimated from carbon monoxide in expired air, were 4.8% and 6.4%, respectively.

Environmental sampling was conducted by the National Institute for Occupational Safety and Health at a number of US border crossing facilities in 1973–74, to investigate the exposure of Federal border inspectors (Kronoveter, 1976). Inspectors are rotated between different work locations through a shift, and the facilities are operated three shifts per day, seven days per week. Mean 8-h average carbon monoxide levels ranged from 2 to 54 ppm (2.3–62 mg/m$^3$) with maximal 8-h average levels of 3–73 ppm (3.4–83.6 mg/m$^3$). Sampling for total particulate matter revealed concentrations from <1.0 to 4.3 mg/m$^3$. Ozone levels ranged from <0.01–0.08 ppm (<0.02–0.16 mg/m$^3$), and concentrations of lead ranged from <10 to 20 µg/m$^3$.

deBruin (1967) measured COHb levels in 13 nonsmoking Dutch customs officers stationed at four remote sites in 1965. The mean concentrations at the four locations studied ranged from 0.8 to 1.5% before work and 1.1 to 3.0% after work.

(iii) *Traffic-control officers*

deBruin (1967) measured COHb levels in nonsmoking and smoking traffic policemen in Rotterdam and Amsterdam, the Netherlands. Results are shown in Table 20. Ambient carbon monoxide levels in Rotterdam at the time of that study averaged 5–15 ppm (6–17 mg/m$^3$) at crossings and crowded streets, ranging up to 50 ppm (60 mg/m$^3$).

Göthe *et al.* (1969) measured COHb levels in 76 traffic policemen in three Swedish towns. Ambient carbon monoxide levels were not given, but in Stockholm nonsmoking officers who had controlled traffic in either the morning or afternoon rush hours had an

Table 20. Carboxyhaemoglobin (COHb) levels in traffic control officers[a]

| Group | No. of subjects | % COHb (mean ± SD) | |
|---|---|---|---|
| | | Before work | After work |
| Rotterdam | | | |
| Exposed nonsmokers (1-4-h average) | 36 | 0.92 ± 0.07 | 1.11 ± 0.07 |
| Control nonsmokers (office) | 16 | 0.85 ± 0.13 | 0.83 ± 0.17 |
| Amsterdam | | | |
| Exposed nonsmokers (4.5-h average) | 10 | 1.43 ± 0.26 | 1.66 ± 0.27 |
| Exposed smokers (4.5-h average) | 14 | 4.62 ± 0.97 | 5.16 ± 0.81 |
| Control nonsmokers (office) | 9 | 1.45 ± 0.22 | 1.40 ± 0.18 |

[a]From deBruin (1967)

average COHb of 1.2% ± 0.39; smokers had a level of 3.5% ± 1.17. In Malmö and Örebro, the levels were 0.8% ± 0.14 and 0.6% ± 0.38 for nonsmokers and 5.0% ± 2.44 and 2.4% ± 1.10 for smokers. The authors noted that unexposed persons in Sweden have an average COHb of 0.5%.

*(iv) Professional drivers*

deBruin (1967) determined COHb levels before and after work in nonsmoking taxi, delivery van and motor hearse drivers in Amsterdam, the Netherlands, in 1965. The mean COHb levels before and after work were 2.0 and 2.15 for 13 taxi drivers exposed for 7 h; 1.5 and 1.65 for six delivery men exposed for 8 h; and 2.0 and 2.45 for four drivers of motor hearses exposed for 6.5 h. The average difference was 0.25%, which was significant ($p < 0.01$).

Maruna and Maruna (1975) investigated δ-aminolaevulinic acid elimination in the urine of 200 taxi drivers in Vienna, Austria, as a means of measuring lead burden. The authors found that 26.5% of the taxi drivers had normal levels (<5.0 mg/l urine), 27% had borderline levels (5.1–7.0 mg/l) and 46.5% had elevated levels (>7.1 mg/l). The authors concluded that the source of the lead was the atmosphere polluted by automobile engine emissions.

del Piano *et al.* (1986), reporting in an abstract, measured hydrocarbons in the breathing zone of the drivers of an Italian bus company. The concentration of aliphatic hydrocarbons ranged from below 0.01 to 51.8 ppm and that of aromatic hydrocarbons, including benzene (<0.01–9.6 ppm; <0.03–31 mg/m$^3$), from below 0.01 to 36.7 ppm. [The Working Group was unable to determine if these workers were exposed mainly to gasoline or to diesel exhausts.]

(v) *Ferry workers*

Purdham *et al.* (1987) studied the potential exposure of stevedores employed in ferry operations to diesel and gasoline exhaust emissions. The constituents considered were total particles, PAHs, aldehydes, nitrogen oxides, sulfur dioxide and carbon monoxide. Exposures to particles averaged 0.50 mg/m³ (range, 0.06–1.72 mg/m³); carbon monoxide levels were detected, in the range of 20–100 ppm (23–115 mg/m³), only when gasoline-powered vehicles were being loaded onto the ferries. The levels of the other constituents did not differ from the background.

Ulfvarson *et al.* (1987) measured personal exposures to airborne contaminants on two types of car ferries during loading and unloading. On the first one, a 2-h route, loading and unloading of vehicles took an average of 20 min; on the second, a 20-min crossing, loading and unloading times were not specified. The results are shown in Table 21.

Table 21. Levels of airborne contaminants measured on Swedish car ferries (mg/m³, unless otherwise specified)[a]

| Contaminant | Car ferry (2-h run)[b] | Car ferry (20-min run) |
|---|---|---|
| Carbon monoxide | 13–100 | 5–190 |
| Nitrogen dioxide | <0.6 | 0.2–0.8 |
| Sulfur dioxide | <1.8 | Not measured |
| Benzene | ≤0.2 | Not measured |
| Toluene | <0.2 | Not measured |
| Formaldehyde | 0.03–0.31 | 0.1–0.3 |
| Acetaldehyde | 0.49–1.5 | 1.02–2.1 |
| Dust | Not measured | 0.1–0.3 |
| Benzo[*a*]pyrene (ng/m³) | <10 | ≤30 |

[a]From Ulfvarson *et al.* (1987)
[b]Loading and unloading of vehicles took an average of 20 min

(vi) *Exhaust system mechanics*

Chambers *et al.* (1984) measured the lead levels in airborne particles and deposited dusts in three centres for the replacement of passenger car exhaust systems. Airborne concentrations of lead collected with environmental and personal samplers ranged from 8.8 to 55.4 $\mu$g/m³, with peak concentrations ranging from 20.2 to 92.7 $\mu$g/m³ when floors were being swept during sampling. Dust concentrations in samples from floors and shelves ranged from 0.14 to 3.02% lead by weight. Dust in samples collected from inside exhaust systems ranged from 0.20 to 58.7% lead by weight, according to site.

(vii) *Motor vehicle inspectors*

An industrial hygiene survey of 38 motor vehicle inspection stations in New Jersey, USA, in 1973–74 indicated that inspectors were exposed to carbon monoxide at a TWA average of 10–24 ppm (11–28 mg/m$^3$); measurements in semi-open and enclosed stations were 11–40 ppm (13–46 mg/m$^3$) and those in outdoor stations, 4–21 ppm (5–24 mg/m$^3$). Average COHb levels in nonsmokers were 2.1% before a shift and 3.7% after a shift ($p <$ 0.01) (Stern *et al.*, 1981).

(viii) *Parking garage attendants*

Ramsey (1967) determined both airborne carbon monoxide levels and blood COHb levels for 38 parking attendants in six garages in Dayton, OH, USA. These garages typically had four floors and a capacity of 300–500 cars. Hourly air sampling revealed a carbon monoxide concentration in the range of 8–275 mg/m$^3$, with a mean of 67.4 ± 28.5 mg/m$^3$ for 18 daily averages. COHb levels were determined in employees prior to and after the work day on Monday; a group of control students was also monitored. The 8:00 and 17.00 h levels were 1.5 ± 0.83 (SD) and 7.3 ± 3.46 for 14 nonsmokers; and 2.9 ± 1.88 and 9.3 ± 3.16 for 24 smokers. In controls, the levels were 0.81 ± 0.54 for ten nonsmokers and 3.9 ± 1.48 for 17 smokers. The differences between 8.00 and 17.00 h levels in garage workers, and between garage workers at 17.00 h and controls are highly significant ($p < 0.0001$).

(ix) *Lumberjacks*

Nilsson *et al.* (1987) studied the composition of exhaust emissions from two-stroke chain-saw engines run on gasoline and estimated operator exposure to chain-saw exhaust under snow-free conditions and with snow on the ground (Table 22). The presence of snow affects techniques used in cutting.

Table 22. Estimated exposure of lumberjacks using chain saws during loggng under snow-free conditions and in the winter with snow on the ground (mg/m$^3$)[a]

| Compound | Snow-free | | With snow | |
|---|---|---|---|---|
| | Time-weighted average | Range | Time-weighted average | Range |
| Total hydrocarbons | 15.0 | 7–40 | 19.0 | 3–74 |
| Benzene | 0.7 | 0.3–1.8 | 0.6 | 0.1–2.4 |
| Formaldehyde | 0.08 | 0.04–0.2 | 0.08 | 0.02–0.1 |
| Tetramethyllead | 0.0008 | 0.0005–0.001 | 0.002 | 0.0004–0.004 |
| 1,2-Dibromoethane | 0.0008 | 0.0004–0.001 | 0.002 | 0.0001–0.005 |
| PAHs | 0.02 | 0.01–0.04 | 0.03 | 0.02–0.04 |
| Carbon monoxide | 34.0 | 24–44 | 20.0 | 10–23 |

[a]From Nilsson *et al.* (1987)

## 2.2 Environmental exposure

In many studies, levels have been reported of combustion products of fossil fuels (including gasoline and diesel fuel) in ambient air. The most frequently determined combustion products have been particles, carbon monoxide, nitrogen oxides, hydrocarbons and lead. These data are difficult to use in assessing the adverse health effects of engine exhausts, for several reasons: (i) the occurrence of these combustion products in ambient air may arise from sources other than engine exhausts; (ii) primary engine emissions may undergo further reactions in the environment at variable rates; and (iii) exposed populations tend to be transient, with variable and poorly characterized exposures (for review, see Holmberg & Ahlborg, 1983). Thus, the occurrence in the environment of the components of engine exhausts has only limited relevance to this monograph and the data have not been reviewed in detail.

Environmental emissions of fossil fuel combustion products from various sources, including engine exhausts, have been estimated for the major categories of pollutants (National Air Pollution Control Administration, 1970; National Research Council, 1972a,b; Howard & Durkin, 1974; National Research Council, 1977a,b; US Environmental Protection Agency, 1979; Bradow, 1980; Cuddihy *et al.*, 1980; Morandi & Eisenbud, 1980; Cuddihy *et al.*, 1981; US Environmental Protection Agency, 1982; Cuddihy *et al.*, 1984; The Motor Vehicle Manufacturers Association of the United States, Inc. and the Engine Manufacturers Association, 1986; US Environmental Protection Agency, 1986).

On the basis of estimates made by the National Research Council (1972a,b, 1977a,b), Hinkle (1980) estimated the environmental contribution of motor vehicle emissions for four categories of air pollutants, as a percentage of total emissions from all sources (and, in parentheses, from man-made sources): carbon monoxide, 7.7% (70%); nitrogen oxides, 2.3% (51%); particles, $1 \times 10^{-6}$% (1.8%); and lead, 98% (98%). It has been estimated that motor vehicle emissions contribute 80% or more of the polynuclear organic matter in the air of some cities (IARC, 1983).

Other authors have placed the contribution of motor vehicle emissions to carbon monoxide and nitrogen oxides in the environment at higher levels, the principal basis for uncertainty being the global input of these oxides from natural sources. In the USA, vehicle engine exhausts were estimated to produce 83% of the carbon monoxide and 44% of the nitrogen oxides from man-made sources in 1976 (US Environmental Protection Agency, 1979, 1982). Very similar estimates were reported for carbon monoxide (86%) and nitrogen oxides (42%) in the UK in 1984, with vehicle exhausts accounting for much higher percentages (up to 85%) of nitrogen oxides at street level in urban environments (Williams, 1987).

Concentrations of a number of engine exhaust components have been measured in ambient air in urban and rural environments. Representative data for particles, hydrocarbons, lead and oxides of nitrogen are given in Table 23. Concentrations of particle-associated PAHs in ambient air have also been reported by others (Sawicki, 1976; Egan *et al.*, 1979; Edwards, 1983; Chuang & Petersen, 1985). Benzo[*a*]pyrene concentrations in the air of over 200 cities in 25 countries worldwide were summarized by Sawicki (1976).

Table 23. Measured concentrations in ambient air of selected pollutants associated with engine exhausts

| Pollutant | Site | Time period | Type of engine exhaust[a] | Concentrations ($\mu g/m^3$) | Reference |
|---|---|---|---|---|---|
| **Particulate matter** | | | | | |
| Suspended | London, UK: Blackwall Tunnel, daytime average | Summers, 1958 and 1959 | Approximately 70% gasoline, 30% diesel | 2250 (daytime) | Waller et al. (1961) |
| Total suspended | Boston, MA, USA: Sumner Tunnel | September 1961 | NS | 588[b] | Larsen & Konopinski (1962) |
| Respirable | Boston, MA: street-level traffic stations, average | Spring, 1971 | NS | 47 | Burgess et al. (1973) |
| Total suspended | Central London, UK: top of County Hall (30 m) | 1975–76 | NS | Summer: 77 Winter: 108 | Ball & Hume (1977) |
| Total suspended | St Louis, MO, USA: annual average for various sectors | 1977 | Mixed | 60–130[c] | Bradow (1980) |
| Inhalable | Watertown, MA, USA (suburb of Boston): high-school athletic field | 1979–81 | NS | Total: 25.9 (3.2)[d] Fine: 17.4 (2.5) Coarse: 8.6 (0.6) | Thurston & Spengler (1985) |
| Inhalable (primarily <15 μm diameter) | Camden, Elizabeth and Newark, NJ, USA | 1981–83 | NS | 45–53[e] | Lioy & Daisey (1986) |
| Nitrogen dioxide | Four major US cities | 1962–71 | NS | Mean, 1962–66: 68 Mean, 1967–71: 72 | US Environmental Protection Agency (1982) |
| | Boston, MA, USA: 16 street-level traffic stations | 1970–71 | NS | Summer: 115 (<10–570)[f] Autumn: 115 (50–340) Winter: 85 (<10–270) Spring: 105 (40–285) | Burgess et al. (1973) |

**Table 23 (contd)**

| Pollutant | Site | Time period | Type of engine exhaust[a] | Concentrations ($\mu g/m^3$) | Reference |
|---|---|---|---|---|---|
| Nitrogen dioxide (contd) | St Louis, MO, USA: 18 regional air monitoring sites within 20 km of the city | 1976 | NS | Annual 1976 means for the 18 sites: 21–62; highest hourly concentrations in 1976 for the 18 sites: 149–676 | US Environmental Protection Agency (1982) |
| | Central London, UK: 40 locations | 1985 | 87% gasoline, 13% diesel | 'Background' sites: 54–75; weekly average values, 90–95; heavy traffic: 140 max | Laxen & Noordally (1987) |
| Nitrogen oxides | Several remote sites in the USA and Australia | 1956–77 | NS | 0.1–3 ppb (background) | Data from several authors summarized by Ritter et al. (1979) |
| Lead | Berlin-Steglitz, FRG At town hall near major traffic intersection Low traffic areas | 1966–67 | NS | >10 0.5 | Lahmann (1969) |
| | New York, NY, USA 1969–73[g] — 40 roof-top sampling stations; 1978 — 27 roof-top stations | 1969–73, 1978 | NS | Annual averages declined from 1.9 in 1970 to 1.1 in 1978 | Nathanson & Nudelman (1980) |
| | Boston, MA, USA: 16 street-level traffic stations | 1970–71 | NS | Summer: 5.4 (1.5–18)[f] Autumn: 6.9 (2.0–19.5) Winter: 6.5 (3.2–11.7) Spring: 4.5 (1.5–15.4) | Burgess et al. (1973) |
| | Central London, UK: top of County Hall (30 m) | 1975–76 | NS | Summer: 0.5 Winter: 1.06 | Ball & Hume (1977) |

Table 23 (contd)

| Pollutant | Site | Time period | Type of engine exhaust[a] | Concentrations ($\mu g/m^3$) | Reference |
|---|---|---|---|---|---|
| Lead (contd) | Jeddah, Saudia Arabia: 2 road traffic areas | 1985 | Gasoline engine (leaded gasoline) | 0.70 (low traffic) 2.38 (high traffic) | Al-Mutaz (1987) |
| | Riyadh, Saudi Arabia Top of a one-storey building in centre of city | 1985 | Gasoline engine (leaded gasoline) | 5.5 | El-Shobokshy (1985) |
| | Top of a building in a new area 12 km from centre of city | | | 2.5 | |
| Polycyclic aromatic hydrocarbons (PAHs) | | | | | |
| Benzo[a]pyrene | Central London, UK: County Hall and St Bartholomews' Hospital | 1949–73 | NS | 0.004–0.046 | Waller (1981) |
| | 122 urban and rural sites in the USA | 1958–59 | NS | Urban: 0.0001–0.061 Rural: 0.00001–0.0019 | Sawicki et al. (1960) |
| | Toronto, Canada: 5 sites ranging from urban to rural | 1972–73 | NS | 0.00011–0.00085 | Pierce & Katz (1975) |
| | FRG industrial city Area with mainly domestic coal heating | 1978–79 | NS | Means: 0.015 | Grimmer et al. (1981) |
| | Area with mainly central oil heating | | | 0.006 | |
| | Tunnel with automobile traffic | | | 0.031 | |
| | Area around a coke plant | | | 0.040 | |

Table 23 (contd)

| Pollutant | Site | Time period | Type of engine exhaust[a] | Concentrations (µg/m³) | Reference |
|---|---|---|---|---|---|
| 15 PAHs | Los Angeles County, CA, USA: 13 sites | 1974–75 | NS | Geometric means: 0.0001–0.003 (benzo[a]pyrene, 0.0005) | Gordon (1976) |
| Cyclopenta[cd]pyrene | FRG industrial city | 1978–79 | NS | Means: | Grimmer et al. (1981) |
| | Area with mainly domestic coal heating | | | 0.003 | |
| | Area with mainly central oil heating | | | 0.002 | |
| | Tunnel with automobile traffic | | | 0.088 | |
| | Area around a coke plant | | | 0.011 | |

[a]NS, not stated

[b] Mean concentration at outlet of tunnel ventilation system

[c]Vehicle contribution (mainly diesel) estimated to be 15% of total fine particles

[d]Numbers in parentheses, estimated contributions from motor vehicles in µg/m³

[e]Vehicle contribution (mainly gasoline) estimated to be 5–10%

[f]Mean (minimum-maximum)

[g]1969–73 data may be underestimated because cellulose filters were used which are less efficient than glass fibre (used in 1978).

Apportionment studies using receptor modelling methods have been used to estimate that the contribution of motor vehicle emissions to inhalable airborne particulate matter (<2.5 μm diameter) is 5–10% (Lioy & Daisey, 1986) or 15% of total fine particles (Bradow, 1980); mutagenicity was 50–74%. These studies were conducted in winter when domestic heating is the other major source of the pollutants in cities (Lewtas & Williams, 1986). Therefore, motor vehicles would be expected to make an even larger contribution to these pollutants during the rest of the year or on an annual average.

In the 1960s and early 1970s, typical average levels of lead in air in the USA ranged from 11.3 μg/m³ or higher near busy motorways, to 1–4 μg/m³ in the central areas of many cities, 0.1–0.5 μg/m³ in suburban and rural areas, and as low as 0.02 μg/m³ in remote areas (National Research Council, 1972b). These ranges appear to be typical for other industrialized nations where leaded gasoline is used in motor vehicles (Lahmann, 1969; Maziarka et al., 1971; Bini, 1973; Fisher & LeRoy, 1975; Ball & Hume, 1977; El-Shobokshy, 1985; Al-Mutaz, 1987). With the increasing use of lead-free gasoline and increasing restrictions on use of leaded gasoline, these levels are declining (Fishbein, 1976; Falk, 1977; US Environmental Protection Agency, 1986).

Motor vehicles have been identified as significant sources of ambient air concentrations of a number of specific volatile hydrocarbons, such as benzene, toluene, xylenes and acetylene (Seifert & Ullrich, 1978; Whitby & Altwicker, 1978; Häsänen et al., 1981; Tsani-Bazaca et al., 1981). The inventory of the Japanese Environmental Agency for total hydrocarbon emissions in 1978 indicates that 39% of hydrocarbon emissions in Japan were from mobile sources (Wadden et al., 1986). In the UK, vehicle emissions were estimated to account for approximately 33% of the volatile organic compounds (mainly hydrocarbons) released to the environment in 1984 (Williams, 1987).

1,2-Dichloroethane and 1,2-dibromoethane are also present in engine exhausts, and the time-dependent concentrations of benzene and 1,2-dibromoethane near roads are reported to be closely correlated (Tsani-Bazaca et al., 1981). Formaldehyde, the principal aldehyde component of engine exhausts, is generally found in ambient air at 12–18 μg/m³, but concentrations of 107–180 μg/m³ have been reported in heavy traffic or photochemical smog (National Research Council, 1981; Grosjean, 1982; Anon., 1984).

Limits have been set on motor vehicle emissions in many parts of the world. The Council of the European Communities (Commission of the European Communities, 1988) has, for example, adopted a phased programme for the implementation of emission standards for carbon monoxide, hydrocarbons and oxides of nitrogen from gasoline- and diesel-powered vehicles. The US Environmental Protection Agency is also proceeding with the phased implementation of standards for gasoline- and diesel-powered vehicles specifying decreasing limits for exhaust emissions of carbon monoxide, hydrocarbons, oxides of nitrogen and particles (diesel only); evaporative hydrocarbon emissions are regulated for gasoline-powered vehicles only (US Environmental Protection Agency, 1987).

## 2.3 Analysis

### (a) Sampling

Vehicle exhaust cannot be sampled correctly at temperatures that occur in or just behind the exhaust pipe because (i) the adsorption/desorption ratio on filter materials is disadvantageous at elevated temperatures and (ii) various exhaust constituents may be converted into artefacts on the filter, depending upon conditions, such as conversion of PAHs into nitroarenes (Pitts *et al.*, 1978; Lee, F.S.-C. *et al.*, 1980; Gibson *et al.*, 1981; Schuetzle & Perez, 1983; Grimmer *et al.*, 1988). Furthermore, exhaust is a heterogeneous material consisting of a gaseous phase and a particulate phase, and different techniques have been used for their collection, which can be classified into dilution tube sampling and raw gas sampling.

Measurements of vehicle emissions are typically made under laboratory conditions using chassis or engine dynamometer testing. Specified driving cycles are used to simulate on-road conditions. The Federal Test Procedure (FTP — also referred to as the LA-4, US-72 and the Urban Cycle; National Research Council, 1982) is the primary cycle used in the USA to approximate urban driving conditions (US Environmental Protection Agency, 1977). A similar test cycle is used in Europe (EEC Regulation 15/04; Commission of the European Communities, 1970).

Emissions collected for the purpose of chemical analysis and bioassays are typically referred to as particulate-phase emissions, gas-phase emissions and condensate emissions. 'Particulate emissions' are defined as all materials collected on a filter from a dilution tube at a dilution ratio of $\simeq 15:1$ and at $\simeq 35°C$ (see below; Hare *et al.*, 1979). 'Gas-phase emissions' are defined as all materials which pass through a filter from the dilution tube under the conditions specified above. 'Condensate/extract' comprises: (i) material extractable by organic solvents (toluene, acetone) from particles collected on filters; (ii) residue obtained by evaporation of condensed water; and (iii) the evaporation residue after washing the condenser with organic solvents. Therefore, 'condensate extract' refers to organic compounds collected from exhaust by this procedure. In general, these compounds are less volatile than naphthalene and do not include nitrogen oxides, sulfur dioxide, $C_1-C_9$ hydrocarbons, benzene, most alkylbenzenes or inorganic substances such as elemental carbon and lead.

#### (i) *Dilution tube sampling*

Vehicle exhaust generated by driving schedules under standard conditions on a chassis dynamometer is diluted with a well-defined quantity of filtered air in a dilution tunnel, from which samples can be taken isokinetically after they have been cooled to about 50°C (Hare & Barnes, 1979). It has been shown that this device (presented schematically in Figure 3) closely simulates the process of dilution (Lee & Schuetzle, 1983; Schuetzle, 1983) under actual atmospheric conditions. The residence time of exhaust in the tunnel before being trapped on filters has been estimated to be less than 5 sec. Particles may be collected on filters, such as Teflon, or by electrostatic precipitators (Lee & Schuetzle, 1983). Hallock *et al.* (1987) recommended a liquid electrostatic aerosol precipitator which preserves

**Fig. 3. Dilution tube used for monitoring and collecting gas- and particulate-phase vehicle emissions**[a]

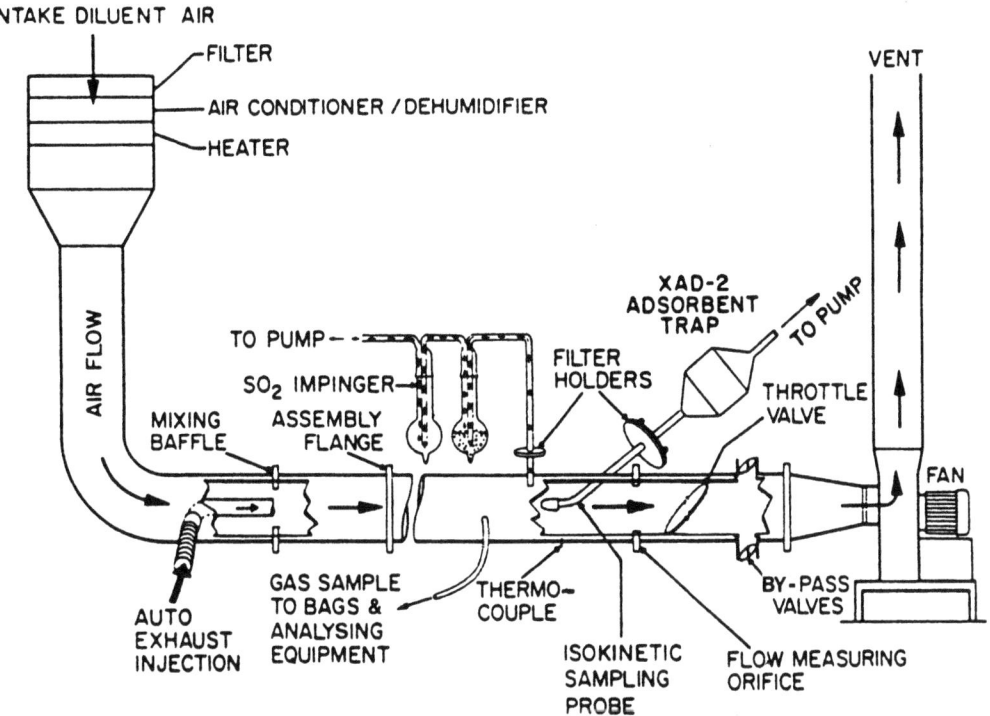

[a]From Schuetzle (1983)

submicronic particle size. Semivolatile compounds in the gaseous phase can be trapped by adsorption filter systems containing inorganic silica or, more satisfactorily, organic materials (e.g., XAD-2, Tenax, Chromosorb 102, Porapak; Jones et al., 1976; Lee et al., 1979; Lee & Schuetzle, 1983; Schuetzle, 1983). Schuetzle (1983) recommended XAD-2, since this material, in contrast to Tenax, does not react with nitrogen oxides.

Gases are sampled in bags either before entering the filter system or after having passed the adsorbent trap (see Figure 3). Stenberg et al. (1983) described a cryogradient technique which allows the separation of NO by cooling with a liquid nitrogen condenser.

(ii) *Raw gas sampling*

In most of these devices, the exhaust is partially condensed before separation by filter combinations. Initially, steel condensers were used (Stenburg et al., 1961); since that time, a collecting device consisting of a vertical glass cooler and a micron filter of impregnated glass fibre with a separation degree of over 99.9% for particle sizes of 0.3–0.5 $\mu$m has been described (Grimmer et al., 1973a; Kraft & Lies, 1981; VDI-Kommision, 1987; see Figure 4).

## Fig. 4. System for collecting undiluted vehicle exhaust[a]

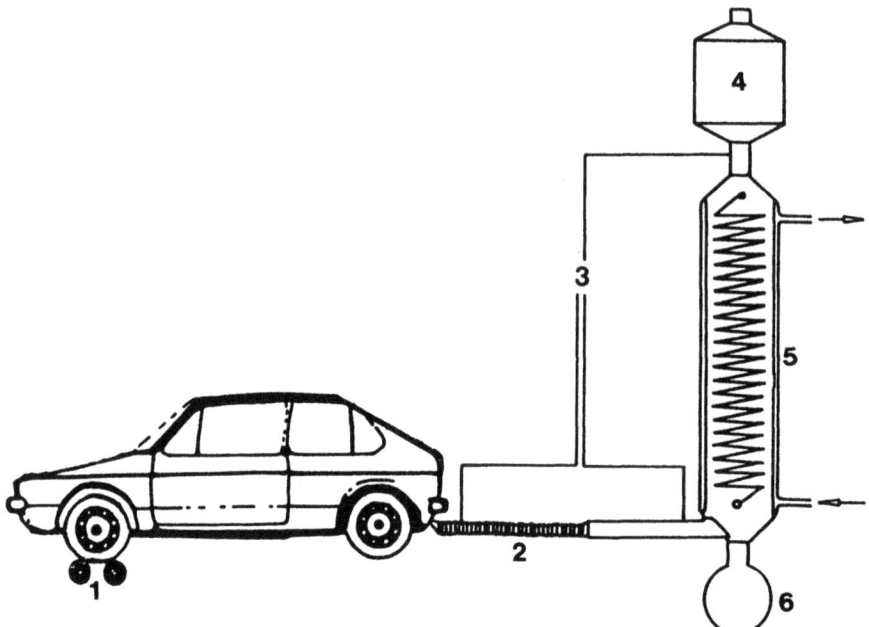

[a]From Grimmer et al. (1988); 1, chassis dynamometer; 2, flexible pipe; 3, thermocouple; 4, glass-fibre filter (silicon bounded, 1 m²); 5, glass cooler; 6, condensate

Proportional raw gas sampling, resulting in samples of more manageable size, has been described (Stenberg et al., 1981; Johnson, 1988). Various filter materials, as such or in combination, have been used to separate particles and semivolatile compounds from exhausts. Quartz and glass fibre, cellulose acetate (Millipore), polyvinylidene fluoride (Duropore), polytetrafluoroethylene (Teflon, Zefluor, Fluoropore), polyvinyl chloride, polyethylene and polycarbonate (Nucleopore) can separate >99.9% of submicrometer particulates (John & Reischl, 1978; Lee, F.S.-C. et al., 1980; Lee & Schuetzle, 1983). Teflon has been cited as being superior to other materials in terms of separation efficiency and chemical inertness (Lee & Schuetzle, 1983; Schuetzle, 1983).

Semivolatile compounds in the gaseous phase can be separated out using polymer materials, such as Tenax, XAD-2 and Porapak, or with Chromosorb. Purification of these materials may be time-consuming since repeated washing (or Soxhlet extraction) with various solvents is required to remove organic impurities which interfere with analysis. Trapping of the gaseous phase can be carried out as in the case of dilution tube sampling, by (i) the cryogradient technique or (ii) gas bag collection.

One of the main problems described in the literature regarding the correct sampling of exhaust is avoidance of chemical conversion of sensitive compounds (e.g., PAHs) to artefacts (e.g., ketones, quinones, phenols, halides and nitroarenes). Losses of pyrene and perylene were studied after direct injection into exhaust near the end of the exhaust pipe, with recoveries of only 20–60% by gas chromatography and high-performance liquid chromatography (Lee et al., 1979). Schuetzle (1983) found that more than 90% of pyrene and benzo[a]pyrene was lost through oxidation under the same conditions.

PAHs can react with nitrogen oxides, ozone or sulfuric acid under sampling conditions. Photooxidation during sample analysis may result in the formation of endoperoxides which then undergo rearrangement to yield hydroquinones and subsequently quinones, or in the formation of exoperoxides which yield ketones (Schuetzle, 1983). In the presence of nitric acid, nitrogen dioxide reacts with PAHs to yield nitroarenes (Pitts et al., 1978; Brorström et al., 1983). On the assumption that nitroarene formation is acid-catalysed, diesel exhaust was collected with and without injection of ammonia during sampling; significantly higher amounts of 1-nitropyrene were found without ammonia injection at a sampling temperature of 100°C. When passed through an exhaust-loaded filter, the particle-free gaseous phase enhanced the concentration of 1-nitropyrene. No such effect was observed when collecting filters were maintained at below 35°C (Grimmer et al., 1988).

The artificial formation of nitroarenes during sampling procedures is still a matter of controversy (Gaddo et al., 1984) and has been critically reviewed (Lee & Schuetzle, 1983).

It should be noted that the invariance of the PAH profile over the collection period is the essential precondition for correct sampling, since certain individual compounds are more sensitive to chemical reactions and/or evaporation effects.

*(b) Extraction*

Extraction of organic material from exhaust collected on filters is often incomplete owing to an inadequate choice of solvent or extraction time (Köhler & Eichhoff, 1967; Stanley et al., 1967; for reviews see Jacob & Grimmer, 1979; Griest & Caton, 1983; Lee & Schuetzle, 1983). The recommended extraction procedure is on a Soxhlet apparatus or hot-solvent extraction with toluene, benzene, xylene (Köhler & Eichhoff, 1967; Grimmer et al., 1982), benzene/ethanol (methanol, propanol; Swarin & Williams, 1980), dichloromethane/methanol (Schuetzle et al., 1985), toluene/ethanol (Schuetzle & Perez, 1981) or toluene/2-propanol (Lee & Schuetzle, 1983). Under these conditions, not only PAHs but also their more polar derivatives exhibit optimal extractability. This method also obviates the artefact formation that can occur with chloroform, dimethyl sulfoxide and other solvents used for extraction. In addition, Soxhlet solvent extraction results in higher recoveries of various PAHs than with cold ultrasonic extraction. If not analysed immediately after collection, the extract should be stored under nitrogen in the dark at 0°C or below.

*(c) Clean-up and fractionation*

After extraction, a small amount of organic material is obtained in a large volume of solvent. In order not to lose low-boiling constituents, the solution must be evaporated carefully. Vacuum rotatory evaporators with vacuum controller or specially designed devices are recommended (Dünges, 1979).

**Fig. 5. One scheme for fractionating automotive exhaust**[a]

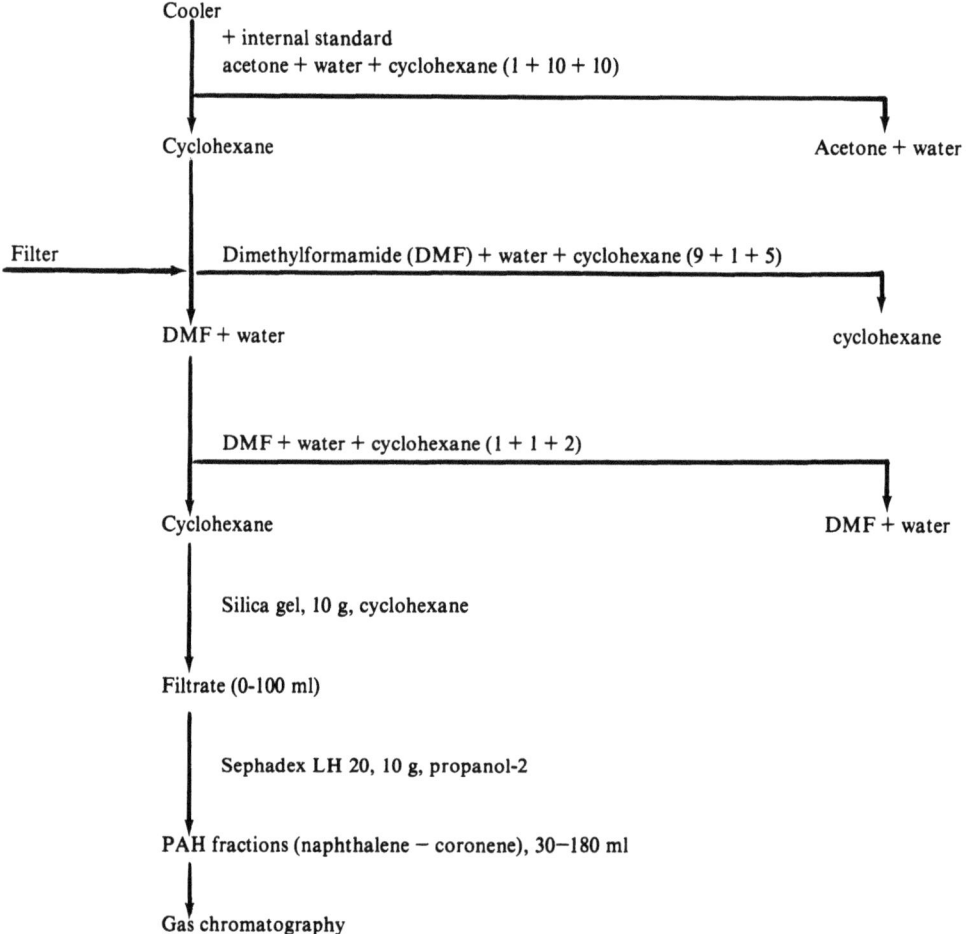

[a]From Grimmer et al. (1977)

A fractionation scheme for vehicle exhaust combining condensed water, cooler washing (acetone) and filter extract (see Figure 5) has been described, which is based on liquid/liquid partition and chromatography on silica gel and Sephadex LH 20 (Grimmer & Böhnke, 1972; Grimmer et al., 1973b, 1977; Lee & Schuetzle, 1983). An additional fractionation step using Sephadex LH 20 partition chromatography may be used. This method has also been used to characterize biologically active fractions; in some cases, the silica gel chromatography step has been deleted (Brune et al., 1978; Grimmer et al., 1984, 1987). A fractionation scheme for the preparation of biologically active fractions from diesel exhaust is given in Figure 6; nitroarenes are also separated by this method. A more complex fractionation

**Fig. 6. One scheme for fractionating diesel exhaust condensate**[a]

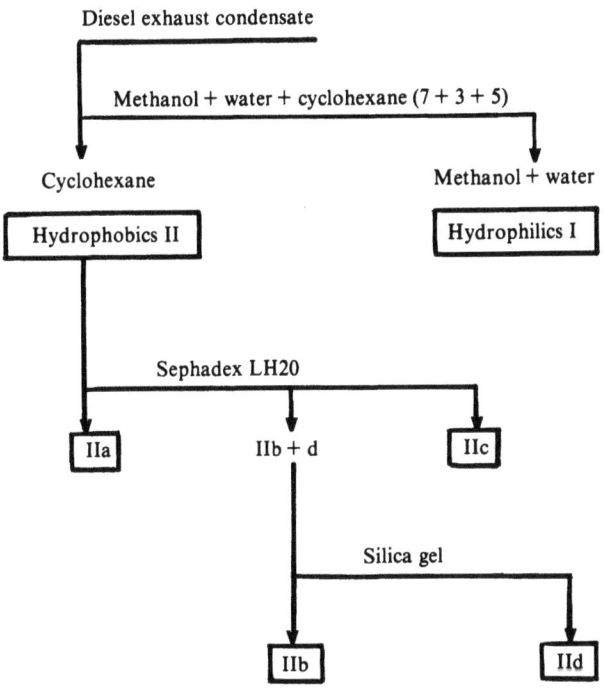

[a]From Grimmer et al. (1987); I, hydrophilic fraction; II, hydrophobic fraction; IIa, nonaromatic compounds and two- and three-ring polycyclic aromatic compounds (PAC); IIb, four- to seven-ring PACs; IIc, polar PACs; IId, nitro-polycyclic aromatic hydrocarbons (PAH)

scheme (Figure 7) can be used to separate the original exhaust extract into aliphatic compounds, aromatic compounds and moderately and highly-polar fractions after the removal of acidic and basic fractions (Petersen & Chuang, 1982). A similar scheme was used by Lee and Schuetzle (1983; see Fig. 1).

Methods for the separation and identification of nitroarenes are given in the monograph on 1-nitropyrene. Organic halides, such as methyl bromide, chloroform, carbon tetrachloride, trichloroethane, tetrachloroethane and various brominated PAHs, have also been analysed in the exhaust of gasoline- and diesel-fueled vehicles (Harsch & Rasmussen, 1977; Alsberg et al., 1985).

**Fig. 7. One scheme for extraction and fractionation of organic material in diesel particulate**[a]

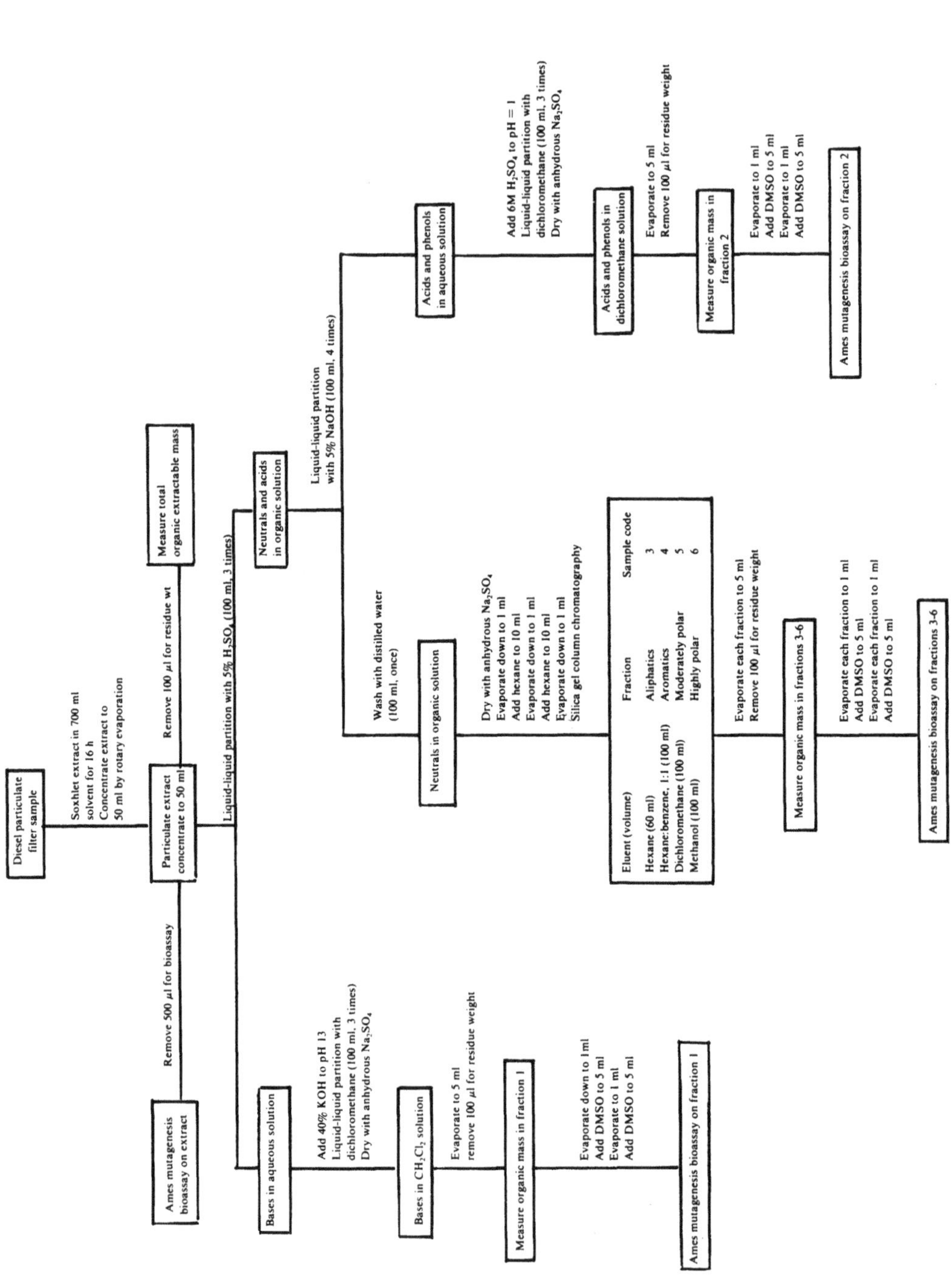

(d) *Chemical analysis*

In order to separate further the various fractions obtained by clean-up methods and to characterize and/or identify individual compounds simultaneously, thin-layer chromatography (TLC), high-performance liquid chromatography (HPLC) and gas chromatography (GC) have been used in combination with ultra-violet, visible and fluorescence spectrophotometry, mass spectrometry (MS) and more or less specific detection methods, such as flame ionization, nitrogen flame ionization and sulfur-specific and electron-capture detectors (Kunte, 1979; Lee & Schuetzle, 1983; Nielsen, 1983; White, 1985).

(i) *Thin-layer chromatography (TLC)*

Two-dimensional cellulose TLC with fluorescence detection is the recommended TLC method for PAH fractions from vehicle exhaust and has given results in good agreement with those obtained by GC (Kraft & Lies, 1981). A simple TLC screening method for the determination of benzo[a]pyrene, which is also applicable to vehicle exhaust, has recently been recommended by the International Union of Pure and Applied Chemistry (Grimmer & Jacob, 1987). The use of TLC for the analysis of PAHs has been reviewed (Daisey, 1983).

(ii) *High-performance liquid chromatography (HPLC)*

The basic advantages and disadvantages of HPLC in comparison to other techniques such as GC have been reviewed (Wise *et al.*, 1980; Wise, 1983). The method has been widely used for the detection and identification of organic constituents of vehicle exhaust, and results of determinations of PAHs in automotive exhaust condensate using HPLC have been compared with those obtained using capillary GC (Doran & McTaggart, 1974). A comparative study of different HPLC methods for the analysis of PAHs in diesel emissions has been carried out (Eisenberg & Cunningham, 1984). Using HPLC/GC-MS, 74 polycyclic aromatic compounds were identified or tentatively identified in diesel particulate extracts (Tong & Karasek, 1984). A normal-phase HPLC method using silica gel columns and *n*-hexane:benzene (3:1) as eluent has been developed to isolate PAHs and their nitro derivatives (Nielsen, 1983). A very precise, routine, on-line reverse-phase HPLC/fluorescence method has been reported for the analysis of nitroarenes in the picogram range by their reduction to highly fluorescent amines (Tejada *et al.*, 1983). A 'pyrenebutyric acid amide phase' has been applied to a multidimensional HPLC method with on-line peak identification by ultra-violet-visible spectrometry, which allows the detection of 1-nitropyrene in the range of 3–100 ng per mg of soot collected on a filter (Lindner *et al.*, 1985). HPLC has been used to compare the concentrations of some PAHs and their nitro derivatives in exhausts from four diesel cars (Gibson *et al.*, 1981). A semipreparative HPLC analysis of a soluble organic fraction of diesel engine exhaust particulates has been reported, together with unsatisfactory results using HPLC/MS coupling (Levine *et al.*, 1982).

(iii) *Gas chromatography (GC) and gas chromatography/mass spectrometry (GC/MS)*

GC methods for the determination of PAHs from exhaust condensates have been reviewed (Olufsen & Björseth, 1983), as have GC and GC/MS analyses of nitroarenes (White, 1985). Collaborative studies have been carried out to analyse PAHs in vehicle exhaust (Janssen, 1976; Metz *et al.*, 1984) in which GC methods were compared with those of HPLC (Metz *et al.*, 1984).

Packed-column GC has been largely replaced by high-resolution glass capillary column GC using fused silica columns and careful sample injection procedures (on-column injection at low temperatures of 50–80°C or thermal desorption cold trap injection procedure). Detection limits down to the picogram level have been reached with GC when single-ion monitoring mass spectrometry is used as the detection system (Ramdahl & Urdal, 1982).

Various classes of organic compounds from vehicle exhausts have been analysed by GC and GC/MS, including paraffins, olefins, PAHs, thia-arenes, aza-arenes, oxo-arenes and aldehyde, phenol, quinone and nitro derivatives of PAHs and their acid anhydrides (Hites *et al.*, 1981; Schuetzle *et al.*, 1981; Lee & Schuetzle, 1983; Alsberg *et al.*, 1984; Ramdahl, 1984; White, 1985). More than 70 individual nitroarenes were found in diesel particulate extracts by means of fused-silica capillary column GC and a nitrogen-specific detector, with detection limits of 0.2–0.5 mg/kg (Paputa-Peck *et al.*, 1983). The emission of PAHs and nitroarenes by diesel engines from PAH-containing and other well defined fuels (hexadecane) were studied using GC/MS and tandem triple-quadrupole MS (Fulford *et al.*, 1982; Henderson *et al.*, 1983, 1984).

The rapid analysis of gaseous and other combustion-related compounds in hot gas streams by atmospheric-pressure chemical ionization/MS has been reported (Sakuma *et al.*, 1981).

(iv) *Other methods*

Photometric, infra-red, colorimetric, electrochemical and chemiluminescence techniques have been used for the analysis of gases such as sulfur dioxide, carbon monoxide, carbon dioxide, nitrogen oxides and formaldehyde (Hare & Baines, 1979; Deutsche Forschungsgemeinschaft, 1985). Test tubes in which various colour reactions are seen are available for the analysis of various constituents of vehicle exhaust such as carbon monoxide, carbon dioxide, sulfur dioxide and nitrogen dioxide (Leichnitz, 1986).

## 3. Biological Data Relevant to the Evaluation of Carcinogenic Risk to Humans

### 3.1 Carcinogenicity studies in animals

*Diesel engine exhaust*

During the past decade, there has been worldwide interest in developing an improved data base for evaluating the potential carcinogenic effects of exposure to diesel exhaust. One of the earliest initiatives in this area was undertaken by the US Environmental Protection Agency (Pepelko & Peirano, 1983). The Working Group took cognizance of these preliminary studies which involved exposure by inhalation of SENCAR or strain A mice to whole diesel exhaust or by intraperitoneal injections of extracts of diesel exhaust particles.

Only increases in the incidence of pulmonary adenomas were measured as the end-point. In some cases, animals were also administered known carcinogens. The Working Group noted that the exposure and observation times in these studies were generally short as compared with those in later studies that yielded positive results.

(a) *Inhalation exposure*

*Mouse*: Heinrich *et al.* (1986a) exposed two groups of 96 female NMRI mice, eight to ten weeks old, to filtered or unfiltered exhaust from a 1.6-l displacement diesel engine operated according to the US-72 (FTP; see p. 80) test cycle to simulate average urban driving, or to clean air, for 19 h per day on five days per week for life. The unfiltered and filtered exhausts were diluted 1:17 with air and contained 4.24 mg/m$^3$ particles. Levels of 1.5 ± 0.3 ppm (3 ± 0.6 (SD) mg/m$^3$) nitrogen dioxide and 11.4 ± 2.1 ppm nitrogen oxides were found in whole exhaust and 1.2 ± 0.26 ppm (2.4 ± 0.5 mg/m$^3$) nitrogen dioxide and 9.9 ± 1.8 ppm nitrogen oxides in filtered exhaust. Exposure to total diesel exhaust and filtered diesel exhaust significantly increased the number of animals with lung tumours (adenomas and carcinomas) to 24/76 (32%) and 29/93 (31%), respectively, as compared to 11/84 (13%) in controls. When the incidences of adenomas and carcinomas were evaluated separately, significantly higher numbers of animals in both diesel exhaust-exposed groups had adenocarcinomas (13 (17%) and 18 (19%), respectively) than in controls (2.4%); no increase was seen in the numbers of animals with adenomas. [The Working Group noted that the incidence of lung tumours in historical controls in this laboratory could reach 32% (Heinrich *et al.*, 1986b).]

Groups of ICR and C57Bl/6N mice (total number of treated and untreated animals combined alive at three months, 315 and 297, respectively) [initial numbers and sex distribution unspecified] were exposed to the exhaust from a small diesel engine (269 cm$^3$ displacement, run at idling speed) used as an electric generator; the exhaust was diluted 1:2 to 1:4 in air (Takemoto *et al.*, 1986). The mice were exposed within 24 h after birth for 4 h per day on four days per week (2–4 mg/m$^3$ particles; size, 0.32 µm; 2–4 ppm, 4–8 mg/m$^3$ nitrogen dioxide). Between months 13 and 28, lung tumours (adenomas and adenocarcinomas) were found in 14/56 exposed ICR mice and in 7/60 controls and in 17/150 treated C57Bl/6N mice and 1/51 controls. The authors reported that the differences were not statistically significant. [The Working Group calculated that the difference in C57Bl/6N mice was statistically significant at $p < 0.05$.]

*Rat*: Karagianes *et al.* (1981) exposed groups of male specific-pathogen-free Wistar rats [numbers unspecified], 18 weeks old, for 6 h per day for 20 months to one of five experimental atmospheres: clean air (controls); 8.3 ± 2.0 (SD) mg/m$^3$ soot from diesel exhaust; 8.3 ± 2.0 mg/m$^3$ soot from diesel exhaust plus 5.8 ± 3.5 mg/m$^3$ coal dust; 6.6 ± 1.9 mg/m$^3$ coal dust; or 14.9 ± 6.2 mg/m$^3$ coal dust. The diesel exhaust was produced by a three-cylinder, 43-brake horse power diesel engine driving a 15 kW electric generator. The fuel injection system of the engine was modified to simulate operating patterns of such engines in mines and was operated on a variable duty cycle (dilution, approximately 35:1). Six rats per group were killed after four, eight, 16 or 20 months of exposure. Complete gross necropsy was performed, and respiratory tract tissues, oesophagus, stomach and other tissues with lesions were examined histopathologically. Significant non-neoplastic lesions were restricted primarily to the respiratory tract and increased in severity with duration of exposure. In the six rats examined from each group after 20 months of exposure, two bronchiolar adenomas were observed — one in the group exposed to diesel exhaust only and one in the group exposed to diesel exhaust and coal dust. None was observed in controls or in the two groups exposed to coal dust only. [The Working Group noted the limited number of animals studied at 20 months.]

Groups of 72 male and 72 female or 144 male Fischer 344 weanling rats were exposed for 7 h per day on five days per week for 24 months to either clean air (controls); 2 mg/m³ coal dust (<7 µm); 2 mg/m³ diesel exhaust particles, with specific limits on gaseous/vapour constituents; or 1 mg/m³ coal dust plus 1 mg/m³ diesel exhaust particles (Lewis et al., 1986). The nitrogen dioxide concentration in the diesel exhaust was $1.5 \pm 0.5$ ppm ($3 \pm 1$ mg/m³); the exhaust was generated by a 7-l displacement, four-cycle, water-cooled, 'naturally aspirated' (open-chamber) diesel engine. The exhaust was diluted by a factor of 27:1 before entering the exposure chambers. Following three, six, 12 and 24 months of exposure, at least ten male rats per group were removed for ancillary studies. After 24 months of exposure, all survivors were killed. The numbers of rats necropsied and examined histologically in each of the four groups were 120–121 males and 71–72 females. No difference in survival was noted among treatment groups, chambers or sexes [data on survival unavailable]. No statistical difference in tumour incidence was noted among the four groups. [The Working Group noted that no detailed information on tumour incidence was available and that the animals were killed at 24 months, a shorter observation period than used in other inhalation studies with rats that gave positive results.][1]

Female specific-pathogen-free Fischer 344 rats [initial number unspecified], aged five weeks, were exposed to diesel exhaust from a small diesel engine (269 cm³ displacement) run at idling speed; rats were treated for 4 h per day on four days per week for 24 months, at which time they were killed or were left untreated (Takemoto et al., 1986). The exhaust was diluted 1:2 to 1:4 with air. The concentration of particulates (size, 0.32 µm) ranged from 2–4 mg/m³, and those of nitrogen dioxide were 2–4 ppm (3–8 mg/m³). No lung tumour was observed in either the 26 treated or 20 control rats; 15 and 12 rats in the two groups, respectively, survived 18–24 months. [The Working Group noted the small group sizes.]

Iwai et al. (1986) exposed two groups of 24 female specific-pathogen-free Fischer 344 rats, seven weeks of age, to either diluted diesel exhaust or diluted filtered diesel exhaust for 8 h per day on seven days a week for 24 months, at which time some rats were sacrificed and the remainder were returned to clean air for a further six months of observation. The diesel exhaust was produced by a 2.4-l displacement small truck engine; it was diluted ten times with clean air and contained $4.9 \pm 1.6$ mg/m³ particles, $1.8 \pm 1.8$ ppm ($3.6 \pm 3.6$ mg/m³) nitrogen dioxide and $30.9 \pm 10.9$ ppm nitrogen oxides. Another group of 24 rats was exposed to fresh air only for 30 months. Incidences of lung tumours, diagnosed as adenomas, adenocarcinomas, squamous-cell carcinomas and adenosquamous carcinomas, were significantly higher in the group exposed to whole diesel exhaust, with or without a subsequent observation period (in 8/19 rats, including five with malignant tumours) than in

---

[1]Subsequent to the meeting, a more detailed report of the study was published (Lewis et al., 1989).

the control group (one adenoma in 1/22 rats; $p < 0.01$). No lung tumour was observed in the group exposed to filtered exhaust (0/16 rats). Incidences of malignant lymphomas and tumours at other sites did not differ among the three groups. [The Working Group noted the small group sizes.]

Ishinishi et al. (1986a) exposed groups of 64 male and 59 female specific-pathogen-free Fischer 344 rats, four weeks of age, to diesel exhaust from either a light-duty 1.8-l displacement, four-cylinder engine (particle concentrations, 0.11, 0.41, 1.08 or 2.32 mg/m$^3$; nitrogen dioxide concentrations, 0.08, 0.26, 0.70 or 1.41 ppm (0.2, 0.5, 1.4 or 2.8 mg/m$^3$); nitrogen oxide concentrations, 1.24, 4.06, 10.14 or 20.34 ppm) or a heavy-duty 11-l displacement, six-cylinder engine (particle concentrations, 0.46, 0.96, 1.84 or 3.72 mg/m$^3$; nitrogen dioxide concentrations, 0.46, 1.02, 1.68 or 3.00 ppm (0.9, 2.1, 3.4 or 6 mg/m$^3$); nitrogen oxide concentrations, 6.17, 13.13, 21.67 or 37.45 ppm). Exposure was for 16 h per day on six days per week for up to 30 months. The diesel emissions were diluted about 10–15 times (v/v) with air. Separate control groups for the light-duty and heavy-duty series were exposed to clean air. The incidence of lung tumours diagnosed as adenocarcinomas, squamous-cell carcinomas or adenosquamous carcinomas was significantly increased only in the highest-dose group (in 5/64 males and 3/60 females) of the heavy-duty diesel exhaust-exposed series compared to controls (in 0/64 males and 1/59 females; $p < 0.05$). The incidences in the next highest-dose group in this series were 3/64 males and 1/59 females. [The Working Group noted that, although this incidence was not statistically different from that in the controls, it suggested an overall positive response for the two highest exposure levels.] No statistically significant increase in the incidence of lung tumours was noted in the groups exposed to light-duty diesel engine exhaust. [The Working Group noted that the highest level of exposure in the light-duty series was approximately one-half of the highest concentration used in the heavy-duty series, and that the incidence (3.3%) of lung tumours in the control animals of the light-duty diesel engine exhaust-exposed series was higher than that in the heavy-duty diesel controls (0.8%).]

Groups of 72 male and 72 female Fischer 344 rats, six to eight weeks old, were exposed to one of three concentrations of diesel engine exhaust or particle-filtered diesel engine exhaust from a 1.5-l displacement engine operated according to the US-72 (FTP) driving cycle which simulates average urban driving; exposure was for 16 h per day on five days per week for two years (Brightwell et al., 1986). The exposure concentrations were reported as a dilution of the exhaust with a constant volume of 800 m$^3$ of air (high dose), a further dilution of this mixture in air of 1:3 (medium dose) and a dilution of 1:9 (low dose). The particle concentrations in the unfiltered diesel exhaust atmosphere were 0.7, 2.2 and 6.6 mg/m$^3$ for the low, medium and high doses (with 8 ± 2 ppm nitrogen oxides in the high dose), respectively. Two control groups of 144 rats of each sex were exposed to conditioned air. Following the exposure period, the animals were maintained for a further six months in clean air. An exposure concentration-related increase in the incidence of primary lung tumours [detailed histopathology unspecified] was reported only in groups exposed to unfiltered diesel exhaust. [The Working Group noted that no information of tumour incidence was given for rats exposed to filtered diesel exhaust.][1]

---

[1]Subsequent to the meeting, a more detailed report of the study was published (Brightwell et al., 1989; see also pp. 93, 98, 99, 104).

Heinrich et al. (1986a) exposed two groups of 96 female Wistar rats, eight to ten weeks old, to filtered or unfiltered exhaust, as described on p. 89. A significantly increased incidence of lung tumours (histologically identified as eight bronchioalveolar adenomas and nine squamous-cell tumours) was observed in rats exposed to unfiltered diesel exhaust (17/95 (18%) versus 0/96 controls). No lung tumour was reported in rats exposed to filtered exhaust.

Mauderly et al. (1986, 1987) exposed groups of 221–230 male and female specific-pathogen-free Fischer 344 rats, 17 weeks old, to one of three concentrations of diesel engine exhaust generated by a 1980 model 5.7-l V8 engine operated according to US FTP cycles; exposure was for 7 h per day on five days per week for up to 30 months. The exposure concentrations were reported as a dilution of the whole exhaust to measured soot concentrations of 0.35 (low), 3.5 (medium) or 7.0 (high dose) mg/m³. Levels of nitrogen dioxide were $0.1 \pm 0.1$ ($0.2 \pm 0.2$), $0.3 \pm 0.2$ ($0.6 \pm 0.4$) and $0.7 \pm 0.5$ ppm ($1.4 \pm 1$ mg/m³), respectively. Sham-exposed controls received filtered air. The soot particles were approximately 0.25 μm mass median diameter, and approximately 12% of their mass was composed of solvent-extractable organics. Subgroups of animals were removed at six, 12, 18 and 24 months for ancillary studies; all rats surviving after 30 months of exposure were killed. All rats that died or were killed were necropsied and examined histologically for lung tumours. Exposures did not significantly affect the survival of animals of either sex. The median survival time ranged from 880 (low) to 897 (medium) days of age for males and from 923 (high) to 962 (low) days for females. A total of 901 rats were examined for lung tumours; four types were found: bronchoalveolar adenomas, adenocarcinomas, squamous cysts (mostly benign) and squamous-cell carcinomas. None of the tumours was found to have metastasized to other organs. The incidences of lung tumours in males and females combined were 0.9% in controls, 1.3% in low-dose, 3.6% in medium-dose and 12.8% in high-dose groups. The authors noted that the prevalences at the medium and high levels were significantly increased ($p < 0.05$). A total of 42 rats developed 46 lung tumours; four females in the high-dose group had two lung tumours each. Lung tumours were found in two male controls, in one low-dose male, in four mid-dose males and in 13 high-dose males; in females, the respective incidences were zero, two, four and 20. Adenomas predominated in the medium-exposure group. Adenocarcinomas, squamous-cell carcinomas and squamous cysts were observed predominantly at the high dose. The tumours were observed late in the study: 81% after two years of exposure. The authors observed no exposure-related difference in cause of death; the tumours were found incidentally at death or at termination of the experiment.

*Hamster*: Groups of 48 female Syrian golden hamsters, eight weeks of age, were exposed to diluted (1:7 air) unfiltered diesel exhaust (mass median particle diameter, 0.1 μm; mean particle concentration, $3.9 \pm 0.5$ mg/m³; nitrogen dioxide, $1.2 \pm 1.7$ ppm ($2.4 \pm 3.4$ mg/m³); nitrogen oxides, $18.6 \pm 5.8$ ppm) or filtered diesel exhaust (nitrogen dioxide, $1.0 \pm 1.5$ ppm ($2 \pm 3$ mg/m³); nitrogen oxides, $19.2 \pm 6.1$ ppm); exposure was for 7–8 h per day on five days per week for life (Heinrich et al., 1982). The exhaust was generated by a 2.4-l displacement engine operating at a steady state. A group of 48 hamsters inhaling clean air served as controls. There was no effect of diesel exhaust on survival; median lifespan was 72–74 weeks in all groups, and no lung tumour was reported in treated or control animals.

Groups of 48 female and 48 male Syrian golden hamsters, eight to ten weeks of age, were exposed to diluted (1:17 air) filtered or unfiltered exhaust as described on p. 89 (Heinrich et al., 1986a). A control group of 48 females and 48 males inhaled clean air. Median lifespan was not significantly influenced by diesel exposure and was 75–80 weeks for females and 80–90 weeks for males. No lung tumour was observed in treated or control animals.

Groups of 52 female and 52 male Syrian hamsters, six to eight weeks of age, were exposed to one of three concentrations of unfiltered or filtered exhaust as described on p. 91 (Brightwell et al., 1986). Two control groups of 104 hamsters of each sex were exposed to clean air only. The authors reported that there was no increase in the incidence of respiratory-tract tumours in treated hamsters. [The Working Group noted the incomplete reporting of tumour incidence and survival.]

*Monkey*: Groups of 15 male cynomolgus monkeys (*Macaca fascicularis*) were exposed by Lewis et al. (1986) to coal dust and/or diesel exhaust particles for 7 h per day on five days per week for 24 months, as described on p. 90. Following the exposure period, all survivors (59/60) were necropsied and examined histologically. No significant difference in tumour incidence was reported among the four groups. [The Working Group noted the short duration and inadequate reporting of the study.]

*(b) Intratracheal or intrapulmonary administration*

*Rat*: Four groups of 31, 59, 27 and 53 female specific-pathogen-free Fischer 344 rats, six weeks of age, received ten weekly intrapulmonary instillations of 1 mg/animal activated carbon or 1 mg/animal diesel exhaust particles [source unspecified] in phosphate buffer with 0.05% Tween 80, 2 ml of buffer alone or were untreated (Kawabata et al., 1986). Rats surviving 18 months constituted the effective numbers. The experiment was terminated 30 months after instillation. The survival rate was 71–83%, with the lowest value in the diesel particle-treated group. The numbers of animals with malignant lung tumours [histological type unspecified] were significantly higher ($p < 0.01$) in the groups treated with activated carbon (7/23) and with diesel particles (20/42) than in untreated (0/44) or vehicle controls (1/23). Similarly, the numbers of animals with benign and malignant lung tumours were also significantly increased in the groups treated with activated carbon (11/23) and diesel particles (31/42). [The Working Group noted the high incidence of pulmonary tumours observed after treatment with activated carbon, a material which is normally considered to be inert.]

Groups of 35 female inbred Osborne-Mendel rats, three months old, received lung implants of organic material from a diesel exhaust or a reconstituted hydrophobic fraction (Grimmer et al., 1987). The organic material was collected from a 3-l diesel passenger car engine, operated under the first cycle of the European test cycle (see p. 80), and was separated by liquid-liquid distribution into a hydrophilic fraction (approximately 25% by weight of the total condensate) and a hydrophobic fraction (approximately 75% by weight). The hydrophobic fraction was separated by column chromatography into several further fractions: (i) nonaromatic compounds plus PAHs with two and three rings (72% by weight of the total condensate), (ii) PAHs with four or more rings (0.8% by weight), (iii) polar PAHs (1.1% by weight) and (iv) nitro-PAHs (0.7% by weight). Animals received 6.7 mg hydrophilic fraction, 20 mg hydrophobic fraction, 19.2, 0.2, 0.3 or 0.2 mg of the four hydrophobic fractions, respectively, or 19.9 mg of reconstituted hydrophobic fraction. Two groups of 35 animals were untreated or received implants of the vehicle (beeswax:trioctanoin, 1:1) only. All animals were observed until spontaneous death (mean survival time, 24–140 weeks). Six lung tumours (squamous-cell carcinomas) were found in animals treated with the hydrophobic subfraction containing PAHs with four to seven rings. Similar carcinogenic potency was seen with the reconstituted hydrophobic subfractions (seven carcinomas) and with the hydrophobic fraction (five carcinomas). A low carcinogenic potential was observed with the subfraction of nitro-PAHs (one carcinoma); the polar PAH produced no tumour; and one bronchiolar-alveolar adenoma was observed in animals treated with the nonaromatic subfraction with two- and three-ring PAHs. One adenoma of the lung occurred in the vehicle control group.

*Hamster*: Shefner *et al.* (1982) gave groups of 50 male Syrian golden hamsters, 12–13 weeks of age, intratracheal instillations once a week for 15 weeks of 1.25, 2.5 or 5 mg diesel particles (obtained from US Environmental Protection Agency; 90% by mass <10 $\mu$m) or diesel particles plus the same amounts of ferric oxide in 0.2 ml propylene glycol/gelatine/-saline; or a dichloromethane extract of diesel particles plus ferric oxide in 0.2 ml propylene glycol/saline once a week for 15 weeks. Ten animals in each group were sacrificed at 12 months. At the time of reporting (61 weeks), one lung adenoma had been found in the group receiving the high dose of diesel particles and one in the group receiving the high dose of diesel particle extract plus ferric oxide. No lung tumour was reported in various untreated or solvent-treated controls. [The Working Group noted the short observation period and the preliminary reporting of the experiment.]

Three groups of 62 male Syrian golden hamsters, eight weeks of age, were given intratracheal instillations of 0.1 ml of a suspension of 0.1, 0.5 or 1 mg of an exhaust extract in Tween 60:ethanol:phosphate buffer (1.5:2.5:30 v/v) from a heavy-duty diesel engine (V6 11-l) once a week for 15 weeks and observed for life (Kunitake *et al.*, 1986). A control group of 59 animals received instillations of the vehicle only and a positive control group of 62 animals received 0.5 mg benzo[*a*]pyrene weekly for 15 weeks. Survival rates were 95%, 92%, 71% and 98% in the three treated groups and the vehicle controls, respectively. No significant difference in the incidences of tumours of the lung, trachea or larynx was observed between untreated control and treated groups; respiratory tumours occurred in 88% benzo[*a*]pyrene-treated hamsters. [The Working Group noted that length of survival was not reported.]

(c) *Skin application*

*Mouse*: A group of 12 male and 40 female C57Bl mice [age unspecified] received skin applications of 0.5 ml of an acetone extract of particles collected from a diesel engine [unspecified] running at zero load during the warm-up phase; treatment was given three times a week for life (Kotin *et al.*, 1955). Groups of 50 male and 25 female strain A mice [age unspecified] received similar applications of an extract of particles derived from the warmed-up engine running at full load. Of the mice in the first group, 16 had died by ten weeks; 33 mice survived to the appearance of the first skin tumour (13 months), and two skin papillomas developed. Of the male strain A mice, eight survived to the appearance of the first skin tumour (16 months), and one papilloma and three squamous-cell carcinomas were observed. Of the female strain A mice, 20 survived to the appearance of the first skin tumour (13 months), and 17 skin tumours [unspecified] were observed between 13 and 17 months. Both experiments were terminated after 22–23 months. No skin tumour occurred in 69 C57Bl controls (37 alive after 13 months) or in 34 (24 female and 10 male) strain A controls.

In a study reported before completion (Depass et al., 1982), groups of 40 male C3H/HeJ mice [age unspecified] received skin applications of 0.25 ml of a 5 or 10% solution in acetone or 5, 10, 25 or 50% dichloromethane extracts of diesel particles collected from a [5.7-l] diesel engine; treatment was given three times per week for life. A positive control group received 0.2% benzo[a]pyrene in acetone, and a negative control group received acetone only. One squamous-cell carcinoma of the skin was observed in the group treated with the highest dose of dichloromethane extract after 714 days of treatment. All 38 mice receiving benzo[a]-pyrene developed skin tumours. [The Working Group noted the inadequate reporting of the study.]

In a series of promotion-initiation studies (Depass et al., 1982), groups of 40 male C3H/HeJ mice received a single initiating dose of 0.025 ml 1.5% benzo[a]pyrene in acetone, followed one week later by repeated applications of the 10% solution of diesel particles in acetone described above, 50% dichloromethane extract, 25% dichloromethane extract, acetone only or 0.015 µg phorbol 12-myristyl 13-acetate (TPA) five times per week for life. An additional group received no further treatment after the initiating dose of benzo[a]-pyrene. In initiation studies, a single initiating dose of 0.025 ml of the 10% solution of diesel particles in acetone, 50% dichloromethane extract, acetone or TPA was followed after one week by of 0.015 µg TPA three times per week. The concentration of TPA used in the initiation and promotion studies was changed after eight months to 1.5 µg. In the promotion study, one mouse receiving the 50% dichloromethane extract had a squamous-cell carcinoma and two mice receiving the 25% extract had one squamous-cell carcinoma and one papilloma. In the initiation study, three (two papillomas, one carcinoma), three (two papillomas, one fibrosarcoma), one (papilloma) and two (one carcinoma, one papilloma) tumours were observed in the groups that received diesel particles, dichloromethane extract, acetone and TPA, respectively. [The Working Group noted the preliminary reporting of the study.]

Nesnow et al. (1982a,b) gave skin applications to groups of 40 male and 40 female SENCAR mice, seven to nine weeks of age, of 0.1, 0.5, 1.0, 2 or 10 mg of dichloromethane extracts of particles obtained from the exhausts of five diesel engines, A, B, C, D and E (E being a heavy duty engine) in 0.2 ml acetone; the 10-mg dose was given in five daily doses. The benzo[a]pyrene content ranged from 1173 ng/mg in the exhaust from engine A to 2 ng/mg in that from engines B and E. One week later, all mice received 2 µg TPA in 0.2 ml acetone twice a week for 24–26 weeks. A control group was treated with TPA only. The sample from engine A produced a dose-related increase in the incidence of skin papillomas, with 5.5 and 5.7 papillomas/mouse, 31% of males and 36% of females at the highest dose having skin carcinomas. With samples from engines B, C and D, responses of 0.1–0.5 papilloma/mouse were observed compared to 0.05–0.08 papilloma/mouse in TPA controls. The sample from engine E produced a response similar to that in controls (0.05–0.2 papilloma/mouse).

Similar groups of 40 male and 40 female SENCAR mice received weekly skin applications of 0.1, 0.5, 1, 2 or 4 mg extracts of particles from the emissions of engines A, B and E for 50–52 weeks (Nesnow et al., 1982b, 1983). The high dose was given in two split doses. At that time, skin carcinomas had occurred in 3% of male and 5% of female mice given the 4-mg dose of the sample from engine A, in 3% of males given the 0.5-mg dose of the sample from engine B and in 3% of females given the 0.1-mg dose of the sample engine E. Doses of 12.6–202 µg per week benzo[a]pyrene produced skin carcinoma responses of 10–93%.

Groups of 50 female specific-pathogen-free ICR mice, aged eight to nine weeks, received skin applications of extracts of diesel particles collected from a V6 11-l heavy-duty displacement diesel engine in 0.1 ml acetone onto shaved back skin every other day for 20 days (total doses, 5, 15 or 45 mg/animal; Kunitake et al., 1986). A further group of 50 mice treated with acetone only served as controls. Beginning one week after the last diesel extract treatment, each animal received applications of 2.5 µg TPA in 0.1 ml acetone three times a week for 25 weeks, at which time they were autopsied. No skin 'cancer' was found in either treated or control groups; skin papillomas were seen in 1/48 and 4/50 surviving animals in the 15- and 45-mg dose groups, respectively [The Working Group noted the short duration of both the treatment and observation time.]

(d) *Subcutaneous administration*

*Mouse*: Groups of 15–30 female specific-pathogen-free C57Bl/6N mice, six weeks of age, received subcutaneous injections into the intrascapular region of suspensions in olive oil containing 5% dimethyl sulfoxide of 10, 25, 50, 100, 200 or 500 mg/kg bw of diesel particles collected from a V6 11-l heavy-duty displacement diesel engine; the treatment was given once a week for five weeks (Kunitake et al., 1986). A control group of 38 mice received injections of the vehicle only. Animals were killed 18 months after the beginning of the experiment. The first tumours were palpated in week 47 (a total dose of 25 mg/kg bw), week 30 (50 mg/kg bw), week 27 (100 mg/kg bw) and week 39 (200 and 500 mg/kg bw) in the five treated groups, respectively. A significant increase in the incidence of subcutaneous tumours, diagnosed as malignant fibrous histiocytomas, was observed only in 5/22 mice receiving the 500-mg/kg bw dose ($p < 0.05$) in comparison with controls (0/38). [The Working Group noted the high dose required to produce a carcinogenic effect.]

(e) *Administration with known carcinogens*

*Rat*: Two groups of female specific-pathogen-free Fischer 344 rats [initial number unspecified], five weeks of age, were exposed to diesel exhaust, as described on p. 89 or to clean air for 4 h per day on four days per week for 24 months (Takemoto et al., 1986). One month after the beginning of treatment, both groups received three weekly intraperitoneal injections of 1 g/kg bw *N*-nitrosodipropanolamine. Rats were killed at six, 12, 18 and 24 months after the start of treatment. A slight but nonsignificant increase in the incidences of lung adenomas and adenocarcinomas was observed in rats exposed to both exhaust and the nitrosamine compared to those exposed to the nitrosamine alone. After 12–24 months of observation, 16 lung tumours (12 adenomas and four carcinomas) were observed in 29 *N*-nitrosodipropanolamine-treated rats and 34 tumours (24 adenomas and 10 carcinomas) were observed in 36 rats exposed to both exhaust and *N*-nitrosodipropanolamine. The authors interpreted this result as an 'overadditive' effect on lung tumour incidence.

Heinrich *et al.* (1986a) gave groups of 48 female specific-pathogen-free Wistar rats, eight to ten weeks of age, 25 weekly subcutaneous injections of 250 or 500 mg/kg bw *N*-nitrosopentylamine during the first 25 weeks of exposure by inhalation to unfiltered diesel engine exhaust, to filtered diesel engine exhaust or to clean air, as described on p. 89. Significant increases in the incidences of squamous-cell carcinomas of the lung were observed in animals treated with the nitrosamine and exposed to total exhaust (22/47 low-dose nitrosamine; 15/48 high-dose nitrosamine compared to 2/46 and 8/48 clean air controls, respectively), although overall lung tumour rates were comparable in the groups exposed to the nitrosamine and to engine exhaust or clean air. The incidence of benign tumours (papillomas) of the upper respiratory tract was significantly reduced in nitrosamine-treated rats exposed to unfiltered or filtered diesel exhaust compared to controls exposed to nitrosamine and clean air.

*Hamster*: Heinrich *et al.* (1982) gave groups of 48–72 female Syrian golden hamsters, eight weeks old, weekly intratracheal instillations of 0.1 or 0.3 mg dibenzo[*a,h*]anthracene for 20 weeks or a single subcutaneous injection of 1.5 or 4.5 mg/kg bw *N*-nitrosodiethylamine (NDEA) and exposed them concomitantly by inhalation to unfiltered or filtered diesel exhaust or clean air, as described on p. 92. The incidence of tumours in the larynx/trachea was increased in animals treated with the higher dose of NDEA and exposed concomitantly to total exhaust (70.2%) or filtered exhaust (66%) as compared to controls (44.7%). The lower dose of NDEA and treatment with dibenzo[*a,h*]anthracene resulted in a lower incidence of these tumours. Only two lung tumours were found: one with the high dose of dibenzo[*a,h*]anthracene and filtered exhaust, the other with the low dose of NDEA and total exhaust.

Groups of 48 male and 48 female Syrian golden hamsters, eight to ten weeks of age, received a single subcutaneous injection of 4.5 mg/kg bw NDEA or 20 intratracheal instillations of 0.25 mg benzo[*a*]pyrene with concomitant exposure by inhalation to filtered or unfiltered diesel engine exhaust or to clean air, as described on p. 89 (Heinrich *et al.*, 1986a). Treatment with NDEA or benzo[*a*]pyrene produced respiratory tract tumour incidences of 10% or 2%, respectively, in animals exposed to clean air; rates were not significantly increased by concomitant exposure to filtered or unfiltered diesel engine exhaust.

Groups of 52 female and 52 male Syrian hamsters, six to eight weeks old, received a single subcutaneous injection of 4.5 mg/kg bw NDEA three days prior to exposure by inhalation to unfiltered or filtered diesel engine exhaust, as described on p. 91 (Brightwell *et al.*, 1986). The authors reported a nonsignificantly increased incidence of tracheal papillomas. [The Working Group noted that no information on tumour incidence was given.]

*Gasoline engine exhaust*

(a) *Inhalation exposure*

*Mouse*: Campbell (1936) exposed two groups of 37 male and 38 female mice [strain unspecified], three months old, by inhalation for 7 h per day on five days per week for about two years to one of two gasoline engine exhaust emissions: A was from a four-cylinder, 23-horse power, ordinary gasoline engine and B from a six-cylinder, 24-horse power engine run on gasoline with tetraethyllead 1:1800. Exposure was to a dilution of 1:145 in air for 4 h in the morning and to a dilution of 1:83 for 3 h in the afternoon. [The total particulate content of the exhaust and the lead concentration were not specified.] Of the animals exposed to exhaust emissions from car A, 9/75 had primary lung tumours compared to 8/74 controls; of those exposed to emissions from car B, primary lung tumours were seen in 12/75 animals compared to 6/70 controls. [Survival data not given.] Other types of tumours observed included mammary tumours and skin cancers among both treated groups and controls. [The Working Group noted the inadequate reporting of the study.]

Two groups of female ICR mice [initial numbers and age unspecified] were either exposed by inhalation to 0.1 mg/m$^3$ gasoline exhaust (1:250 dilution of emission from a small gasoline engine; carbon monoxide, 300 ± 50 ppm (350 ± 60 mg/m$^3$); nitric oxide, 0.21 ppm (0.3 mg/m$^3$); nitrogen dioxide, 0.08 ppm (0.16 mg/m$^3$) [total particulate concentration unspecified]) for 2 h per day on three days per week for six to 12 months, or were administered urethane (0.01%) in the drinking-water until sacrifice (Yoshimura, 1983). No untreated control group was included. Lung adenomas were found in 2/19 exposed mice killed between seven and 12 months; the incidence of tumours (adenomas and adenocarcinomas) in the urethane-treated group was 21/25. [The Working Group noted the short period of treatment, the short observation time and the absence of a control group.]

*Rat*: Groups of 72 male and 72 female Fischer 344 rats, six to eight weeks old, were exposed to one of three dilutions of gasoline engine exhaust from a 1.6-l displacement engine operated according to the US-72 (FTP) driving cycle; exposure was for 16 h per day on five days per week for two years (Brightwell *et al.*, 1986). Further groups were exposed to exhaust from a gasoline engine fitted with a three-way catalytic converter. The exhaust was diluted by a constant volume of 800 m$^3$ air or at further dilutions of 1:3 or 1:9 of this mixture in air; the particulate concentration was less than the detection limit of 0.2 mg/m$^3$. The concentration of nitrogen oxides in the high dose of exhaust from the engine without a converter was 49 ± 5 ppm and that of carbon monoxide was 224 ± 32 ppm (260 ± 36 mg/m$^3$). Two control groups of 144 rats of each sex were exposed to conditioned air. After the exposure period, animals were maintained for a further six months in clean air. No increase in lung tumour incidence was reported among rats exposed to gasoline engine exhaust as compared with controls. [The Working Group noted the inadequate reporting of the study.]

Three groups of 80–83 female Bor:WISW rats, ten to 12 weeks old, were exposed by inhalation to 1:61 or 1:27 dilutions with clean air of leaded gasoline engine exhaust generated by a 1.6-l engine operated according to the US-72 (FTP) driving cycle or to clean air (Heinrich *et al.*, 1986c). The lead content of the fuel was 0.3–0.56 g/l. Mean concentrations of exhaust components measured in the inhalation chambers were (high [low]): carbon monoxide, $350 \pm 24$ [$177.5 \pm 12.5$] mg/m$^3$; nitric oxide, $28 \pm 3$ [$13.7 \pm 1.5$] mg/m$^3$; nitrogen dioxide, $1.9 \pm 0.4$ [$1.0 \pm 0.2$] mg/m$^3$; particles, $95.8 \pm 16.5$ [$47.9 \pm 20.2$] 25g/m$^3$. About 35% of the particulate mass was lead. Exposure was for 18–19 h per day on five days per week for two years, followed by a maximal observation period of six months in clean air. Mean survival time of exposed and control animals was 105 weeks. Exposure to either concentration (1:61 or 1:27) of gasoline exhaust did not produce a significant increase in lung tumour incidence: 1/83 exposed to 1:61 had a squamous-cell carcinoma and 3/78 exposed to 1:27 had two squamous-cell carcinomas and one adenoma; 1/78 controls had an adenoma. In addition, one animal in each of the three exposure groups showed a tumour in the nasal cavities. [The Working Group noted that the nonlead particulate concentration was less than 1/20 the lowest level of particulates that produced an excess of lung tumours in the studies of diesel exhaust. The highest levels of gasoline engine exhaust that can be tested are limited by the toxicity of carbon monoxide.]

*Hamster*: Three groups of 80–83 female Syrian golden hamsters, ten to 12 weeks old, were exposed to gasoline engine exhaust, as described above but without the six-month observation period (Heinrich *et al.*, 1986c). Median survival in treated and control groups was 70 weeks. One of 75 animals exposed to the high concentration of exhaust (1:27) and three of 80 exposed to the low concentration (1:61) had a tumour of the respiratory tract. No respiratory tract tumour occurred in the 83 controls. [The Working Group noted that the nonlead particulate concentration was less than 1/20 the lowest level of particulates that produced an excess of lung tumours in the studies of diesel exhaust. The highest levels of gasoline engine exhaust that can be tested are limited by the toxicity of carbon monoxide.]

Brightwell *et al.* (1986) exposed groups of 52 male and 52 female Syrian hamsters, six to eight weeks of age, to gasoline engine exhaust, as described on p. 98. Two control groups of 104 hamsters of each sex were exposed to conditioned air only. The authors reported that respiratory tract tumours in treated hamsters were rare and not related to treatment. [The Working Group noted the inadequate reporting of the data.]

*Dog*: Stara *et al.* (1980) exposed seven groups of 12 female beagle dogs, four months of age, to exhaust from a six-cylinder, 2.4-l gasoline engine run on leaded fuel and operated to simulate urban driving, and to specific pollutants found in gasoline engine exhaust (dilution, 1:570 in air). The groups were exposed to nonirradiated exhaust, to exhaust irradiated with ultra-violet, to sulfur dioxide and sulfuric acid, to nonirradiated exhaust plus sulfur dioxide and sulfuric acid, to exhaust irradiated with ultra-violet plus sulfur dioxide and sulfuric acid, to nitrogen oxides with high nitrogen dioxide and to nitrogen oxides with high nitric oxide. A group of 20 dogs was exposed to clean air. The exhaust contained 100 ppm (115 mg/m$^3$) carbon monoxide and 24–30 ppm hydrocarbon expressed as methane. The irradiated exhaust contained 0.5–1.0 ppm (1–2 mg/m$^3$) nitrogen dioxide, 0.1 ppm (0.12 mg/m$^3$) nitric oxide and 0.2–0.4 ppm oxygen expressed as $O_3$. The concentration of lead measured in the different exposure atmospheres was 14—26 µg/m³. The dogs were exposed for 16 h per day for 68 months and then held in clean air for 29—36 months. Complete necropsies were performed on 85 dogs. No lung tumour was observed in the 40 exposed or 17 control dogs. [The Working Group noted that the concentrations of particles in the exposure atmospheres were not given.]

*(b) Intratracheal or intrapulmonary administration*

*Rat*: Groups of 34—35 inbred female Osborne-Mendel rats, three months old, received a single implantation of 5.0 or 10.0 mg/animal of gasoline engine exhaust condensate, 4.36, 8.73 or 17.45 mg/animal of a PAH-free fraction, 0.50, 0.99 or 1.98 mg/animal of a fraction of PAHs with two to three rings, 0.14, 0.28 or 0.56 mg/animal of a fraction of PAHs with more than three rings, or 0.03, 0.10 or 0.30 mg benzo[*a*]pyrene in beeswax:trioctanoin (1:1) into the left lobe of the lung and were observed until natural death (Grimmer *et al.*, 1984). The exhaust was produced by a 1.5-l passenger car engine operated on the European test cycle. One control group of 34 rats received an injection of the vehicle only, and another control group of 35 animals remained untreated. At death, animals were autopsied and lungs were examined histopathologically. Mean survival times in the treated groups and controls were similar, ranging from 80—111 weeks. Only the fraction containing PAHs with more than three rings produced lung tumour (carcinomas and sarcomas) incidences comparable to those induced by total exhaust condensate (4/35, 17/34 and 24/35 *versus* 7/35 and 20/35). No lung tumour was observed in the untreated or vehicle controls. A dose-response relationship was obtained with the total condensate and with the fraction of PAHs with more than three rings.

*Hamster*: In an experiment by Mohr *et al.* (1976) and Reznik-Schüller and Mohr (1977), two groups of six male Syrian golden hamsters, 12 weeks old, each received intratracheal instillations of 2.5 or 5 mg gasoline exhaust condensate, prepared from emissions of a common German passenger car operating according to the European test cycle and containing 340 µg/g benzo[*a*]pyrene, in Tris-HCl and EDTA solution. Treatment was every two weeks for life. Moribund animals were killed and their lungs examined histologically for tumours. A further group of six animals was treated with solvent only and were sacrificed after the last exhaust condensate-treated animal had died. Survival times ranged from 30—60 weeks, during which time animals had received 15—30 instillations of condensate. All condensate-treated animals developed pulmonary adenomas.

Groups of 30 male Syrian golden hamsters, 16 weeks of age, received intratracheal instillations of 0.2 ml of a gasoline exhaust condensate from a 1.5-l engine, its fractions, including the methanol phase, the cyclohexane phase II and the nitromethane phase, a reconstitution product of these fractions, a synthetic mixture of pure carcinogenic PAHs or 40 µg benzo[*a*]pyrene in Tris-buffer/saline; treatment was every two weeks until natural death (Künstler, 1983). One group of 30 untreated animals and one group of 30 solvent-treated animals served as controls. Tracheas and lungs of all hamsters were examined histologically by light microscopy. Survival time was 68—87 weeks. No lung tumour was found in animals treated with the condensate or its fractions. In the benzo[*a*]pyrene-treated group, one mucoepidermoidal carcinoma of the respiratory tract and one lung adenoma were found; one animal treated with cyclohexane phase II (0.13 mg/animal; 10.7 μg benzo[a]pyrene equivalents) had a lung adenoma.

(c) *Skin application*

*Mouse*: A group of 108 C57Bl mice [age and sex unspecified] received skin applications of a concentrated benzene extract of particles from a V8 gasoline engine [procedures unspecified] (Kotin *et al.*, 1954). Among 86 mice surviving at the appearance of the first skin tumour (390 days), 38 developed 68 skin tumours, including 22 skin carcinomas. Among 69 benzene-treated controls, 42 survived to the time of appearance of the first skin tumour in treated mice; no skin tumour was reported.

Wynder and Hoffmann (1962) gave groups of 50 female Swiss (Millerton) mice, six weeks of age, skin applications of 5, 10, 25, 33 or 50% solutions in acetone of the 'tar' from a V8 gasoline engine (Hoffmann & Wynder, 1962b) exhaust extracted with benzene. Treatment was given three times a week for 15 months; the mice were observed for a further three months, at which time they were killed. Thirty mice painted with acetone served as controls. The numbers of mice with skin papillomas at 18 months were 0, 4, 50, 60 and 60% in the control, 5, 10, 25 and 33% dose groups, respectively; the corresponding incidences of skin carcinomas were 0, 4, 32, 48 and 54, respectively. In the high-dose group, all mice had died by ten months; 70% had skin papillomas and 4% had skin carcinomas.

In similar studies by Hoffmann *et al.* (1965), the incidence of skin papillomas and carcinomas was higher in 20 Swiss ICR mice treated with extracts of exhaust from a V8 engine that used approximately 1 l of engine oil/200 miles (0.3 l/100 km) than in those treated with exhausts from an engine that used approximately 1 l of oil/1600 miles (0.04 l/100 km).

Brune *et al.* (1978) gave groups of 50 or 80 female random-bred CFLP mice, approximately 12 weeks of age, skin applications of an exhaust condensate produced from a 1.5-l gasoline engine during a European test cycle, fractions of this condensate or benzo[a]pyrene in 0.1 ml dimethyl sulfoxide:acetone (3:1) twice a week for life. The groups treated with the total condensate received doses of 0.526, 1.579 or 4.737 mg/animal (0.15, 0.45 or 1.35 μg/animal benzo[a]pyrene equivalents) per treatment; the two groups treated with the methanol phase (66% of the total condensate) received doses of 1.389 or 4.168 mg/animal (0.60 or 1.80 μg/animal benzo[a]pyrene equivalents); those treated with the cyclohexane phases I and II (34% and 17% of the total condensate), the nitromethane phase (17% of the total condensate) and a reconstitution of the fractions received 0.30 and 0.90 μg/animal benzo[a]pyrene equivalents. Three further groups of 50 mice received applications of 1.92, 3.84 or 7.68 μg/animal benzo[a]pyrene. One control group received applications of the vehicle alone and another remained untreated. Animals with advanced malignant tumours were killed; all other animals were observed until natural death. Statistical analysis of the results revealed a linear relationship between the percentage of animals with local tumours (squamous-cell papillomas or carcinomas) and dose for the nitromethane phase (16.4 and 68.9%), the cyclohexane phase I (13.7 and 68.8%), the reconstitution (7.9 and 54.7%) and the total condensate (3.9, 35.1 and 76.9%). Local tumour rates in mice treated with total condensate were significantly higher than those in mice treated with benzo[a]pyrene (19.5, 15.2 and 60%) or the PAH-free fractions (methanol phase (2.6 and 5.9%) and cyclohexane phase II (2.8 and 1.5%)), which did not differ significantly from controls (1.3 and 0%). A second experiment by the same group using 40 mice per group gave similar results; however, local tumour incidences were significantly higher in the first experiment, probably due to minor differences in experimental techniques.

Grimmer *et al.* (1983a) gave groups of 65 or 80 female CFLP mice, seven weeks old, dermal applications of extracts of an exhaust condensate from a 1.5-l gasoline engine run on the European test cycle, its fractions or benzo[a]pyrene in 0.1 ml dimethyl sulfoxide:acetone (1:3) solvent; treatment was given twice a week for 104 weeks. Doses administered were: total condensate — 0.292, 0.875 or 2.626 mg/animal (0.12, 0.36 or 1.09 $\mu$g/animal benzo[a]pyrene equivalents); benzo[a]pyrene, 0.0039, 0.0077 or 0.0154 mg/animal; the methanol phase (PAH-free fraction), 0.97 or 2.9 mg/animal (0.48 or 1.45 $\mu$g/animal benzo[a]pyrene equivalents); the PAH-fraction containing PAHs with two and three rings, 0.152 or 0.455 mg/animal (0.46 or 1.39 $\mu$g/animal benzo[a]pyrene equivalents); the PAH-fraction containing PAHs with more than three rings, 0.02 or 0.06 mg/animal (0.24 or 0.73 $\mu$g/animal benzo[a]pyrene equivalents); and a mixture of 15 PAHs in a ratio corresponding to that of the automobile exhaust, 0.003 or 0.009 mg/animal (0.24 or 0.73 $\mu$g/animal benzo[a]pyrene equivalents). One group treated with 0.1 ml of the solvent only and one untreated group served as controls. Animals with advanced tumours were killed; the remaining animals were observed until natural death. The PAH-free fraction (methanol phase) and the fraction of PAHs with two or three rings produced low rates of skin tumours (carcinomas and papillomas): 11 [13.9%] and one [1.3%] animals with local tumours, respectively, in the high-dose groups. Clear dose-response relationships were demonstrated for tumour incidence in the groups treated with total condensate (six [7.7%], 34 [44.3%] and 65 [83.3%]), in those given the fraction containing PAHs with more than three rings (seven [8.9%] and 50 [63.5%]), in those given the mixture of 15 PAHs (one [1.3%] and 29 [38.7%]) and in benzo[a]pyrene-treated animals (22 [34.4%], 39 [60.9%] and 56 [89.1%]). No local skin tumour was seen in controls. Similar results were obtained by Grimmer *et al.* (1983b).

Groups of 40 male and 40 female SENCAR mice, seven to nine weeks of age, received single skin applications in 0.2 ml acetone of 0.1, 0.5, 1, 2 or 3 mg of dichloromethane extracts of particulates collected from the emission of an unleaded gasoline engine (of a 1977 model passenger car [engine volume unspecified]) with a catalytic converter (Nesnow *et al.*, 1982a). One week later, all mice received 2 $\mu$g TPA in 0.2 ml acetone twice weekly for 24–26 weeks. At that time, the percentages of mice with papillomas and the numbers of papillomas/mouse in TPA-treated controls were 8% and 0.08 in males and 5% and 0.05 in females, respectively. In the groups treated with both TPA and the gasoline extract, the respective percentages and numbers were: males — 5% and 0.05 (0.1 mg), 13% and 0.15 (0.5 mg), 18% and 0.18 (1 mg), 22% and 0.24 (2 mg) and 18% and 0.24 (3 mg); females — 13% and 0.23 (0.1 mg), 18% and 0.24 (0.5 mg), 10% and 0.13 (1 mg), 21% and 0.23 (2 mg) and 23% and 0.28 (3 mg).

(d) *Subcutaneous administration*

*Mouse*: Groups of 87 or 88 female NMRI mice [age unspecified] received a single subcutaneous injection in 0.5 ml tricaprylin of 20 or 60 mg exhaust condensate from a gasoline engine [unspecified] (Pott *et al.*, 1977). A third group of 45 mice was injected three times with 60 mg condensate containing 0.163 $\mu$g/mg benzo[a]pyrene. A group of 89 mice that received 0.5 ml tricaprylin alone and a further group of 87 untreated mice served as controls. Animals that developed tumours up to 10 mm in diameter at the application site were killed. The mean survival time in the low- and medium-dose groups was in the range of that of the control groups (80–88 weeks), but was 57 weeks in the high-dose group. The numbers of animals with sarcomas at the injection site were 10/87 (11.5%), 6/88 (6.8%) and 5/45 (11.1%) in the condensate-treated groups and 3.4% in the tricaprylin-treated group.

(e) *Administration with known carcinogens*

*Mouse*: Groups of 60 female NMRI mice, eight to ten weeks old, received ten intratracheal instillations of 100 $\mu$g benzo[a]pyrene, 20 intratracheal instillations of 50 $\mu$g benzo[a]pyrene or ten intratracheal instillations of 50 $\mu$g dibenzo[a,h]anthracene, with concomitant exposure to gasoline engine exhaust, as described on p. 99, for 53 weeks only and were observed for a further 40 weeks (Heinrich *et al.*, 1986c). Administration of benzo[a]pyrene or dibenzo[a,h]anthracene with clean air induced a high basic lung tumour rate of 70–90% (adenomas and adenocarcinomas). Mean survival times (75–85 weeks) of exhaust-exposed animals were clearly shorter, with the exception of the groups treated ten times with 100 $\mu$g benzo[a]pyrene, in which gasoline exhaust exposure induced a higher incidence of adenocarcinomas (22/38 and 28/40 in the 1:27 and 1:61 dilution groups) but a significantly reduced incidence of adenomas (4/38 and 3/40) compared to clean air controls (20/42 adenocarcinomas, 16/42 adenomas). The total numbers of tumour-bearing animals in clean air and exhaust-exposed groups were not, however, significantly different. In the groups exposed 20 times to 50 $\mu$g benzo[a]pyrene, adenocarcinoma induction by the exhaust was inhibited significantly (3/35, 5/36, 15/42 in the 1:27, 1:61 and control groups, respectively). Additional groups of 61–83 newborn NMRI mice received a single subcutaneous injection of 4 $\mu$g (females and males) or 10 $\mu$g (females only) dibenzo[a,h]anthracene followed by inhalation exposure to one of the two dilutions of gasoline exhaust for six months, after which they were killed; the number of lung tumours per animal was not significantly different from that in controls exposed simultaneously to clean air.

Groups of 86–90 female NMRI mice [age unspecified] were injected subcutaneously with 10, 30 or 90 $\mu$g benzo[a]pyrene alone or together with 6.6 or 20 mg exhaust condensate from a gasoline engine [unspecified] (Pott *et al.*, 1977). The dose-response relationship for local sarcomas produced by benzo[a]pyrene (20%, 54%, 76%) was reduced significantly by the addition of both doses of the condensate. The difference was seen most clearly 30 weeks after treatment.

*Rat*: Two groups of female Sprague-Dawley rats [initial numbers unspecified] were either administered *N*-nitrosodiisopropanolamine in the drinking-water (0.01%) or were exposed concomitantly by inhalation for 2 h per day on three days per week to gasoline engine (generator EM300) exhaust diluted 1:250 in air for six to 12 months, at which time the animals were killed (Yoshimura, 1983). In animals killed between seven and 12 months, the number of lung tumours (11/37) in the combined treatment group (one adenoma and ten undifferentiated carcinomas, squamous-cell carcinomas, adenocarcinomas and mixed tumours) was significantly greater than that in the 24 nitrosamine controls (two carcinomas; $p < 0.05$).

Groups of 60 female Bor:WISW rats, ten to 12 weeks old, received 25 daily subcutaneous injections of 0.25 or 0.5 g/kg bw $N$-nitrosodipentylamine and were exposed to gasoline engine exhaust, as described on p. 99 (Heinrich *et al.*, 1986c). The treatments induced significant increases in the incidences of benign tumours of the whole respiratory tract (in 9/47 and 14/48 rats given the 1:27 and 1:61 dilutions of exhaust and receiving 0.5 g/kg bw nitrosamine, and in 15/50 and 14/45 rats given the 1:27 and 1:61 dilutions and receiving 0.25 g/kg bw nitrosamine, respectively) compared with clean air controls (5/48 and 4/46 rats), but decreases in the incidences of malignant tumours (33/47 and 34/48, respectively, compared to 43/48 controls; and 13/50 and 18/45 rats, compared to 29/46 in the groups receiving 0.5 and 0.25 g/kg bw nitrosamine). When lung tumour rates were evaluated separately, the incidences of malignant tumours (mostly squamous-cell carcinomas and adenocarcinomas) were also reduced in nitrosamine-treated rats by exposure to either concentration of exhaust (in 24/48, 25/49 and 40/49 rats in the 0.5 g/kg bw groups and in 11/54, 14/47 and 26/48 rats in the 0.25 g/kg bw groups exposed to 1:27 and 1:61 dilutions and clean air, respectively), whereas the incidence of benign tumours remained unchanged. Rats given the low dose of $N$-nitrosodipentylamine exposed to 1:61 or 1:27 dilutions of gasoline exhaust showed overall lung tumour rates of 15/47 and 13/54, respectively, *versus* 27/48 rats treated with nitrosamine but exposed to clean air. In animals given the high dose of $N$-nitrosodipentylamine, these rates were 33/49 and 28/48, respectively, *versus* 44/49 controls.

*Hamster*: Groups of 80–81 female Syrian golden hamsters, ten to 12 weeks old, received a single subcutaneous injection of 3 mg/kg bw $N$-nitrosodiethylamine (NDEA) or 20 intratracheal instillations of 0.25 mg benzo[*a*]pyrene and were exposed to gasoline engine exhaust, as described on p. 99 (Heinrich *et al.*, 1986c). Administration of NDEA or benzo[*a*]pyrene to hamsters exposed to clean air resulted in basic rates of benign respiratory tract tumours of 12.8 and 6.5% of animals, respectively; one malignant tumour of the paranasal cavity was also seen in the group exposed to benzo[*a*]pyrene. The basic tumour rate was not significantly increased by exposure to either dilution of exhaust. Tumour rates in NDEA- and benzo[*a*]pyrene-treated animals inhaling the 1:27 dilution of exhaust were approximately 50% lower than those in treated animals inhaling the 1:61 dilution or clean air.

Groups of 52 male and 52 female Syrian hamsters, six to eight weeks old, received a single subcutaneous injection of 4.5 mg/kg bw NDEA three days prior to exposure by inhalation to gasoline engine exhaust, as described on p. 98 (Brightwell *et al.*, 1986). The authors reported that NDEA-treated hamsters had a nonsignificantly increased incidence of tracheal papillomas. [The Working Group noted the inadequate reporting of the data.]

## 3.2 Other relevant data

(a) *Experimental systems*

(i) *Deposition, clearance, retention and metabolism*

Engine exhaust contains material in gaseous, vapour and particulate phases, and the absorption, distribution and excretion of individual constituents is influenced by the phase in which they occur and by the properties of each compound. After inhalation, highly soluble compounds in the gaseous phase, such as sulfur dioxide, are absorbed in the upper airways and do not penetrate significantly beyond the level of the bronchioles. Compounds that interact biochemically with the body are also retained in significant quantities; thus, processes such as binding of carbon monoxide to haemoglobin normally occur in the gas-exchange (pulmonary) region of the lung. Retention characteristics of materials not associated with the particulate phase are highly compound-specific. The factors affecting the uptake of a wide variety of vapours and gases have been summarized (Davies, 1985).

As described on p. 47, a proportion of a compound in the vapour phase condenses onto the particulate material produced in the engine exhaust. The association of a compound with the particulate phase modifies the deposition pattern and affects its lung retention; the lung burden of a compound following continuous exposure to that compound coated on particles may be many times that of continuous exposure to the compound alone (Bond *et al.*, 1986).

Deposition in the respiratory tract is a function of particle size. The median particle size in a variety of long-term exposure systems has been between 0.19 and 0.54 $\mu$m (Yu & Xu, 1986), representative of that in an urban environment (Cheng *et al.*, 1984). However, some of the carbonaceous mass in environmental samples results from airborne suspension of material collected in automobile exhaust pipes and is >5 $\mu$m in size (Chamberlain *et al.*, 1978); such particles are unlikely to be produced in a static exposure system. Dilution has little effect on the size distribution of particles used in long-term studies (0.3–7 mg/m$^3$; Cheng *et al.*, 1984), although rapid dilution (<1 sec) can lead to a smaller size (0.10–0.15 $\mu$m; Chan *et al.*, 1981). The presence of sulfates in the particulate phase (Lies *et al.*, 1986) may lead to enlargement of individual particles in the high humidity of the respiratory tract, thereby altering the deposition pattern (Pritchard, 1987).

### Diesel engine exhaust

*Deposition*: Studies of the deposition of diesel engine exhaust, representative of fresh urban exhaust, are summarized in Table 24; the particle sizes used were in the lower part of the range found in long-term exposure chambers. Deposition following nose-only exposure was measured by radiotracer technique. Data are quoted as a proportion of the amount of inhaled aerosol, which is based on estimates of ventilation rates. [The Working Group noted that the data on deposition of diesel particles in rats are in broad agreement with data for other particulate materials of similar size (Raab *et al.*, 1977; Wolff *et al.*, 1984).]

Table 24. Experimental deposition in the respiratory tract of diesel engine exhaust particles

| Species | Mass median particle diameter ($\mu$m) | % total deposition of inhaled exhaust particles | Reference |
|---|---|---|---|
| Rat | 0.1–0.15 | 15–17 | Chan et al. (1981) |
| Rat | 0.16–0.19 | 10–17 | Dutcher et al. (1984) |
| Rat | 0.12 | 17[a] (calculated) 20[a] (estimated) | Lee et al. (1983) |
| Guinea-pig | 0.12 | 20[a] (initial deposition) | Lee et al. (1983) |

[a]Mean values

A model for the deposition of diesel exhaust particles predicts that, as the median size increases from 0.08 to 0.30 $\mu$m, total deposition in rats falls from 25 to 15%, tracheobronchial deposition from 5 to 2% and pulmonary deposition from 12 to 5%; upper respiratory tract deposition remains constant at 8% (Yu & Xu, 1986). The model predicts that pulmonary deposition will vary only with (body weight)$^{-0.14}$, since diffusion is the predominant mechanism (Xu & Yu, 1987). [The Working Group noted that this model is in good agreement with the observed deposition of other particles (e.g., Raab et al., 1977; Wolff et al., 1981, 1984)].

Following exposure of rats for six, 12, 18 and 24 months to 0.4, 3.5 and 7.1 mg/m³ diesel exhaust particles, there was no significant effect of length of exposure or exposure concentration on the deposition of 0.1 $\mu$m gallium oxide particles (Wolff et al., 1987).

*Mucociliary clearance*: The clearance of particles from the lung following a single exposure to radiolabelled diesel particles is summarized in Table 25. The fast phase of clearance is conventionally assumed to be due to mucociliary action, the remainder (slow phase) to pulmonary clearance. The variation in the fraction of the lung deposit cleared by mucociliary action (i.e., the tracheobronchial deposit) is linked to particle size and hence deposition pattern. [The Working Group noted that Gutwein et al. (1974) give no information on particle size and that, without this, the high tracheobronchial deposit cannot be accounted for.]

In rats exposed for short periods (4–100 h) to diesel exhaust with particulate concentrations in the range 0.9–17 mg/m³, a dose-dependent reduction in mucociliary clearance occurred, although the effect was less marked on exposure to the gas phase alone (Battigelli et al., 1966). No such effect occurred in sheep exposed for 30 min to concentrations of 0.4–0.5 mg/m³ of resuspended diesel particles, i.e., in the absence of the gas phase (Abraham et al., 1980). Exposure-related differences in tracheal mucociliary clearance have also been reported over 1–12 weeks in rats exposed to 1 and 4.4 mg/m³ particulates in diesel exhaust. However, in another study, there was no effect on tracheal

Table 25. Clearance of diesel exhaust particles from rat lung following single exposures

| Fraction of lung deposit clearance (%) | | Half-time of slow phase (days) | Reference |
|---|---|---|---|
| Fast phase | Slow phase | | |
| 34 | 66 | 62 | Chan et al. (1981) |
| 6 | 35 | 6[a] | Lee et al. (1983) |
|  | 59 | 80[a] | |
| b | b | 77 | Chan et al. (1984) |
| 75 | 25 | b | Gutwein et al. (1974) |

[a]Three clearance phases are given: fast clearance with a half-time of one day (cf. Chan et al., 1981), a clearance phase with a half-time of six days and a slow phase with a half-time of 80 days.

[b]Data not available

mucociliary clearance of exposures of six to 24 months to particulate concentrations of 0.4–7.1 mg/m³ (Wolff et al., 1987). [The Working Group noted that there may be some impairment of mucociliary clearance, possibly caused by the gas phase of engine exhaust, but that its effect is of limited significance in the long term.]

*Pulmonary (alveolar) clearance*: The pulmonary clearance of diesel particles is very much slower than the mucociliary clearance (see Table 25). On the basis of these data, the lung burden of rats during protracted exposure should tend exponentially toward an equilibrium value at 12 months. In rats exposed to diesel exhaust with a particulate concentration of 0.3 mg/m³, there was evidence of equilibration after 12 months (only a 2.5-fold increase over 24 months); however, with exposures of 3.5 and 7.0 mg/m³, lung burdens increased steadily (five to 11 fold) over 24 months. This has been referred to as the 'overload' phenomenon (Wolff et al., 1987). The clearance rate of insoluble particles following prolonged exposure to diesel exhaust at a variety of concentrations and durations also indicates impaired long-term clearance (Wolff et al., 1984). Thus, it appears that the normal clearance mechanisms become seriously impaired, leading to very long-term retention of material in the lung, usually referred to as 'sequestration'.

Results of studies on particulate clearance in rats following repeated exposures to diesel exhaust are summarized in Table 26. Lung clearance was estimated either by exposure to a pulse of $^{14}$C-labelled diesel exhaust particles at the end of the cumulative exposure (Chan et al., 1984; Lee et al., 1987) or by measuring the lung burden of soot spectrophotometrically (Griffis et al., 1983). Also included are data on the clearance of a pulse of radiolabelled fused aluminosilicate particles following exposure to diesel exhaust for two years at particulate concentrations between 0.4 and 7.0 mg/m³ (Wolff et al., 1987). [The Working Group noted that pulse techniques measure only the clearance of the material that has most recently entered the lung. Since there is no difference between this and total soot measurements,

Table 26. Pulmonary clearance in rats of insoluble particles following exposure to diesel exhaust

| Exposure | | | Pulmonary clearance | | Reference |
|---|---|---|---|---|---|
| Concentration (mg/m$^3$) | Duration (weeks) | h per day × days/week | Material studied | Half-time (days) | |
| 0 | 0 | 0 | Diesel exhaust | 77 | Chan et al. (1984) |
| 0.25 | 7 | 20 × 7 | | 90 | |
| 0.25 | 16 | 20 × 7 | | 92 | |
| 6.00 | 1 | 20 × 7 | | 166 | |
| 6.00 | 9 | 20 × 7 | | 562 | |
| 6.00 | 16 | 20 × 7 | | [>1000] | |
| 0.15 | 18 | 7 × 5 | Diesel exhaust | 87 | Griffis et al. (1983) |
| 0.94 | 18 | 7 × 5 | | 99 | |
| 4.10 | 18 | 7 × 5 | | 165 | |
| 6.00 | 1 | 20 × 7 | Diesel exhaust | 61 | Lee et al. (1987) |
| 6.00 | 3 | 20 × 7 | | 124 | |
| 6.00 | 6 | 20 × 7 | | 192 | |
| 0 | 0 | 0 | FAP[a] | 79 | Wolff et al. (1987) |
| 0.35 | 104 | 7 × 5 | | 81 | |
| 3.50 | 104 | 7 × 5 | | 264 | |
| 7.00 | 104 | 7 × 5 | | 240 | |

[a]FAP, radiolabelled ($^{134}$Cs) fused aluminosilicate particles

deposition, and hence ventilation, must continue to occur in those areas where clearance is impaired, confirming the findings of Wolff et al. (1987) that deposition is unaffected by prolonged exposure to diesel exhaust.]

Pulmonary clearance as a function of contemporary lung burden has also been considered (McClellan, 1986). In an analysis of the published data, Wolff et al. (1986) concluded that in rats sequestration becomes a significant burden at a certain level [about 1 mg/lung] and is related to the rate of accumulation; i.e., short exposure to a high concentration produces an effect at a lower lung burden than more protracted exposure at a lower concentration. Thus, there is no strong relationship between the half-time of clearance and cumulative exposure.

[The relationship between half-times for pulmonary clearance of diesel exhaust particles and other insoluble particles in the rat following exposure to diesel exhaust and an 'exposure rate', calculated by the Working Group from cumulative exposure, mg/m$^3$ × weeks × (h/week)/168, is plotted in Figure 8. The Working Group noted that there is an effect on clearance at 'exposure rates' above 10 mg/m$^3$ × week (i.e., continuous exposure to 0.2 mg/m$^3$ or exposure for 40 h per week to 0.8 mg/m$^3$ for one year) and a strong suggestion that impaired clearance occurs over the whole range of 'exposure rates' studied.]

**Fig. 8. Pulmonary clearance in rats of diesel exhaust particles and other insoluble particles following exposure to diesel exhaust**

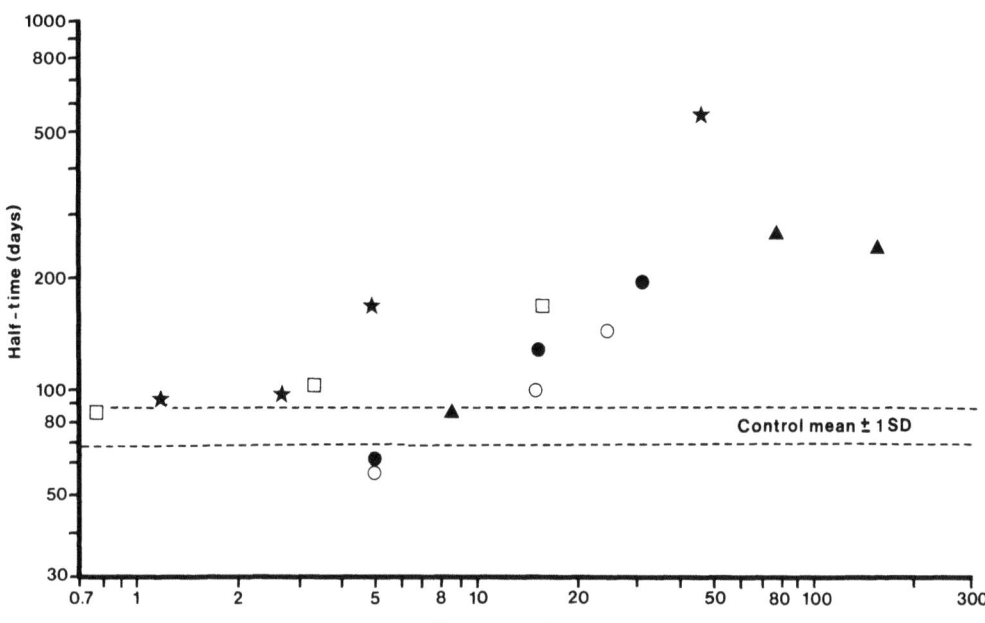

□, Griffis et al. (1983), spectrophotometric technique; ★, Chan et al. (1984), pulse technique; ●, Lee et al. (1987), pulse technique; ○, Lee et al. (1987), carbon black; ▲, Wolff et al. (1987), radiolabelled ($^{134}$Cs) fused aluminosilicate particles. Exposure rate = (mg × week/m³) × (h/week)/168

Studies in rats on the effect of exposure to diesel exhaust on the clearance of metal oxide particles containing a γ-emitting isotope are summarized in Table 27 (Bellmann et al., 1983; Heinrich et al., 1986a; Lewis et al., 1986; Wolff et al., 1987). The control animals cleared the metal oxide particles much faster than they did diesel particles or fused aluminosilicate particles (see Table 26; Wolff et al., 1987). [The Working Group noted that this suggests that clearance of metal oxides involves a significant soluble component.]

[The relationship between half-times for pulmonary clearance of metal oxide particles in rats following exposure to diesel exhaust and an 'exposure rate' calculated by the Working Group is plotted in Figure 9. The Working Group noted that impaired clearance of metal oxide particles does not become apparent until significantly higher values of 'exposure rate' than in the studies on diesel and fused aluminosilicate particles and considered that the differences in the results could be explained by continuing solubility masking an impairment in mechanical clearance, implying that sequestration is primarily a mechanical effect. For comparison, data for gasoline from Bellmann et al. (1983) have been added.]

After only two months' exposure of rats to a diesel exhaust particulate concentration of 2 mg/m³, clearance of metal oxide particles was significantly faster than in controls,

**Table 27. Pulmonary clearance in rats of metal oxide particles following exposure to diesel engine exhausts**

| Exposure | | | Pulmonary clearance | | Reference |
|---|---|---|---|---|---|
| Concentration (mg/m³) | Duration (weeks) | h/day × days/week | Material | Half-time (days) | |
| 0 | 0 | 0 | $^{59}Fe_2O_3$ | 50[a] | Bellmann et al. (1983) |
| 0 | 0 | 0 | | 47[b] | |
| 0 | 0 | 0 | | 43[c] | |
| 3.90 | 52 | 7 × 5 | | 127 | |
| 3.90 | 78 | 7 × 5 | | 92 | |
| 3.90 | 104 | 7 × 5 | | 54 | |
| 0 | 0 | 0 | $^{59}Fe_3O_4$ | 47 | Lewis et al. (1986) |
| 2 | 9 | 7 × 5 | | 37 | |
| 0 | 0 | 0 | $^{67}Ga_2O_3$ | 36[d] | Wolff et al. (1987) |
| 0 | 0 | 0 | | 48[a] | |
| 0 | 0 | 0 | | 47[b] | |
| 0 | 0 | 0 | | 36[c] | |
| 0.35 | 26 | 7 × 5 | | 53 | |
| 0.35 | 52 | 7 × 5 | | 36 | |
| 0.35 | 78 | 7 × 5 | | 72 | |
| 0.35 | 104 | 7 × 5 | | 40 | |
| 3.50 | 26 | 7 × 5 | | 37 | |
| 3.50 | 52 | 7 × 5 | | 60 | |
| 3.50 | 78 | 7 × 5 | | 82 | |
| 3.50 | 104 | 7 × 5 | | 79 | |
| 7.00 | 26 | 7 × 5 | | 151 | |
| 7.00 | 52 | 7 × 5 | | 121 | |
| 7.00 | 78 | 7 × 5 | | 84 | |
| 7.00 | 104 | 7 × 5 | | 121 | |
| 0 | 0 | 0 | $Fe_2O_3$ | 49[e] | Heinrich et al. (1986a) |
| 4 | 13 | 19 × 5 | | 170 | |
| 4 | 35 | 19 × 5 | | 170 | |
| 4 | 52 | 19 × 5 | | 95 | |
| 4 | 82 | 19 × 5 | | 125 | |

[a]Control animals (17 weeks of age at start) after 26 weeks

[b]Control animals after 52 weeks

[c]Control animals after 78 weeks

[d]Control animals after 164 weeks

[e]Average of controls aged 26–104 weeks

**Fig. 9. Pulmonary clearance of metal oxide particles in rats following exposure to engine exhaust**

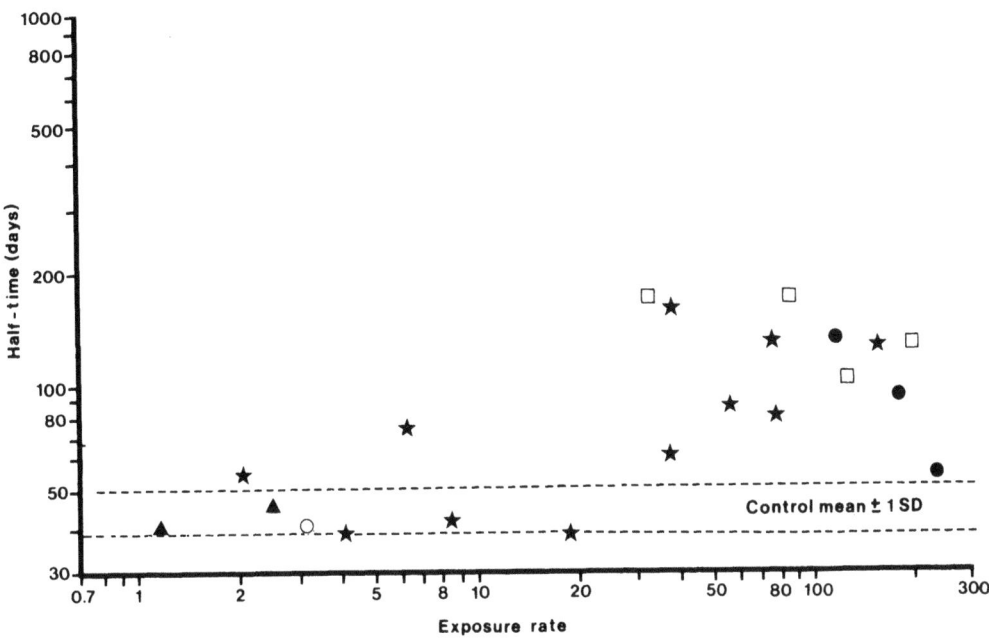

□, Heinrich et al. (1986a), diesel exhaust; ★, Wolff et al. (1987), diesel exhaust; ●, Bellmann et al (1983), diesel exhaust; o, Lewis et al. (1986), diesel exhaust; Δ, Bellmann et al. (1983), gasoline exhaust. Exposure rate = (mg × week/m³) × (h/week)/168

suggesting a stimulated lung response; no such effect was observed subsequently (Oberdoerster et al., 1984; Lewis et al., 1986). [The Working Group noted that overloading had probably occurred.]

The rate of clearance of ferric oxide in hamsters was slightly lower (75 ± 40 days) following one year's exposure to diesel exhaust particles (4 mg/m³) than that in clean-air controls (55 ± 17 days; Heinrich et al., 1986a). In another study, only 10% clearance of ¹⁴C-labelled diesel particles was observed 400 days after a single exposure of guinea-pigs (Lee et al., 1983). Six months after a three-month exposure of mice, rats and hamsters to diesel exhaust (particles, 1.5 mg/m³), the mice appeared to have a slower clearance than rats and hamsters (Kaplan et al., 1982).

The gas phase alone appears to have no effect on pulmonary clearance in rats or hamsters (Heinrich et al., 1986a). Clearance of diesel particles following prolonged exposure to a carbon black aerosol of similar size showed a pattern of impairment similar to that observed after diesel exposure (see Fig. 8), strongly suggesting that dust overloading *per se* impairs mechanical clearance (Lee et al., 1987). [The Working Group noted that the half-time lung clearance of carbon black is shorter than that of diesel exhaust at similar 'exposure rates'. This may reflect a local effect of diesel particles on the alveolar macrophages which mediate mechanical clearance; diesel particles depress the phagocytic capacity of macrophages, whereas coal dust activates them (see below and Castranova *et al.*, 1985).]

The majority of the particles that are cleared by macrophages from the pulmonary region leave *via* the ciliated epithelium and are excreted *via* the gut. However, a proportion penetrate the lymphatic system, borne by macrophages, and are filtered by the lymph nodes to form aggregates of particles (Vostal *et al.*, 1981). It has been estimated that one-third of clearance occurred *via* this route during the first 28 days after exposure of rats to diesel exhaust (Chan *et al.*, 1981). [The Working Group noted that there is no information on how this proportion changes with time or with prolonged exposure.]

*Retention*: The retention of the organic compounds associated with exhaust particles has been reviewed (McClellan *et al.*, 1982; Vostal *et al.*, 1982; Holmberg & Ahlborg, 1983; Vostal, 1983; Wolff *et al.*, 1986). Organic compounds adsorbed on exhaust particles can be extracted by biological fluids, as has been observed in assays for mutagenesis (Claxton, 1983; Lewtas & Williams, 1986; see p. 121). The half-time of the slow phase of lung clearance for $^{14}$C derived from labelled diesel exhaust was 25 days in rats (Sun & McClellan, 1984), and that for $^{3}$H-benzo[*a*]pyrene coated on diesel particles was 18 days (Sun *et al.*, 1984). The retention of 1-nitropyrene adsorbed onto diesel exhaust particles is described in the monograph on that compound.

No data were available on changes in the retention of individual compounds after prolonged exposure to diesel exhaust.

*Metabolism*: The metabolism of several components of engine exhausts has been reported previously: some polycyclic aromatic hydrocarbons (IARC, 1983), formaldehyde (IARC, 1982a), lead (IARC, 1980), nitroarenes (IARC, 1984) and benzene (IARC, 1982b). The metabolism of 1-nitropyrene associated with diesel exhaust particles is described in the monograph on that compound.

The metabolism of benzo[*a*]pyrene coated on diesel exhaust particles has been studied in different experimental systems. Fischer 344 rats were exposed for 30 min by nose-only inhalation to $^{3}$H-benzo[*a*]pyrene adsorbed onto diesel engine exhaust particles. The majority (65–76%) of the radioactivity retained in the lungs (as determined by high-performance liquid chromatography) 30 min and 20 days after exposure was associated with benzo[*a*]pyrene. Smaller amounts of benzo[*a*]pyrene-phenols (13–18%) and benzo[*a*]-pyrene-quinones (5–18%) were also detected. No other metabolite was found (Sun *et al.*, 1984).

The pulmonary macrophages of dogs metabolized 1 $\mu$M $^{14}$C-benzo[*a*]pyrene, either in solution or coated on diesel particles, into benzo[*a*]pyrene-7,8-, -4,5- and -9,10-dihydrodiols (major metabolites) as well as into benzo[*a*]pyrene-phenols and benzo[*a*]pyrene-quinones (minor metabolites). The total quantity of metabolites did not differ when macrophages were incubated with either benzo[*a*]pyrene in solution or benzo[*a*]pyrene coated on diesel particles (Bond *et al.*, 1984).

Fischer 344 rats were exposed to diesel engine exhaust (7.1 mg/m³ particles) for about 31 months. After sacrifice, DNA was extracted from the right lung lobe and analysed for adducts by $^{32}$P-postlabelling: more DNA adducts were found in the exhaust-exposed group than in the unexposed group (Wong et al., 1986).

Fischer 344 rats and Syrian golden hamsters were exposed to different dilutions of diesel engine exhaust for six months to two years, when blood samples were analysed for levels of haemoglobin adducts (2-hydroxyethylvaline and 2-hydroxypropylvaline) by gas chromatography-mass spectrometry. A dose-dependent increase in the level of haemoglobin adducts was found, corresponding to the metabolic conversion of about 5–10% of inhaled ethylene and propylene to ethylene oxide and propylene oxide, respectively (Törnqvist et al., 1988).

### Gasoline engine exhaust

*Deposition*: In a study on the deposition of particles from inhaled gasoline exhausts (mass median diameter, 0.5 µm) in rats, mean total deposition of particles was 30.5%. Most deposition occurred in the alveolar region and in the nasal passages (Morgan & Holmes, 1978). In this study, the concentration of carbon monoxide in the gasoline exhaust was reduced before inhalation, and the particles were larger than those of the diesel exhausts reported. [The Working Group noted that the greater deposition of gasoline exhaust particles is consistent with the larger size of the particles and does not imply any fundamental difference in deposition between diesel and gasoline exhausts particles.]

*Clearance*: The results of a study on pulmonary clearance of ferric oxide by rats and hamsters following exposure to gasoline engine particles (0.04 and 0.09 mg/m³) for two years are summarized in Table 28 (Bellmann et al., 1983). Clearance was similar to that in controls and in animals exposed to diesel exhaust (see Table 27). [The Working Group noted that, on the basis of the data concerning exposure to diesel exhaust, clearance of metal oxide particles would not be impaired by exposures to such low concentrations.]

Table 28. Pulmonary clearance by rats and hamsters of ferric oxide particles following exposure to gasoline engine exhausts[a]

| Exposure | | | Pulmonary clearance (half-time in days) | |
|---|---|---|---|---|
| Concentration (mg/m³) | Duration (months) | h/day × days/week | Rats | Hamsters |
| 0 | 0 | 0 | 34 | 86 |
| 0.04 | 12 | 19 × 5 | 39 | 64 |
| 0.09 | (US–72 cycle) | 19 × 5 | 44 | 86 |

[a]From Bellmann et al. (1983)

*Metabolism*: As reported in an abstract, crude extracts of gasoline exhaust were applied topically to male BALB/c mice over a period of one to two weeks and DNA was isolated from the treated skin for analysis by $^{32}$P-postlabelling. The major DNA adduct derived from benzo[*a*]pyrene-7,8-dihydrodiol-9,10-epoxide was found in exposed mice (Randerath *et al.*, 1985).

Fischer 344 rats and Syrian golden hamsters were exposed to different dilutions of gasoline engine exhaust for six months to two years, and blood samples were analysed for levels of 2-hydroxyethylvaline and 2-hydroxypropylvaline in haemoglobin by gas chromatography-mass spectrometry. A dose-dependent increase in the level of haemoglobin adducts was found, corresponding to the metabolic conversion of about 5–10% of inhaled ethylene and propylene to ethylene oxide and propylene oxide, respectively (Törnqvist *et al.*, 1988).

(ii) *Toxic effects*

**Diesel engine exhaust**

After about 480 days, NMRI mice exposed to unfiltered, diluted (1:17) diesel exhaust (particles, 4 mg/m$^3$; carbon monoxide 14.3 ± 2.5 mg/m$^3$) had lost body weight in comparison with animals exposed to filtered exhaust (carbon monoxide, 12.7 ± 2.2 mg/m$^3$) or with controls. Under the same circumstances, rats had a lower weight increase (Heinrich *et al.*, 1986a).

The livers of Syrian golden hamsters exposed for five months to diesel exhaust diluted 1:5 and 1:10 in air had enlarged sinusoids with activated Kupffer's cells. Nucleoli were frequently fragmented or irregularly shaped. Fat deposition was observed in the sinusoids. Mitochondria from animals exposed to the 1:5 dilution had frequently lost cristae. Giant microbodies were observed in hepatocytes, and gap junctions between hepatocytes were disturbed (Meiss *et al.*, 1981).

In an initiation-promotion assay in rat liver using induction of γ-glutamyl transpeptidase-positive foci as the endpoint, Pereira *et al.* (1981a) exposed partially hepatectomized Sprague-Dawley rats to diesel exhaust (particles, 6 mg/m$^3$) for up to six months. The animals were also fed choline-supplemented or choline-deficient diets. Exposure to diesel exhaust did not alter the number of foci or induce 'remarkable' liver toxicity.

*Lung function*: Short-term exposure to diesel exhaust (28 days) led to a 35% increase in pulmonary air flow resistance in Hartley guinea-pigs (Wiester *et al.*, 1980) but increased vital capacity and total lung capacity in Sprague-Dawley rats (Pepelko, 1982a).

Prolonged exposure of rats to diluted diesel exhaust has led to impairment of lung function in some studies (Gross, 1981; Heinrich *et al.*, 1986a; McClellan, 1986) but not in others (Green *et al.*, 1983). No significant impairment of lung function was reported in hamsters (Heinrich *et al.*, 1986a).

A classic pattern of restrictive lung disease was observed in cats after 124 weeks of exposure to diesel exhaust (weeks 1–61: dilution factor, air:diesel, 18; particles, ~6 mg/m$^3$;

weeks 62–124: dilution factor, 9; particles, ~12 mg/m$^3$; Moorman et al., 1985). No such effect was observed during the first 61 weeks of the study (Pepelko et al., 1980, 1981; Moorman et al., 1985).

*Lung morphology, biochemistry and cytology*: After two years of exposure, the wet and dry weights of lungs from both mice and rats exposed to unfiltered, diluted (1:17) diesel exhaust (particles, 4 mg/m$^3$; carbon monoxide, 14.3 ± 2.5 mg/m$^3$) were two to three times higher than those of controls. The lung weights of Syrian golden hamsters exposed similarly had increased by 50 and 70% (Heinrich et al., 1986a). An increased lung to body weight ratio was also observed in guinea-pigs following an eight-week exposure to a dilution of 1:13 (Wiester et al., 1980).

Exposure of rats for 30 months to diesel exhaust (particles, 1–4 mg/m$^3$) resulted in dose-dependent irregularity, shortening and loss of cilia in ciliated epithelia, particularly the trachea and the main bronchi (Ishinishi et al., 1986a).

Increased numbers of alveolar macrophages containing diesel particles and of type II pneumocytes and accumulation of inflammatory cells within the alveoli and septal walls were observed after a 24-h exposure of Fischer 344 rats to high concentrations of diesel exhaust (particles, 6 mg/m$^3$; White & Garg, 1981). Macrophage aggregates were still present six weeks after a two-week exposure (Garg, 1983).

Following prolonged exposure of rats to diesel exhausts (particles, 2–5 mg/m$^3$), particle-containing alveolar macrophages and type II cell hyperplasia were observed (Heinrich et al., 1986a; Iwai et al., 1986; Vallyathan et al., 1986). Increases in both the number and size of macrophages and in the number of polymorphonuclear leukocytes were also observed in rats and hamsters (Chen et al., 1980; Vostal et al., 1982; Strom, 1984; Heinrich et al., 1986a). Elevated levels of lymphocytes have also been reported in rats and hamsters (Strom, 1984; Heinrich et al., 1986a). Particle accumulation and cellular proliferation have been observed in guinea-pigs (Chen et al., 1980; Wiester et al., 1980; Barnhart et al., 1981; Weller et al., 1981), and granulocyte counts were increased dramatically (up to ten-fold) in hamsters (Heinrich et al., 1986a).

In Fischer 344 rats exposed to diesel engine exhaust (particles, 2 mg/m$^3$) for two years, depressed chemiluminescence and decreased surface ruffling of alveolar macrophage membranes were observed, indicating a depression of the phagocytic activity of the macrophages (Castranova et al., 1985).

In specific-pathogen-free Wistar rats exposed to diesel exhaust (soot, 8.3 ± 2.0 mg/m$^3$) continuously for up to 20 months, slight focal and diffuse macrophage accumulation and alveolar cell hypertrophy were observed after four months. After 20 months' exposure, focal macrophage accumulation was moderate and diffuse accumulation was slight to moderate. Alveolar cell hypertrophy was more marked (up to severe), and interstitial fibrosis and alveolar emphysema were more pronounced than after four months. Alveolar bronchiolization was seen in one group at four months, but was present in four of six groups up to a moderate degree after 20 months (Karagianes et al., 1981). In a long-term inhalation study with pathogen-free Fischer 344 rats exposed for up to 30 months to whole exhaust diluted to contain soot concentrations of 0.35, 3.5 or 7.0 mg/m$^3$, focal accumulation of soot was dose-dependent and was paralleled by an active inflammation involving alveolar macrophages adjacent to terminal bronchioli. Progressive fibrosis was present in areas of soot accumulation. Epithelial hyperplasia and squamous metaplasia occurred adjacent to fibrotic foci (Mauderly *et al.*, 1987). However, although there was accumulation of particles, no histopathological sign of fibrotic change was observed after 12 or 24 months' exposure of Fischer 344 rats to diesel emissions (particles, 2 mg/m$^3$; Green *et al.*, 1983; Vallyathan *et al.*, 1986).

Fibrotic changes in the lungs of Hartley guinea-pigs exposed to diesel exhaust (particles, 0.25–6 mg/m$^3$) began after six months' exposure at a particulate concentration of about 0.75 mg/m$^3$; ultrastructural changes were concentration-dependent and started to appear after two weeks of exposure at this level. Alveolar septa were thickened following exposures above 0.25 mg/m$^3$ particles (Barnhart *et al.*, 1981, 1982).

After exposure of cats to diesel exhaust for 27 months (particles, 6 mg/m$^3$ for weeks 1–61; 12 mg/m$^3$ for weeks 62–124), bronchiolar epithelial metaplasia and peribronchial fibrosis were observed; the latter became more severe after an additional six months' exposure to clean air, but the bronchiolar epithelium returned to normal (Hyde *et al.*, 1985).

Biochemical changes in the lung associated with the changes described have been discussed by McClellan (1986). Lavage fluids from hamsters and rats after one and two years' exposure to unfiltered, diluted (1:17) diesel exhaust (particles, 4 mg/m$^3$; carbon monoxide, 14.3 ± 2.5 mg/m$^3$) contained increased levels of lactate dehydrogenase, alkaline and acid phosphatase, and glucose-6-phosphate dehydrogenase and of collagen and total protein (Heinrich *et al.*, 1986a). In contrast, acid phosphatase activity was reduced in rats and guinea-pigs exposed for one day to 12 months to diesel engine exhaust (particles, 0.25–6 mg/m$^3$); the effects were directly related to duration and levels of exposure (Weller *et al.*, 1981). Protein content and $\beta$-glucuronidase and acid phosphatase activities were elevated in lavage fluid cells from rats exposed to diesel exhaust for 48 weeks (particles, 1.5 mg/m$^3$) or 52 weeks (particles, 0.75 mg/m$^3$; Strom, 1984). Rats exposed to filtered diesel exhaust showed only small increases in glucose-6-phosphate dehydrogenase activity, collagen and protein content, while hamsters showed no increase (Heinrich *et al.*, 1986a). The total lung collagen level was elevated in the lungs of cats six months after exposure to diesel exhaust for 27 months. The cross-linked collagen content was more than doubled at the end of the exposure to air, and the collagen aldehydes:hydroxyproline ratio was elevated (Hyde *et al.*, 1985).

Sequestration (discussed above, p. 107) can be correlated with histopathological changes observed after prolonged exposure. Strom (1984) concluded that the apparent threshold of exposure of rats for increased influx of cells into the lung, beginning with alveolar macrophages, followed by polymorphonuclear leukocytes and lymphocytes, was 0.25–0.75 mg/m$^3$ for 28 weeks. [The Working Group noted that this would correspond to a calculated 'exposure rate' of 9 mg/m$^3$ × week, 110 h/week, which is not dissimilar to the point at which marked sequestration occurs (see Fig. 8).]

In Fischer 344 rats, DNA synthesis in lung tissue was increased four-fold after two days of continuous exposure by inhalation to diesel exhaust (particles, 6 mg/m$^3$). DNA synthesis returned to control levels one week after exposure. The labelling index of type II cells was significantly greater than that in controls after two and three days of exposure to diesel exhaust. After one day of exposure, palmitic acid incorporation into phosphatidylcholine in lung tissue increased by three fold when tissue palmitic acid content decreased. Total lung fatty acid content decreased by 23% after one day of exposure (Wright, 1986).

*Effects on metabolism*: Exposure to diesel particles or diesel particulate extracts has been reported to have no effect (Chen & Vostal, 1981; Rabovsky *et al.*, 1984) or a moderate (<two-fold change) effect (Lee, I.P. *et al.*, 1980; Pepelko, 1982b; Dehnen *et al.*, 1985; Chen, 1986) on aryl hydrocarbon hydroxylase activity in the lung and liver of mice and rats and in the lung of hamsters.

Exposure of Fischer 344/Crl rats by inhalation to diesel engine exhaust (particles, 7.4 mg/m$^3$) for four weeks doubled the rate of 1-nitropyrene metabolism in both nasal tissue and perfused lung. In addition, the amount of $^{14}$C covalently bound to lung macromolecules was increased four fold (Bond *et al.*, 1985). (See also the monograph on 1-nitropyrene.)

One week after instillation, there was significantly more residual benzo[*a*]pyrene in the lungs of A/Jax mice exposed to diesel engine exhaust (particles, 6 mg/m$^3$) for nine months, probably because benzo[*a*]pyrene had bound to exhaust particles. The amounts of free benzo[*a*]pyrene and of different unconjugated and conjugated metabolite fractions in lungs, liver and testis were similar to those in diesel exhaust-exposed and control mice (Cantrell *et al.*, 1981; Tyrer *et al.*, 1981).

*Immunology and infection*: In guinea-pigs exposed to diesel engine exhaust (particles, 1.5 mg/m$^3$) for up to eight weeks, B- and T-cell counts in lymph nodes were not altered (Dziedzic, 1981). No change was observed in the immunological function of splenic B- or T-cells from Fischer 344 rats exposed for up to 24 months to diesel engine exhaust (particles, 2 mg/m$^3$; Mentnech *et al.*, 1984).

CD-1 mice and Fischer 344 rats exposed to high (particles, 7 mg/m$^3$), medium (particles, 3.5 mg/m$^3$) or low (particles, 0.35 mg/m$^3$) levels of diesel engine exhaust for up to 24 months had exposure-related pathological changes in lung-associated lymph nodes, including enlargement, with histiocytes containing particles in the peripheral sinusoids and within the cortex. The total number of lymphoid cells in lung-associated lymph nodes was significantly increased after six months of exposure. In groups of mice and rats immunized at six-monthly intervals by intratracheal instillation of sheep red blood cells and analysed for IgM antibodies in lymphoid cells in rats and mice and for IgM, IgC and IgA antibodies in serum of rats, mice had an increased number of antibody-forming cells in lymph nodes from six months, but differences from controls were not statistically significant. In rats, the total number of IgM antibody-forming cells in lymph nodes was significantly elevated after six months of exposure to the high level of diesel exhaust and after 12 months of exposure to all levels. Antibody titres to sheep red cells in rat serum were not altered (Bice *et al.*, 1985).

The IgE antibody response of BDF$_1$ mice was increased after five intranasal inoculations at intervals of three weeks of varying doses of a suspension of diesel engine exhaust particles in ovalbumin solution. Antiovalbumin IgE antibody titres, assayed by passive cutaneous anaphylaxis, were enhanced by doses as low as 1 $\mu$g particles given at a three-week interval (Takafuji *et al.*, 1987).

Exposure to diesel engine exhaust may increase the susceptibility of mice to infection (Campbell *et al.*, 1981; Hahon *et al.*, 1985).

### Gasoline engine exhaust

Lifetime exposure of specific-pathogen-free Sprague-Dawley rats to gasoline engine exhaust (carbon monoxide, 57 mg/m$^3$; nitrogen oxides, 23 ppm) reduced body weight (Stupfel *et al.*, 1973). Body growth rate was also reduced among Sprague-Dawley rats exposed for up to 88 days to exhaust (dilution, 1:11) from a gasoline engine operated with (carbon monoxide, 80 mg/m$^3$) or without (carbon monoxide, 240 mg/m$^3$) a catalytic converter (Cooper *et al.*, 1977).

Haematocrit and haemoglobin and erythrocyte counts were increased in Wistar rats exposed to gasoline engine exhaust (carbon monoxide, 583 mg/m$^3$) for five weeks (Massad *et al.*, 1986). Sprague-Dawley rats were exposed to diluted (~1:10) exhaust from a gasoline engine with and without a catalytic converter (particles, ~1.2 mg/m$^3$ irradiated, 1.1 mg/m$^3$ nonirradiated; carbon monoxide, 47 and 53 mg/m$^3$; and particles, 0.77 mg/m$^3$ nonirradiated, 3.59 mg/m$^3$ irradiated; carbon monoxide, 631 and 640 mg/m$^3$, respectively) for seven days. Haematocrit and serum lactate dehydrogenase activities were elevated in both groups exposed to emissions generated without a catalyst; no such change was observed in the groups exposed to emissions generated with a catalyst. No change was observed in serum glutamate oxaloacetate transaminase activity (Lee *et al.*, 1976).

Beagle dogs exposed for 61 months to gasoline engine exhaust (carbon monoxide, 114 mg/m$^3$; Malanchuk, 1980) developed arrhythmia and bradycardia (Lewis & Moorman, 1980).

*Lung function*: Long-lasting functional disturbances of the lung were observed in beagle dogs after exposure to raw or irradiated gasoline engine exhaust (carbon monoxide, 114–126 mg/m$^3$) for 68 months (Lewis *et al.*, 1974; Gillespie, 1980). In contrast, no impairment in lung function was detected in Crl:COBS CD(SD)BR rats exposed for 45 or 90 days to diluted (1:10) exhaust from a catalyst-equipped gasoline engine (particles, 11.32 ± 1.27 mg/m$^3$; carbon monoxide, 19.5 ± 3.5 mg/m$^3$; Pepelko *et al.*, 1979).

*Lung morphology, biochemistry and cytology*: In several reports of studies in beagle dogs, atypical epithelial hyperplasia was observed in animals exposed for 68 months to raw or irradiated gasoline engine exhaust (carbon monoxide, 114 mg/m$^3$). Increases in alveolar air space and cilia loss were observed after a long recovery period following exposure to irradiated exhaust (Hyde *et al.*, 1980). The collagen content of lung tissues following exposure to raw or irradiated exhaust, with and without a 2.5-3-year recovery period was not significantly different from that in unexposed animals; prolyl hydroxylase levels in the lung were highest in groups exposed to irradiated exhaust. Exposure to a mixture of sulfur oxides and irradiated exhaust also increased the level of this enzyme (Orthoefer *et al.*, 1976; Bhatnagar, 1980). Phosphatidyl ethanolamine content was lower in liver tissues of some dogs exposed for 68 months, and lung tissue phosphatidyl ethanolamine content was 90% of the mean control value. Lysobisphosphatidic acid and phosphatidyl glycerol levels in the lungs were increased (Rouser & Aloia, 1980).

*Effects on metabolism*: Extracts of gasoline engine particles instilled into hamster lungs increased aryl hydrocarbon hydroxylase activity of lung tissue by three to five fold (Dehnen *et al.*, 1985).

*Immunology and infection*: Increased sensitivity to infection has been demonstrated following exposure of mice to the exhaust of a gasoline engine with a catalytic converter, but the effect was less than that in mice following similar exposure to diesel engine exhaust (Campbell *et al.*, 1981).

(iii) *Effects on reproduction and prenatal toxicity*

**Diesel engine exhaust**

A three-fold increase in sperm abnormalities was observed in male Chinese hamsters exposed to diesel engine exhaust [dose unspecified] for six months, as compared to controls exposed to fresh air (Pereira *et al.*, 1981b). As reported in an abstract, a statistically significant dose-related increase in sperm abnormalities was observed in male (C57Bl/6 × C3H)$F_1$ mice receiving 50, 100 or 200 mg/kg bw diesel engine exhaust particles by intraperitoneal injection for five days. An eight-fold increase in sperm abnormalities over the spontaneous level was observed in mice receiving the highest dose. A significant decrease in the number of sperm was observed only at the highest dose; testicular weight was not affected (Quinto & De Marinis, 1984).

**Gasoline engine exhaust**

Fertilized white Leghorn eggs were incubated with diluted (1:11, exhaust:air) light-irradiated or unirradiated exhaust from a gasoline engine operated with and without a catalytic converter. Exposure was maintained for about 14 days at particulate levels of approximately 0.7 or 15 mg/$m^3$. Exposure to unirradiated exhaust resulted in decreased survival and embryonic weight; irradiated exhaust had a less pronounced effect. Similar effects were seen with the catalytic converter, but they were less pronounced (Hoffman & Campbell, 1977, 1978).

Two studies have shown decreased fertility in mice following exposure to irradiated automobile exhaust [unspecifed] (Hueter *et al.*, 1966; Lewis *et al.*, 1967).

(iv) *Genetic and related effects*

The genetic and related effects of diesel and gasoline engine exhausts have been reviewed (Lewtas, 1982; Claxton, 1983; Holmberg & Ahlborg, 1983; Ishinishi *et al.*, 1986b; Lewtas & Williams, 1986).

Since engine exhaust is difficult to administer in short-term tests, studies have been conducted on several components and fractions of exhausts. Early studies were conducted on exhaust condensates; recent dilution sampling methods have permitted the collection of soot particles. Biological studies have been conducted on collected particles and on various extracts of particles, primarily extractable or soluble organic matter. Several solvents are effective for extracting organic material from diesel and gasoline particles (Claxton, 1983);

dichloromethane is that used most commonly. More volatile organic compounds are collected on adsorbent resins and extracted for bioassay. Only limited studies have been conducted on direct exposure to gaseous and whole exhausts.

Studies of genotoxicity are thus conducted on particles, particulate extracts, volatile organic condensates or whole emissions, and the results are expressed as activity per unit mass. In order to compare different emissions, genotoxicity is often expressed as emission rate or genotoxicity per unit distance driven or per mass of fuel consumed. Thus, for example, the mutagenic activity in *Salmonella typhimurium* TA98 of several gasoline particulate extracts is greater than that of diesel particulate extracts per unit mass of organic extract, while the mutagenic emission factor per kilometre driven for gasoline automobiles is less than that for diesel engines (Lewtas & Williams, 1986). The data on gasoline engine exhausts are considered together, whether or not the engine used was equipped with a catalyst and regardless of the type of fuel used (e.g., leaded or unleaded). When this information was available to the Working Group, however, it is noted in the text.

The genotoxic activity of diesel particulate extracts is generally decreased by the addition of a metabolic activation system (e.g., Aroclor 1254-induced or uninduced liver $9000 \times g$ supernatant (S9), lung S9, microsomal preparations). In contrast, the genotoxicity of gasoline particulate extracts is generally increased by the addition of metabolic activation (Claxton, 1983; Lewtas & Williams, 1986).

**Diesel engine exhaust**

The soluble organic matter extracted from diesel particles obtained from the exhaust of several types of diesel engines induced DNA damage in *Bacillus subtilis* in the absence of an exogenous metabolic system at doses of 60–500 $\mu$g/ml (Dukovich *et al.*, 1981).

The majority of studies on the mutagenicity of diesel exhaust have been conducted in *S. typhimurium* on soluble or extractable organic matter removed from soot particles. The dichloromethane extractable organic matter from soot particles collected from two diesel engines was mutagenic to *S. typhimurium* TA1537, TA1538, TA98 and TA100 in the presence and absence of an exogenous metabolic system from Aroclor 1254-induced rat liver. In the presence of activation, one soot extract was weakly mutagenic to TA1535 (Huisingh *et al.*, 1978). Other studies of particulate extracts from the exhausts of various diesel engines and vehicles also induced mutation in *S. typhimurium* TA1537, TA1538, TA98 and TA100 with and without an exogenous metabolic system, but not in TA1535 (Clark & Vigil, 1980; Clark *et al.*, 1981; Claxton, 1981; Claxton & Kohan, 1981; Dukovich *et al.*, 1981; Belisario *et al.*, 1984). Diesel engine exhaust particulate extracts were also mutagenic in *S. typhimurium* TM677 and TA100 in a forward mutation assay using 8-azaguanine resistance (Claxton & Kohan, 1981; Liber *et al.*, 1981) and in mutagenesis assays in *Escherichia coli* WP2 and K12 (Lewtas, 1983; Lewtas & Williams, 1986). In these assays, except in *E. coli* K12 where metabolic activation was required, the particulate extracts were mutagenic both in the absence and presence of an exogenous metabolic system.

Fractionation of diesel engine exhaust particulate extracts resulted in fractions (aliphatic hydrocarbons in a paraffin fraction) that were not mutagenic to *S. typhimurium*

TA1535, TA1537, TA1538, TA98 or TA100, as well as in fractions that were highly mutagenic and contained most of the activity (moderately polar and highly polar neutral fractions; Huisingh *et al.*, 1978). Similar studies in *S. typhimurium* TA98 using different fractionation procedures showed that most of the mutagenic activity of diesel engine exhaust particulate extracts was in neutral and acidic fractions (Petersen & Chuang, 1982; Pitts *et al.*, 1982; Handa *et al.*, 1983; Schuetzle, 1983; Austin *et al.*, 1985). Separation of the neutral fraction on the basis of polarity resulted in concentration of the mutagenic activity in the aromatic, moderately polar and highly polar oxygenated fractions (Huisingh *et al.*, 1978; Rappaport *et al.*, 1980; Pederson & Siak, 1981; Petersen & Chuang, 1982; Schuetzle, 1983; Austin *et al.*, 1985).

Chemical characterization by the use of bioassays has been reviewed (Schuetzle & Lewtas, 1986). Such studies have shown that nitrated PAHs contribute to the mutagenicity of diesel particulate extracts. The first evidence for the presence of nitroarenes in diesel particulate extracts was provided when a decrease in mutagenicity was observed in nitroreductase-deficient strains of *S. typhimurium* (Claxton & Kohan, 1981; Löfroth, 1981a; Pederson & Siak, 1981; Rosenkranz *et al.*, 1981; Pitts *et al.*, 1982). The contribution of mono- and dinitro-PAHs to the mutagenicity of these extracts (20–55%) was estimated by measuring both nitro-PAH and mutagenicity in *S. typhimurium* TA98 in the same diesel particulate extracts (Nishioka *et al.*, 1982; Salmeen *et al.*, 1982; Nakagawa *et al.*, 1983; Schuetzle, 1983; Tokiwa *et al.*, 1986). Other oxidized PAHs in diesel particulate extracts, such as PAH epoxides (Stauff *et al.*, 1980), pyrene-3,4-dicarboxylic acid anhydride (Rappaport *et al.*, 1980) and 5*H*-phenanthro[4,5-*bcd*]pyran-5-one (Pitts *et al.*, 1982), have been shown to be mutagenic to *S. typhimurium*. The formation of both nitro- and oxidized PAH has been reviewed (Pitts, 1983).

The use of the *S. typhimurium* mutagenesis assay to investigate the bioavailability of mutagens has also been reviewed (Claxton, 1983; Lewtas & Williams, 1986). Diesel particles dispersed in dipalmitoyl lecithin, a component of pulmonary surfactant, in saline were mutagenic to *S. typhimurium* TA98 (Wallace *et al.*, 1987). One diesel soot particulate sample collected by electrostatic precipitation from a diesel automobile was directly mutagenic to *S. typhimurium* TA98, TA100, TA1538 and TA1537 in the absence and presence of an exogenous metabolic system from Aroclor 1254-induced rat liver when particles were added directly to the top agar (1–20 mg/plate) without prior extraction or suspension in dimethyl sulfoxide. The sample was not mutagenic to *S. typhimurium* TA1535 when tested at up to 20 mg/plate (Belisario *et al.*, 1984). Diesel soot particles were either not mutagenic or weakly mutagenic to *S. typhimurium* when incubated with physiological fluids such as serum, saline, albumin, lung surfactant and lung lavage fluid (Brooks *et al.*, 1980; King *et al.*, 1981; Siak *et al.*, 1981). Serum and lung cytosol (proteinaceous fluids) inhibited mutagenicity of diesel particulate extracts in *S. typhimurium* (King *et al.*, 1981). Engulfment and incubation of diesel particles with lung macrophages decreased their mutagenic activity (King *et al.*, 1983).

Filtered diesel exhaust was mutagenic to *S. typhimurium* TA100 and to *E. coli* WP2*uvr*A/pkM101 in the absence but not in presence of an exogenous metabolic system; a marginal response was obtained in *S. typhimurium* TA104 in the presence of an Aroclor

1254-induced liver metabolic system (Matsushita et al., 1986). Gaseous emissions from diesel exhaust collected by condensation after dilution and filtration of the particles were mutagenic to *S. typhimurium* TA98 and TA100 in the absence of an exogenous metabolic system; addition of an Aroclor-induced liver metabolic system reduced their mutagenic activity (Rannug, 1983; Rannug et al., 1983). These two approaches to testing the gaseous emissions from diesel engine exhaust thus both show that they are mutagenic to *S. typhimurium* TA98 and TA100 in the absence of an exogenous metabolic system. The studies differ in the quantitative estimates of the contribution that the gaseous emissions make to the total mutagenicity of diesel exhaust: direct testing of gaseous emissions suggests that the gas phase contributes at least 30 times more to the total mutagenicity than the particles (Matsushita et al., 1986); testing of the condensation extract indicated that the gaseous emissions contributed less (up to 30%) than the particles to the total mutagenicity (Rannug, 1983). [The Working Group noted that the latter procedure could result in loss of some volatile components during sampling, extraction or preparation for bioassay.]

The urine of female Swiss mice exposed for 8 h per day on five days per week to whole diesel exhaust (dilution, 1:18; particles, 6–7 mg/m$^3$) for seven weeks (Pereira et al., 1981c) or of Fischer 344 rats exposed to diesel exhaust particles (1.9 mg/m$^3$) for three to 24 months (Green et al., 1983; Ong et al., 1985) was not mutagenic to *S. typhimurium*. However, positive responses were obtained with the urine of Sprague-Dawley rats given 1000–2000 mg/kg bw diesel exhaust particles by gastric intubation or by intraperitoneal or subcutaneous administration (Belisario et al., 1984, 1985). [The Working Group noted that this result can be taken as evidence for the bioavailability of mutagens from diesel particles.]

Particulate extracts of diesel engine exhaust emissions increased the number of mitotic recombinants in *Saccharomyces cerevisiae* D3 (Lewtas & Williams, 1986). Mitchell et al. (1981) also found a slight elevation in the number of recombinants with concentrations of 100–2000 µg/ml diesel exhaust, but the authors concluded that the results overall were negative. An 8-h exposure to an approximately five-fold dilution of exhaust (particles, 2.2 mg/m$^3$) from a diesel engine did not increase the incidence of sex-linked recessive lethal mutations in *Drosophila melanogaster* (Schuler & Niemeier, 1981).

Extracts from the emissions of diesel engines (up to 250 µg/ml) did not induce DNA damage in cultured Syrian hamster embryo cells, as determined by alkaline sucrose gradient centrifugation (Casto et al., 1981). However, diesel exhaust particles (1 and 2 mg/ml) induced unscheduled DNA synthesis in tracheal ring cultures prepared from female Fischer 344 rats (Kawabata et al., 1986).

As reported in an abstract, diesel engine emission particles and particulate extracts were more cytotoxic for excision repair-deficient xeroderma pigmentosum fibroblasts than for normal human fibroblasts (McCormick et al., 1980).

Particulate extracts (2.5–150 µg/ml) from the exhaust of one light-duty diesel engine induced mutation to ouabain resistance in mouse BALB/c 3T3 cells in the absence and presence of an exogenous metabolic system, while no significant increase in mutation frequency was found with particulate extracts from another light-duty or from a heavy-duty diesel engine (Curren et al., 1981). Another diesel engine exhaust extract induced mutation in the absence of metabolic activation (Lewtas & Williams, 1986).

In two separate studies, particulate extracts of diesel engine emissions from several passenger cars and one heavy-duty engine all induced mutations in mouse lymphoma L5178Y TK$^{+/-}$ cells. Maximal increases in mutation frequency occurred at concentrations of 20–300 µg/ml (Rudd, 1980; Mitchell et al., 1981).

Particulate extracts (60 µg/ml) from the exhaust emission of five light-duty diesel passenger cars induced mutations to 6-thioguanine resistance in Chinese hamster CHO cells both in the absence and presence of an exogenous metabolic system from Aroclor 1254-induced rat liver (Li & Royer, 1982). In another study, similar particulate extracts from two light-duty diesel engines (tested at 25–100 and 100–400 µg/ml) induced mutation in Chinese hamster CHO cells, but no mutagenic activity was observed with samples from one light-duty (up to 300 µg/ml) or one heavy-duty diesel engine (up to 750 µg/ml; Casto et al., 1981). In a third study, extracts from the exhaust of a light-duty diesel engine (25–75 µg/ml) induced mutation in Chinese hamster CHO cells in the presence, but not in the absence, of an exogenous metabolic system (Brooks et al., 1984). In a study on whole particles from diesel engines (500–750 µg/ml), mutations were induced in Chinese hamster CHO cells in the absence of an exogenous metabolic system (Chescheir et al., 1981).

Diesel particulate extracts (100–200 µg/ml) from emissions of light-duty and heavy-duty diesel engines induced 8-azaguanine and ouabain resistance in Chinese hamster V79 cells. The light-duty samples were more mutagenic than the heavy-duty samples (Morimoto et al., 1986). In another study, particulate extracts (up to 100 µg/ml) generated by a light-duty diesel engine did not induce mutation to 6-thioguanine, 8-azaguanine or ouabain resistance in Chinese hamster V79 cells (Rudd, 1980). [The Working Group noted the small number of plates used.]

Particulate extracts (100 µg/ml) of diesel exhaust induced mutation to trifluorothymidine and 6-thioguanine resistance in human TK6 lymphoblasts in the presence, but not in the absence of an exogenous metabolic system (Liber et al., 1980; Barfknecht et al., 1981).

Particulate extracts of emissions from three light-duty and one heavy-duty diesel engines (100–400 µg/ml) induced sister chromatid exchange in Chinese hamster CHO cells (Mitchell et al., 1981; Brooks et al., 1984).

When whole diesel exhaust was bubbled through cultures of human peripheral lymphocytes from four healthy nonsmokers, sister chromatid exchange was induced in two of the samples (Tucker et al., 1986). Sister chromatid exchange was also induced in cultured human lymphocytes by a light-duty diesel particulate extract (5–50 µg/ml; Lockard et al., 1982) and by diesel particulate extracts (10–200 µg/ml) from emissions of light-duty and heavy-duty diesel engines (Morimoto et al., 1986). In the last study, light-duty samples were more potent in inducing sister chromatid exchange than heavy-duty samples.

A particulate extract (20–80 µg/ml) from the exhaust emission of one light-duty diesel engine induced structural chromosomal abnormalities in Chinese hamster CHO cells (Lewtas, 1982), but an extract from a similar engine did not (Brooks et al., 1984).

A particulate extract (0.1–100 µg/ml) from the exhaust of a light-duty diesel engine induced chromosomal aberrations in cultured human lymphocytes in the absence of an exogenous metabolic system. In the presence of metabolic activation, no increase in the total percentage of cells with aberrations was observed, although an increase in the number of chromosomal fragments and dicentrics was observed (Lewtas, 1982, 1983).

Particulate extracts (2.5–100 µg/ml) from the exhaust of one light-duty diesel engine induced morphological transformation in BALB/c 3T3 cells in the absence, but not in the presence, of an exogenous metabolic system from Aroclor 1254-induced rat liver (Curren *et al.*, 1981). Similar extracts from two other light-duty diesel engines and a heavy-duty diesel engine did not induce morphological transformation in these cells in the absence or presence of a metabolic system (Curren *et al.*, 1981, up to 300 µg/ml; Zamora *et al.*, 1983, up to 40 µg/ml). An extract from a light-duty diesel engine (2–10 µg/ml) induced morphological transformation in BALB/c 3T3 cells initiated by treatment with 3-methylcholanthrene (Zamora *et al.*, 1983).

Particulate extracts (31–500 µg/ml) from the emissions of three light-duty diesel engines enhanced transformation of Syrian hamster embryo cells in the presence of SA7 virus. No significant enhancement of transformation was observed with the corresponding extract (up to 500 µg/ml) from a heavy-duty engine (Casto *et al.*, 1981).

A particulate extract (5–10 µg/ml) of exhaust from a light-duty engine inhibited intercellular communication, as measured by metabolic cooperation in Chinese hamster V79 lung cells (Zamora *et al.*, 1983).

Primary cultures of 12-day-old hamster embryos from pregnant Syrian hamsters that received intraperitoneal injections of the neutral fractions of light-duty or heavy-duty diesel particulate extracts (2000–4000 mg/kg bw) on day 11 of gestation had an increased number of 8-azaguanine-resistant mutations (Morimoto *et al.*, 1986).

Exposure of B6C3F1 mice to whole diesel engine exhaust emission (12 mg/m$^3$ particles) for one month did not induce sister chromatid exchange in bone-marrow cells, but injection [unspecified] of either diesel particles (300 mg/kg bw) or their extract (800 mg/kg bw) resulted in an increased incidence of sister chromatid exchange in the bone marrow of mice sacrificed two days after treatment (Pereira, 1982).

No increase in the frequency of sister chromatid exchange was observed in the peripheral lymphocytes of Fischer 344 rats exposed to whole diesel engine exhaust emission (1.9 mg/m$^3$ particles) for three months (Ong *et al.*, 1985), and no significant increase was observed in bone-marrow cells of rats exposed to 4 mg/kg whole emissions from light- or heavy-duty diesel engines for up to 30 months (Morimoto *et al.*, 1986). [The Working Group could not determine the accumulated dose.]

Intratracheal instillation of diesel engine exhaust particles (6–20 mg) in male Syrian hamsters increased the incidence of sister chromatid exchange in lung cells, as did exposure of Syrian hamsters for 3.5 months to whole diesel engine exhaust emissions (particles, 12 mg/m$^3$; Guerrero *et al.*, 1981). Exposure of pregnant Syrian hamsters to whole diesel engine exhaust emissions (particles, 12 mg/m$^3$) from day 1 of gestation, or intraperitoneal administration of diesel engine exhaust particles at the $LD_{50}$ (300 mg/kg bw) on day 12 of gestation, did not result in increased frequencies of sister chromatid exchange in fetal liver, as determined on day 13. However, an increase was seen after intraperitoneal administration on day 12 of a dichloromethane extract of the particles (Pereira, 1982; Pereira et al., 1982).

No increase in the frequency of micronuclei in bone marrow was found in male ICR mice exposed to whole exhaust emission from a light-duty diesel engine at particulate concentrations of 0.4 and 2.0 mg/m$^3$ for up to 18 months (Morimoto et al., 1986), or in Swiss-Webster CD-1 mice or Fischer 344 rats exposed to whole emission (particles, 1.9 mg/m$^3$) for six months and two years, respectively (Ong et al., 1985), or in B6C3F1 and Swiss mice and Chinese hamsters exposed to exhaust emissions for one to six months (particles, 6 mg/m$^3$) or for one month (particles, 12 mg/m$^3$); however, an increase was observed in Chinese hamsters exposed to 6 mg/m$^3$ for six months. There was a slight increase in the number of micronucleated bone-marrow cells in B6C3F1 mice, but not in Chinese hamsters, administered an extract of diesel particles (800 and 1000 mg/kg bw) intraperitoneally (Pereira et al., 1981b,c; Pereira, 1982; Pepelko & Peirano, 1983). As reported in an abstract, extracts of diesel engine exhaust particles given intraperitoneally at concentrations of up to 1000 mg/kg bw to Chinese hamsters did not increase the frequencies of chromosomal aberrations, micronuclei or sister chromatid exchange in bone-marrow cells (Heidemann & Miltenburger, 1983).

No increase in the incidence of dominant lethal mutations was found when male T-stock mice exposed for 7.5 weeks to diesel exhaust (particulates, 6 mg/m$^3$; 8 h/day, 7 days/week) were mated with (101×C3H)F$_1$, (SEC×C57Bl)F$_1$, (C3H×C57Bl)F$_1$ or T-stock female mice or when female (101×C3H)F$_1$ mice were similarly exposed for 7 weeks prior to mating with untreated males. No increase in the frequency of heritable point mutations was found after T-stock males were similarly exposed to diesel exhaust [length of exposure not given] prior to mating, and no oocyte killing was observed in (SEC×C57Bl)F$_1$ female mice after exposure for eight weeks prior to mating (Pepelko & Peirano, 1983).

### Gasoline exhaust

Gasoline exhaust emissions from both catalyst and noncatalyst automobiles, collected using several standard methods, were mutagenic to *S. typhimurium* TA98 and TA100 (Claxton & Kohan, 1981; Löfroth, 1981a,b; Ohnishi et al., 1982; Zweidinger, 1982; Clark et al., 1983; Handa et al., 1983; Rannug, 1983; Rannug et al., 1983; Brooks et al., 1984; Norpoth et al., 1985; Westerholm et al., 1988). Addition of a catalyst, however, significantly decreases the rate of emission from gasoline engine vehicles of material that is mutagenic to these strains (Ohnishi et al., 1980; Zweidinger, 1982; Rannug, 1983; Rannug et al., 1983; Lewtas, 1985).

Extracts of particles collected from the exhaust pipes of gasoline automobiles [assumed to be noncatalyst, using leaded fuel] were mutagenic to *S. typhimurium* TA1537, TA98 and TA100 both in the absence and presence of an exogenous metabolic system from Aroclor-induced rat liver (Wang et al., 1978). Particulate and condensate extracts of the exhausts of a noncatalyst gasoline engine and a catalyst (oxidizing) gasoline vehicle were mutagenic to *S. typhimurium* TA1538, TA98 and TA100 in the presence of an exogenous metabolic system from Aroclor-induced rat liver. The samples were either not mutagenic or weakly mutagenic to *S. typhimurium* TA1535 (Ohnishi *et al.*, 1980). Dichloromethane extracts of soot particles from a gasoline catalyst vehicle were mutagenic to *S. typhimurium* TA98 and TA100 in the absence and presence of an exogenous metabolic system but were not mutagenic to *S. typhimurium* TA1535 (Claxton, 1981). Particulate extracts of gasoline catalyst engine (unleaded fuel) emissions were mutagenic to *S. typhimurium* TA98 in the absence and presence of an exogenous metabolic system and in *S. typhimurium* TA100 only in the presence of an exogenous metabolic system (Westerholm *et al.*, 1988).

Gas-phase emissions collected from catalyst and noncatalyst engines by condensation after dilution and filtration were mutagenic to *S. typhimurium* TA98 and TA100 in the absence of an exogenous metabolic system, and the contribution of the gas phase to the total mutagenicity ranged from 50–90% in the absence of activation. In the presence of a metabolic system, the mutagenicity was decreased (Rannug, 1983; Rannug *et al.*, 1983; Westerholm *et al.*, 1988).

After fractionation of gasoline engine exhaust particulate and condensate extracts, the neutral aromatic fraction, which contains the PAHs, was found to be mutagenic to *S. typhimurium* TA98 in the presence of an exogenous metabolic system (Löfroth, 1981b; Handa *et al.*, 1983); the highest dose-dependent increase in mutagenicity was induced by the four- to seven-ring PAH fraction in *S. typhimurium* TA98 and TA100 (Norpoth *et al.*, 1985). Handa *et al.* (1983) found the acidic fraction to be significantly more mutagenic in *S. typhimurium* TA98 in the absence than in the presence of an exogenous metabolic system.

Nitro-PAH are either not detectable or present at much lower concentrations in particulate extracts from gasoline engine exhausts than in diesel particle extracts (Nishioka *et al.*, 1982; Handa *et al.*, 1983). In studies using strains of *S. typhimurium* that do not respond to nitro-PAH, gasoline engine exhaust particulate extracts (Brooks *et al.*, 1984) and whole catalyst gasoline engine emissions (Jones *et al.*, 1985) were less mutagenic than in TA98 (in the absence of activation), suggesting the presence of nitroaromatic compounds. Löfroth (1981a), however, using similar techniques, did not see a decrease in mutagenicity attributable to nitro-PAHs. [The Working Group noted that these results are not necessarily inconsistent, since different strains and sampling methods were used.]

Several studies of exhaust emissions from vehicles run on gasoline blended with alcohol (10–23% ethanol or methanol) have shown either no significant change or a decreased emission rate of material mutagenic to *S. typhimurium* TA98 and TA100 (Clark *et al.*, 1983; Rannug, 1983; Clark *et al.*, 1984).

Particulate extracts of one unleaded gasoline catalyst engine exhaust emission tested at up to 1500 $\mu$g/ml did not induce mitotic recombination in *S. cerevisiae* D3 (Mitchell *et al.*, 1981).

An extract of emissions from an unleaded gasoline catalyst engine (250 $\mu$g/ml) induced DNA damage in cultured Syrian hamster embryo cells, as measured by alkaline sucrose gradients, in the absence of an exogenous metabolic system (Casto *et al.*, 1981).

Particulate extracts from the exhaust of an unleaded gasoline catalyst engine (2.5–500 µg/l) induced mutation to ouabain resistance in mouse BALB/c 3T3 cells in the absence and presence of an exogenous metabolic system (Curren *et al.*, 1981). Particulate extracts from unleaded gasoline catalyst automobiles and leaded gasoline noncatalyst automobiles (20–350 µg/ml) were mutagenic to mouse lymphoma L5178Y $TK^{+/-}$ cells. Metabolic activation increased the mutagenic activity (Mitchell *et al.*, 1981; Lewtas, 1982). Particulate extracts from the exhaust emission from a gasoline engine with catalytic converter (50–400 µg/ml) induced mutations to 6-thioguanine resistance in CHO cells in the absence of an exogenous metabolic system (Casto *et al.*, 1981). In another study, extracts from an unleaded gasoline catalyst engine (25–75 µg/ml) induced mutations to 6-thioguanine resistance in the *hgpt* locus in Chinese hamster CHO cells only in the presence of an exogenous metabolic system (Brooks *et al.*, 1984).

Particulate extracts of unleaded gasoline catalyst engine emissions (10–200 µg/ml) induced sister chromatid exchange in Chinese hamster CHO cells in the absence of an exogenous metabolic system (Mitchell *et al.*, 1981). Extracts from another unleaded gasoline catalyst engine exhaust (10–50 µg/ml) also induced sister chromatid exchange in Chinese hamster CHO cells both in the absence and presence of an exogenous metabolic system (Brooks *et al.*, 1984). Leaded gasoline noncatalyst engine exhaust particulate extracts induced sister chromatid exchange in Chinese hamster CHO cells in the presence of an exogenous metabolic system (Lewtas & Williams, 1986). [The Working Group noted that no data were provided on responses in the absence of an exogenous metabolic system.]

Extracts from an unleaded gasoline catalyst engine exhaust (20–60 µg/ml) induced chromosomal aberrations in Chinese hamster CHO cells in the presence of an exogenous metabolic system (Brooks *et al.*, 1984). Particulate extract [type of fuel and presence of catalyst unspecified] (0.6–5 µg/ml) induced aneuploidy and polyploidy in Chinese hamster V79 cells in the absence of an exogenous metabolic system (Hadnagy & Seemayer, 1986) and induced disturbance of the spindle apparatus (Seemayer *et al.*, 1987).

Dichloromethane particulate extracts from the exhaust of an unleaded gasoline catalyst engine (2.5–500 µg/ml) increased the frequency of morphological transformation of BALB/c 3T3 cells in both the absence and presence of an exogenous metabolic system from Aroclor 1254-induced rat liver (Curren *et al.*, 1981). Dichloromethane extracts of the particulate emissions of an unleaded gasoline catalyst engine (31–500 µg/ml) enhanced morphological transformation of Syrian hamster embryo cells in the presence of SA7 virus (Casto *et al.*, 1981).

In male BALB/c mice exposed to whole gasoline engine exhaust [type of fuel and presence of catalyst unspecified] emissions for 8 h per day for ten days and killed 18 h after the last exposure period, an increased frequency of micronucleated bone-marrow cells was found (Massad *et al.*, 1986).

(b) *Humans*

(i) *Deposition, clearance, retention and metabolism*

The factors affecting the uptake of gases and vapours, including model calculations for their absorption in the different regions of the human respiratory tract, have been summarized (Davies, 1985).

**Diesel engine exhaust**

No data on the deposition, clearance, retention or metabolism of diesel engine exhaust were available to the Working Group. A model has been developed to predict the deposition of diesel exhaust in humans (Yu & Xu, 1986; Xu & Yu, 1987; Yu & Xu, 1987).

**Gasoline engine exhaust**

The results of two laboratory experiments in which human volunteers inhaled the exhaust from an engine run on gasoline containing $^{203}$Pb-tetraethyllead are summarized in Table 29. In one of the experiments, the exhaust was contained in a 600-l chamber; the concentrations of carbon monoxide and carbon dioxide were reduced using chemical traps; median particulate size was about 0.4 μm (Chamberlain *et al.*, 1975) or 0.35 and 0.7 μm, resulting in an aerosol considered typical of urban environments (Chamberlain *et al.*, 1978). In the other experiment, the exhaust was rapidly diluted in a wind tunnel which prevented coagulation of the primary exhaust particles and resulted in aerosols with median particulate sizes of 0.02–0.09 μm. Both experiments were conducted with a variety of breathing patterns, which were monitored but not controlled. Total deposition was relatively constant at 30% over a wide range of breathing patterns for sizes typical of urban aerosols (Chamberlain, 1985). However, as the size of the primary particles decreased (below 0.1 μm), deposition increased sharply, and the length of the respiratory cycle (time between the start of successive breaths) significantly affected deposition. [The Working Group noted that these data are in broad agreement with those for other particulate materials of similar size (Heyder *et al.*, 1983; Schiller *et al.*, 1986.]

In a separate analysis of the same data, deposition was shown to increase with respiratory cycle in an approximately linear fashion — ranging from 10% at 3 sec to 55% at 20 sec; the slope of this line was somewhat dependent on tidal volume. A small, but significant effect of expiratory reserve volume on deposition was observed: total deposition dropped by a factor of 1.2 for an increase in expiratory reserve volume of 2.5 l (Wells *et al.*, 1977).

In a third study, measurements of total deposition were performed in the field by comparing inhaled and exhaled airborne lead concentrations; the method was found to give results comparable to experimental measurements involving $^{203}$Pb. Total deposition was measured for inhalation at an average breathing pattern of 0.8 l and a respiratory cycle of 5.2 sec in persons seated by a motorway (61%), by a roundabout (64%), in an urban street (48%) and in a car park (48%). Median particulate sizes in the breath of persons near quickly moving traffic (0.04 μm) were found to be much smaller than those in persons in the urban

Table 29. Total deposition (%) of leaded gasoline particles as a function of size and breathing pattern[a]

| Particulate diameter ($\mu$m) | Tidal volume in litres (respiratory cycle in seconds) | | | | | | | | | | |
|---|---|---|---|---|---|---|---|---|---|---|---|
| | 0.5 (2) | 0.5 (4) | 1.0 (4) | 1.5 (4) | 0.5 (6) | 1.0 (6) | 1.5 (6) | 0.5 (8) | 1.0 (8) | 2.0 (8) | 1.5 (12) |
| 0.02 | 53 | 64 | | 86 | | 82 | | 86 | | | 86 |
| 0.04 | | | 42 | | 40 | 58 | 56 | | 55 | 61 | |
| 0.09 | | 35 | | | | 32 | | 27 | | | |
| 0.35 | | | | | | | | | | 38 | |
| ~0.4[b] | | 32 | 26 | | 42 | 46 | 36 | | 37 | 62 | 62 |
| 0.70 | | | | | | | 40 | | | 50 | |

[a]Compiled by the Working Group from Chamberlain et al. (1978), except where noted

[b]From Chamberlain et al. (1975); individual data grouped by the Working Group according to breathing pattern and particle size

environment or in a car park (0.3 $\mu$m), although the air near roundabouts also contained a large proportion by mass of adventitious particles (2 $\mu$m) (Chamberlain et al., 1978).

Lung clearance was best described by a four-component exponential clearance. The first two phases (half-times, 0.7 and 2.5 h) were similar for exhaust particles, lead nitrate (which is soluble) and lead oxide (which is insoluble), and therefore probably represent mucociliary clearance (Chamberlain et al., 1975, 1978). On average, 40% of lung deposition of 0.35-$\mu$m aerosols was in the pulmonary region and 60% in the tracheobronchial region. The removal of lead compounds from the pulmonary region was described by a two-component exponential with half-times of 9 and 44 h; one exception was the removal of lead from highly carbonaceous particles, which exhibited half times of 24 and 220 h (Chamberlain et al., 1978; Chamberlain, 1985).

No data on the metabolism in humans of gasoline engine exhaust were available to the Working Group.

(ii) *Toxic effects*

Early studies involving human volunteers showed that exposure to gasoline engine exhaust may cause headache, nausea and vomiting (Henderson et al., 1921). Sayers et al. (1929) monitored the carbon monoxide content of gasoline engine exhaust gas-air mixtures and found a relationship between increasing carbon monoxide concentration, carboxyhaemoglobin (COHb) level and reports of headache in six men exposed to atmospheres containing 229–458 mg/m$^3$ carbon monoxide. In a more recent study of ten patients with angina (Aronow et al., 1972), significant increases in COHb levels and significant reductions in exercise performance until onset of angina symptoms were observed in persons driving for 90 min in heavy traffic, as compared with tests both before the experiment and after breathing purified air for 90 min.

Among six volunteers exposed for 3.7 h to diesel engine exhaust gases containing about 4 mg/m$^3$ nitrogen dioxide, there was no increase in urinary thioether concentration (Ulfvarson et al., 1987).

Effects of exposure to diesel engine exhaust on the lung have been reviewed (Calabrese et al., 1981). Although bus garage and car ferry workers, exposed occupationally to mixtures of gasoline and diesel engine exhausts, had lower mean levels of respiratory function (forced respiratory volume in 1 sec ($FEV_1$) and forced vital capacity (FVC)) than expected, they showed no change in these measures over working shifts (for exposure measurements, see Tables 17 and 21, respectively). In contrast, workers on roll-on roll-off ships, exposed mainly to diesel engine fumes, showed statistically significant reductions in $FEV_1$ and FVC during working shifts (for exposure measurements, see Table 18). These reductions were reversible, however, the levels returning to normal after a few days with no exposure. The work-shift concentrations of nitrogen dioxide and carbon monoxide in these three groups averaged 0.54 mg/m$^3$ and 1.1 mg/m$^3$, respectively (Ulfvarson et al., 1987). A small reduction in $FEV_1$/FVC and in $FEF_{25-75\%}$ (forced expiratory flow at 25–75% of forced vital capacity) was also observed at the end of a work shift among a group of chain-saw operators (Hagberg et al., 1983; for exposure measurements, see Table 22). Concentrations of diesel engine emissions in coal mines, involving, on average, 0.6 mg/m$^3$ nitrogen dioxide and 13.7 mg/m$^3$ carbon monoxide, were not associated with decrements in the miners' ventilatory function (Ames et al., 1982).

Studies in which changes in COHb levels were investigated over the course of a work shift are summarized in section 2 (pp. 69–73).

Possible effects on the lung of chronic occupational exposures to low levels of diesel engine exhaust emissions were studied cross-sectionally in railroad engine house workers (Battigelli et al., 1964), in iron ore miners (Jörgensen & Svensson, 1970), in potash miners (Attfield et al., 1982), in coal miners (Reger et al., 1982; for exposure measurements, see Table 15), in salt miners (Gamble et al., 1983), in coal miners exposed to oxides of nitrogen generated (in part) by diesel engine emissions underground (Robertson et al., 1984) and in bus garage workers (Gamble et al., 1987b). Effects of relatively high concentrations of automobile emissions have been described among bridge and road tunnel workers in two large cities (Speizer & Ferris, 1963; Ayres et al., 1973; for exposure measurements, see Table 19). Changes in lung function over a five-year period have also been studied longitudinally among coal miners working underground in mines with and without diesel engines (Ames et al., 1984). Some, but not all, of the results from these various studies showed decrements in lung function and increased prevalence of respiratory symptoms in subgroups exposed to engine emissions.

Exposure to engine exhaust has also been associated with irritation of the eyes (Waller et al., 1961; Battigelli, 1965; Hamming & MacPhee, 1967; Hagberg et al., 1983).

A 15-year follow-up of 34 156 members of a heavy construction equipment operators' union showed a highly significant overall excess of deaths certified as due to emphysema (116 observed, 70.2 expected), and this excess appeared to be higher among men with longer membership in the union (Wong et al., 1985). No data on smoking habits were included in the mortality analyses, and the authors noted that they were unable to estimate the degree to which exposure to diesel engine emissions (as distinct from other occupational factors, such as exposure to dust) might have contributed to the excess mortality from emphysema.

Another cohort study, of 1558 white motor vehicle examiners, yielded a slight excess of deaths from cardiovascular disease (124 observed, 118.4 expected) in a 29-year follow-up. The excess was more pronounced for deaths occurring during the first ten years of employment (28 oberved, 20.9 expected; Stern *et al.*, 1981). [The Working Group noted that the excesses observed are easily attributable to chance ($p > 0.1$).] A 32-year follow-up of 694 Swedish bus garage employees also showed a small, statistically nonsignificant, excess of deaths from cardiovascular disease (121 observed, 115.9 expected) which showed no pattern to indicate a relation to probable intensity or duration of exposure to diesel emissions (Edling *et al.*, 1987). Moreover, Rushton *et al.* (1983) found no excess of deaths from cerebrovascular or ischaemic heart disease among maintenance workers in London bus garages. A 27-year follow-up of 3886 potash miners and millers also showed no excess mortality that could be attributed to the presence of diesel engines in some of the mines that were studied; in only two of eight mines had diesel engines been used (Waxweiler *et al.*, 1973). None of these four analyses of mortality included adjustments for the men's smoking habits. However, the authors noted that the US potash workers whom they had studied included a greater proportion of cigarette smokers than among all US males.

(iii) *Effects on reproduction and prenatal toxicity*

No data were available to the Working Group.

(iv) *Genetic and related effects*

The frequency of chromosomal aberrations in cultured lymphocytes from 14 male miners exposed to diesel engine exhaust (five were smokers) was no greater than in 15 male office workers (five smokers; Nordenson *et al.*, 1981). The incidence of chromosomal changes was also investigated in four groups of 12 men: drivers of diesel-engine trucks, drivers of gasoline-engine trucks, automobile inspectors and a reference group, matched with respect to age, smoking habits and length in the jobs. The frequencies of gaps, breaks and sister chromatid exchange in lymphocyte preparations were not significantly different in the four groups (Fredga *et al.*, 1982). [The Working Group noted the small number of subjects in both of these studies.]

Among workers with relatively heavy exposure to diesel engine exhaust — in particular, crews of roll-on roll-off ships and car ferries and bus garage staff (the latter two groups also having exposure to gasoline engine exhausts) — no difference in mutagenicity to *S. typhimurium* TA98 or *E. coli* WP2 *uvrA* was observed between urine collected during exposed periods and that collected during unexposed periods. Similarly, no increase in urinary mutagenicity was found among six volunteers before and after an experimental exposure to diesel engine exhaust gases from an automobile run for 3.7 h at 60 km/h, 2580 revolutions/min (Ulfvarson *et al.*, 1987).

## 3.3 Epidemiological studies of carcinogenicity to humans

*(a) Introduction*

Although population-based studies to detect a possible association between exposure to engine exhausts and cancer in humans are the most direct methods for detecting human carcinogenesis, for low levels of risk the approach is complicated by several factors. These factors can be divided broadly into problems related to the documentation of levels of exposure and the potential for unidentified confounding factors to influence the results.

Nonoccupational exposure to engine exhaust is nearly ubiquitous in urban areas and in the vicinity of vehicles. Because emissions are diluted in the nonoccupational environment, it is unlikely that investigations of the general population would reveal risks when groups with heavy exposure show only a small risk.

'Unexposed' reference populations used in epidemiological studies are likely to contain a substantial number of subjects who are exposed nonoccupationally to engine exhausts. The 'exposed' group is often defined on the basis of job title, which may be an inadequate surrogate for exposure to exhaust emissions, and this may lead to an underestimation of risk. The situation is further complicated by the presence of possible confounding factors, such as smoking and other exposures (e.g., asbestos in railroad yards), which may influence results, especially when lung and bladder cancers are being studied. In addition, in many studies of the occupational setting, there is an inextricable link between exposure to exhaust emissions and to vapours from the fuels themselves. Some occupational groups, such as car-park attendants and toll-booth workers, which might be thought to be a source of more direct information due to their heavy exposure, are usually too small and/or too transient for a population-based study of cancer to be feasible.

Another important consideration is that occupational cohorts tend to have below-average mortality, both from all causes and from various major categories of specific causes. These deficits are, typically, manifestations of a selection process based on health status, referred to as the 'healthy worker effect'. In view of this overall deficit in cancer mortality in working cohorts, conventional statistical evaluation of site-specific standardized mortality ratios (SMRs) is usually conservative. That is, comparison of the SMR with an 'expected' value of 100 derived from the general population - rather than from some defined internal unexposed comparison group — may result in an underestimation of the true magnitude of any occupation-related increase in risk for specific cancers.

In the studies reviewed, retrospective assessment of an individual's exposure to engine exhausts is necessarily indirect, since there are generally no systematic or quantitative records of work-place or ambient exposures. In some studies, the title of a job or occupation with known or presumed exposure is used as a simple surrogate measure of exposure, and the cancer risk of groups of individuals in such jobs is compared with that of the general population or of persons in unrelated jobs. In some other studies, mainly of case-control design, each individual's past exposure is assessed by the use of a job-exposure matrix. In its simplest form, a job-exposure matrix is a two-way table in which each job or occupation is assigned a code indicating the presence (and sometimes the magnitude) of substances to which persons in that job would be exposed, on the basis of contemporary measurements and knowledge of working practices. The job history obtained from the subject is then used to construct his or her record of past exposure from the matrix. Among the limitations of this approach is the fact that individual exposures may differ widely even within narrowly defined occupations, because of differences in working practices between individuals and work sites, from country to country and over time. It should be noted, however, that while such problems in exposure assessment reduce the precision with which any effect can be measured, they are not likely to give rise to a spurious association where none exists; consistency of results between different studies of this kind is therefore of particular importance in assessing the relationship between exposure and disease.

Several of the available case-control studies are hospital-based rather than population-based; i.e., the control group consists of subjects hospitalized for diseases different from those of the cases. Because little is known about the etiology of many diseases, some of which may be associated with exposure to engine exhaust, it is difficult to rule out bias resulting from the choice of specific sets of controls.

*(b) Mortality and morbidity statistics*

The Working Group noted that surveys of mortality or morbidity statistics suffer from many limitations, which reduce their usefulness in the evaluation of carcinogenic risks. Comparison of the results of different studies is complicated by the varying definitions and groupings of occupations and cancer sites. Generally, these studies have been designed to generate hypotheses about potentially exposed groups. For example, a striking difference in the male:female sex ratio for tumours unrelated to hormonal status within a specific geographical region might suggest an area that should be explored in either cohort or case-control studies, in which exposure can be assessed more readily.

Studies of this type that may relate to exposure to exhaust fumes include the following: Menck and Henderson (1976), Decouflé *et al.* (1977), Office of Population Censuses and Surveys (1978), Petersen and Milham (1980), Howe and Lindsay (1983), Milham (1983), Dubrow and Wegman (1984), Malker and Weiner (1984), Baxter and McDowall (1986) and Olsen and Jensen (1987).

*(c) Cohort studies*

(i) *Railroad workers*

Kaplan (1959) evaluated 6506 deaths among railroad workers from the medical records of the Baltimore and Ohio Railroad relief department between 1953 and 1958, 818 of which were due to cancer and 154 of which were lung cancer. The cases were categorized into three groups by exposure to diesel exhaust. In comparison with national death rates, none of the groups had an excess risk for lung cancer. [The Working Group noted that, since changeover to diesel engines began in 1935 and was 95% complete by 1959 (Garshick *et al.*, 1988), few if any of the lung cancer deaths could have occurred in workers with more than ten years' exposure to diesel exhaust; in addition, smoking habits were not considered.]

Howe *et al.* (1983) studied a cohort of 43 826 male pensioners of the Canadian National Railway Company consisting of retired railroad workers who were known to be alive in 1965 plus those who retired between 1965 and 1977. Of the total of 17 838 deaths that occurred in 1965-77, 16 812 (94.4%) were successfully linked to a record in the Canadian mortality data base. The expected number of cancer deaths was estimated from that of the total Canadian population, adjusted for age and calendar period. Available information included birth date, province of residence, date of retirement and occupation at time of retirement. Occupational exposures were classified into three types: 'diesel fumes', coal dust and other. The two statistically significant results for the whole cohort were deficits in deaths from all causes (SMR, 95 [95% confidence interval (CI), 93-96]) and from leukaemia (SMR, 80 [95% CI, 65-97]). For exposure to diesel engine exhaust, the risk for cancer of the trachea, bronchus and lung increased with likelihood of exposure: the relative risks were 1.0 for unexposed, 1.2 [1.1-1.3] for 'possibly exposed' and 1.4 [1.2-1.5] for 'probably exposed' ($p$ for trend $< 0.001$). The SMR for bladder cancer was 103 [88-119]. Similar results were found for the risk for cancer of the trachea, bronchus and lung from exposure to coal dust. Since there was considerable overlap in exposures to diesel fumes and coal dust, the risk was evaluated by calendar time during which one of these exposures predominated. The risk was largely accounted for by exposure to diesel exhaust. Since exposure to asbestos occurs during locomotive maintenance, workers thought to have had such exposure were removed from the analysis, with little effect on the risk associated with exposure to diesel engine exhaust. Exclusion of workers exposed to welding fumes did not alter the result. The authors noted that the data presented and the risks observed probably represent an underestimate of the true risk, for at least two reasons: exposure misclassification because of the use of job held last and failure to determine the cause of death for 5.6% of cases. [The Working Group noted that no data were available on duration of exposure, usual occupation or smoking habits and recognized the potential for competing biases in the way in which the cohort was composed.]

Garshick *et al.* (1988) studied a cohort of 55 407 white male railroad workers aged 40-64 in 1959 who had started railroad service ten to 20 years earlier. The cohort was traced from records of the pension scheme for US railway workers through to 1980; it was estimated that less than 2% left the industry during the period covered by the study. Death certificates were available for 88% of the 19 396 deaths, of which 1694 were from lung cancer; decedents for whom a death certificate was not obtained were classified as having died of unknown causes. Records of railroad jobs from 1959 through to death, retirement or 1980 were also available from the records of the pension scheme. Jobs were divided into regular exposure to diesel exhausts (train crews, workers in diesel repair shops) and no exposure (clerks, ticket and station agents, and signal maintenance workers). Job categories with recognized asbestos exposure, such as car repair and construction trades, were excluded from those selected for study. Information was available on duration of exposure. There was a significant excess risk for lung cancer in the groups exposed to diesel engine exhaust; this risk was highest in those who had the longest exposure: aged 40-44 (relative risk, 1.5; 95% CI, 1.1-1.9) and 45-49 (1.3; 1.0-1.7) and exposed to diesel exhaust in 1959. The groups aged 50-54 and 55-59 in 1959 also had excess risks, of 1.1 and 1.2, respectively, although these were not statistically significant. When workers with further potential asbestos exposure (shop workers) were excluded, similarly elevated lung cancer rates were observed. Although smoking habits were not considered directly, the authors pointed out that there was no difference in smoking habits by job title in comparison studies of current workers or in a case-control study in which smoking was assessed. [The Working Group noted that exclusion of shop workers would also have excluded men exposed to welding fumes.]

As part of this study, exposure was assessed on the basis of several hundred time-weighted samples of respirable dust taken in the early 1980s both at stationary sites in parts of four existing, smaller railroad yards and with personal samplers carried by railroad workers in different job categories (Woskie *et al.*, 1988a). Samples were taken from workers in 39/155 Interstate Commerce Commission job codes, and the results were used to classify the jobs; these 39 categories were subsequently combined into 13 job groups, which could be further combined into five: clerks, signal maintenance, engineers/firers, brakers/-conductors and shop workers. The nicotine content was used to adjust the extractable respirable particulate content of each sample to account for the portion contributed by cigarette smoking. Mean exposure levels by national career groups in the five major categories of exposure suggested a five-fold range of exposure to respirable particles between clerks and shop workers (Woskie *et al.* 1988b). These values confirmed the a-priori assignment of the categories of diesel exposure used in the cohort study (Garshick *et al.*, 1988) and the assignment to appropriate exposure categories for the case-control study (Garshick *et al.*, 1987; see p. 140).

(ii) *Bus company employees*

Raffle (1957) determined deaths, retirements and transfers due to lung cancer in London Transport employees aged 45–64 years in jobs with presumably different exposures to exhaust fumes in 1950–54 and compared the figures with those for lung cancer mortality for men in England and Wales or in Greater London. No relationship between presumed exposure and lung cancer incidence was noted. In a subgroup of bus and trolley bus engineering staff aged 55–64, 30 deaths from lung cancer occurred while 21.2 were expected (observed:expected, 1.4) on the basis of the experience of other London Transport employees. [The Working Group noted that no information on smoking habits was available, and that all the deaths occurred in men over 55 years of age.] Waller (1981) compared lung cancer deaths and retirements or transfers to alternative jobs due to lung cancer in men aged 45–64 employed within five job categories of London Transport (bus drivers, bus conductors, engineers (garages), engineers (central works) and motor men and guards) to lung cancer mortality (age- and calendar time-adjusted) for men in Greater London. The study covered 25 years, ending in 1974, thus including some of the data described by Raffle (1957). A total of 667 cases of lung cancer were observed; although the risk was not elevated for any of the five job categories, the highest SMR occurred in the group that was presumably most heavily exposed to diesel exhaust (bus garage workers). [The Working Group noted that no data on smoking habits were available, and neither duration nor latency was examined.]

Rushton *et al.* (1983) examined a cohort of 8684 men employed as maintenance workers in 71 bus garages in London for at least one year in 1967–75. Follow-up until 31 December 1975 was completed for 8490 (97.8%) workers, and cause of death was known for 701 of 705 who had died. The SMRs were 84 [95% CI, 78–91] for all causes and 95 [83–109] for all neoplasms, 101 [82–122] for lung and pleural cancer, 151 [60–307] for leukaemia, 121 [49–250] for central nervous system tumours and 139 [72–244] for bladder cancer. None of the rates for cancer at individual sites was statistically significantly increased. The authors noted the short follow-up period.

Edling *et al.* (1987) studied 694 men, five of whom (0.7%) were lost to follow-up, who had been employed as clerks, bus drivers or bus garage workers in five bus companies in south-eastern Sweden at any time between 1950 and 1959, and followed for 1951–83. The SMRs, based on age-, sex- and calendar time-adjusted national rates, were 80 (195 deaths observed; 95% CI, 70–90) for deaths from all causes and 70 (50–90) for deaths from malignancy. Dividing the data by exposure category, exposure time or latency did not appreciably change the risk ratios. The small sample size did not allow detailed examination of cancers at specific sites, although six lung cancer cases were observed compared to nine expected. [The Working Group noted that smoking habits were not addressed.]

(iii) *Professional drivers and some other groups exposed to vehicle exhausts*

Ahlberg *et al.* (1981) identified a cohort of Swedish drivers said by the authors to be exposed to diesel exhaust (1865 or 1856 [*sic*] fuel oil tanker drivers and 34 027 other truck drivers) from the national census of 1960. In this cohort, 1143 cancers were registered within the Swedish Cancer Registry in 1961–73. The reference population consisted of 686 708 blue-collar workers from the 1960 census who were thought to have had no exposure to petroleum products or chemicals. The data were adjusted for age and residence. The relative risk for lung cancer was elevated in the whole cohort (1.3; 95% CI, 1.1–1.6) and in Stockholm truck drivers in particular (1.6; 1.2–2.3). From a questionnaire study of 470 professional drivers in Stockholm, it was noted that 78% of fuel truck drivers and 31% of other truck drivers smoked. The authors cited an unpublished study indicating that the comparable smoking rate in Stockholm was 40% and concluded that the results could not be explained by smoking.

Wong *et al.* (1985) studied a cohort of 34 156 male members of a heavy construction equipment operators' union in the USA with potential exposure to diesel exhaust. Cohort members had to have been a union member for at least one year between 1 January 1964 and 31 December 1978, by which time 3345 had died and 1765 (5.2%) could not be traced. Death certificates were obtained for all but 102 (3.1%) decedents. No information was available for jobs held before 1967 and limited information was available on jobs held between 1967 and 1978. The SMRs, based on national figures, adjusted for age, sex, race and calendar time, were 81 (95% CI, 79–84) for all causes, 93 (87–99.6) for all cancers, 99 (88–110) for lung cancer (ICD7 162–163) and 118 (78–172) for bladder cancer. The data were also analysed by duration of union membership, latent period, retirement status, job category and exposure status. Significant upward trends in risk were detected for lung cancer with duration of union membership, used as a surrogate for duration of potential exposure to diesel exhaust, with SMRs for lung cancer of 45 [22–83], 75 [49–111], 108 [81–141], 102 [78–132] and 107 [91–125] for workers with <5, 5–9, 10–14, 15–19 and ≥20 years of union membership, respectively. A significant upward trend was also noted for lung cancer with latent period. Mortality from cancers of the digestive system (SMR, 142; 116–173) and respiratory system (SMR, 162; 138–190) and from lymphosarcoma and reticulosarcoma (SMR, 231; 111–425) was elevated in retirees. Exclusion of early retirees did not remove the risks for respiratory cancer or lymphatic cancer. In general, groups with jobs with presumed high exposure to diesel fumes did not show the excesses reported above. A random sample of union members was surveyed to determine smoking habits, and no significant difference between members and the general population was revealed.

In a review, Steenland (1986) presented data on a preliminary study of the mortality experience of about 10 000 teamsters (truck drivers, dock workers, mechanics and jobs outside the trucking industry) who had died in 1982–83 and had worked for at least ten years in a teamster job. Using occupational data on death certificates, proportionate mortality ratios were calculated for lung cancer for 255 mechanics (226; 95% CI, 162–309), 5834 truck drivers (154; 144–166), 490 dock workers (132; 99–175) and 1064 others (116; 95–142). [The Working Group noted that this was an interim report and that judgement should be reserved until the final results are available.]

Gustafsson et al. (1986) studied 6071 Swedish 'dockers' assumed by the authors to have been exposed to diesel exhaust and first employed before 1974 for at least six months. The group had been followed for death from 1 January 1961 or from the date of first employment (if this date occurred later) through to 1 January 1981. Age-, calendar time- and region-specific rates were used to generate expected numbers of deaths. The SMRs were 89 (95% CI, 84–94) for all causes, 103 for all cancers, 132 for lung cancer (105–166) and 110 (85–142) for urogenital tract cancer. Cancer morbidity was determined among 6063 workers who had been alive and without cancer on 1 January 1961 and were followed through to 1 January 1980; a standard morbidity ratio of 110 (101–120; 452 cases) was seen for cancers at all sites and of 168 (136–207; 86 cases) for lung cancer. [The Working Group noted that there was no consideration of duration, intensity or latency of exposure or of smoking habits in this study.]

Stern et al. (1981) examined mortality patterns among 1558 white male vehicle examiners who had been employed in New Jersey, USA, for at least six months between 1944 and 1973. The vital status of all but eight (0.5%) of these was ascertained as of 31 August 1973; these eight were assumed to be alive. Approximately 63% of the cohort members had begun employment prior to 1957. A modified life-table analysis was used to generate the expected number of cause-specific deaths on the basis of national rates, adjusting for age and calendar time. There were 52 deaths from cancer (47.8 expected [SMR, 109; 95% CI, 81–143]). The SMRs for malignant disease increased significantly with latency: 0–9 years, 69 [25–151]; 10–19 years, 98 [56–159]; 20–29 years, 107 [62–171]; >30 years, 189 [101–323]. Cancer at no specific organ site accounted for this excess. The exposure of interest was carbon monoxide, but the authors speculated that other components of automobile exhaust might have been responsible. No information on smoking habits was available for deceased workers, but COHb levels in currently nonsmoking workers increased during the work shift, indicating exposure to exhaust.

In a cohort study of white men enlisted in the US Navy (Garland et al., 1988), 143 cases of testicular cancer were identified in the period 1974–79; age-specific incidence rates were similar to those for the US population, derived from the US National Cancer Institute

Surveillance, Epidemiology and End Results (SEER) programme for 1973−77. Of 110 occupational groups in the Navy, three involving maintenance of gasoline and diesel engines and daily exposure to their exhaust emissions (aviation support equipment technicians, enginemen and construction mechanics) had significantly high standardized incidence ratios for testicular cancer: 3.4 (95% CI, 1.9−5.6) in comparison to SEER rates, and 3.8 (2.1−6.3) in comparison to men in the US Navy as a whole, based on 15 cases. The authors noted that this was a hypothesis-generating study and that the men also had potential daily exposure to solvents and other chemicals.

(iv) *Miners*

Although diesel engines have been used in many mines for a number of years, the Working Group decided not to consider all groups of miners because they may be exposed concurrently to other potential lung carcinogens such as radon decay products, heavy metals and silica, and there was no way that the possible confounding effects of such factors could be determined from the data available in published reports.

Waxweiler *et al.* (1973) studied potash miners and millers, who are exposed to no known carcinogens in the ore, who had been employed for at least one year between January 1940 and July 1967 by eight companies. The vital status of the cohort was identified to July 1967. Of a total of 3886 men, 31 could not be traced and were assumed to be alive. Causes of death were compared with those of the general US population, standardized for age, race, sex and calendar time. Of the cohort, 2743 men had worked at least one year underground and less than one year on the surface and 1143 men had worked at least one year on the surface and less than one year underground. In only two of the eight mines were diesel engines used; one mine changed to diesel in 1949 and the other in 1957. Death certificates were available for 433 of the 438 workers who had died. The effect of smoking was taken into account. No excess mortality from lung cancer was seen in either surface or underground miners. Mortality rates did not differ between the mines with diesel vehicles and those without. The authors noted the short follow-up, the small expected numbers of deaths and the broad classification of causes of death.

(*d*) *Case-control studies*

(i) *Lung cancer*

Williams *et al.* (1977) examined cancer incidence and its relationship to occupation and industry in a study based on the US Third National Cancer Survey. In this study, detailed personal interviews were sought for 13 179 cancer patients (a random 10% sample of all incident invasive tumours occurring in three years in eight areas in the USA) and obtained for 7518 (57%). The numbers of cases of cancer at various anatomical sites were compared with that of cases at all other sites combined. The interview included occupational history (main employment and recent employment), other demographic data and information on smoking and drinking habits; the analysis also controlled for age, sex, race and geographical location. A statistically nonsignificant lung cancer excess (odds ratio, 1.5; [CI could not be calculated]) was observed for truck drivers, which could not be accounted for by smoking.

Intensity, duration of exposure and latency were not evaluated. [The Working Group noted the potential for bias due to the relatively low level of compliance with the questionnaire.]

In a population-based case-control study, Coggon et al. (1984) used the data on occupation on the death certificates of all men under the age of 40 years in England and Wales who had died of tracheobronchial carcinoma during the period 1975-79; 598 cases were detected, 582 of which were matched with two and the rest with one control who had died from any other cause, for sex, year of death, local authority district of residence and year of birth. Occupations were coded using the Office of Population Census and Surveys 1970 classification of occupations, and a job-exposure matrix was constructed by an occupational hygienist, in which the occupations were grouped according to likely exposure to each of nine known or putative carcinogens. All occupations entailing exposure to diesel fumes were associated with an elevated odds ratio for bronchial carcinoma (1.3; 95% CI, 1.0-1.6); however, for occupations with presumed high exposure, the odds ratio was 1.1 (0.7-1.8). [The Working Group noted the limited information on occupation from death certificates, the young age of the subjects and the consequent short times of exposure and latency, and the lack of information on smoking habits and on the possible confounding effects of other carcinogenic exposures.]

In a hospital-based case-control study (Hall & Wynder, 1984) in 18 hospitals in six US cities, 502 men with histologically confirmed primary lung cancer (20-80 years old) and 502 control patients, matched for age, race and hospital were identified. Patients were interviewed between December 1980 and November 1982. Half of the controls had cancer; patients with tobacco-related diseases were excluded. The questionnaire included items on smoking habits, demographic variables and usual occupation. Occupations were grouped either dichotomously as exposed to diesel exhaust (warehousemen, bus drivers, truck drivers, railroad workers and heavy equipment repairmen and operators) or nonexposed, or, in a separate evaluation, in three presumed categories of frequency of exposure in the job (high, moderate, little). Using the dichotomous division, the exposed group had a significantly elevated odds ratio (2.0; 95% CI, 1.2-3.2), which, however, decreased to 1.4 (0.8-2.4; not significant) when adjusted for smoking. The crude odds ratios were 1.7 (0.6-4.6) for a high probability of exposure to diesel exhaust and 0.7 (0.4-1.3) for a moderate probability of exposure. [The Working Group questioned the possible consequences on risk estimates of excluding patients with tobacco-related diseases from the control group.]

In a hypothesis-generating case-control study, Buiatti et al. (1985) investigated the occupational histories of histologically confirmed cases of primary lung cancer among residents of metropolitan Florence, Italy, diagnosed during 1981-83 in the regional general hospital and referral centre for lung cancers in the Province of Florence. For the 376 cases (340 men, 36 women), 892 controls (817 men, 75 women), matched by sex, age, date of admission and smoking status in seven categories, were selected from the medical service of the same hospital, excluding patients with lung cancer, attempted suicides and patients not resident in metropolitan Florence. Each case and control completed a structured questionnaire on demographic variables and on all jobs held for more than one year. The jobs were classified into 21 major classes and 251 subclasses, using the International Labour Office classification. Odds ratios for industries and occupations (ever *versus* never worked) were calculated using logistic regression, in which age and smoking status were included. Taxi drivers had an elevated relative risk for lung cancer after adjusting for tobacco smoking (1.8; 95% CI, 1.0–3.4). [The Working Group noted that multiple comparisons were made, increasing the probability that statistically significant results would be found.]

In a case-control study in northern Sweden, Damber and Larsson (1987) analysed the association between lung cancer and occupation. The cases were 604 male lung cancers reported to the Swedish Cancer Registry during 1972–77 and who had died before May 1979. For each case, a control was drawn from the National Registry for Causes of Deaths, and was matched for sex, year of death, age and municipality; cases of lung cancer and attempted suicide were excluded as controls. In addition, for each case, one living control (less than 80 years old) was drawn from the National Population Registry, matched for sex, year of birth and municipality. Information on residence, occupation, employment and smoking habits was collected by a questionnaire mailed to surviving relatives and to living controls; the response rates were 98% for cases and 96% and 97% for dead and living controls, respectively. Information was requested on all jobs held for at least one year and on lifetime smoking history. A linear logistic regression model, using three discrete levels of employment (<1 year, 1–20 years, and >20 years) and four levels of lifetime tobacco consumption, was used to calculate odds ratios. For professional drivers with more than 20 years' employment, the unmatched odds ratio was 1.5 (95% CI, 0.9–2.6) in comparison with dead controls; this was reduced to 1.2 (0.6–2.2) after adjustment for smoking. The figures obtained in comparison with living controls were 1.7 (0.9–3.2) and 1.1 (0.6–2.2), respectively.

Garshick *et al.* (1987) performed a case-control study on lung cancer deaths among employed and retired US male railroad workers with ten or more years of service, who had been born on 1 January 1900 or after and who had died between 1 March 1981 and February 1982. Cases of primary lung cancer (1256) were matched to two controls by age and date of death. Workers who had died from cancer, suicide, accident or unknown causes were not included among controls. Potential exposure to diesel exhaust was assigned on the basis of an industrial hygiene evaluation of the >150 railroad jobs and areas described by the US Interstate Commerce Commission. Job codes for each worker were available from the US Railroad Retirement Board starting in 1959 and ending with death or retirement. For workers who had retired between 1955 and 1959, the last railroad job held was available. Asbestos exposure prior to 1959 was categorized by job held in 1959 (end of steam locomotive era) or by the last job before retirement, if this was before 1959. Smoking history was obtained by questionnaire from the next-of-kin. Using multiple conditional logistic regression analysis to adjust for smoking and asbestos exposure, workers 64 years of age or younger at time of death who had worked in a diesel exhaust-exposed job for 20 years had a significantly elevated odds ratio for lung cancer (1.4; 95% CI, 1.1–1.9). No such effect was observed among older workers (0.91; 0.71–1.2), many of whom had retired shortly after the transition to diesel-powered locomotives and were therefore not exposed.

In a population-based case-control study (Lerchen *et al.*, 1987), all white and Hispanic white residents of New Mexico, USA, aged 25–84 years, with primary lung cancer, excluding bronchioalveolar carcinoma, diagnosed between 1 January 1980 and 31 December 1982, were identified from the New Mexico Tumor Registry. The cases (333 men and 173 women) were frequency matched with controls selected randomly from the telephone directory or, for persons 65 years or older, from the roster of participants in a health insurance scheme, for sex, ethnic group and ten-year age band at a ratio of approximately 1.5 controls per case (449 men and 272 women). Detailed occupational and smoking histories were obtained by personal interview, with response rates of 89% for cases and 83% for controls. Next-of-kin provided interviews for 50% of the male and 43% of the female cases and for 2% of the controls; the authors recognized the possible bias introduced by this practice. The odds ratio for exposure to diesel exhaust fumes, adjusted for age, ethnic group and smoking, was 0.6 (95% CI, 0.2–1.6). [The Working Group noted the possible bias in choosing controls from the telephone directory when cases are not required to have a telephone or to be listed.]

In a case-control study of lung cancer in France (Benhamou *et al.*, 1988), 1625 histologically confirmed cases and 3091 controls, matched for sex, age at diagnosis, hospital admission and interviewer, completed a questionnaire on residence, education, occupation, and smoking and drinking habits. All occupations held for more than one year were recorded and coded without knowledge of the case status of the patient, using the International Standard Classification of Occupations and according to chemical or physical exposures. The analysis was limited to men (1260 cases and 2084 controls); adjustment was made for age at starting smoking, amount smoked and duration of smoking. Several occupations were associated with increased odds ratios for lung cancer, including miners and quarry men (2.1; 95% CI, 1.1–4.3) and transport equipment operators (1.4; 1.1–1.8); the subcategory of motor vehicle drivers also had an increased risk (1.4; 1.1–1.9).

(ii) *Bladder cancer*

In a population-based case-control study in Canada (Howe *et al.*, 1980), all patients with bladder cancer newly diagnosed in three Canadian provinces between April 1974 and June 1976 were identified; 77% of the patients were interviewed, and for each patient one neighbourhood control, individually matched for age and sex, was interviewed. In the analysis, 632 case-control pairs (480 male and 152 female) were included. Lifetime smoking and employment histories were obtained, and exposure to dusts and fumes was elucidated. Elevated odds ratios were observed for railroad workers [not further defined] (9.0; 95% CI, 1.2–394.5; nine exposed cases) and for exposure to diesel and traffic exhaust (2.8; 0.8–11.8; 11 exposed cases).

In a death certificate-based case-control study (Coggon *et al.*, 1984; for details, see description on p. 139), the occupations of 291 bladder cancer cases and 578 hospital controls were compared. The odds ratio for all diesel fume-exposed occupations was 1.0 (95% CI, 0.7–1.3) and that for occupations with high exposure was 1.7 (0.9–3.3). [The Working Group had the same reservations about this study as expressed on p. 139.]

In a population-based case-control study, the relationship between truck driving and bladder cancer was investigated (Hoar & Hoover, 1985). Cases consisted of all white residents of New Hampshire and Vermont, USA, who had died from bladder cancer in

1975—79. One control per case was selected randomly from all other deaths among residents, excluding suicides, and matched for state, sex, age, race and year of death. A second control per case was selected with the additional matching criterion of county of residence. There were 230 and 210 eligible cases in the two states, respectively; the rate of response to interview was 87% for New Hampshire and 58% for Vermont, and the non-respondents were similar to the respondents with respect to case-control status, sex, age and county of residence. The odds ratio for ever having been a truck driver was 1.5 (95% CI, 0.9—2.6), and there was a significant trend between bladder cancer risk and number of years of truck driving: odds ratios, 1.4 (0.6—3.3), 2.9 (1.2—6.7) and 1.8 (0.8—4.1) for those employed as truck drivers for 1—4, 5—9 and >10 years, respectively. Additional adjustment for age, county, coffee drinking or cigarette smoking (six categories) did not alter these crude odds ratios. [The Working Group noted the nonlinearity of the trend.]

In a hospital-based case-control study in Turin, Italy (Vineis & Magnani, 1985), 512 male cases and 596 male controls randomly selected from among other patients in the main hospital of the city of Turin between 1978 and 1983 were interviewed for lifetime occupational and smoking histories. Occupations were coded using the International Labour Office classification, and associations between specific chemicals and bladder cancer were studied using a job exposure matrix. Adjusting for age and smoking, the odds ratio for bladder cancer for truck drivers was 1.2 (95% CI, 0.6—2.5).

In a hospital-based case-control study, Wynder *et al.* (1985) examined the occupational histories and life style factors (smoking, alcohol and coffee consumption, demographic factors) of 194 male cases of histologically confirmed bladder cancer, 20—80 years of age, diagnosed during two-and-a-half years (January 1981—May 1983) in 18 hospitals in six US cities, and of 582 controls, matched by age, race, year of interview and hospital of admission, hospitalized during the same period for diseases not related to tobacco use. The participation rate among eligible subjects was 75% among cases and 72% among controls. 'Usual' occupation was coded according to an abbreviated list of the US Bureau of Census codes. No significant association was detected between bladder cancer and occupations presumed to involve exposure to diesel exhaust: warehousemen and materials handlers, bus and truck drivers, railroad workers, heavy equipment operators and mechanics (odds ratio, 0.87; 95% CI, 0.47—1.6). [The Working Group questioned the possible consequences on risk estimates of excluding patients with tobacco-related diseases from the control group.]

Data from all ten areas of the US National Bladder Cancer Study were used to evaluate the association of motor exhausts with bladder cancer (Silverman *et al.*, 1986). The study group comprised 1909 white male cases with histologically confirmed bladder carcinoma or papilloma not specified as benign and 3569 frequency-matched controls. Significantly elevated age- and smoking-adjusted odds ratios for bladder cancer were observed for truck drivers or delivery men, and for taxi drivers or chauffeurs: 1.5 (95% CI, 1.1—2.0) and 6.3 (1.6—29.3) for 'usual' occupation, 1.3 (1.1—1.4) and 1.6 (1.2—2.2) for 'ever' occupation. For bus drivers, the odds ratios did not reach significance (1.3, 0.9—1.9 and 1.5, 0.6—3.9 for 'ever' and 'usual', respectively). When allowance was made for a 50-year latency, a significant trend with increasing duration of employment as a truck driver was observed: 1.2, 1.4, 2.1 and 2.2 for a duration of employment of <5, 5—9, 10—24 and >25 years, respectively

($p<0.0001$). Information on subsets of this cohort has been published elsewhere (Silverman et al., 1983; Schoenberg et al., 1984; Smith et al., 1985). In the Detroit subset (Silverman et al., 1983), the adjusted odds ratio for bladder cancer for truck drivers who had never driven a vehicle with a diesel engine was 1.4 (0.7–2.9) and that for men who had ever driven a vehicle with a diesel engine was 11.9 (2.3–61.1).

Occupational risk factors were investigated as part of a population-based case-control study in Copenhagen, Denmark (Jensen et al., 1987). Between May 1979 and April 1981, a total of 412 live patients with bladder cancer (invasive tumours and papillomas) were reported in the study, 389 of whom were interviewed. Live controls were selected at random from the municipalities where the cases lived, and the sample was stratified to match the cases with regard to sex and age in five-year groups. Among the 1052 controls approached, the overall participation rate was 75%. Cases and controls were interviewed for information on occupational history coded according to the Danish version of the International Standard Industrial Classification. Cigarette smoking was adjusted for in the analysis by using two dichotomous variables (ever/never smoked, current/noncurrent smoker) and a continuous variable (logarithm of pack-years smoked). The adjusted odds ratio for bladder cancer was elevated in land transport workers (1.6; 95% CI, 1.1–2.3). The adjusted odds ratios for bladder cancer for bus, taxi and truck drivers were 0.7 (0.4–1.5), 1.6 (0.8–3.4), 3.5 (1.1–11.6) and 2.4 (0.9–6.6) for durations of employment of 1–9, 10–19, 20–29 and >30 years, respectively, representing a significant trend with duration of employment. The trend was not significant for land transport workers.

In a hospital-based case-control study in Argentina (Iscovich et al., 1987), 120 patients with histologically confirmed bladder carcinoma admitted to ten general hospitals in Greater La Plata between March 1983 and December 1985 were identified. The 117 patients who could be interviewed represented approximately 60% of all incident cases. For each case, a hospital control from the same establishment was selected (patients with diseases associated with tobacco smoking constituted 12% of the control group); a neighbourhood control, matched for age and sex, was also selected. Information on smoking and past and present occupations was collected by questionnaire. An exposure index based on a job-exposure matrix was generated. The adjusted odds ratio for truck and railway drivers was 4.3 [95% CI, 2.1–29.6].

Covering the period 1960–82, Steenland et al. (1987) identified 731 male bladder cancer (ICD-9 188) deaths in the Hamilton County, Ohio, region, where there is a known high bladder cancer rate. Six controls were matched to each case on sex and residence in the county at the time of death, year of death, age of death and race. Death certificates and city directories for all residents over 18 were used to identify job history. The first two controls that were listed in the directory within at least five years of the first listing of the cases were selected. Of the 648 cases (89%) listed in the directories, all but 21 had two controls; the remaining 21 had one control. A comparable analysis of all 731 cases and two controls per case was carried out using usual lifetime occupation from the death certificate. A significant increase in the frequency of bladder cancer was found for men with more than 20 years' duration of employment, identified through the city directories as truck drivers (odds ratio, 12.0 [95% CI, 2.3–62.9]; six cases, one control) and railroad workers (odds ratio, 2.2

[95% CI, 1.2—4.0]). Notably, those workers identified as 'drivers not otherwise specified' for ≥20 years had an odds ratio of 0.15 [95% CI, 0—0.8]. In contrast, on the basis of job ever held identified from either the death certificate or the city directory (without taking duration into account), none of the above findings was significant. [The Working Group noted that this study involved application of a new methodology for exposure ascertainment, which requires further validation.]

In a case-control study of bladder cancer incidence in Edmonton, Calgary and Toronto and Kingston, Canada (Risch *et al.*, 1988), 826 cases of histologically verified bladder cancer were compared with 792 population-based controls matched for age, sex and area of residence. Cases were aged 35—79 and had been ascertained between 1979 and 1982. Information was collected by questionnaire, administered by personal interview, covering family, medical, occupational, residential, smoking and dietary histories. Analysis of the occupational data included adjustment for lifetime smoking habits. Among other findings related to occupation and industry was that the 309 men who had had jobs with exposure to engine exhausts had an odds ratio of 1.5 (95% CI, 1.2—2.0) for 'ever' exposure and an odds ratio of 1.7 (1.2—2.3) for exposure during the period eight to 28 years prior to diagnosis. The authors also calculated that there was a significant increase in trend with duration of exposure for each ten years (1.2; 1.1—1.4). This relationship was not seen for women, but only 19 had been exposed. The relationship was also not seen when an analysis was undertaken by exposure to 18 categories of substances, including engine exhaust. [The Working Group found it difficult to interpret the differences in risk seen when exposure was defined in various ways.]

(iii) *Other and multiple sites*

In a hypothesis-generating, hospital-based case-control study in Sweden, Flodin *et al.* (1987) analysed the association between occupation and multiple myeloma. The cases were in persons diagnosed between 1973 and 1983 and still alive during 1981—83. From comparisons with cancer registry data, it was concluded that the cases represented one-third of all cases diagnosed in the area. Controls were drawn randomly from population registers. There were 131 cases and 431 controls for analysis. Information on occupational history, X-ray treatment and smoking habits were obtained by a mailed questionnaire. The crude odds ratio for occupational exposure to engine exhaust was 2.3 (95% CI, 1.4—3.7); this association remained significant after adjusting for confounding variables. In a study using the same set of controls (431) and source of cases, Flodin *et al.* (1988) investigated the association with occupational exposures for 111 cases of chronic lymphatic [lymphocytic] leukaemia. The crude odds ratio for occupational exposure to engine exhausts was 2.5 (95% CI, 1.5—4.0); the association remained significant after adjustment for confounding variables. [The Working Group noted that the study population and control of confounding were not clearly described, and that exposure to engine exhausts was self-reported and not further defined by the authors.]

In a large, hypothesis-generating, population-based case-control study in Canada (Siemiatycki *et al.*, 1988), the associations between ten types of engine exhaust and combustion products and cancers at 12 different sites were evaluated. The 3726 cancer patients diagnosed in any of the 19 participating hospitals in Montreal were interviewed (rate of response, 82%). The patients were all men aged 35–70 years. For each cancer site, patients with cancers at other sites comprised the control group. The interview elicited a detailed job history, and a team of chemists and industrial hygienists translated each job into a list of potential exposures (Gérin *et al.*, 1985). The probability of exposure ('possible', 'probable', 'definite'), the frequency of exposure (<5, 5–30, >30% working time) and the level of exposure (low, medium, high) were estimated. Separate analyses were performed for oat-cell, squamous-cell, adenocarcinoma and other carcinomas of the lungs. After stratifying for age, socioeconomic status, ethnic group, cigarette smoking and blue-/white-collar job history, an elevated odds ratio was observed for squamous-cell cancer of the lung and exposure to gasoline engine exhaust (OR, 1.2; 90% CI, 1.0–1.4). In a detailed analysis in which all covariables that changed the estimate of the disease-exposure odds ratio by more than 10% were included as confounders, further associations were revealed: long-term high-level exposure to gasoline engine exhaust (1.4; 1.1–1.8) and short-term high-level exposure to diesel engine exhaust (1.5; 0.9–2.7) were associated with squamous-cell cancer of the lung. The odds ratio for squamous-cell cancer of the lung (1.5; 0.9–2.5) was also elevated for bus, truck and taxi drivers (classified as exposed to gasoline engine exhaust) and for mining and quarrying (classified as exposed to diesel engine exhaust; 2.8, 1.4–5.8), but analyses by duration and intensity of exposure did not support a causal association. Marginally elevated odds ratios were also seen for colon cancer and exposure to diesel engine exhaust (1.3; 1.1–1.6); for cancer of the rectum (1.6; 1.1–2.3) and kidney (1.4; 1.0–2.0) with long-term high-level exposure to gasoline engine exhaust; for colon cancer (1.7; 1.2–2.5) with long-term high-level exposure to diesel engine exhaust; and for rectal cancer (1.5; 1.0–2.2) in bus, truck and taxi drivers. [The Working Group noted that 90% CI were used and that, at the 95% level, most of the intervals would have included unity.]

(*e*) *Childhood cancer*

Studies have been carried out to examine the hypothesis that exposure of adults to engine exhaust may result in mutations in germ cells, direct intrauterine exposure or early postnatal exposure.

In a case-control study in Québec, Canada (Fabia & Thuy, 1974), occupation of the father at time of birth was ascertained from the birth certificates of 386 children (out of 402 patients ascertained from death certificates, hospital insurance data and hospital records) who had died from malignant disease before the age of five years in 1965–70 and of 772 control children whose birth registration immediately preceded or followed that of the case in the official records. The occupation of the father was not known for 30 cases or for 56 controls. Father's occupation was recorded as motor vehicle mechanic or service station attendant for 29 (7.5%) cases and 29 (3.8%) controls [odds ratio, 2.1 (95% CI, 1.2–3.4)] and as driver for 19 (4.9%) cases and 49 (6.4%) controls [0.76 (0.4–1.3)].

In a case-control study in Finland (Hakulinen *et al.*, 1976), all 1409 incident cases of cancer in children under 15 years reported to the Cancer Registry in 1959–68 were ascertained. Paternal occupation was obtained from antenatal clinic records for the first trimester of pregnancy. After excluding twins and cases for which the father's occupation was unobtainable, 852 cases were available for analysis. For each case, a child with date of birth immediately before that of the case and who had been born in the same maternity welfare district was chosen as a control. Leukaemias and lymphomas (339 pairs; 158 under five years of age), brain tumours (219 pairs; 77 under five years of age) and other tumours (294 pairs; 160 under five years of age) were analysed separately; analyses were carried out separately for the whole group (children under 15 years of age) and for children under five years of age at the time of diagnosis. Paternal occupation as a motor vehicle driver was not more frequent in any group of cases than in controls: the odds ratio for leukaemia in children under five (based on 14 cases) was 0.74 (95% CI, 0.34—1.6); that for leukaemia and lymphoma in the whole group (35 cases), 1.1 (0.63—1.8); that for brain tumours in children under five (four cases), 0.17 (0.00—1.4); and that for brain tumours in the whole group (16 cases), 0.67 (0.29—1.5). [The Working Group noted that only 60% of cases were available for analysis.]

In a case-control study in Connecticut, USA (Kantor *et al.*, 1979), paternal occupation was ascertained from birth certificates for all 149 cases of Wilms' tumour (aged 0—19 years) reported to the Connecticut Tumor Registry in 1935—73 and for 149 controls selected from State Health Department files and matched for sex, race and year of birth. The father's occupation was recorded as driver for eight cases and four controls [odds ratio, 2.1 (95% CI, 0.6—6.7)], as motor vehicle mechanic for six cases and one control [6.2 (0.8—49.8)] and as service station attendant for three cases and no control.

In a case-control study on the association between paternal occupation and childhood cancer (Kwa & Fine, 1980), 692 children born in 1947—57 or 1963—67 and who had died of cancer before the age of 15 in Massachusetts, USA, were identified from the National Center for Health Statistics. Two controls were selected from the registry of births for each case — one born immediately before the case and the other immediately after. Paternal occupation was taken from birth certificates and classified into one of nine categories on the basis of the type of chemical exposures involved. Mechanic/service station attendant was recorded as the father's occupation for 21 (4.9%) leukaemia/lymphoma cases [odds ratio, 1.1 (95% CI, 0.7—1.5)], six (4.5%) cases of neurological cancer [1.02 (0.4—2.4)], four (11.8%) cases of urinary tract cancer [2.9 (1.0—8.1); significant], four (4.2%) cases of all other cancers [0.93 (0.34—2.6)] and 61 (4.4%) controls. No excess of leukaemia/lymphoma, neurological cancer, urinary tract cancer or all other cancer was observed in the children of fathers who were motor vehicle drivers.

In a case-control study on associations between childhood cancer and parental occupation (Zack *et al.*, 1980), the parents of 296 children with cancer followed at a haematology clinic in Houston, TX, USA, from March 1976 to December 1977 and three sets of controls were interviewed for demographic information and job history in the year preceding the birth of the child until diagnosis of cancer. The first set of controls comprised 283 fathers and stepfathers and 283 mothers and stepmothers of children without cancer in the same clinic; the second set consisted of siblings of the parents of the case (413 uncles and 425 aunts), matched by age and number of children; and the third set was selected from among residents in the neighbourhood of the cases (228 fathers and 237 mothers). The proportion of cases with paternal occupation as motor vehicle mechanic, service station attendant or driver did not differ from that in any control group [crude odds ratio in comparison with the first control group, 0.59 (95% CI, 0.28−1.2); that in comparison with the second control group, 0.79 (0.38−1.6); and that in comparison with neighbourhood controls, 0.92 (0.40−2.1)]. [The Working Group noted that the selection criteria were not given for either cases or controls, that it was unclear whether information on exposure was obtained from mothers or fathers or both, and that confounding factors were not taken into consideration.]

Hemminki *et al.* (1981) obtained data from the Finnish Cancer Registry on children less than 15 years old with cancer diagnosed in 1959−75 and on parental occupation, as in the study of Hakulinen *et al.* (1976; see pp. 145−146). The odds ratio for the father of a child with leukaemia in 1969−75 being a professional driver was 1.9 [95% CI, 1.1−3.7].

In a proportionate mortality study in England and Wales (Sanders *et al.*, 1981), paternal occupations recorded on the death certificates of children under 15 years of age during the years 1959−63 and 1970−72 (167 646 deaths; 6920 deaths from neoplasms) were investigated. Proportionate mortality ratios for neoplasms were not elevated for children of fathers employed as 'drivers of stationary engines, cranes, etc.', as transport workers or as warehousemen.

Associations between paternal occupation and childhood leukaemia and brain tumours were investigated in a case-control study in Maryland, USA (Gold *et al.*, 1982). Children under the age of 20 with leukaemia (diagnosed in 1969−74) or brain tumours (diagnosed in 1965−74) were ascertained in the Baltimore Standard Metropolitan Statistical Area from hospital records, death certificates, hospital tumour registries and from the pathology, radiotherapy and clinical oncology records of 21 of 23 Baltimore hospitals. There were two control groups: one consisted of children with no malignant disease, selected from birth certificates at the Maryland State Health Department and matched for sex, date of birth and race; the other group consisted of children with malignancies other than leukaemia or brain cancer, matched for sex, race, date of diagnosis and age at diagnosis. Information on occupational exposures of both parents before the birth of the child and between birth and diagnosis was collected by interviewing the mother. A total of 43 children had leukaemia and 70 had brain tumours. The paternal occupational category that included driver, motor vehicle mechanic, service station attendant or railroad worker was not more frequent for children with leukaemia or brain tumours than for the control children. [The Working Group noted the small numbers involved and found the results difficult to interpret.]

In a case-control study on childhood leukaemia and neuroblastoma (Vianna *et al.*, 1984), children born in 1949−78 who were diagnosed with acute leukaemia during the first year of life and reported to the Tumor Registry of the New York State Health Department or with neuroblastoma up to 12 years of age at diagnosis were identified. Using information from birth certificates, two sets of controls were selected: one was matched by year of birth, sex, race and county of residence; the other was additionally matched for age of the mother and birth order of the child. Information on parental age, race, education and occupation, and medical, obstetrical and therapeutic histories were obtained by telephone interview of the mothers. Of 65 eligible cases of leukaemia, 60, with two controls each, were finally included in the analysis. The odds ratio for acute leukaemia for children with 'high' presumed paternal exposure to motor exhaust fumes (service station attendants, automobile or truck repairmen, aircraft maintenance personnel) was 2.5 [1.2−5.3] in comparison with the first control group and 2.4 [1.1−3.7] in comparison with the second. For 'lower' presumed exposure (taxi drivers, travelling salesmen, truck or bus drivers, railroad workers, toll-booth attendants, highway workers, police officers), the odds ratio was 3.4 [1.4−10.2] in comparison with the first control group and 1.3 [0.8−2.1] in comparison with the second. For the 103 cases of neuroblastoma, there was no significant difference from controls in the number of fathers who had had 'high' exposure. [The Working Group questioned the categorization of exposures as 'high' and 'lower' on the basis of the jobs listed.]

In a case-control study on paternal occupation and Wilms' tumour (Wilkins & Sinks, 1984), 105 patients were identified through the Columbus, OH, USA, Children's Hospital Tumor Registry during the period 1950−81. For each case, two controls were selected from Ohio birth certificate files; the first control series was individually matched for sex, race and year of birth, and the second series was additionally matched for mother's county of residence when the child was born. Due to changes in birth certification, the study included only the 62 cases and their matched controls for which father's occupation was recorded. The crude odds ratio for Wilms' tumour in children with paternal occupation as motor vehicle mechanic, service station attendant or driver/heavy equipment operator was 1.1 [95% CI, 0.36−3.5 compared to both controls taken together].

## 4. Summary of Data Reported and Evaluation

### 4.1 Exhaust composition and exposure data

Internal combustion engines have been used in cars, trucks, locomotives and other motorized machinery for about 100 years. Engine exhausts contain thousands of gaseous and particulate substances. The major gaseous products of both diesel- and gasoline-fuelled engines are carbon dioxide and water, but lower percentages of carbon monoxide, sulfur dioxide and nitrogen oxides as well as low molecular weight hydrocarbons and their derivatives are also formed. Submicron-size particles are present in the exhaust emissions of internal combustion engines. The particles present in diesel engine exhaust are composed mainly of elemental carbon, adsorbed organic material and traces of metallic compounds. The particles emitted from gasoline engines are composed primarily of metallic compounds (especially lead, if present in the fuel), elemental carbon and adsorbed organic material. Soluble organic fractions of the particles contain primarily polycyclic aromatic hydrocarbons, heterocyclic compounds, phenols, nitroarenes and other oxygen- and nitrogen-containing derivatives.

The composition and quantity of the emissions from an engine depend mainly on the type and condition of the engine, fuel composition and additives, operating conditions and emission control devices. Particles emitted from engines operating with gasoline are different from diesel engine exhaust particles in terms of their size distribution and surface properties. Emissions of organic compounds from gasoline (leaded and unleaded) and diesel engines are qualitatively similar, but there are quantitative differences: diesel engines produce two to 40 times more particulate emissions and 20–30 times more nitroarenes than gasoline engines with a catalytic converter in the exhaust system when the engines have similar power output. Gasoline engines without catalytic converters and diesel engines of similar power output produce similar quantities of polycyclic aromatic hydrocarbons per kilometre; catalytic converters of the type used with gasoline vehicles reduce emissions of polycyclic aromatic hydrocarbons by more than ten times. Lead and halogenated compounds are also typically found in emissions from engines using leaded gasoline.

In urban areas, exposures to low levels and short-term peak levels of engine exhausts are ubiquitous. Higher exposures to engine exhausts may occur in some occupations, such as transportation and garage work, underground mining, vehicle maintenance and examination, traffic control, logging, firefighting and heavy equipment operation. The components of exhaust most often quantified in an occupational setting are particles, carbon monoxide and oxides of nitrogen; polycyclic aromatic compounds and aldehydes from engine exhausts have also been measured in work environments.

The exhausts of engines share similar physical and chemical characteristics with airborne materials from many sources. This makes it difficult to quantify the portion of an individual's exposure from the general environment that derives directly from engine exhausts and also complicates assessment of occupational exposures to engine exhausts.

## 4.2 Experimental data

Many studies have been carried out, using several animal species, to evaluate the potential carcinogenicity of exposure to whole exhaust and to components of exhaust from diesel- and gasoline-fuelled internal combustion engines. The studies are considered within six subgroupings: (i) whole diesel engine exhaust; (ii) gas-phase diesel engine exhaust (with particles removed); (iii) diesel engine exhaust particles or extracts of diesel engine exhaust particles; (iv) whole gasoline engine exhaust; (v) condensates/extracts of gasoline engine exhaust; and (vi) engine exhausts in combination with known carcinogens.

*Whole diesel engine exhaust*

Mice, rats, Syrian hamsters and monkeys (*Macaca fascicularis*) were exposed by inhalation to a range of concentrations of whole diesel engine exhaust, with observations in some studies extending to the lifespan of the animals. Five studies conducted using two different strains of rats showed an increased incidence of benign and malignant lung tumours that was related to the exposure concentration. Four of the studies involved exhaust from light-duty engines, and one the exhaust from a heavy-duty engine. One study of rats exposed to exhaust from a light-duty engine did not show a tumorigenic effect. Of three studies in Syrian hamsters, two did not show induction of lung tumours; the other was considered to be inadequate for an evaluation of carcinogenicity. In two studies in mice, the incidences of lung tumours, including adenocarcinomas, were increased over that in concurrent controls; however, in one study, the total incidence of lung tumours was not elevated over that in historical controls. Monkeys exposed for two years to diesel exhaust did not develop lung tumours, but the short duration of the experiment rendered it inadequate for an evaluation of carcinogenicity.

*Gas-phase diesel engine exhaust (with particles removed)*

Three studies in which rats and Syrian hamsters were exposed to diesel engine exhaust from which soot particles had been removed by filtration did not show induction of lung tumours. In one study, mice exposed to filtered diesel engine exhaust had an increased incidence of lung tumours, including adenocarcinomas, compared to concurrent controls, a result similar to that seen with exposure to whole exhaust. However, the total incidence of lung tumours in this study was similar to that of historical controls.

*Diesel engine exhaust particles or extracts of diesel engine exhaust particles*

In other studies, organic extracts of diesel engine exhaust particles were used to evaluate the effects of concentrates of the organic compounds associated with carbonaceous soot particles. These extracts were applied to the skin or administered by intratracheal instillation or intrapulmonary implantation to mice, rats or Syrian hamsters. An excess of skin tumours was observed in mice in one study by skin painting and in one series of studies on tumour initiation using extracts of particles from several different diesel engines. An excess of lung tumours was observed in one study in rats following intrapulmonary implantation of beeswax pellets containing extracts of diesel engine exhaust particles.

In one study, an excess of tumours at the injection site was observed following subcutaneous administration of diesel engine exhaust particles to mice.

*Whole gasoline engine exhaust*

In one study in which rats were exposed by inhalation to whole leaded gasoline engine exhaust for up to two years and observed for up to an additional six months, the incidence of lung tumours was not different from that in controls. A similar study in Syrian hamsters also showed no induction of lung tumours. In a third study, dogs exposed to whole leaded gasoline exhaust for 68 months and held for an additional 32–36 months did not develop lung tumours.

*Condensates/extracts of gasoline engine exhaust*

Condensates/extracts of gasoline engine exhaust have been tested by skin painting, subcutaneous injection, intratracheal instillation or implantation into the lung. An excess of skin tumours was produced in five studies in mice by skin painting and in one series of tumour-initiation studies. An excess of lung tumours was observed in one study in rats that were given intrapulmonary implants of beeswax pellets containing condensates/extracts of gasoline engine exhaust. In one study, an excess of lung adenomas was observed in Syrian hamsters given intratracheal instillations of condensates/extracts of gasoline engine exhaust. Subcutaneous injections of condensates/extracts of gasoline engine exhaust also produced an excess of tumours at the injection site in one study in mice.

*Engine exhausts in combination with known carcinogens*

In studies in which known carcinogens were given to animals exposed either to diesel or gasoline engine exhausts or administered organic compounds from gasoline engine exhaust, inconclusive and inconsistent results were obtained.

## 4.3 Human data

*Studies of workers whose predominant engine exhaust exposure is that from diesel engines*

In the two most informative cohort studies (of railroad workers), one in the USA and one in Canada, the risk for lung cancer in those exposed to diesel engine exhaust increased significantly with duration of exposure in the first study and with increased likelihood of exposure in the second (in which smoking was not considered). Three further studies of cohorts with less certain exposure to diesel engine exhaust were also considered; two studies of London bus company employees showed elevated lung cancer rates that were not statistically significant, but a third, of Swedish dockers, showed a significantly increased risk for lung cancer.

In only two case-control studies of lung cancer (one of US railroad workers and one in Canada) could exposure to diesel engine exhaust be distinguished satisfactorily from exposures to other exhausts; modest increases in risk for lung cancer were seen in both, and in the first the increase was significant. In three further case-control studies, in which exposure to diesel engine exhaust in professional drivers and lung cancer risks were addressed, the Working Group considered that the possibility of mixed exposure to engine exhausts could not be excluded. None of these studies showed a significant increase in risk for lung cancer, although the risk was elevated in two.

In the three cohort studies (on railroad workers, bus company workers and 'dockers', respectively) in which bladder cancer rates were reported, the risk was elevated, although not significantly so. Four of the case-control studies of bladder cancer were designed to examine groups whose predominant engine exhaust exposure was assumed to be to that from diesel engines. Three showed a significantly increased risk for bladder cancer. In one of these, the large US study, a significant trend was also seen with duration of exposure; and in an analysis of one subset of self-reported diesel truck drivers, a substantial, significant relative risk was seen for bladder cancer.

*Studies of workers whose predominant engine exhaust exposure is that from gasoline engines*

Only one cohort study addressed workers exposed predominantly to gasoline engine exhaust (vehicle examiners). The risk for cancer increased with latency; no particular site accounted for this increase. In one case-control study, exposure to gasoline engine exhaust was isolated from that to diesel engine exhaust, but no consistent increase in risk was observed.

*Studies of workers whose predominant engine exhaust exposure cannot be defined*

In a cohort of Swedish drivers, a statistically significantly elevated risk for lung cancer was reported. A second cohort study of heavy construction equipment drivers showed significant increasing trends in lung cancer risk with duration of exposure, but the trend in risk for other smoking-related diseases was also increased. Increased risks for lung cancer were seen in three case-control studies of persons with mixed occupational exposures to engine exhausts in the USA, Italy and France; in two of these, the increase was significant.

In the one cohort study that addressed risk for bladder cancer, the risk was elevated, although not significantly so. In three case-control studies of bladder cancer in the USA, Italy and Denmark, modest increases in risk were seen; two showed significant trends with duration of exposure. In two further studies using the same set of controls, significant associations were also seen with multiple myeloma and chronic lymphocytic leukaemia. Three occupational groups in the US Navy with presumed exposure to engine exhausts were found to have a significantly high incidence of testicular cancer, although the influence of other exposures could not be assessed.

Possible associations between parental exposure to engine exhausts and cancer in children were considered in ten studies. No clear pattern of risk emerged.

## 4.4 Other relevant data

No relevant data were available on the toxic effects or metabolism of engine exhausts in humans, and there was no adequate study to evaluate whether diesel and gasoline engine exhausts induce chromosomal effects in humans.

Prolonged exposure of experimental animals to diesel engine exhaust leads to a number of effects related to the concentration to which they are exposed, including particle accumulation in macrophages, changes in the lung cell population, fibrotic effects and squamous metaplasia, which appear to be correlated with impaired pulmonary clearance. It has also caused exposure-related pathological changes in regional lymph nodes in mice and rats and an apparent increase in immunoglobulin M antibody response.

Prolonged exposure to diesel engine exhaust resulted in DNA adduct formation in rats and protein adduct formation in rats and hamsters.

Exposure of rodents to whole diesel engine exhaust induced sister chromatid exchange but not germ-cell mutations, micronuclei or dominant lethal mutations. Whole diesel engine exhaust induced sister chromatid exchange in cultured human cells. It did not induce sex-linked recessive lethal mutations in *Drosophila melanogaster* and gave inconclusive results in an assay for recombination in yeast. Particles or their extracts induced somatic gene mutations and sister chromatid exchange in rodents *in vivo* but did not induce micronuclei. They induced chromosomal aberrations, sister chromatid exchange and gene mutations in cultured human cells and cell transformation, sister chromatid exchange, gene mutations and DNA damage in rodent cells *in vitro* and inhibited intercellular communication. Particles or their extracts were weakly recombinogenic in yeast and induced mutations and DNA damage in bacteria. The gaseous phase was also mutagenic to bacteria.

Prolonged exposure to gasoline engine exhaust caused protein adduct formation in rats and hamsters.

Whole gasoline engine exhaust induced micronuclei in mice. Gasoline engine exhaust particle extracts induced cell transformation, aneuploidy, chromosomal aberrations, sister chromatid exchange, gene mutations and DNA damage in cultured animal cells but were not recombinogenic in yeast. Whole gasoline engine exhaust, particle extracts and the gaseous phase were mutagenic to bacteria.

## 4.5 Evaluation[1]

There is *sufficient evidence* for the carcinogenicity in experimental animals of whole diesel engine exhaust.

There is *inadequate evidence* for the carcinogenicity in experimental animals of gas-phase diesel engine exhaust (with particles removed).

There is *sufficient evidence* for the carcinogenicity in experimental animals of extracts of diesel engine exhaust particles.

There is *inadequate evidence* for the carcinogenicity in experimental animals of whole gasoline engine exhaust.

There is *sufficient evidence* for the carcinogenicity in experimental animals of condensates/extracts of gasoline engine exhaust.

There is *limited evidence* for the carcinogenicity in humans of diesel engine exhaust.

There is *inadequate evidence* for the carcinogenicity in humans of gasoline engine exhaust.

There is *limited evidence* for the carcinogenicity in humans of engine exhausts (unspecified as from diesel or gasoline engines).

### Overall evaluation

Diesel engine exhaust *is probably carcinogenic to humans (Group 2A)*.

Gasoline engine exhaust *is possibly carcinogenic to humans (Group 2B)*.

---

[1]For definitions of the italicized terms, see Preamble, pp. 25–28.

# Summary table of genetic and related effects of diesel and gasoline engine exhausts

| | Nonmammalian systems | | | | | | | | | | | | | Mammalian systems | | | | | | | | | | | | | | | | | | | | | | |
|---|---|---|---|---|---|---|---|---|---|---|---|---|---|---|---|---|---|---|---|---|---|---|---|---|---|---|---|---|---|---|---|---|---|---|---|
| | Proka-ryotes | | Lower eukaryotes | | | Plants | | | | Insects | | | | In vitro | | | | | | | | | | | | | | | | | In vivo | | | | | |
| | | | | | | | | | | | | | | Animal cells | | | | | | | | Human cells | | | | | | | | Animals | | | | | | | Humans | | | | | |
| | D | G | D | G | R | A | D | G | C | A | R | G | C | A | D | G | S | M | C | A | T | I | D | G | S | M | C | A | T | I | D | G | S | M | C | DL | A | D | S | M | C | A |
| Diesel engine exhaust | +ib | +ab | | ?bc | | | | | | | | | | -c | +b | +b | +b | ?b | +b | +b | | +ib | +b | +bc | | | | | | +ib | +ic | * | +bc | -bc | | -ic | | | ?c | | ?c | |
| Gasoline engine exhaust | +abc | -ib | | | | | | | | | | | | | +ib | +b | +b | | +ib | +b | | | | | | | | | | | | | | +ic | | | | | ?c | | ?c | |

A, aneuploidy; C, chromosomal aberrations; D, DNA damage; DL, dominant lethal mutation; G, gene mutation; I, inhibition of intercellular communication; M, micronuclei; R, mitotic recombination and gene conversion; S, sister chromatid exchange; T, cell transformation

*In completing the tables, the following symbols indicate the consensus of the Working Group with regard to the results for each endpoint:*
+ considered to be positive for the specific endpoint and level of biological complexity
+! considered to be positive, but only one valid study was available to the Working Group
− considered to be negative
−! considered to be negative, but only one valid study was available to the Working Group
? considered to be equivocal or inconclusive (e.g., there were contradictory results from different laboratories; there were confounding exposures; the results were equivocal)

[a] gas
[b] particles or extracts thereof
[c] whole exhaust
*positive in somatic cells[c], negative in germ cells[c]

## 5. References

Abraham, W.M., Kim, C.S., Januszkiewicz, A.J., Welker, M., Mingle, M.A. & Schreck, R. (1980) Effects of a brief low-level exposure to the particulate fraction of diesel exhaust on pulmonary function of conscious sheep. *Arch. environ. Health*, 35, 77–80

Ahlberg, J., Ahlbom, A., Lipping, H., Norell, S. & Österblom, L. (1981) Cancer among professional drivers — a problem-oriented register-based study (Swed.). *Läkartidningen*, 78, 1545–1546

Al-Mutaz, I.S. (1987) Automotive emission problem in Saudi Arabia. *Environ. int.*, 13, 335–338

Alsberg, T., Westerholm, R., Stenberg, U., Strandell, M. & Jansson, B. (1984) Particle associated organic halides in exhausts from gasoline and diesel fueled vehicles. In: Cooke, M. & Dennis, A.J., eds, *Polynuclear Aromatic Hydrocarbons, 8th International Symposium: Mechanisms, Methods and Metabolism*, Columbus, OH, Battelle, pp. 87–97

Alsberg, T., Stenberg, U., Westerholm, R., Strandell, M., Rannug, U., Sundvall, A., Romert, L., Bernson, V., Pettersson, B., Toftgård, R., Franzén, B., Jansson, M., Gustafsson, J.A., Egebäck, K.E. & Tejle, G. (1985) Chemical and biological characterization of organic material from gasoline exhaust materials. *Environ. Sci. Technol.*, 19, 43–50

Ames, R.G., Attfield, M.D., Hankinson, J.L., Hearl, F.J. & Reger, R.B. (1982) Acute respiratory effects of exposure to diesel emissions in coal miners. *Am. Rev. respir. Dis.*, 125, 39–42

Ames, R.G., Hall, D.S. & Reger, R.B. (1984) Chronic respiratory effects of exposure to diesel emissions in coal mines. *Arch. environ. Health*, 39, 389–394

Anon. (1984) Report on the consensus workshop on formaldehyde. *Environ. Health Perspect.*, 58, 323–381

Apol, A.G. (1983) *Health Hazard Evaluation Report No. HETA-82-137-1264, Regional Transportation District, Denver, CO*, Cincinnati, OH, National Institute for Occupational Safety and Health

Aronow, W.S., Harris, C.N., Isbell, M.W., Rokaw, S.N. & Imparato, B. (1972) Effect of freeway travel on angina pectoris. *Ann. intern. Med.*, 77, 669–676

Attfield, M.D., Trabant, G.D. & Wheeler, R.W. (1982) Exposure to diesel fumes and dust at six potash mines. *Ann. occup. Hyg.*, 26, 817–831

Austin, A.C., Claxton, L.D. & Lewtas, J. (1985) Mutagenicity of the fractionated organic emissions from diesel, cigarette smoke condensate, coke oven, and roofing tar in the Ames assay. *Environ. Mutagenesis*, 7, 471–487

Ayres, S.M., Evans, R., Licht, D., Griesbach, J., Reimold, F., Ferrand, E.F. & Criscitiello, A. (1973) Health effects of exposure to high concentrations of automotive emissions. Studies in bridge and tunnel workers in New York City. *Arch. environ. Health*, 27, 168–178

Ball, D.J. (1987) Particulate carbon emissions and diesel vehicles. In: *Proceedings of the Institution of Mechanical Engineers: Vehicle Emissions and their Impact in European Air Quality, March 1987 (C337/87)*, Edmonds, Surrey, Automobile Division of the Institution of Mechanical Engineers, pp. 83–87

Ball, D.J. & Hume, R. (1977) The relative importance of vehicular and domestic emissions of dark smoke in greater London in the mid-1970s, the significance of smoke shade measurements, and an explanation of the relationship of smoke shade to gravimetric measurements of particulate. *Atmos. Environ.*, 11, 1065–1073

Barfknecht, T.R., Andon, B.M., Thilly, W.G. & Hites, R.A. (1981) Soot and mutation in bacteria and human cells. In: Cooke, M. & Dennis, A.J., eds, *Polynuclear Aromatic Hydrocarbons, 5th International Symposium: Chemical Analysis and Biological Fate*, Columbus, OH, Battelle, pp. 231–242

Barnhart, M.I., Chen, S.-T., Salley, S.O. & Puro, H. (1981) Ultrastructure and morphometry of the alveolar lung of guinea pigs chronically exposed to diesel engine exhaust: six months' experience. *J. appl. Toxicol., 1*, 88–103

Barnhart, M.I., Salley, S.O., Chen, S.-T. & Puro, H. (1982) Morphometric ultrastructural analysis of alveolar lungs of guinea pigs chronically exposed by inhalation to diesel exhaust (DE). In: Lewtas, J., ed., *Toxicological Effects of Emissions from Diesel Engines*, Amsterdam, Elsevier, pp. 183–200

Battigelli, M.C. (1965) Effects of diesel exhaust. *Arch. environ. Health, 10*, 165–167

Battigelli, M.C., Mannella, R.J. & Hatch, T.F. (1964) Environmental and clinical investigation of workmen exposed to diesel exhaust in railroad engine houses. *Ind. Med. Surg., 33*, 121–124

Battigelli, M.C., Hengstenberg, F., Mannella, R.J. & Thomas, A.P. (1966) Mucociliary activity. *Arch. environ. Health, 12*, 460–466

Baxter, P.J. & McDowall, M.E. (1986) Occupation and cancer in London: an investigation into nasal and bladder cancer using the Cancer Atlas. *Br. J. ind. Med., 43*, 44–49

Begeman, C.R. & Colucci, J.M. (1962) Apparatus for determining the contribution of the automobile to the benzene-soluble organic matter in air. *Natl Cancer Inst. Monogr., 9*, 17–57

Belisario, M.A., Buonocore, V., De Marinis, E. & De Lorenzo, F. (1984) Biological availability of mutagenic compounds adsorbed onto diesel exhaust particulate. *Mutat. Res., 135*, 1–9

Belisario, M.A., Farina, C. & Buonocore, V. (1985) Evaluation of concentration procedures of mutagenic metabolites from urine of diesel particulate-treated rats. *Toxicol. Lett., 25*, 81–88

Bellmann, B., Muhle, H. & Heinrich, U. (1983) Lung clearance after long time exposure of rats to airborne pollutants. *J. Aerosol Sci., 14*, 194–196

Benhamou, S., Benhamou, E. & Flamant, R. (1988) Occupational risk factors of lung cancer in a French case-control study. *Br. J. ind. Med., 45*, 231–233

Bhatnagar, R.S. (1980) Collagen and prolyl hydroxylase levels in lungs in dogs exposed to automobile exhaust and other noxious gas mixtures. In: Stara, J.F., Dungworth, D.L., Orthoefer, J.G. & Tyler, W.S., eds, *Long-term Effects of Air Pollutants: in Canine Species (EPA-600/8-80-014)*, Washington DC, US Environmental Protection Agency, pp. 71–77

Bice, D.E., Mauderly, J.L., Jones, R.K. & McClellan, R.O. (1985) Effects of inhaled diesel exhaust on immune responses after lung immunization. *Fundam. appl. Toxicol., 5*, 1075–1086

Bini, G. (1973) Lead in the urban environment. 2. *Int. J. environ. Stud., 5*, 131–135

Bjørseth, A., ed. (1983) *Handbook of Polycyclic Aromatic Hydrocarbons*, New York, Marcel Dekker

Bond, J.A., Butler, M.M., Medinsky, M.A., Muggenburg, B.A. & McClellan, R.O. (1984) Dog pulmonary macrophage metabolism of free and particle-associated [$^{14}$C]benzo[a]pyrene. *J. Toxicol. environ. Health, 14*, 181–189

Bond, J.A., Mauderly, J.L., Henderson, R.F. & McClellan, R.O. (1985) Metabolism of 1-[$^{14}$C]nitropyrene in respiratory tract tissue of rats exposed to diesel exhaust. *Toxicol. appl. Pharmacol., 79*, 461–470

Bond, J.A., Sun, J.D., Medinsky, M.A., Jones, R.K. & Yeh, H.C. (1986) Deposition, metabolism, and excretion of 1-[$^{14}$C]nitropyrene and 1-[$^{14}$C]nitropyrene coated on diesel exhaust particles as influenced by exposure concentration. *Toxicol. appl. Pharmacol.*, 85, 102–117

Bradow, R.L. (1980) Diesel particle emissions. *Bull. N.Y. Acad. Med.*, 56, 797–811

Brightwell, J., Fouillet, X., Cassano-Zoppi, A.-L., Bernstein, D., Gatz, R. & Duchosal, F. (1986) Neoplastic and functional changes in rodents after chronic inhalation of engine exhaust emissions. In: Ishinishi, N., Koizumi, A., McClellan, R.O. & Stöber, W., eds, *Carcinogenic and Mutagenic Effects of Diesel Engine Exhaust*, Amsterdam, Elsevier, pp. 471–485

Brightwell, J., Fouillet, X., Cassano-Zoppi, A.-L., Bernstein, D., Crawley, F., Duchosal, F., Gatz, R., Perczel, S. & Pfeifer, H. (1989) Tumours of the respiratory tract in rats and hamsters following chronic inhalation of engine exhaust emissions. *J. appl. Toxicol.*, 9, 23–31

Brooks, A.L., Wolff, R.K., Royer, R.E., Clark, C.R., Sanchez, A. & McClellan, R.O. (1980) Biological availability of mutagenic chemicals associated with diesel exhaust particles. In: Pepelko, W.E., Danner, R.M. & Clarke, N.A., eds, *Health Effects of Diesel Engine Emissions (EPA-600/9-80-057a)*, Cincinnati, OH, US Environmental Protection Agency, pp. 345–358

Brooks, A.L., Li, A.P., Dutcher, J.S., Clark, C.R., Rothenberg, S.J., Kiyoura, R., Bechtold, W.E. & McClellan, R.O. (1984) A comparison of genotoxicity of automotive exhaust particles from laboratory and environmental sources. *Environ. Mutagenesis*, 6, 651–668

Brorström, E., Grennfelt, P., Lindskog, A., Sjödin, A. & Nielsen, T. (1983) Transformation of polycyclic aromatic hydrocarbons during sampling in ambient air by exposure to different oxidized nitrogen compounds and ozone. In: Cooke, M. & Dennis, A.J., eds, *Polynuclear Aromatic Hydrocarbons, 7th International Symposium: Formation, Metabolism and Measurement*, Colombus, OH, Battelle, pp. 201–210

deBruin, A. (1967) Carboxyhemoglobin levels due to traffic exhaust. *Arch. environ. Health*, 15, 384–389

Brune, H., Habs, M. & Schmähl, D. (1978) The tumor-producing effect of automobile exhaust condensate and fractions thereof. Part II: Animal studies. *J. environ. Pathol. Toxicol.*, 1, 737–746

Buiatti, E., Kriebel, D., Geddes, M., Santucci, M. & Pucci, N. (1985) A case control study of lung cancer in Florence, Italy. I. Occupational risk factors. *J. Epidemiol. Commun. Health*, 39, 244–250

Burgess, W.A., DiBerardinis, L. & Speizer, F.E. (1973) Exposure to automobile exhaust. III. An environmental assessment. *Arch. environ. Health*, 26, 325–329

Burgess, W.A., DiBerardinis, L. & Speizer, F.E. (1977) Health effects of exposure to automobile exhaust — V. Exposure of toll booth operators to automobile exhaust. *Am. ind. Hyg. Assoc. J.*, 38, 184–191

Cadle, S.H. & Mulawa, P.A. (1980) Low molecular weight aliphatic amines in exhaust from catalyst-equipped cars. *Environ. Sci. Technol.*, 14, 718–723

Calabrese, E.J., Moore, G.S., Guisti, R.A., Rowan, C.A. & Schulz, E.N. (1981) A review of human health effects associated with exposure to diesel fuel exhaust. *Environ. int.*, 5, 473–477

Campbell, J.A. (1936) The effects of exhaust gases from internal combustion engines and of tobacco smoke upon mice, with special reference to incidence of tumours of the lung. *Br. J. exp. Pathol.*, 17, 146–158

Campbell, K.I., George, E.L. & Washington, I.S., Jr (1981) Enhanced susceptibility to infection in mice after exposure to dilute exhaust from light duty diesel engines. *Environ. int.*, 5, 377–382

Cantrell, E.T., Tyrer, H.W., Peirano, W.B. & Danner, R.M. (1981) Benzo(a)pyrene metabolism in mice exposed to diesel exhaust: II. Metabolism and excretion. *Environ. int.*, 5, 313–316

Cantrell, B.K., Zeller, H.W., Williams, K.L. & Cocalis, J. (1986) Monitoring and measurement of in-mine aerosol: diesel emissions. In: *Diesels in Underground Mines, Proceedings of the Bureau of Mines Technology Transfer Seminar, Louisville KY, 21 April 1987 and Denver CO, 23 April 1987 (BOM Information Circular 9141)*, Washington DC, US Department of the Interior, Bureau of Mines, pp. 18–40

Carey, P.M. (1987) *Air Toxics Emissions from Motor Vehicles (Technical Report) (EPA-AA-TSS-PA-86-5)*, Washington DC, US Environmental Protection Agency

Casto, B.C., Hatch, G.G., Huang, S.L., Lewtas, J., Nesnow, S. & Waters, M.D. (1981) Mutagenic and carcinogenic potency of extracts of diesel and related environmental emissions: in vitro mutagenesis and oncogenic transformation. *Environ. int.*, 5, 403–409

Castranova, V., Bowman, L., Reasor, M.J., Lewis, T., Tucker, J. & Miles, P.R. (1985) The response of rat alveolar macrophages to chronic inhalation of coal dust and/or diesel exhaust. *Environ. Res.*, 36, 405–419

Chamberlain, A.C. (1985) Prediction of response of blood lead to airborne and dietary lead from volunteer experiments with lead isotopes. *Proc. R. Soc. Lond. B.*, 224, 149–182

Chamberlain, A.C., Clough, W.S., Heard, M.J., Newton, D., Stott, A.N.B. & Wells, A.C. (1975) Uptake of lead by inhalation of motor exhaust. *Proc. R. Soc. Lond. B.*, 192, 77–110

Chamberlain, A.C., Heard, M.J., Little, P., Newton, D., Wells, A.C. & Wiffen, R.D. (1978) *Investigations into Lead from Motor Vehicles (Harwell Laboratory Report AERE-R9198)*, London, Her Majesty's Stationery Office

Chambers, D., Farrant, G.B. & Mendham, J. (1984) Lead levels in exhaust replacement centres. *Sci. total Environ.*, 33, 31–36

Chan, T.L., Lee, P.S. & Hering, W.E. (1981) Deposition and clearance of inhaled diesel exhaust particles in the respiratory tract of Fischer rats. *J. appl. Toxicol.*, 1, 77–82

Chan, T.L., Lee, P.S. & Hering, W.E. (1984) Pulmonary retention of inhaled diesel particles after prolonged exposures to diesel exhaust. *Fundam. appl. Toxicol.*, 4, 624–631

Chen, K.C. (1986) Induction of aryl hydrocarbon hydroxylase in rat tissue following intratracheal instillation of diesel particulate extract and benzo[*a*]pyrene. *J. appl. Toxicol.*, 6, 259–262

Chen, K.C. & Vostal, J.J. (1981) Aryl hydrocarbon hydroxylase activity induced by injected diesel particulate extract vs inhalation of diluted diesel exhaust. *J. appl. Toxicol.*, 1, 127–131

Chen, S., Weller, M.A. & Barnhart, M.I. (1980) Effects of diesel engine exhaust on pulmonary alveolar macrophages. *Scanning Electron Microsc.*, 3, 327–338

Cheng, Y.S., Yeh, H.C., Mauderly, J.L. & Mokler, B.V. (1984) Characterization of diesel exhaust in a chronic inhalation study. *Am. ind. Hyg. Assoc. J.*, 45, 547–555

Chescheir, G.M., III, Garrett, N.E., Shelburne, J.D., Lewtas Huisingh, J. & Waters, M.D. (1981) Mutagenic effects of environmental particulates in the CHO/HGPRT system. In: Waters, M.D., Sandhu, S.S., Lewtas Huisingh, J., Claxton, L. & Nesnow, S., eds, *Short-term Bioassays in the Analysis of Complex Environmental Mixtures, II*, New York, Plenum, pp. 337–350

Chuang, C.C. & Petersen, B.A. (1985) *Review of Sampling and Analysis Methodology for Polynuclear Aromatic Compounds in Air from Mobile Sources (EPA 600/4-85-045; US NTIS PB85-227759)*, Research Triangle Park, NC, US Environmental Protection Agency

Clark, C.R. & Vigil, C.L. (1980) Influence of rat lung and liver homogenates on the mutagenicity of diesel exhaust particulate extracts. *Toxicol. appl. Pharmacol.*, 56, 110–115

Clark, C.R., Royer, R.E., Brooks, A.L., McClellan, R.O., Marshal, W.F., Naman, T.M. & Seizinger, D.E. (1981) Mutagenicity of diesel exhaust particle extracts: influence of car type. *Fundam. appl. Toxicol.*, 1, 260–265

Clark, C.R., Henderson, T.R., Royer, R.E., Brooks, A.L., McClellan, R.O., Marshall, W.F. & Naman, T.M. (1982a) Mutagenicity of diesel exhaust particle extracts: influence of fuel composition in two diesel engines. *Fundam. appl. Toxicol.*, 2, 38–43

Clark, C.R., Dutcher, J.S., Brooks, A.L., McClellan, R.O., Marshall, W.F. & Naman, T.M. (1982b) Mutagenicity of diesel exhaust particle extracts: influence of driving cycle and environmental temperature. *Fundam. appl. Toxicol.*, 2, 153–157

Clark, C.R., McClellan, R.O., Marshall, W.F., Naman, T.M. & Seizinger, D.E. (1982c) Mutagenicity of diesel exhaust particle extracts: influence of non-petroleum fuel extenders. *Arch. environ. Contam. Toxicol.*, 11, 749–752

Clark, C.R., Dutcher, J.S., McClellan, R.O., Naman, T.M. & Seizinger, D.E. (1983) Influence of ethanol and methanol gasoline blends on the mutagenicity of particulate exhaust extracts. *Arch. environ. Contam. Toxicol.*, 12, 311–317

Clark, C.R., Dutcher, J.S., Henderson, T.R., McClellan, R.O., Marshall, W.F., Naman, T.M. & Seizinger, D.E. (1984) Mutagenicity of automotive particulate exhaust: influence of fuel extenders, additives and aromatic content. *Adv. mod. environ. Toxicol.*, 6, 109–122

Claxton, L.D. (1981) Mutagenic and carcinogenic potency of diesel and related environmental emissions: *Salmonella* bioassay. *Environ. int.*, 5, 389–391

Claxton, L.D. (1983) Characterization of automotive emissions by bacterial mutagenesis bioassay: a review. *Environ. Mutagenesis*, 5, 609–631

Claxton, L.D. & Barnes, H.M. (1981) The mutagenicity of diesel-exhaust particle extracts collected under smog-chamber conditions using the *Salmonella typhimurium* test system. *Mutat. Res.*, 88, 255–272

Claxton, L.D. & Kohan, M. (1981) Bacterial mutagenesis and the evaluation of mobile-source emissions. In: Waters, M.D., Sandhu, S.S., Lewtas Huisingh, J., Claxton, L. & Nesnow, S., eds, *Short-term Bioassays in the Analysis of Complex Environmental Mixtures, II*, New York, Plenum, pp. 299–317

Coggon, D., Pannett, B. & Acheson, E.D. (1984) Use of job-exposure matrix in an occupational analysis of lung and bladder cancers on the basis of death certificates. *J. natl Cancer Inst.*, 72, 61–65

Cohen, S.I., Dorion, G., Goldsmith, J.R. & Permutt, S. (1971) Carbon monoxide uptake by inspectors at a United States-Mexico border station. *Arch. environ. Health*, 22, 47–54

Commission of the European Communities (1970) Council Directive of 20 March 1970 concerning the approximation of the laws of the Member States relating to measures to take against air pollution by gases from ignition engines of motor vehicles (70/220/CEE). *Off. J. Eur. Communities*, L76, 1–23

Commission of the European Communities (1988) Council Directive of 3 December 1987 amending Directive 70/220/EEC on the approximation of the laws of the Member States relating to measures to be taken against air pollution by gases from the engines of motor vehicles (88/76/EEC). *Off. J. Eur. Communities*, L36, 1–61

Cooper, G.P., Lewkowski, J.P., Hastings, L. & Malanchuk, M. (1977) Catalytically and noncatalytically treated automobile exhaust: biological effects in rats. *J. Toxicol. environ. Health*, 3, 923–934

Cornwell, R.J. (1982) *Health Hazard Evaluation Determination Report No. MHETA-81-108-9004; Climax Molybdenum Company, Climax, CO (PB84-14850 1)*, Morgantown, WV, National Institute for Occupational Safety and Health

Cuddihy, R.G., Seiler, F.A., Griffith, W.C., Scott, B.R. & McClellan, R.O. (1980) *Potential Health and Environmental Effects of Diesel Light Duty Vehicles (LMF-82)*, Springfield, VA, National Technical Information Service, US Department of Commerce

Cuddihy, R.G., Griffith, W.C., Clark, C.R. & McClellan, R.O. (1981) *Potential Health and Environmental Effects of Light Duty Diesel Vehicles. II (LMF-89)*, Springfield, VA, National Technical Information Service, US Department of Commerce

Cuddihy, R.G., Griffith, W.C. & McClellan, R.O. (1984) Health risks from light-duty diesel vehicles. *Environ. Sci. Technol.*, *18*, 14A–21A

Curren, R.D., Kouri, R.E., Kim, C.M. & Schechtman, L.M. (1981) Mutagenic and carcinogenic potency of extracts from diesel related environmental emissions: simultaneous morphological transformation and mutagenesis in BALB/c 3T3 cells. *Environ. int.*, *5*, 411–415

Currie, L.A. & Klouda, G.A. (1982) Counters, accelerators, and chemistry. In: Currie, L.A., ed., *Nuclear and Chemical Dating Techniques, Interpreting the Environmental Record (ACS Symposium Series 176)*, Washington DC, American Chemical Society, pp. 159–166

Daisey, J.M. (1983) Analysis of polycyclic aromatic hydrocarbons by thin-layer chromatography. In: Bjørseth, A., ed., *Handbook of Polycyclic Aromatic Hydrocarbons*, New York, Marcel Dekker, pp. 397–437

Damber, L.A. & Larsson, L.G. (1987) Occupation and male lung cancer: a case-control study in northern Sweden. *Br. J. ind. Med.*, *44*, 446–453

Daniel, J.H., Jr (1984) *Diesels in Underground Mining: a Review and an Evaluation of an Air Quality Monitoring Methodology (RI-8884; US NTIS PB84-214444)*, Washington DC, US Department of the Interior, Bureau of Mines

Davies, C.N. (1985) Absorption of gases in the respiratory tract. *Ann. occup. Hyg.*, *29*, 13–25

Decouflé, P., Stanislawczyk, K., Houten, L., Bross, J.D.J. & Viadana, E. (1977) *A Retrospective Survey of Cancer in Relation to Occupation (DHEW (NIOSH) Publ. No. 77-178)*, Cincinnati, OH, US Department of Health, Education, and Welfare

Dehnen, W., Tomingas, R., Kouros, M. & Mönch, W. (1985) Comparative study on the behaviour of particles from diesel and gasoline engines in the lungs of rodents: elimination rate and induction of benzo[a]pyrene hydroxylase and ethoxycoumarin deethylase (Ger.). *Zbl. Bakt. Hyg., I. Abt. Orig. B.*, *180*, 351–358

Depass, L.R., Chen, K.C. & Peterson, L.G. (1982) Dermal carcinogenesis bioassays of diesel particulates and dichloromethane extract of diesel particulates in C3H mice. In: Lewtas, J., ed., *Toxicological Effects of Emissions from Diesel Engines*, Amsterdam, Elsevier, pp. 321–327

Deutsche Forschungsgemeinschaft (German Research Association) (1985) *Air Analysis* (Ger.), Weinheim, VCH Verlagsgesellschaft mbH

Doran, T. & McTaggart, N.G. (1974) The combined use of high efficiency liquid and capillary gas chromatography for the determination of polycyclic aromatic hydrocarbons in automotive exhaust condensates and other hydrocarbon mixtures. *J. chromatogr. Sci.*, *12*, 715–721

Draper, W.M. (1986) Quantitation of nitro- and dinitropolycyclic aromatic hydrocarbons in diesel exhaust particulate matter. *Chemosphere*, *15*, 437–447

Dubrow, R. & Wegman, D.H. (1984) Cancer and occupation in Massachusetts: a death certificate study. *Am. J. ind. Med., 6*, 207–230

Dukovich, M., Yasbin, R.E., Lestz, S.S., Risby, T.H. & Zweidinger, R.B. (1981) The mutagenic and SOS-inducing potential of the soluble organic fraction collected from diesel particulate emissions. *Environ. Mutagenesis, 3*, 253–264

Duleep, K.G. & Dulla, R.G. (1980) Survey and analysis of automotive particulate sampling. In: Pepelko, W.E., Danner, R.M. & Clarke, N.A., eds, *Health Effects of Diesel Engine Emissions: Proceedings of an International Symposium, December 3-5, 1979 (EPA-600/9-80-057A)*, Springfield, VA, US Environmental Protection Agency, pp. 93–112

Dünges, W. (1979) Prä-chromatographische Mikromethoden. $\mu$l-Techniken für die Biomedizinische Spureanalytik [Pre-chromatographic Micromethods. $\mu$l-Techniques for Biomedical Trace Analysis], Heidelberg, A. Hüthig Verlag

Dutcher, J.S., Sun, J.D., Lopez, J.A., Wolf, I., Wolff, R.K. & McClellan, R.O. (1984) Generation and characterization of radiolabelled diesel exhaust. *Am. ind. Hyg. Assoc. J., 45*, 491–498

Dziedzic, D. (1981) Differential counts of B and T lymphocytes in the lymph nodes, circulating blood and spleen after inhalation of high concentrations of diesel exhaust. *J. appl. Toxicol., 1*, 111–115

Edling, C., Anjou, C.-G., Axelson, O. & Kling, H. (1987) Mortality among personnel exposed to diesel exhaust. *Int. Arch. occup. environ. Health, 59*, 559–565

Edwards, N.T. (1983) Polycyclic aromatic hydrocarbons (PAH's) in the terrestrial environment. A review. *J. environ. Qual., 12*, 427–441

Egan, H., Castegnaro, M., Bogovski, P., Kunte, H. & Walker, E.A., eds (1979) *Environmental Carcinogens. Selected Methods of Analysis, Vol. 3, Analysis of Polycyclic Aromatic Hydrocarbons in Environmental Samples (IARC Scientific Publications No. 29)*, Lyon, International Agency for Research on Cancer

Eisenberg, W.C. & Cunningham, D.L.B. (1984) Analysis of polycyclic aromatic hydrocarbons in diesel emissions using high performance liquid chromatography: a method development study. In: Cooke, M. & Dennis, A.J., eds, *Polynuclear Aromatic Hydrocarbons. 8th International Symposium: Mechanisms, Methods and Metabolism*, Columbus, OH, Battelle, pp. 379–393

El Batawi, M.A. & Noweir, M.H. (1966) Health problems resulting from prolonged exposure to air pollution in diesel bus garages. *Ind. Health, 4*, 1–10

El-Shobokshy, M.S. (1985) Atmospheric lead pollution in areas of children's schools in the city of Riyadh. In: *Proceedings of the 78th Annual Meeting of the Air Pollution Control Association, Detroit, MI, June 16–21, 1985, Vol. 5, paper (85-59B.3)*, Pittsburg, PA, Air Pollution Control Association

Fabia, J. & Thuy, T.D. (1974) Occupation of father at time of birth of children dying of malignant dieseases. *Br. J. prev. soc. Med., 28*, 98-100

Falk, H.L. (1977) Conclusions of the Committee on Human Health: consequences of lead exposure from automobile emissions. *Environ. Health Perspect., 19*, 243–246

Fishbein, L. (1976) Environmental metallic carcinogens: an overview of exposure levels. *J. Toxicol. environ. Health, 2*, 77–109

Fisher, A. & LeRoy, P. (1975) Particulate lead concentrations in Melbourne air. *Clean Air, August*, 56–57

Flodin, U., Fredriksson, M. & Persson, B. (1987) Multiple myeloma and engine exhausts, fresh wood, and creosote: a case-referent study. *Am. J. ind. Med., 12*, 519–529

Flodin, U., Fredriksson, M., Persson, B. & Axelson, O. (1988) Chronic lymphatic leukaemia and engine exhausts, fresh wood, and DDT: a case-referent study. *Br. J. ind. Med.*, *45*, 33–38

Fredga, K., Dävring, L., Sunner, M., Bengtsson, B.O., Elinder, C.-G., Sigtryggsson, P. & Berlin, M. (1982) Chromosome changes in workers (smokers and nonsmokers) exposed to automobile fuels and exhaust gases. *Scand. J. Work Environ. Health*, *8*, 209–221

Froines, J.R., Hinds, W.C., Duffy, R.M., Lafuente, E.J. & Liu, W.-C.V. (1987) Exposure of firefighters to diesel emissions in fire stations. *Am. ind. Hyg. Assoc. J.*, *48*, 202–207

Fulford, J.E., Sakuma, T. & Lane, D.A. (1982) Real-time analysis of exhaust gases using triple quadrupole mass spectrometry. In: Cooke, M., Dennis, A.J. & Fisher, G.L., eds, *Polynuclear Aromatic Hydrocarbons, 6th International Symposium: Physical and Biological Chemistry*, Columbus, OH, Battelle, pp. 297–303

Gaddo, P., Settis, M. & Giacomelli, L. (1984) *Artifact formation during diesel particulate collection.* In: Cooke, M. & Dennis, A.J., eds, *Polynuclear Aromatic Hydrocarbons, 8th International Symposium: Mechanisms, Methods and Metabolism*, Columbus, OH, Battelle, pp. 437–449

Gamble, J., Jones, W. & Hudak, J. (1983) An epidemiological study of salt miners in diesel and nondiesel mines. *Am. J. ind. Med.*, *4*, 435–458

Gamble, J., Jones, W. & Minshall, S. (1987a) Epidemiological-environmental study of diesel bus garage workers: acute effects of $NO_2$ and respirable particulate on the respiratory system. *Environ. Res.*, *42*, 201–214

Gamble, J., Jones, W. & Minshall, S. (1987b) Epidemiological-environmental study of diesel bus garage workers: chronic effects of diesel exhaust on the respiratory system. *Environ. Res.*, *44*, 6–17

Garg, B.D. (1983) Histologic quantitation of macrophage aggregates in the lungs of diesel exhaust exposed rats. *Acta stereol.*, *2 (Suppl. I)*, 235–238

Garland, F.C., Gorham, E.D., Garland, C.F. & Ducatman, A.M. (1988) Testicular cancer in US Navy personnel. *Am. J. Epidemiol.*, *127*, 411–414

Garshick, E., Schenker, M.B., Muñoz, A., Segal, M., Smith, T.J., Woskie, S.R., Hammond, K.S. & Speizer, F.E. (1987) A case-control study of lung cancer and diesel exhaust exposure in railroad workers. *Am. Rev. respir. Dis.*, *135*, 1242–1248

Garshick, E., Schenker, M.B., Muñoz, A., Segal, M., Smith, T.J., Woskie, S.R., Hammond, S.K. & Speizer, F.E. (1988) A retrospective cohort study of lung cancer and diesel exhaust exposure in railroad workers. *Am. Rev. respir. Dis.*, *137*, 820–825

Gérin, M., Siemiatycki, J., Kemper, H. & Bégin, D. (1985) Obtaining occupational exposure histories in epidemiologic case-control studies. *J. occup. Med.*, *27*, 420–426

Gibson, T.L., Ricci, A.I. & Williams, R.L. (1981) Measurement of polynuclear aromatic hydrocarbons, their derivatives, and their reactivity in diesel automobile exhaust. In: Cooke, M. & Dennis, A.J., eds, *Polynuclear Aromatic Hydrocarbons, 5th International Symposium: Chemical Analysis and Biological Fate*, Columbus, OH, Battelle, pp. 707–717

Gillespie, J.R. (1980) Review of the cardiovascular and pulmonary function studies on beagles exposed for 68 months to auto exhaust and other air pollutants. In: Stara, J.F., Dungworth, D.L., Orthoefer, J.G. & Tyler, W.S., eds, *Long-term Effects of Air Pollutants: in Canine Species (EPA-600/8-80-014)*, Washington DC, US Environmental Protection Agency, pp. 115–148

Goff, E.U., Coombs, J.R., Fine, D.H. & Baines, T.M. (1980) Determination of *N*-nitrosamines from diesel engine crankcase emissions. *Anal. Chem.*, *52*, 1833–1836

Gold, E.B., Diener, M.D. & Szklo, M. (1982) Parental occupations and cancer in children. A case-control study and review of the methodologic issues. *J. occup. Med.*, 24, 578–584

Gordon, R.J. (1976) Distribution of airborne polycyclic aromatic hydrocarbons throughout Los Angeles. *Environ. Sci. Technol.*, 10, 370–373

Göthe, C.-J., Fristedt, B., Sundell, L., Kolmodin, B., Ehrner-Samuel, H. & Göthe, K. (1969) Carbon monoxide hazard in city traffic. An examination of traffic policemen in three Swedish towns. *Arch. environ. Health*, 19, 310–314

Green, F.H.Y., Boyd, R.L., Danner-Rabovsky, J., Fisher, M.J., Moorman, W.J., Ong, T.-M., Tucker, J., Vallyathan, V., Whong, W.-Z., Zoldak, J. & Lewis, T. (1983) Inhalation studies of diesel exhaust and coal dust in rats. *Scand. J. Work Environ. Health*, 9, 181–188

Griest, W.H. & Caton, J.E. (1983) Extraction of polycyclic aromatic hydrocarbons for quantitative analysis. In: Björseth, A., ed., *Handbook of Polycyclic Aromatic Hydrocarbons*, New York, Marcel Dekker, pp. 95–148

Griffis, L.C., Wolff, R.K., Henderson, R.F., Griffith, W.C., Mokler, B.V. & McClellan, R.O. (1983) Clearance of diesel soot particles from rat lung after a subchronic diesel exhaust exposure. *Fundam. appl. Toxicol.*, 3, 99–103

Grimmer, G. & Böhnke, H. (1972) Determination of polycyclic aromatic hydrocarbons in automobile exhaust and air dust by capillary-gas-chromatography (Ger.). *Z. anal. Chem.*, 261, 310–314

Grimmer, C. & Jacob, J. (1987) Recommended method for a thin-layer chromatographic screening method for the determination of benzo(a)pyrene in smoked food. *Pure appl. Chem.*, 59, 1735–1738

Grimmer, G., Hildebrandt, A. & Böhnke, H. (1973a) Investigations on the carcinogenic burden by air pollution in man. II. Sampling and analysis of polycyclic aromatic hydrocarbons in automobile exhaust gas. 1. Optimization of the collecting arrangement. *Zbl. Bakt. Hyg., I. Abt. Orig. B.*, 158, 22–34

Grimmer, G., Hildebrandt, A. & Böhnke, H. (1973b) Investigations on the carcinogenic burden by air pollution in man. III. Sampling and analytics of polycyclic aromatic hydrocarbons in automobile exhaust gas. 2. Enrichment of the PNA and separation of the mixture of all PNA. *Zbl. Bakt. Hyg., I. Abt. Orig. B.*, 158, 35–49

Grimmer, G., Böhnke, H. & Glaser, A. (1977) Investigation on the carcinogenic burden by air pollution in man. XV. Polycyclic aromatic hydrocarbons in automobile exhaust gas — an inventory. *Zbl. Bakt. Hyg., I. Abt. Orig. B.*, 164, 218–234

Grimmer, G., Naujack, K.-W. & Schneider, D. (1981) Comparison of the profiles of polycyclic aromatic hydrocarbons in different areas of a city by glass-capillary-gas-chromatography in the nanogram-range. *Int. J. environ. anal. Chem.*, 10, 265–276

Grimmer, G., Naujack, K.-W. & Schneider, D. (1982) Profile analysis of polycyclic aromatic hydrocarbons by glass capillary gas chromatography in atmospheric suspended particulate matter in the nanogram range collecting 10 m³ of air. *Fresenius Z. anal. Chem.*, 311, 475–484

Grimmer, G., Brune, H., Deutsch-Wenzel, R., Naujack, K.-W., Misfeld, J. & Timm, J. (1983a) On the contribution of polycyclic aromatic hydrocarbons to the carcinogenic impact of automobile exhaust condensate evaluated by local application onto mouse skin. *Cancer Lett.*, 21, 105–113

Grimmer, G., Naujack, K.-W., Dettbarn, G., Brune, H., Deutsch-Wenzel, R. & Misfeld, J. (1983b) Characterization of polycyclic aromatic hydrocarbons as essential carcinogenic constituents of coal combustion and automobile exhaust using mouse-skin painting as a carcinogen-specific detector. *Toxicol. environ. Chem.*, 6, 97–107

Grimmer, G., Brune, H., Deutsch-Wenzel, R., Dettbarn, G. & Misfeld, J. (1984) Contribution of polycyclic aromatic hydrocarbons to the carcinogenic impact of gasoline engine exhaust condensate evaluated by implantation into the lungs of rats. *J. natl Cancer Inst.*, 72, 733–739

Grimmer, G., Brune, H., Deutsch-Wenzel, R., Dettbarn, G., Jacob, J., Naujack, K.-W., Mohr, U. & Ernst, H. (1987) Contribution of polycyclic aromatic hydrocarbons and nitro-derivatives to the carcinogenic impact of diesel engine exhaust condensate evaluated by implantation into the lungs of rats. *Cancer Lett.*, 37, 173–180

Grimmer, G., Jacob, J., Dettbarn, G. & Naujack, K.-W. (1988) Effect of the pH-value of diesel exhaust on the amount of filter-collected nitro-PAH. In: Cooke, M. & Dennis, A.J., eds, *Polynuclear Aromatic Hydrocarbons, 10th International Symposium: A Decade of Progress*, Columbus, OH, Battelle, pp. 341–351

Grosjean, D. (1982) Formaldehyde and other carbonyls in Los Angeles ambient air. *Environ. Sci. Technol.*, 16, 254–262

Gross, K.B. (1981) Pulmonary function testing of animals chronically exposed to diluted diesel exhaust. *J. appl. Toxicol.*, 1, 116–123

Guerrero, R.R., Rounds, D.E. & Orthoefer, J. (1981) Genotoxicity of Syrian hamster lung cells treated *in vivo* with diesel exhaust particulates. *Environ. int.*, 5, 445–454

Gustafsson, L., Wall, S., Larsson, L.-G. & Skog, B. (1986) Mortality and cancer incidence among Swedish dock workers — a retrospective cohort study. *Scand. J. Work Environ. Health*, 12, 22–26

Gutwein, E.E., Landolt, R.R. & Brenchley, D.L. (1974) Barium retention in rats exposed to combustion products from diesel fuel containing a barium-based antismoke additive. *J. Air Pollut. Control Assoc.*, 24, 40–43

Hadnagy, W. & Seemayer, N.H. (1986) Induction of C-type metaphases and aneuploidy in cultures of V79 cells exposed to extract of automobile exhaust particulates. *Mutagenesis*, 1, 445–448

Hagberg, M., Kolmodin-Hedman, B., Lindahl, R., Nilsson, C.-A. & Norström, Å. (1983) *Sampling and Analysis of Chain Saw Exhaust. III. Lung Function, Carboxyhaemoglobin and Complaints among Chain Saw Operators after Exposure to Exhaust* (Swed.) (*Arbete och Hälsa 1983:7*), Solna, Arbetarskyddsstyrelsen, pp. 75–104

Hahon, N., Booth, J.A., Green, F. & Lewis, T.R. (1985) Influenza virus infection in mice after exposure to coal dust and diesel engine emissions. *Environ. Res.*, 37, 44–60

Hakulinen, T., Salonen, T. & Teppo, L. (1976) Cancer in the offspring of fathers in hydrocarbon-related occupations. *Br. J. prev. soc. Med.*, 30, 138–140

Hall, N.E.L. & Wynder, E.L. (1984) Diesel exhaust exposure and lung cancer: a case-control study. *Environ. Res.*, 34, 77–86

Hallock, M., Smith, T.S., Hammond, K., Beck, B. & Brain, J.D. (1987) A new technique for collecting ambient diesel particles for bioassays. *Am. ind. Hyg. Assoc. J.*, 48, 487–493

Hamming, W.J. & MacPhee, R.D. (1967) Relationship of nitrogen oxides in auto exhaust to eye irritation — further results of chamber studies. *Atmos. Environ.*, 1, 577–584

Hammond, S.K., Smith, T.J., Woskie, S., Schenker, M.B. & Speizer, F.E. (1984) Characterization of diesel exhaust exposures for a mortality study. In: Cooke, M. & Dennis, A.J., eds, *Polynuclear Aromatic Hydrocarbons, 8th International Symposium: Mechanisms, Methods and Metabolism*, Columbus, OH, Battelle, pp. 533–541

Hampton, C.V., Pierson, W.R., Schuetzle, D. & Harvey, T.M. (1983) Hydrocarbon gases emitted from vehicles on the road. 2. Determination of emission rates from diesel and spark-ignition vehicles. *Environ. Sci. Technol.*, *17*, 699–708

Handa, T., Yamauchi, T., Ohnishi, M., Hisamatsu, Y. & Ishii, T. (1983) Detection and average content levels of carcinogenic and mutagenic compounds from the particulates on diesel and gasoline engine mufflers. *Environ. int.*, *9*, 335–341

Hare, C.T. & Baines, T.M. (1979) *Characterization of Particulate and Gaseous Emissions from Two Diesel Automobiles as Functions of Fuel and Driving Cycle (Technical Paper Series 790424)*, Warrendale, PA, Society of Automotive Engineers

Hare, C.T., Springer, K.J. & Bradow, R.L. (1979) *Fuel and Additive Effects on Diesel Particulate — Development and Demonstration of Methodology (SAE-paper No. 760130)*, Warrendale, PA, Society of Automotive Engineers

Harris, G.W., Mackay, G.I., Iguchi, T., Schiff, H.I. & Schuetzle, D. (1987) Measurement of $NO_2$ and $HNO_3$ in diesel exhaust gas by tunable diode laser absorption spectrometry. *Environ. Sci. Technol.*, *21*, 299–304

Harsch, D.E. & Rasmussen, R.A. (1977) Identification of methyl bromide in urban air. *Anal. Lett.*, *10*, 1041–1047

Häsänen, E., Karlsson, V., Leppämaki, E. & Juhula, M. (1981) Benzene, toluene and xylene concentrations in car exhausts and in city air. *Atmos. Environ.*, *15*, 1755–1757

Heidemann, A. & Miltenburger, H.G. (1983) Investigations on the mutagenic activity of fractions from diesel exhaust particulate matter in mammalian cells *in vivo* and *in vitro* (Abstract No. 15). *Mutat. Res.*, *113*, 339

Heino, M., Ketola, R., Mäkelä, P., Mäkinen, R., Niemelä, R., Starck, J. & Partanen, T. (1978) Work conditions and health of locomotive engineers. I. Noise, vibration, thermal climate, diesel exhaust constituents, ergonomics. *Scand. J. Work Environ. Health, 4 (Suppl. 3)*, 3–14

Heinrich, U., Peters, L., Funcke, W., Pott, F., Mohr, U. & Stöber, W. (1982) Investigations of toxic and carcinogenic effects of diesel exhaust in long-term inhalation exposure of rodents. In: Lewtas, J., ed., *Toxicological Effects of Emissions from Diesel Engines*, Amsterdam, Elsevier, pp. 225–242

Heinrich, U., Muhle, H., Takenaka, S., Ernst, E., Fuhst, R., Mohr, U., Pott, F. & Stöber, W. (1986a) Chronic effects on the respiratory tract of hamsters, mice and rats after long-term inhalation of high concentrations of filtered and unfiltered diesel engine emissions. *J. appl. Toxicol.*, *6*, 383–395

Heinrich, U., Pott, F., Mohr, U., Fuhst, R. & König, J. (1986b) Lung tumours in rats and mice after inhalation of PAH-rich emissions. *Exp. Pathol.*, *29*, 29–34

Heinrich, U., Peters, L., Mohr, U., Bellmann, B., Fuhst, R., Ketkar, M.B., König, J., König, H. & Pott, F. (1986c) *Investigation of Subacute and Chronic Effects of Gasoline Engine Exhaust on Rodents* (Ger.) (*FAT Series No. 55*), Frankfurt/Maine, Forschungsvereinigung Automobiltechnik e.V.

Hemminki, K., Saloniemi, I., Salonen, T., Partanen, T. & Vainio, H. (1981) Childhood cancer and parental occupation in Finland. *J. Epidemiol. Commun. Health*, *35*, 11–15

Henderson, Y., Haggard, H.W., Teague, M.C., Prince, A.L. & Wunderlich, R.M. (1921) Physiological effects of automobile exhaust gas and standards of ventilation for brief exposures. *J. ind. Hyg.*, *3*, 79–92, 137–146

Henderson, T.R., Sun, J.D., Royer, R.E., Clark, C.R., Li, A.P., Harvey, T.M., Hunt, D.H., Fulford, J.E., Lovette, A.M. & Davidson, W.R. (1983) Triple-quadrupole mass spectrometry studies of nitroaromatic emissions from different diesel engines. *Environ. Sci. Technol.*, *17*, 443–449

Henderson, T.R., Sun, J.D., Li, A.P., Hanson, R.L., Bechtold, W.E., Harvey, T.M., Shabanowitz, J. & Hunt, D.F. (1984) GC/MS and MS/MS studies of diesel exhaust mutagenicity and emissions from chemically defined fuels. *Environ. Sci. Technol.*, *18*, 428–434

Heyder, J., Gebhart, J., Roth, C., Scheuch, G. & Stahlhofen, W. (1983) Diffusional transport of aerosol particles. *J. Aerosol Sci.*, *14*, 279–280

Hinkle, L.E., Jr (1980) Automobile emissions in the perspective of human health: health benefits and social costs of pollution control. *Bull. N.Y. Acad. Med.*, *56*, 948–979

Hites, R.A., Yu, M.-L. & Thilly, W.G. (1981) Compounds associated with diesel exhaust particulates. In: Cooke, M. & Dennis, J.D., eds, *Polynuclear Aromatic Hydrocarbons, 5th International Symposium: Chemical Analysis and Biological Fate*, Columbus, OH, Battelle, pp. 455–466

Hoar, S.K. & Hoover, R. (1985) Truck driving and bladder cancer mortality in rural New England. *J. natl Cancer Inst.*, *74*, 771–774

Hobbs, J.R., Walter, R.A., Hard, T. & Devoe, D. (1977) *Train Generated Air Contaminants in the Train Crew's Working Environment (FRA/ORD-77/08: US NTIS PB265-355)*, Springfield, VA, National Technical Information Service, US Department of Commerce

Hoffman, D.J. & Campbell, K.I. (1977) Embryotoxicity of irradiated and nonirradiated catalytic converter-treated automotive exhaust. *J. Toxicol. environ. Health*, *3*, 705–712

Hoffman, D.J. & Campbell, K.I. (1978) Embryotoxicity of irradiated and nonirradiated automotive exhaust and carbon monoxide. *Environ. Res.*, *15*, 100–107

Hoffmann, D. & Wynder, E.L. (1962a) A study of air pollution carcinogenesis. II. The isolation and identification of polynuclear aromatic hydrocarbons from gasoline engine exhaust condensate. *Cancer*, *15*, 93–102

Hoffmann, D. & Wynder, E.L. (1962b) Analytical and biological studies on gasoline engine exhaust. *Natl Cancer Inst. Monogr.*, *9*, 91–112

Hoffmann, D., Theisz, E. & Wynder, E.L. (1965) Studies on the carcinogenicity of gasoline exhaust. *J. Air Pollut. Control Assoc.*, *15*, 162–165

Holland, W.D. (1978) *Determination of Breathing Zone Concentrations of Contaminants from Emissions from Diesel Powered Vehicles in Underground Mines (BuMines OFR 24-80; US NTIS PB80-150766)*, Washington DC, US Department of the Interior, Bureau of Mines

Holmberg, B. & Ahlborg, U., eds (1983) Consensus report: mutagenicity and carcinogenicity of car exhausts and coal combustion emissions. *Environ. Health Perspect.*, *47*, 1–30

Howard, P.H. & Durkin, P.R. (1974) *Benzene, Environmental Sources of Contamination, Ambient Levels, and Fate (EPA 560/5-75-005; US NTIS PB-244-139)*, Washington DC, US Environmental Protection Agency

Howe, G.R. & Lindsay, J.P. (1983) A follow-up study of a ten-percent sample of the Canadian labor force. I. Cancer mortality in males, 1965–73. *J. natl Cancer Inst.*, *70*, 37–44

Howe, G.R., Burch, J.D., Miller, A.B., Cook, G.M., Estève, J., Morrison, B., Gordon, P., Chambers, L.W., Fodor, G. & Winsor, G.M. (1980) Tobacco use, occupation, coffee, various nutrients, and bladder cancer. *J. natl Cancer Inst.*, *64*, 701–713

Howe, G.R., Fraser, D., Lindsay, J., Presnal, B. & Yu, S.Z. (1983) Cancer mortality (1965–77) in relation to diesel fume and coal exposure in a cohort of retired railway workers. *J. natl Cancer Inst.*, *70*, 1015–1019

Hueter, F.G., Contner, G.L., Busch, K.A. & Hinners, R.G. (1966) Biological effects of atmospheres contaminated by auto exhaust. *Arch. environ. Health*, *12*, 553–560

Huisingh, J.L., Bradow, R., Jungers, R., Claxton, L., Zweidinger, R., Tejada, S., Bumgarner, J., Duffield, F., Waters, M., Simmon, V.F., Hare, C., Rodriguez, C. & Snow, L. (1978) Application of bioassay to the characterization of diesel particle emissions. In: Waters, M.D., Nesnow, S., Huisingh, J.L., Sandhu, S.S. & Claxton, L., eds, *Application of Short-term Bioassays in the Fractionation and Analysis of Complex Environmental Mixtures*, New York, Plenum, pp. 381–418

Huisingh, J.L., Coffin, D.L., Bradow, R., Claxton, L., Austin, A., Zweidinger, R., Walter, R., Sturm, J. & Jungers, R.J. (1981) Comparative mutagenicity of combustion emissions of a high quality no. 2 diesel fuel derived from shale oil and a petroleum derived no. 2 diesel fuel. In: Griest, W.H., Guerin, M.R. & Coffin, D.L., eds, *Health Effects Investigations of Oil Shale Development*, Ann Arbor, MI, Ann Arbor Science, pp. 201–207

Hyde, D., Orthoefer, J.G., Dungworth, D., Tyler, W., Carter, R. & Lum, H. (1980) Morphometric and morphologic evaluation of pulmonary lesions in beagle dogs chronically exposed to high ambient levels of air pollutants. In: Stara, J.F., Dungworth, D.L., Orthoefer, J.G. & Tyler, W.S., eds, *Long-term Effects of Air Pollutants: in Canine Species (EPA-600/8-80-014)*, Washington DC, US Environmental Protection Agency, pp. 195–227

Hyde, D.M., Plopper, C.G., Weir, A.J., Murnane, R.D., Warren, D.L., Last, J.A. & Pepelko, W.E. (1985) Peribronchiolar fibrosis in lungs of cats chronically exposed to diesel exhaust. *Lab. Invest.*, *52*, 195–206

IARC (1980) *IARC Monographs on the Evaluation of the Carcinogenic Risk of Chemicals to Humans*, Vol. 23, *Some Metals and Metallic Compounds*, Lyon, pp. 325–415

IARC (1982a) *IARC Monographs on the Evaluation of the Carcinogenic Risk of Chemicals to Humans*, Vol. 29, *Some Industrial Chemicals and Dyestuffs*, Lyon, pp. 345–389

IARC (1982b) *IARC Monographs on the Evaluation of the Carcinogenic Risk of Chemicals to Humans*, Vol. 29, *Some Industrial Chemicals and Dyestuffs*, Lyon, pp. 93–148

IARC (1983) *IARC Monographs on the Evaluation of the Carcinogenic Risk of Chemicals to Humans*, Vol. 32, *Polynuclear Aromatic Compounds, Part 1, Chemical, Environmental and Experimental Data*, Lyon

IARC (1984) *IARC Monographs on the Evaluation of the Carcinogenic Risk of Chemicals to Humans*, Vol. 33, *Polynuclear Aromatic Compounds, Part 2, Carbon Blacks, Mineral Oils and Some Nitroarenes*, Lyon, pp. 171–222

IARC (1987a) *IARC Monographs on the Evaluation of Carcinogenic Risks to Humans*, Suppl. 7, *Overall Evaluations of Carcinogenicity: An Updating of* IARC Monographs *Volumes 1 to 42*, Lyon

IARC (1987b) *IARC Monographs on the Evaluation of the Carcinogenic Risk of Chemicals to Humans*, Vol. 42, *Silica and Some Silicates*, Lyon, pp. 39–143

IARC (1988) *IARC Monographs on the Evaluation of Carcinogenic Risks to Humans*, Vol. 43, *Man-made Mineral Fibres and Radon*, Lyon, pp. 173–259

IARC (1989) *IARC Monographs on the Evaluation of Carcinogenic Risks to Humans*, Vol. 45, *Occupational Exposures in Petroleum Refining; Crude Oil and Major Petroleum Fuels*, Lyon, pp. 159–201, 219–237

Iscovich, J., Castelletto, R., Estève, J., Muñoz, N., Colanzi, R., Coronel, A., Deamezola, I., Tassi, V. & Arslan, A. (1987) Tobacco smoking, occupational exposure and bladder cancer in Argentina. *Int. J. Cancer*, 40, 734–740

Ishinishi, N., Kuwabara, N., Nagase, S., Suzuki, T., Ishiwata, S. & Kohno, T. (1986a) Long-term inhalation studies on effects of exhaust from heavy and light duty diesel engines on F344 rats. In: Ishinishi, N., Koizumi, A., McClellan, R.O. & Stöber, W., eds, *Carcinogenic and Mutagenic Effects of Diesel Engine Exhaust*, Amsterdam, Elsevier, pp. 329–348

Ishinishi, N., Koizumi, A., McClellan, R.O. & Stöber, W., eds (1986b) *Carcinogenic and Mutagenic Effects of Diesel Engine Exhaust*, Amsterdam, Elsevier

Iwai, K., Udagawa, T., Yamagishi, M. & Yamada, H. (1986) Long-term inhalation studies of diesel exhaust on F344 SPF rats. Incidence of lung cancer and lymphoma. In: Ishinishi, N., Koizumi, A., McClellan, R.O. & Stöber, W., eds, *Carcinogenic and Mutagenic Effects of Diesel Engine Exhaust*, Amsterdam, Elsevier, pp. 349–360

Jacob, J. & Grimmer, G. (1979) Extraction and enrichment of polycyclic aromatic hydrocarbons (PAH) from environmental matter. In: Egan, H., Castegnaro, M., Bogovski, P., Kunte, H. & Walker, E.A., eds, *Environmental Carcinogens. Selected Methods of Analysis*, Vol. 3, *Analysis of Polycyclic Aromatic Hydrocarbons in Environmental Samples (IARC Scientific Publications No. 29)*, Lyon, International Agency for Research on Cancer, pp. 79–89

Janssen, O. (1976) *Experiences of Collaborative Studies for Analysis of PAH* (Ger.) (*Erdöl & Kohle, Erdgas, Petrochemie Compendium 1975/1976*), Leinfelden, Hernhaussen KG, pp. 624–638

Jensen, O.M., Wahrendorf, J., Knudsen, J.B. & Sørensen, B.L. (1987) The Copenhagen case-referent study on bladder cancer. Risks among drivers, painters and certain other occupations. *Scand. J. Work Environ. Health*, 13, 129–134

John, W. & Reischl, G. (1978) Measurements of the filtration efficiencies of selected filter types. *Atmos. Environ.*, 12, 2015–2019

Johnson, B.L., Cohen, H.H., Struble, R., Setzer, J.V., Anger, W.K., Gutnik, B.D., McDonough, T. & Hauser, P. (1974) Field evaluation of carbon monoxide exposed toll collectors. In: *Behavioral Toxicology, Early Detection of Occupational Hazards (DHEW (NIOSH) Publ. No. 74-126)*, Cincinnati, OH, National Institute for Occupational Safety and Health, pp. 306–328

Johnson, J. (1988) Automotive emissions. In: Watson, A.Y., Bates, R.R. & Kennedy, D., eds, *Air Pollution, the Automobile, and Public Health*, Washington DC, National Academy Press

Johnson, R.L., Shah, J.J., Cary, R.A. & Huntzicker, J.J. (1981) An automated thermal-optical method for the analysis of carbonaceous aerosol. In: Macias, E.S. & Hopke, P.K., eds, *Atmospheric Aerosol: Source/Air Quality Relationships (ACS Symposium Series No. 167)*, Washington CD, American Chemical Society, pp. 223–233

Jones, E., Richold, M., May, J.H. & Saje, A. (1985) The assessment of the mutagenic potential of vehicle engine exhaust in the Ames *Salmonella* assay using a direct exposure method. *Mutat. Res.*, 155, 35–40

Jones, P.W., Giammar, R.D., Strup, P.E. & Stanford, T.B. (1976) Efficient collection of polycyclic organic compounds from combustion effluents. *Environ. Sci. Technol.*, 10, 806–810

Jörgensen, H. & Svensson, Å. (1970) Studies on pulmonary function and respiratory tract symptoms of workers in an iron ore mine where diesel trucks are used underground. *J. occup. Med.*, *12*, 348–354

Kantor, A.F., McCrea Curnen, M.G., Meigs, J.W. & Flannery, J.T. (1979) Occupations of fathers of patients with Wilms's tumour. *J. Epidemiol. Commun. Health*, *33*, 253–256

Kaplan, I. (1959) Relationship of noxious gases to carcinoma of the lung in railroad workers. *J. Am. med. Assoc.*, *171*, 97–101

Kaplan, H.L., MacKenzie, W.F., Springer, K.J., Schreck, R.M. & Vostal, J.J. (1982) A subchronic study of the effects of exposure of three species of rodents to diesel exhaust. In: Lewtas, J., ed., *Toxicological Effects of Emissions from Diesel Engines*, Amsterdam, Elsevier, pp. 161–182

Karagianes, M.T., Palmer, R.F. & Busch, R.H. (1981) Effects of inhaled diesel emissions and coal dust in rats. *Am. ind. Hyg. Assoc. J.*, *42*, 382–391

Kawabata, Y., Iwai, K., Udagawa, T., Tukagoshi, K. & Higuchi, K. (1986) Effects of diesel soot on unscheduled DNA synthesis of tracheal epithelium and lung tumor formation. In: Ishinishi, N., Koizumi, A., McClellan, R.O. & Stöber, W., eds, *Carcinogenic and Mutagenic Effects of Diesel Engine Exhaust*, Amsterdam, Elsevier, pp. 213–222

King, L.C., Kohan, M.J., Austin, A.C., Claxton, L.D. & Lewtas Huisingh, J. (1981) Evaluation of the release of mutagens from diesel particles in the presence of physiological fluids. *Environ. Mutagenesis*, *3*, 109–121

King, L.C., Loud, K., Tejada, S.B., Kohan, M.J. & Lewtas, J. (1983) Evaluation of the release of mutagens and 1-nitropyrene from diesel particles in the presence of lung macrophages in culture. *Environ. Mutagenesis*, *5*, 577–588

Köhler, M. & Eichhoff, H.-J. (1967) Quick method for determination of aromatic hydrocarbons in air dust (Ger.). *Z. anal. Chem.*, *232*, 401–409

Kotin, P., Falk, H.L. & Thomas, M. (1954) Aromatic hydrocarbons. II. Presence in the particulate phase of gasoline-engine exhausts and the carcinogenicity of exhaust extracts. *Arch. ind. Hyg. occup. Med.*, *9*, 164–177

Kotin, P., Falk, H.L. & Thomas, M. (1955) Aromatic hydrocarbons. III. Presence in the particulate phase of diesel-engine exhausts and the carcinogenicity of exhaust extracts. *Arch. ind. Health*, *11*, 113–120

Kraft, J. & Lies, K.-H. (1981) *Polycyclic Aromatic Hydrocarbons in the Exhaust of Gasoline and Diesel Vehicles (Technical Paper Series No. 810082)*, Warrendale, PA, Society of Automotive Engineers

Kronoveter, K.J. (1976) *Industrial Hygiene Surveys at US Border Crossing Stations During August 1973–June 1974 (DHEW (NIOSH) Publ. No. 76-135)*, Cincinnati, OH, National Institute for Occupational Safety and Health

Kunitake, E., Shimamura, K., Katayama, H., Takemoto, K., Yamamoto, A., Hisanaga, A., Ohyama, S. & Ishinishi, N. (1986) Studies concerning carcinogenesis of diesel particulate extracts following intratracheal instillation, subcutaneous injection, or skin application. In: Ishinishi, N., Koizumi, A., McClellan, R.O. & Stöber, W., eds, *Carcinogenic and Mutagenic Effects of Diesel Engine Exhaust*, Amsterdam, Elsevier, pp. 235–252

Künstler, K. (1983) Failure to induce tumors by intratracheal instillation of automobile exhaust condensate and fractions thereof in Syrian golden hamsters. *Cancer Lett.*, *18*, 105–108

Kunte, H. (1979) Separation, detection and identification of polycyclic aromatic hydrocarbons. In: Egan, H., Castegnaro, M., Bogovski, P., Kunte, H. & Walker, E.A., eds, *Environmental Carcinogens. Selected Methods of Analysis*, Vol. 3, *Analysis of Polycyclic Aromatic Hydrocarbons in Environmental Samples (IARC Scientific Publications No. 29)*, Lyon, International Agency for Research on Cancer, pp. 91–99

Kwa, S.-L. & Fine, L.J. (1980) The association between parental occupation and childhood malignancy. *J. occup. Med.*, 22, 792–794

Lahmann, E. (1969) *Untersuchungen über Luftverunreinigungen durch den Kraftverkehr* [Air Pollution by Automobiles] *(Schriftenreihe des Vereins für Wasser-, Boden- und Lufthygiene No. 28)*, Stuttgart, Gustav Fischer Verlag

Lang, J.M., Snow, L., Carlson, R., Black, F., Zweidinger, R. & Tejada, S. (1981) *Characterization of Particulate Emissions from In-use Gasoline-fuelled Motor Vehicles (Technical Paper Series No. 811186)*, Warrendale, PA, Society of Automotive Engineers

Larsen, R.I. & Konopinski, V.J. (1962) Sumner Tunnel air quality. *Arch. environ. Health*, 5, 597–608

Lassiter, D.V. & Milby, T.H. (1978) *Health Effects of Diesel Exhaust Emissions: A Comprehensive Literature Review, Evaluation and Research Gaps Analysis (US NTIS PB-282-795)*, Washington DC, American Mining Congress

Lawter, J.R. & Kendall, D.A. (1977) *Effects of Diesel Engine Emissions on Coal Mine Air Quality (BuMines OFR 46-78; US NTIS PB-282-377)*, Washington DC, US Department of the Interior, Bureau of Mines

Laxen, D.P.H. & Noordally, E. (1987) Nitrogen dioxide distribution in street canyons. *Atmos. Environ.*, 21, 1899–1903

Lee, F.S.-C. & Schuetzle, D. (1983) Sampling, extraction and analysis of polycyclic aromatic hydrocarbons from internal combustion engines. In: Bjørseth, A., ed., *Handbook of Polycyclic Aromatic Hydrocarbons*, New York, Marcel Dekker, pp. 27–94

Lee, S.D., Malanchuk, M. & Finelli, V.N. (1976) Biological effects of auto emissions. I. Exhaust from engine with and without catalytic converter. *J. Toxicol. environ. Health*, 1, 705–712

Lee, F.S.-C., Prater, T.J. & Ferris, F. (1979) PAH emissions from a stratified-charge vehicle with and without oxidation catalyst: sampling and analysis evaluation. In: Jones, P.W. & Leber, P., eds, *Polynuclear Aromatic Hydrocarbons, 3rd International Symposium: Chemistry and Biology. Carcinogenesis and Mutagenesis*, Ann Arbor, MI, Ann Arbor Science, pp. 83–110

Lee, F.S.-C., Pierson, W.R. & Ezike, J. (1980) The problem of PAH degradation during filter collection of airborne particulates. An evaluation of several commonly used filter media. In: Björseth, A. & Dennis, A.J., eds, *Polynuclear Aromatic Hydrocarbons, 4th International Symposium: Chemistry and Biological Effects*, Columbus, OH, Battelle, pp. 543–563

Lee, I.P., Suzuki, K., Lee, S.D. & Dixon, R.L. (1980) Aryl hydrocarbon hydroxylase induction in rat lung, liver and male reproductive organs following inhalation exposure to diesel emission. *Toxicol. appl. Pharmacol.*, 52, 181–184

Lee, P.S., Chan, T.L. & Hering, W.E. (1983) Long-term clearance of inhaled diesel exhaust particles in rodents. *J. Toxicol. environ. Health*, 12, 801–813

Lee, P.S., Gorski, R.A., Hering, W.E. & Chan, T.L. (1987) Lung clearance of inhaled particles after exposure to carbon black generated from a resuspension system. *Environ. Res.*, 43, 364–373

Leichnitz, K. (1986) *Gefahrstoff-Analytik* [Dangerous Substances Analysis], Landsberg, Ecomed Verlagsgesellschaft mbH

Lerchen, M.L., Wiggins, C.L. & Samet, J.M. (1987) Lung cancer and occupation in New Mexico. *J. natl Cancer Inst.*, *79*, 639—645

Levine, S.P., Skewes, L.M., Abrams, L.D. & Palmer, A.G., III (1982) High performance semi-preparative liquid chromatography and liquid chromatography-mass spectrometry of diesel engine emission particulate extracts. In: Cooke, M., Dennis, A.J. & Fisher, G.L., eds, *Polynuclear Aromatic Hydrocarbons, 6th International Symposium: Physical and Biological Chemistry*, Columbus, OH, Battelle, pp. 439—448

Lewis, T.R. & Moorman, W.J. (1980) Pulmonary and cardiovascular physiology studies during exposure. In: Stara, J.F., Dungworth, D.L., Orthoefer, J.G. & Tyler, W.S., eds, *Long-term Effects of Air Pollutants: in Canine Species (EPA-600/8-80-014)*, Washington DC, US Environmental Protection Agency, pp. 97—108

Lewis, T.R., Hueter, F.G. & Busch, K.A. (1967) Irradiated automobile exhaust. Its effects on the reproduction in mice. *Arch. environ. Health*, *15*, 26—35

Lewis, T.R., Moorman, W.J., Yang, Y.-Y. & Stara, J.F. (1974) Long-term exposure to auto exhaust and other pollutant mixtures. Effects on pulmonary funciton in the beagle. *Arch. environ. Health*, *29*, 102—106

Lewis, T.R., Green, F.H.Y., Moorman, W.J., Burg, J.A.R. & Lynch, D.W. (1986) A chronic inhalation toxicity study of diesel engine emissions and coal dust, alone and combined. In: Ishinishi, N., Koizumi, A., McClellan, R.O. & Stöber, W., eds, *Carcinogenic and Mutagenic Effects of Diesel Engine Exhaust*, Amsterdam, Elsevier, pp. 361—380

Lewis, T.R., Green, F.H.Y., Moorman, W.J., Burg, J.R. & Lynch, D.W. (1989) A chronic inhalation toxicity study of diesel engine emissions and coal dust, alone and combined. *J. Am. Coll. Toxicol.*, *8*, 345—375

Lewtas, J. (1982) *Mutagenic activity of diesel emissions*. In: Lewtas, J., ed., *Toxicological Effects of Emissions from Diesel Engines*, Amsterdam, Elsevier, pp. 243—264

Lewtas, J. (1983) Evaluation of the mutagenicity and carcinogenicity of motor vehicle emissions in short-term bioassays. *Environ. Health Perspect.*, *47*, 141—152

Lewtas, J. (1985) Combustion emissions: characterization and comparison of their mutagenic and carcinogenic activity. In: Stich, H.F., ed., *Carcinogens and Mutagens in the Environment*, Vol. V, *The Workplace: Sources of Carcinogens*, Boca Raton, FL, CRC Press, pp. 59—74

Lewtas, J. & Williams, K. (1986) A retrospective view of the value of short-term genetic bioassays in predicting the chronic effects of diesel soot. In: Ishinishi, N., Koizumi, A., McClellan, R.O. & Stöber, W., eds, *Carcinogenicity and Mutagenic Effects of Diesel Engine Exhaust*, Amsterdam, Elsevier, pp. 119—140

Li, A.P. & Royer, R.E. (1982) Diesel-exhaust-particle extract enhancement of chemical-induced mutagenesis in cultured Chinese hamster ovary cells: possible interaction of diesel exhaust with environmental carcinogens. *Mutat. Res.*, *103*, 349—355

Liber, H.L., Andon, B.M., Hites, R.A. & Thilly, W.G. (1980) Diesel soot: mutation measurements in bacterial and human cells. In: Pepelko, W.E., Danner, R.M. & Clarke, N.A., eds, *Health Effects of Diesel Engine Emissions (EPA-600/9-80-057a)*, Cincinnati, OH, US Environmental Protection Agency, pp. 404—412

Liber, H.L., Andon, B.M., Hites, R.A. & Thilly, W.G. (1981) Diesel soot: mutation measurements in bacterial and human cells. *Environ. int.*, *5*, 281—284

Liberti, A., Ciccioli, P., Cecinato, A., Brancaleoni, E. & Di Palo, C. (1984) Determination of nitrated-polyaromatic hydrocarbons (nitro-PAHs) in environmental samples by high resolution chromatographic techniques. *J. high Resolut. Chromatogr. Chromatogr. Commun.*, *7*, 389—397

Lies, K.-H., Hartung, A., Postulka, A., Gring, H. & Schuetzle, J. (1986) Composition of diesel exhaust with particular reference to particle bound organics including formation of artifacts. In: Ishinishi, N., Koizumi, A., McClellan, R.O. & Stöber, W., eds, *Carcinogenic and Mutagenic Effects of Diesel Engine Exhaust*, Amsterdam, Elsevier, pp. 65–82

Lindner, W., Posch, W., Wolfbeis, O.S. & Tritthart, P. (1985) Analysis of nitro-PAHs in diesel exhaust particulate extracts with multicolumn HPLC. *Chromatographia, 20*, 213–218

Lioy, P.J. & Daisey, J.M. (1986) Airborne toxic elements and organic substances. *Environ. Sci. Technol., 20*, 8–14

Lockard, J.M., Kaur, P., Lee-Stephens, C., Sabharwal, P.S., Pereira, M.A., McMillan, L. & Mattox, J. (1982) Induction of sister-chromatid exchanges in human lymphocytes by extracts of particulate emissions from a diesel engine. *Mutat. Res., 104*, 355–359

Löfroth, G. (1981a) Comparison of the mutagenic activity in carbon particulate matter and in diesel and gasoline engine exhaust. In: Waters, M.D., Sandhu, S.S., Lewtas Huisingh, J., Claxton, L. & Nesnow, S., eds, *Short-term Bioassays in the Analysis of Complex Environmental Mixtures, II*, New York, Plenum, pp. 319–336

Löfroth, G. (1981b) *Salmonella*/microsome mutagenicity assays of exhaust from diesel and gasoline powered motor vehicles. *Environ. int., 5*, 255–261

Malanchuk, M. (1980) Exposure chamber atmospheres. Sampling and analysis. In: Stara, J.F., Dungworth, D.L., Orthoefer, J.G. & Tyler, W.S., eds, *Long-term Effects of Air Pollutants: in Canine Species (EPA-6008-80-014)*, Washington DC, US Environmental Protection Agency, pp. 41–54

Malker, H. & Weiner, J. (1984) *Cancer-miljöregistret. Exempel på Utnyuttjande av Registerepidemiologi inom Arbetsmiljöområdet* [The Cancer-Environment Registry 1961-1973. Examples of the Use of Register Epidemiology in Studies in the Work Environment] (*Arbete och Hälsa 1984:9*), Solna, Arbetarskyddsstyrelsen

Manabe, Y., Kinouchi, T. & Ohnishi, Y. (1985) Identification and quantification of highly mutagenic nitroacetoxypyrenes and nitrohydroxypyrenes in diesel-exhaust particles. *Mutat. Res., 158*, 3–18

Maruna, R.F.L. & Maruna, H. (1975) Lead load in taxi drivers characterized by delta aminolaevulinic acid in the urine (Ger.). *Wien. med. Wochenschr., 125*, 615–620

Massad, E., Saldiva, P.H.N., Saldiva, C.D., Pires do Rio Caldeira, M., Cardoso, L.M.N., Méri Steves de Morais, A., Calheiros, D.F., da Silva, R. & Böhm, G.M. (1986) Toxicity of prolonged exposure to ethanol and gasoline autoengine exhaust gases. *Environ. Res., 40*, 479–486

Matsushita, H., Goto, S., Endo, O., Lee, J.-H. & Kawai, A. (1986) Mutagenicity of diesel exhaust and related chemicals. In: Ishinishi, N., Koizumi, A., McClellan, R.O. & Stöber, W., eds, *Carcinogenic and Mutagenic Effects of Diesel Engine Exhaust*, Amsterdam, Elsevier, pp. 103–118

Mauderly, J.L., Jones, R.K., McClellan, R.O., Henderson, R.F. & Griffith, W.C. (1986) Carcinogenicity of diesel exhaust inhaled chronically by rats. In: Ishinishi, N., Koizumi, A., McClellan, R.O. & Stöber, W., eds, *Carcinogenic and Mutagenic Effects of Diesel Engine Exhaust*, Amsterdam, Elsevier, pp. 397–409

Mauderly, J.L., Jones, R.K., Griffith, W.C., Henderson, R.F. & McClellan, R.O. (1987) Diesel exhaust is a pulmonary carcinogen in rats exposed chronically by inhalation. *Fundam. appl. Toxicol., 9*, 208–221

Maziarka, S., Strusiński, A. & Wyszyńska, H. (1971) Lead compounds in the atmosphere of Polish towns (Pol.). *Roczn. Panstw. Zakl. Hig.*, *22*, 399–406

McClellan, R.O. (1986) Health effects of diesel exhaust: a case study in risk assessment. *Am. ind. Hyg. Assoc. J.*, *47*, 1–13

McClellan, R.O., Brooks, A.L., Cuddihy, R.G., Jones, R.K., Mauderly, J.L. & Wolff, R.K. (1982) Inhalation toxicology of diesel exhaust particles. In: Lewtas, J., ed., *Toxicological Effects of Emissions from Diesel Engines*, Amsterdam, Elsevier, pp. 99–120

McCormick, J.J., Zator, R.M., DaGue, B.B. & Maher, V.M. (1980) Studies on the effects of diesel particulate on normal and xeroderma pigmentosum cells. In: Pepelko, W.E., Danner, R.M. & Clarke, N.A., eds, *Health Effects of Diesel Engine Emissions (EPA-600/9-80-057a)*, Cincinnati, OH, US Environmental Protection Agency, pp. 413–415

Meiss, R., Robenek, H., Schubert, M., Themann, H. & Heinrich, U. (1981) Ultrastructural alterations in the livers of golden hamsters following experimental chronic inhalation of diluted diesel exhaust emission. *Int. Arch. occup. environ. Health*, *48*, 147–157

Menck, H.R. & Henderson, B.E. (1976) Occupational differences in rates of lung cancer. *J. occup. Med.*, *18*, 797–801

Mentnech, M.S., Lewis, D.M., Olenchock, S.A., Mull, J.C. & Koller, W.A. (1984) Effects of coal dust and diesel on immune competence in rats. *J. Toxicol. environ. Health*, *13*, 31–41

Metz, N., Lies, K.-H. & Hartung, A. (1984) Polynuclear aromatic hydrocarbons in diesel soot: round robin test results from eight European laboratories of the Committee of Common Market Automobile Constructors (CCMC). In: Cooke, M. & Dennis, A.J., eds, *Polynuclear Aromatic Hydrocarbons, 8th International Symposium: Mechanisms, Methods and Metabolism*, Columbus, OH, Battelle, pp. 899–912

Milham, S., Jr (1983) *Occupational Mortality in Washington State 1950-1979 (DHHS (NIOSH) Publ. No. 83-116)*, Cincinnati, OH, US Department of Health and Human Services

Mitchell, A.D., Evans, E.L., Jotz, M.M., Riccio, E.S., Mortelmans, K.E. & Simmon, V.F. (1981) Mutagenic and carcinogenic potency of extracts of diesel and related environmental emissions: in vitro mutagenesis and DNA damage. *Environ. int.*, *5*, 393–401

Mohr, U., Reznik-Schüller, H., Reznik, G., Grimmer, G. & Misfeld, J. (1976) Investigations on the carcinogenic burden by air pollution in man. XIV. Effects of automobile exhaust condensate on the Syrian golden hamster lung. *Zbl. Bakt. Hyg., I. Abt. Orig. B*, *163*, 425–432

Moore, W., Orthoefer, J., Burkart, J. & Malanchuk, M. (1978) Preliminary findings of the deposition and retention of automotive diesel particulate in rat lungs. In: *Proceedings of the 71st Annual Meeting of the Air Pollution Control Association*, Vol. 3, Pittsburg, PA, Air Pollution Control Association, pp. 3–15

Moorman, W.J., Clark, J.C., Pepelko, W.E. & Mattox, J. (1985) Pulmonary function responses in cats following long-term exposure to diesel exhaust. *J. appl. Toxicol.*, *5*, 301–305

Morandi, M. & Eisenbud, M. (1980) Carbon monoxide exposure in New York City: a historical overview. *Bull. N.Y. Acad. Med.*, *56*, 817–828

Morgan, A. & Holmes, A. (1978) The fate of lead in petrol-engine exhaust particulates inhaled by the rat. *Environ. Res.*, *15*, 44–56

Morimoto, K., Kitamura, M., Kondo, H. & Koizumi, A. (1986) Genotoxicity of diesel exhaust emissions in a battery of in-vitro short-term and in-vivo bioassays. In: Ishinishi, N., Koizumi, A., McClellan, R.O. & Stöber, W., eds, *Carcinogenic and Mutagenic Effects of Diesel Engine Exhaust*, Amsterdam, Elsevier, pp. 85–101

The Motor Vehicle Manufacturers Association of the United States and The Engine Manufacturers Association (1986) *Analysis of the Environmental Protection Agency's 'Diesel Particulate Study' and a Diesel Particulate Emission Projection*, Detroit, MI

Nakagawa, R., Kitamori, S., Horikawa, K., Nakashima, K. & Tokiwa, H. (1983) Identification of dinitropyrenes in diesel-exhaust particles: their probable presence as the major mutagens. *Mutat. Res., 124*, 201–211

Nathanson, B. & Nudelman, H. (1980) Ambient lead concentrations in New York City and their health implications. *Bull. N.Y. Acad. Med., 56*, 866–875

National Air Pollution Control Administration (1970) *Air Quality Criteria for Hydrocarbons (AP-64; US NTIS PB190-489)*, Washington DC, US Department of Health, Education, and Welfare

National Research Council (1972a) *Biological Effects of Atmospheric Pollutants: Particulate Polycyclic Organic Matter*, Washington DC, National Academy of Sciences

National Research Council (1972b) *Biological Effects of Atmospheric Pollutants: Lead*, Washington DC, National Academy of Sciences

National Research Council (1977a) *Medical and Biological Effects of Environmental Pollutants: Carbon Monoxide*, Washington DC, National Academy of Sciences

National Research Council (1977b) *Medical and Biological Effects of Environmental Pollutants: Nitrogen Oxides*, Washington DC, National Academy of Sciences

National Research Council (1981) *Formaldehyde and Other Aldehydes*, Washington DC, National Academy of Sciences

National Research Council (1982) *Diesel Technology — Impacts of Diesel-powered Light-duty Vehicles*, Washington DC, National Academy of Sciences

National Research Council (1983) *Feasibility of Assessment of Health Risks from Vapor-phase Organic Chemicals in Gasoline and Diesel Exhaust*, Washington DC, National Academy of Sciences

Nesnow, S., Triplett, L.L. & Slaga, T.J. (1982a) Comparative tumor-initiating activity of complex mixtures from environmental particulate emissions on SENCAR mouse skin. *J. natl Cancer Inst., 68*, 829–834

Nesnow, S., Evans, C., Stead, A., Creason, J., Slaga, T.J. & Triplett, L.L. (1982b) Skin carcinogenesis studies of emission extracts. In: Lewtas, J., ed., *Toxicological Effects of Emissions from Diesel Engines*, Amsterdam, Elsevier, pp. 295–320

Nesnow, S., Triplett, L.L. & Slaga, T.J. (1983) Mouse skin tumor initiation-promotion and complete carcinogenesis bioassays: mechanisms and biological activities of emission samples. *Environ. Health Perspect., 47*, 255–268

Nielsen, T. (1983) Isolation of polycyclic aromatic hydrocarbons and nitro derivatives in complex mixtures by liquid chromatography. *Anal. Chem., 55*, 286–290

Nilsson, C.-A., Lindahl, R. & Norström, Å. (1987) Occupational exposure to chain saw exhausts in logging operations. *Am. ind. Hyg. Assoc. J., 48*, 99–105

Nishioka, M.G., Petersen, B.A. & Lewtas, J. (1982) Comparison of nitro-aromatic content and direct-acting mutagenicity of diesel emissions. In: Cooke, M., Dennis, A.J. & Fisher, G.L., eds, *Polynuclear Aromatic Hydrocarbons, 6th International Symposium: Physical and Biological Chemistry*, Columbus, OH, Battelle, pp. 603–613

Nishioka, M.G., Petersen, B.A. & Lewtas, J. (1983) Comparison of nitro-aromatic content and direct-acting mutagenicity of passenger car engine emissions. In: Rondia, D., Cooke, M. & Haroz, R.K., eds, *Mobile Source Emissions Including Polycyclic Organic Species*, Dordrecht, D. Reidel, pp. 197–210

Nordenson, I., Sweins, A., Dahlgren, E. & Beckman, L. (1981) A study of chromosomal aberrations in miners exposed to diesel exhausts. *Scand. J. Work Environ. Health, 7*, 14–17

Norpoth, K., Jacob, J., Grimmer, G. & Mohtashamipur, E. (1985) Determination of mutagenic activities in different fractions of automobile exhaust condensate by the *Salmonella*/oxygenase mutagenicity test system. *Zbl. Bakt. Hyg., I. Abt. Orig B, 180*, 540–547

Oberdoerster, G., Green, F.H.Y. & Freedman, A.P. (1984) Clearance of $^{59}Fe_3O_4$ particles from the lungs of rats during exposure to coal mine dust and diesel exhaust. *J. Aerosol Sci., 15*, 235–237

Office of Population Censuses and Surveys (1978) *Occupational Mortality. The Registrar General's Decennial Supplement for England and Wales 1970–1972 (Series DS No. 1)*, London, Her Majesty's Stationery Office

Ohnishi, Y., Kachi, K., Sato, K., Tahara, I., Takeyoshi, H. & Tokiwa, H. (1980) Detection of mutagenic activity in automobile exhaust. *Mutat. Res., 77*, 229–240

Ohnishi, Y., Okazaki, H., Wakisaka, K., Kinouchi, T., Kikuchi, T. & Furuya, K. (1982) Mutagenicity of particulates in small engine exhaust. *Mutat. Res., 103*, 251–256

Olsen, J.H. & Jensen, O.M. (1987) Occupation and risk of cancer in Denmark. An analysis of 93 810 cancer cases, 1970-1979. *Scand. J. Work Environ. Health, 13 (Suppl. 1)*

Olufsen, B.S. & Bjørseth, A. (1983) Analysis of polycyclic aromatic hydrocarbons by gas chromatography. In: Bjørseth, A., ed., *Handbook of Aromatic Hydrocarbons*, New York, Marcel Dekker, pp. 257–300

Ong, T., Whong, W.-Z., Xu, J., Burchell, B., Green, F.H.Y. & Lewis, T. (1985) Genotoxicity studies of rodents exposed to coal dust and diesel emission particulates. *Environ. Res., 37*, 399–409

Orthoefer, J.G., Bhatnagar, R.S., Rahman, A., Yang, Y.Y., Lee, S.D. & Stara, J.F. (1976) Collagen and prolyl hydroxylase levels in lungs of beagles exposed to air pollutants. *Environ. Res., 12*, 299–305

Paputa-Peck, M.C., Marano, R.S., Schuetzle, D., Riley, T.L., Hampton, C.V., Prater, T.J., Skewes, L.M., Jensen, T.E., Ruehle, P.H., Bosch, L.C. & Duncan, W.P. (1983) Determination of nitrated polynuclear aromatic hydrocarbons in particulate extracts by capillary column gas chromatography with nitrogen selective detection. *Anal. Chem., 55*, 1946–1954

Pederson, T.C. & Siak, J.-S. (1981) The role of nitroaromatic compounds in the direct-acting mutagenicity of diesel particle extracts. *J. appl. Toxicol., 1*, 54–60

Pepelko, W.E. (1982a) Effects of 28 days exposure to diesel engine emissions in rats. *Environ. Res., 27*, 16–23

Pepelko, W.E. (1982b) EPA studies on the toxicological effects of inhaled diesel engine emissions. In: Lewtas, J., ed., *Toxicological Effects of Emissions from Diesel Engines*, Amsterdam, Elsevier, pp. 121–142

Pepelko, W.E. & Peirano, W.B. (1983) Health effects of exposure to diesel engine emissions. A summary of animal studies conducted by the US Environmental Protection Agency's Health Effects Research Laboratory at Cincinnati, OH. *J. Am. Coll. Toxicol., 2*, 253–306

Pepelko, W.E., Orthoefer, J.G. & Yang, Y.-Y. (1979) Effects of 90 days exposure to catalytically treated automobile exhaust in rats. *Environ. Res., 19*, 91–101

Pepelko, W.E., Mattox, J.K., Yang, Y.-Y. & Moore, W., Jr (1980) Pulmonary function and pathology in cats exposed 28 days to diesel exhaust. *J. environ. Pathol. Toxicol.*, *4*, 449–458

Pepelko, W.E., Mattox, J., Moorman, W.J. & Clark, J.C. (1981) Pulmonary function evaluation of cats after one year of exposure to diesel exhaust. *Environ. int.*, *5*, 373–376

Pereira, M.A. (1982) Genotoxicity of diesel exhaust emissions in laboratory animals. In: Lewtas, J., ed., *Toxicological Effects of Emissions from Diesel Engines*, Amsterdam, Elsevier, pp. 265–276

Pereira, M.A., Shinozuka, H. & Lombardi, B. (1981a) Test of diesel exhaust emissions in the rat liver foci assay. *Environ. int.*, *5*, 455–458

Pereira, M.A., Sabharwal, P.S., Kaur, P., Ross, C.B., Choi, A. & Dixon, T. (1981b) In vivo detection of mutagenic effects of diesel exhaust by short-term mammalian bioassays. *Environ. int.*, *5*, 439–443

Pereira, M.A., Connor, T.H., Meyne, J. & Legator, M.S. (1981c) Metaphase analysis, micronuclei assay, and urinary mutagenicity assay of mice exposed to diesel emissions. *Environ. int.*, *5*, 435–438

Pereira, M.A., McMillan, L., Kaur, P., Gulati, D.K. & Sabharwal, P.S. (1982) Effect of diesel exhaust emissions, particulates, and extract on sister chromatid exchange in transplacentally exposed fetal hamster liver. *Environ. Mutagenesis*, *4*, 215–220

Petersen, B.A. & Chuang, C.C. (1982) Methodology of fractionation and partition of diesel exhaust particulate samples. In: Lewtas, J., ed., *Toxicological Effects of Emissions from Diesel Engines*, Amsterdam, Elsevier, pp. 51–67

Petersen, G.R. & Milham, S., Jr (1980) *Occupational Mortality in the State of California 1959-61 (DHEW (NIOSH) Publ. No. 80-104)*, Cincinnati, OH, US Department of Health, Education, and Welfare

del Piano, M., Gaudiuso, M., Rimatori, V., Sessa, R. & Bellanti, M. (1986) Exposure of workers to chemical pollutants in a public transport company (Abstract). In: *Proceedings of the International Congress on Industrial Hygiene, Rome, October 5–9 1986*, Rome, Pontificia Università Urbaniana, pp. 125–127

Pierce, R.C. & Katz, M. (1975) Dependency of polynuclear aromatic hydrocarbon content on size distribution of atmospheric aerosols. *Environ. Sci. Technol.*, *9*, 347–353

Pierson, W.R. & Brachaczek, W.W. (1983) Particulate matter associated with vehicles on the road. II. *Aerosol Sci. Technol.*, *2*, 1–40

Pierson, W.R., Gorse, R.A., Jr, Szkarlat, A.C., Brachaczek, W.W., Japar, S.M., Lee, F.S.-C., Zweidinger, R.B. & Claxton, L.D. (1983) Mutagenicity and chemical characteristics of carbonaceous particulate matter from vehicles on the road. *Environ. Sci. Technol.*, *17*, 31–44

Pitts, J.N., Jr (1983) Formation and fate of gaseous and particulate mutagens and carcinogens in real and simulated atmospheres. *Environ. Health Perspect.*, *47*, 115–140

Pitts, J.N., Jr, Van Cauwenberghe, K.A., Grosjean, D., Schmid, J.P., Fitz, D.R., Belser, W.L., Jr, Knudson, G.B. & Hynds, P.M. (1978) Atmospheric reactions of polycyclic aromatic hydrocarbons: facile formation of mutagenic nitro derivatives. *Science*, *202*, 515–519

Pitts, J.N., Jr, Lokensgard, D.M., Harger, W., Fisher, T.S., Mejia, V., Schuler, J.J., Scorziell, G.M. & Katzenstein, Y.A. (1982) Mutagens in diesel exhaust particulate: identification and direct activities of 6-nitrobenzo[a]pyrene, 9-nitroanthracene, 1-nitropyrene and 5H-phenanthro[4,5-bcd]pyran-5-one. *Mutat. Res.*, *103*, 241–249

Pott, F., Tomingas, R. & Misfeld, J. (1977) Tumours in mice after subcutaneous injection of automobile exhaust condensates. In: Mohr, U., Schmähl, D. & Tomatis, L., eds, *Air Pollution and Cancer in Man (IARC Scientific Publications No. 16)*, Lyon, International Agency for Research on Cancer, pp. 79—87

Pritchard, J.N. (1987) *Particle growth in the airways and the influence of airflow*. In: Newman, S.P., Morén, F. & Crompton, G.K., eds, *A New Concept in Inhalation Therapy*, Bussum, Medicom, pp. 3—24

Pryor, P. (1983) *Trailways Bus System, Denver, CO (Health Hazard Evaluation Report No. HETA 81-416-1334)*, Cincinnati, OH, National Institute for Occupational Safety and Health

Purdham, J.T., Holness, D.L. & Pilger, C.W. (1987) Environmental and medical assessment of stevedores employed in ferry operations. *Appl. ind. Hyg.*, 2, 133—139

Quinto, J. & De Marinis, E. (1984) Sperm abnormalities in mice exposed to diesel particulate. *Mutat. Res.*, 130, 242

Raab, O.G., Yeh, H.-C., Newton, G.J., Phalen, R.F. & Velasquez, D.J. (1977) Deposition of inhaled monodisperse aerosols in small rodents. In: Walton, W.H., ed., *Inhaled Particles*, IV, Part 1, Oxford, Pergamon, pp. 3—21

Rabovsky, J., Petersen, M.R., Lewis, T.R., Marion, K.J. & Groseclose, R.D. (1984) Chronic inhalation of diesel exhaust and coal dust: effect of age and exposure on selected enzyme activities associated with microsomal cytochrome P-450 in rat lung and liver. *J. Toxicol. environ. Health*, 14, 655—666

Raffle, P.A.B. (1957) The health of the worker. *Br. J. ind. Med.*, 14, 73—80

Ramdahl, T. (1984) Polycyclic aromatic ketones in source emissions and ambient air. In: Cooke, M. & Dennis, A.J., eds, *Polynuclear Aromatic Hydrocarbons, 8th International Symposium: Mechanisms, Methods and Metabolism*, Columbus, OH, Battelle, pp. 1075—1087

Ramdahl, T. & Urdal, K. (1982) Determination of nitrated polycyclic aromatic hydrocarbons by fused silica capillary gas chromatography/negative ion chemical ionization mass spectrometry. *Anal. Chem.*, 54, 2256—2260

Ramsey, J.M. (1967) Carboxyhemoglobinemia in parking garage employees. *Arch. environ. Health*, 15, 580—583

Randerath, E., Reddy, M.V., Avitts, T.A. & Randerath, K. (1985) $^{32}$P-Postlabeling test for genotoxicity of environmental carcinogens/mutagens in condensates of cigarette smoke, gasoline exhaust and diesel exhaust (Abstract No. 332). *Proc. Am. Assoc. Cancer Res.*, 26, 84

Rannug, U. (1983) Data from short-term tests on motor vehicle exhausts. *Environ. Health Perspect.*, 47, 161—169

Rannug, U., Sundvall, A., Westerholm, R., Alsberg, T. & Stenberg, U. (1983) Some aspects of mutagenicity testing of the particulate phase and the gas phase of diluted and undiluted automobile exhaust. *Environ. Sci. Res.*, 27, 3—16

Rappaport, S.M., Wang, Y.Y., Wei, E.T., Sawyer, R., Watkins, B.E. & Rapoport, H. (1980) Isolation and identification of a direct-acting mutagen in diesel-exhaust particulates. *Environ. Sci. Technol.*, 14, 1505—1509

Reger, R., Hancock, J., Hankinson, J., Hearl, F. & Merchant, J. (1982) Coal miners exposed to diesel exhaust emissions. *Ann. occup. Hyg.*, 26, 799—815

Reznik-Schüller, H. & Mohr, U. (1977) Pulmonary tumorigenesis in Syrian golden hamsters after intratracheal instillations with automobile exhaust condensate. *Cancer*, 40, 203—210

Risch, H.A., Burch, J.D., Miller, A.B., Hill, G.B., Steele, R. & Howe, G.R. (1988) Occupational factors and the incidence of cancer of the bladder in Canada. *Br. J. ind. Med.*, *45*, 361–367

Ritter, J.A., Stedman, D.H. & Kelly, T.J. (1979) Ground level measurements of nitric oxide, nitrogen dioxide and ozone in rural air. In: Grosjean, D., ed., *Nitrogenous Air Pollutants, Proceedings of a Symposium, 175th National Meeting, American Chemical Society, Anaheim, California, March 12–17, 1978*, Ann Arbor, MI, Ann Arbor Science, pp. 325–343

Robertson, A., Dodgson, J., Collings, P. & Seaton, A. (1984) Exposure to oxides of nitrogen: respiratory symptoms and lung function in British coalminers. *Br. J. ind. Med.*, *41*, 214–219

Rosenkranz, H.S., McCoy, E.C., Mermelstein, R. & Speck, W.T. (1981) A cautionary note on the use of nitroreductase-deficient strains of *Salmonella typhimurium* for the detection of nitroarenes as mutagens in complex mixtures including diesel exhausts. *Mutat. Res.*, *91*, 103–105

Rouser, G. & Aloia, R. (1980) The effects of air pollutants on membrane lipids. In: Stara, J.F., Dungworth, D.L., Orthoefer, J.G. & Tyler, W.S., eds, *Long-term Effects of Air Pollutants: in Canine Species (EPA-600/8-80-014)*, Washington DC, US Environmental Protection Agency, pp. 87–91

Rudd, C.J. (1980) Diesel particulate extract in cultured mammalian cells. In: Pepelko, W.E., Danner, R.M. & Clarke, N.A., eds, *Health Effects of Diesel Engine Emissions (EPA-600/9-80-057a)*, Cincinnati, OH, US Environmental Protection Agency, pp. 385–403

Rushton, L., Alderson, M.R. & Nagarajah, C.R. (1983) Epidemiological survey of maintenance workers in London Transport executive bus garages and Chiswick works. *Br. J. ind. Med.*, *40*, 340–345

Sakuma, T., Davidson, W.R., Lane, D.A., Thomson, B.A., Fulford, J.E. & Quan, E.S.K. (1981) The rapid analysis of gaseous PAH and other combustion related compounds in hot gas streams by APCI/MS and APCI/MS/MS. In: Cooke, M. & Dennis, A.J., eds, *Polynuclear Aromatic Hydrocarbons, 5th International Symposium: Chemical Analysis and Biological Fate*, Columbus, OH, Battelle, pp. 179–188

Salmeen, I., Durisin, A.M., Prater, T.J., Riley, T. & Schuetzle, D. (1982) Contribution of 1-nitropyrene to direct-acting Ames assay mutagenicities of diesel particulate extracts. *Mutat. Res.*, *104*, 17–23

Sanders, B.M., White, G.C. & Draper, G.J. (1981) Occupations of fathers of children dying from neoplasms. *J. Epidemiol. Commun. Health*, *35*, 245–250

Sawicki, E. (1976) Analysis of atmospheric carcinogens and their cofactors. In: Rosenfeld, C. & Davis, W., eds, *Environmental Pollution and Carcinogenic Risks (IARC Scientific Publications No. 13)*, Lyon, International Agency for Research on Cancer, pp. 297–354

Sawicki, E., Elbert, W.C., Hauser, T.R., Fox, F.T. & Stanley, T.W. (1960) Benzo(a)pyrene content of the air of American communities. *Am. ind. Hyg. Assoc. J.*, *21*, 443–451

Sawicki, E., Meeker, J.E. & Morgan, M.J. (1965) Polynuclear aza compounds in automotive exhaust. *Arch. environ. Health*, *11*, 773–775

Sayers, R.R., Yant, W.P., Levy, E. & Fulton, W.B. (1929) *Effect of Repeated Daily Exposure of Several Hours to Small Amounts of Automobile Exhaust Gas (Public Health Bulletin No. 186)*, Washington DC, US Government Printing Office

Schiller, C.F., Gebhart, J., Heyder, J., Rudolf, G. & Stahlhofen, W. (1986) Factors influencing total deposition of ultrafine aerosol particles in the human respiratory tract. *J. Aerosol Sci.*, *17*, 328–332

Schoenberg, J.B., Stemhagen, A., Mogielnicki, A.P., Altman, R., Abe, T. & Mason, T.J. (1984) Case-control study of bladder cancer in New Jersey. I. Occupational exposures in white males. *J. natl Cancer Inst.*, *72*, 973–981

Schuetzle, D. (1983) Sampling of vehicle emissions for chemical analysis and biological testing. *Environ. Health Perspect.*, *47*, 65–80

Schuetzle, D. & Frazier, J.A. (1986) Factors influencing the emission of vapor and particulate phase components from diesel engines. In: Ishinishi, N., Koizumi, A., McClellan, R.O. & Stöber, W., eds, *Carcinogenic and Mutagenic Effects of Diesel Engine Exhaust*, Amsterdam, Elsevier, pp. 41–63

Schuetzle, D. & Jensen, T.E. (1985) Analysis of nitrated polycyclic aromatic hydrocarbons (nitro-PAH) by mass spectrometry. In: White, C., ed., *Nitrated Polycyclic Aromatic Hydrocarbons*, Heidelberg, A. Hüthig Verlag, pp. 121–167

Schuetzle, D. & Lewtas, J. (1986) Bioassay-directed chemical analysis in environmental research. *Anal. Chem.*, *58*, 1060A–1075A

Schuetzle, D. & Perez, J.M. (1981) A CRC cooperative comparison of extraction and HPLC techniques for diesel particulate emissions (Paper 81-56.4). In: *Proceedings of the 74th Annual Meeting of the Air Pollution Control Association, Philadelphia, PA, June 16-21 1981*, Pittsburg, PA, Air Pollution Control Association

Schuetzle, D. & Perez, J.M. (1983) Factors influencing the emissions of nitrated-polynuclear aromatic hydrocarbons (nitro-PAH) from diesel engines. *J. Air Pollut. Control Assoc.*, *33*, 751–755

Schuetzle, D., Lee, F.S.-C., Prater, T.J. & Tejada, S.B. (1981) The identification of polynuclear aromatic hydrocarbon (PAH) derivatives in mutagenic fractions of diesel particulate extracts. *Int. J. environ. anal. Chem.*, *9*, 93–144

Schuetzle, D., Riley, T.L., Prater, T.J., Salmeen, I. & Harvey, T.M. (1982) The identification of mutagenic chemical species in air particulate samples. In: Albaiges, J., ed., *Analytical Techniques in Environmental Chemistry*, Vol. 2, Oxford, Pergamon, pp. 259–280

Schuetzle, D., Jensen, T.E. & Ball, J.C. (1985) Polar polynuclear aromatic hydrocarbon derivatives in extracts of particulates: biological characterization and techniques for chemical analysis. *Environ. int.*, *11*, 169

Schuler, R.L. & Niemeier, R.W. (1981) A study of diesel emissions on *Drosophila*. *Environ. int.*, *5*, 431–434

Seemayer, N.H., Hadnagy, W. & Tomingas, R. (1987) The effect of automobile exhaust particulates on cell viability, plating efficiency and cell division of mammalian tissue culture cells. *Sci. total Environ.*, *61*, 107–115

Seifert, B. & Ullrich, D. (1978) Concentration of inorganic and organic air pollutants at a traffic intersection in Berlin (Ger.). *Staub-Reinhalt. Luft*, *38*, 359–363

Shefner, A.M., Collins, B.R., Dooley, L., Fiks, A., Graf, J.L. & Preache, M.M. (1982) Respiratory carcinogenicity of diesel fuel emissions. Interim results. In: Lewtas, J., ed., *Toxicological Effects of Emissions from Diesel Engines*, Amsterdam, Elsevier, pp. 329–350

Siak, J.S., Chan, J.L. & Lee, P.S. (1981) Diesel particulate extracts in bacterial test systems. *Environ. int.*, *5*, 243–248

Siemiatycki, J., Gérin, M., Stewart, P., Nadon, L., Dewar, R. & Richardson, L. (1988) Associations between several sites of cancer and ten types of exhaust and combustion products: results from a case-referent study in Montreal. *Scand. J. Work Environ. Health*, *14*, 79–90

Silverman, D.T., Hoover, R.N., Albert, S. & Graff, K.M. (1983) Occupation and cancer of the lower urinary tract in Detroit. *J. natl Cancer Inst.*, 70, 237–245

Silverman, D.T., Hoover, R.N., Mason, T.J. & Swanson, G.M. (1986) Motor exhaust-related occupations and bladder cancer. *Cancer Res.*, 46, 2113–2116

Smith, E.M., Miller, E.R., Woolson, R.F. & Brown, C.K. (1985) Bladder cancer risk among auto and truck mechanics and chemically related occupations. *Am. J. publ. Health*, 75, 881–883

Speizer, F.E. & Ferris, B.G., Jr (1963) The prevalence of chronic nonspecific respiratory disease in road tunnel employees. *Am. Rev. respir. Dis.*, 88, 205–212

Stanley, T.W., Meeker, J.E. & Morgan, M.J. (1967) Extraction of organics from airborne particulates. Effects of various solvents and conditions on the recovery of benzo(*a*)pyrene, benz(*c*)acridine, and 7*H*-benz(*de*)anthracen-7-one. *Environ. Sci. Technol.*, 1, 927–931

Stara, J.F., Dungworth, D.L., Orthoefer, J.G. & Tyler, W.S., eds (1980) *Long-term Effects of Air Pollutants: in Canine Species (EPA-600/8-80-014)*, Cincinnati, OH, US Environmental Protection Agency

Stauff, J., Tsai, W.-L., Stärk, G. & Miltenburger, H. (1980) Chemiluminescence and mutagenic activity of exhaust gas after combustion (Ger.). *Staub-Reinhalt. Luft*, 40, 284–289

Steenland, K. (1986) Lung cancer and diesel exhaust: a review. *Am. J. ind. Med.*, 10, 177–189

Steenland, K., Burnett, C. & Osorio, A.M. (1987) A case-control study of bladder cancer using city directories as a source of occupational data. *Am. J. Epidemiol.*, 126, 247–257

Stenberg, U., Alsberg, T. & Bertilsson, B.M. (1981) *A Comparison of the Emission of Polynuclear Aromatic Hydrocarbons from Automobiles Using Gasoline or a Methanol/Gasoline Blend (SAE Technical Paper No. 810441)*, Warrendale, PA, Society of Automotive Engineers

Stenberg, U., Alsberg, T. & Westerholm, R. (1983) Applicability of a cryogradient technique for the enrichment of PAH from automobile exhausts: demonstration of methodology and evaluation experiments. *Environ. Health Perspect.*, 47, 43–51

Stenburg, R.L., von Lehmden, D.J. & Hangebrauck, R.P. (1961) Sample collection techniques for combustion sources — benzopyrene determination. *Am. ind. Hyg. Assoc. J.*, 22, 271–275

Stern, F.B., Curtis, R.A. & Lemen, R.A. (1981) Exposure of motor vehicle examiners to carbon monoxide: a historical prospective mortality study. *Arch. environ. Health*, 36, 59–66

Strom, K.A. (1984) Response of pulmonary cellular defenses to the inhalation of high concentrations of diesel exhaust. *J. Toxicol. environ. Health*, 13, 919–944

Stupfel, M., Magnier, M., Romary, F., Tran, M.-H. & Moutet, J.-P. (1973) Lifelong exposure of SPF rats to automotive exhaust gas. Dilution containing 20 ppm of nitrogen oxides. *Arch. environ. Health*, 26, 264–269

Sun, J.D. & McClellan, R.O. (1984) Respiratory tract clearance of $^{14}$C-labelled diesel exhaust compounds associated with diesel particles or as a particle-free extract. *Fundam. appl. Toxicol.*, 4, 388–393

Sun, J.D., Wolff, R.K., Kanapilly, G.M. & McClellan, R.O. (1984) Lung retention and metabolic fate of inhaled benzo(*a*)pyrene associated with diesel exhaust particles. *Toxicol. appl. Pharmacol.*, 73, 48–59

Swarin, S.J. & Williams, R.L. (1980) Liquid chromatographic determination of benzo[*a*]pyrene in diesel exhaust particulate: verification of the collection and analytical methods. In: Bjørseth, A. & Dennis, A.J., eds, *Polynuclear Aromatic Hydrocarbons, 4th International Symposium: Chemistry and Biological Effects*, Columbus, OH, Battelle, pp. 771–806

Takafuji, S., Suzuki, S., Koizumi, K., Tadokoro, K., Miyamoto, T., Ikemori, R. & Muranaka, M. (1987) Diesel-exhaust particulates inoculated by the intranasal route have an adjuvant activity for IgE production in mice. *J. Allerg. clin. Immunol.*, 79, 639–645

Takemoto, K., Yoshimura, H. & Katayama, H. (1986) Effects of chronic inhalation exposure to diesel exhaust on the development of lung tumors in di-isopropanol-nitrosamine-treated F344 rats and newborn C57BL and ICR mice. In: Ishinishi, N., Koizumi, A., McClellan, R.O. & Stöber, W., eds, *Carcinogenic and Mutagenic Effects of Diesel Engine Exhaust*, Amsterdam, Elsevier, pp. 311–327

Tejada, S.B., Zweidinger, R.B. & Sigsby, J.E., Jr (1983) *Analysis of Nitroaromatics in Diesel and Gasoline Car Emissions (SAE Technical Paper No. 820775)*, Warrendale, PA, Society of Automotive Engineers

Thurston, G.D. & Spengler, J.D. (1985) A quantitative assessment of source contributions to inhalable particulate matter pollution in metropolitan Boston. *Atmos. Environ.*, 19, 9–25

Tokiwa, H., Otofuji, T., Nakagawa, R., Horikawa, K., Maeda, T., Sano, N., Izumi, K. & Otsuka, H. (1986) Dinitro derivatives of pyrene and fluoranthene in diesel emission particulates and their tumorigenicity in mice and rats. In: Ishinishi, N., Koizumi, A., McClellan, R.O. & Stöber, W., eds, *Carcinogenic and Mutagenic Effects of Diesel Engine Exhaust*, Amsterdam, Elsevier, pp. 253–270

Tong, H.Y. & Karasek, F.W. (1984) Quantitation of polycyclic aromatic hydrocarbons in diesel exhaust particulate matter by high-performance liquid chromatography fractionation and high-resolution gas chromatography. *Anal. Chem.*, 56, 2129–2134

Törnqvist, M., Kautiainen, A., Gatz, R.N. & Ehrenberg, L. (1988) Hemoglobin adducts in animals exposed to gasoline and diesel exhausts. 1. Alkenes. *J. appl. Toxicol.*, 8, 159–170

Tsani-Bazaca, E., McIntyre, A.E., Lester, J.N. & Perry, R. (1981) Concentrations and correlations of 1,2-dibromoethane, 1,2-dichloroethane, benzene and toluene in vehicle exhaust and ambient air. *Environ. Technol. Lett.*, 2, 303–316

Tucker, J.D., Xu, J., Stewart, J., Baciu, P.C. & Ong, T.-M. (1986) Detection of sister chromatid exchanges induced by volatile genotoxicants. *Teratog. Carcinog. Mutagenesis*, 6, 15–21

Tyrer, H.W., Cantrell, E.T., Horres, R., Lee, I.P. & Peirano, W.B. & Danner, R.M. (1981) Benzo(*a*)pyrene metabolism in mice exposed to diesel exhaust: I. Uptake and distribution. *Environ. int.*, 5, 307–311

Ulfvarson, U., Alexandersson, R., Aringer, L., Anshelm-Olson, B., Ekholm, U., Hedenstierna, G., Hogstedt, C., Holmberg, B., Lindstedt, G., Randma, E., Rosén, G., Sorsa, M. & Svensson, E. (1985) *Hälsoeffekter vid Exponering för Motoravgaser* [Health Effects of Exposure to Motor Exhaust Gases] (*Arbete och Hälsa 1985:5*), Solna, Arbetarskyddsstyrelsen

Ulfvarson, U., Alexandersson, R., Aringer, L., Svensson, E., Hedenstierna, G., Hogstedt, C., Holmberg, B., Rosén, G. & Sorsa, M. (1987) Effects of exposure to vehicle exhaust on health. *Scand. J. Work Environ. Health*, 13, 505–512

Ungers, L.J. (1984) *Measurement of Exhaust Emissions from Diesel-powered Forklifts during Operations in Ammunition Storage Magazines (Phase I (AD-A141-792)*, Cincinnati, OH, PEDCo Environmental

Ungers, L.J. (1985) *Measurement of Exhaust Emissions from Diesel-powered Forklifts during Operations in Ammunition Storage Magazines (Phase II (AD-A153-092)*, Cincinnati, OH, PEI Associates

US Environmental Protection Agency (1977) Protection of the environment, Chapter 1, Part 8B, Subpart B, section 86. *US Code fed. Regul., Title 40*, 113–178

US Environmental Protection Agency (1979) *Air Quality Criteria for Carbon Monoxide* (*Report No. EPA 600/8-79-022; US NTIS PB81-244840*), Research Triangle Park, NC, Environmental Criteria and Assessment Office

US Environmental Protection Agency (1982) *Air Quality Criteria for Oxides of Nitrogen. Final Report* (*Report No. EPA 600/8-82-026F; US NTIS Pb83-163337*), Research Triangle Park, NC, Environmental Criteria and Assessment Office

US Environmental Protection Agency (1986) *Air Quality for Lead, Volume 4* (*EPA-600/8-83-028dF; US NTIS PB87-142378*), Research Triangle Park, NC, Environmental Criteria and Assessment Office

US Environmental Protection Agency (1987) *USEPA Mobile Source Emission Standards Summary*, Bethesda, MD, Office of Air and Radiation

Vallyathan, V., Virmani, R., Rochlani, S., Green, F.H.Y. & Lewis, T. (1986) Effect of diesel emissions and coal dust inhalation on heart and pulmonary arteries of rats. *J. Toxicol. environ. Health, 19*, 33–41

VDI-Kommision (1987) *Emission Measurement. Measurement of Polycyclic Aromatic Hydrocarbons (PAH). Measurement of PAH in the Exhaust Gas from Gasoline and Diesel Engines of Passenger Cars — Gas Chromatographic Determination* (Ger.) (*VDI-Handbuch Reinhaltung der Luft Vol. 5*), Düsseldorf, VDI (Verein Deutscher Ingenieure)-Verlag GmbH

Vianna, N.J., Kovasznay, B., Polan, A. & Ju, C. (1984) Infant leukemia and paternal exposure to motor vehicle exhaust fumes. *J. occup. Med., 26*, 679–682

Vineis, P. & Magnani, C. (1985) Occupation and bladder cancer in males: a case-control study. *Int. J. Cancer, 35*, 599–606

Vostal, J.J. (1983) Bioavailability and biotransformation of the mutagenic component of particulate emissions present in motor exhaust samples. *Environ. Health Perspect., 47*, 269–281

Vostal, J.J., Chan, T.L., Garg, B.D., Lee, P.S. & Strom, K.A. (1981) Lymphatic transport of inhaled diesel particles in the lungs of rats and guinea pigs exposed to diluted diesel exhaust. *Environ. int., 5*, 339–347

Vostal, J.J., White, H.J., Strom, K.A., Siak, J.-S., Chen, K.-C. & Dziedzic, D. (1982) Response of the pulmonary defense system to diesel particulate exposure. In: Lewtas, J., ed., *Toxicological Effects of Emissions from Diesel Engines*, Amsterdam, Elsevier, pp. 201–221

Wadden, R.A., Uno, I. & Wakamatsu, S. (1986) Source discrimination of short-term hydrocarbon samples measured aloft. *Environ. Sci. Technol., 20*, 473–483

Wallace, W.E., Keane, M.J., Hill, C.A., Xu, J. & Ong, T.-M. (1987) Mutagenicity of diesel exhaust particles and oil shale particles dispersed in lecithin surfactant. *J. Toxicol. environ. Health, 21*, 163–171

Waller, R.E. (1981) Trends in lung cancer in London in relation to exposure to diesel fumes. *Environ. int., 5*, 479–483

Waller, R.E., Commins, B.T. & Lawther, P.J. (1961) Air pollution in road tunnels. *Br. J. ind. Med., 18*, 250–259

Waller, R.E., Hampton, L. & Lawther, P.J. (1985) A further study of air pollution in diesel bus garages. *Br. J. ind. Med., 42*, 824–830

Wang, Y.Y., Rappaport, S.M., Sawyer, R.F., Talcott, R.E. & Wei, E.T. (1978) Direct-acting mutagens in automobile exhaust. *Cancer Lett.*, 5, 39–47

Waxweiler, R.J., Wagoner, J.K. & Archer, V.E. (1973) Mortality of potash workers. *J. occup. Med.*, 15, 486–489

Weller, M.A., Chen, S.-T. & Barnhart, M.I. (1981) Acid phosphatase in alveolar macrophages exposed *in vivo* to diesel engine exhaust. *Micron*, 12, 89–90

Wells, A.C., Venn, J.B. & Heard, M.J. (1977) Deposition in the lung and uptake to blood of motor exhaust labelled with $^{203}$Pb. In: Walton, W.H., ed., *Inhaled Particles*, IV, Part 1, Oxford, Pergamon, pp. 175–189

Westerholm, R.N., Alsberg, T.E., Frommelin, A.B., Strandell, M.E., Rannug, U., Winquist, L., Grigoriadis, V. & Egebäck, K.E. (1988) Effect of fuel polycyclic aromatic hydrocarbons content on the emissions of polycyclic aromatic hydrocarbons and other mutagenic substances from a gasoline-fueled automobile. *Environ. Sci. Technol.*, 22, 925–930

Wheeler, R.W., Hearl, F.J. & McCawley, M. (1981) An industrial hygiene characterization of exposure to diesel emissions in an underground coal mine. *Environ. int.*, 5, 485–488

Whitby, R.A. & Altwicker, E.R. (1978) Acetylene in the atmosphere: sources, representative ambient concentrations and ratios to other hydrocarbons. *Atmos. Environ.*, 12, 1289–1296

White, C.M. (1985) Analysis of nitrated polycyclic aromatic hydrocarbons by gas chromatography. In: White, C.M., ed., *Nitrated Polycyclic Aromatic Hydrocarbons*, Heidelberg, A. Hüthig Verlag, pp. 1–86

White, H.J. & Garg, B.D. (1981) Early pulmonary response of the rat lung to inhalation of high concentration of diesel particles. *J. appl. Toxicol.*, 1, 104–110

Wiester, M.J., Iltis, R. & Moore, W. (1980) Altered function and histology in guinea pigs after inhalation of diesel exhaust. *Environ. Res*, 22, 285–297

Wilkins, J.R., III & Sinks, T.H., Jr (1984) Paternal occupation and Wilms' tumour in offspring. *J. Epidemiol. Commun. Health*, 38, 7–11

Williams, M.L. (1987) The impact of motor vehicles on air pollutant emissions and air quality in the UK — an overview. *Sci. total Environ.*, 59, 47–61

Williams, R.L. & Swarin, S.J. (1979) *Benzo[a]pyrene Emissions from Gasoline and Diesel Automobiles (Technical Paper Series No. 790419)*, Warrendale, PA, Society of Automotive Engineers

Williams, R.R., Stegens, N.L. & Goldsmith, J.R. (1977) Associations of cancer site and type with occupation and industry from the Third National Cancer Survey interview. *J. natl Cancer Inst.*, 59, 1147–1185

Wise, S.A. (1983) High-performance liquid chromatography for the determination of polycyclic aromatic hydrocarbons. In: Bjørseth, A., ed., *Handbook of Polycyclic Aromatic Hydrocarbons*, New York, Marcel Dekker, pp. 183–256

Wise, S.A., Bonnett, W.J. & May, W.E. (1980) Normal- and reverse-phase liquid chromatographic separations of polycyclic aromatic hydrocarbons. In: Bjørseth, A. & Dennis, A.J., eds, *Polynuclear Aromatic Hydrocarbons, 4th International Symposium: Chemistry and Biological Effects*, Columbus, OH, Battelle, pp. 791–806

Wolff, R.K., Kanapilly, G.M., DeNee, P.B. & McClellan, R.O. (1981) Deposition of 0.1 $\mu$m chain aggregate aerosols in beagle dogs. *J. Aerosol Sci.*, 12, 119–129

Wolff, R.K., Kanapilly, G.M., Gray, R.H. & McClellan, R.O. (1984) Deposition and retention of inhaled aggregate $^{67}Ga_2O_3$ particles in beagle dogs, Fischer-344 rats, and CD-1 mice. *Am. ind. Hyg. Assoc. J.*, *45*, 377–381

Wolff, R.K., Henderson, R.F., Snipes, M.B., Sun, J.D., Bond, J.A., Mitchell, C.E., Mauderly, J.L. & McClellan, R.O. (1986) Lung retention of diesel soot and associated organic compounds. In: Ishinishi, N., Koizumi, A., McClellan, R.O. & Stöber, W., eds, *Carcinogenic and Mutagenic Effects of Diesel Engine Exhaust*, Amsterdam, Elsevier, pp. 199–211

Wolff, R.K., Henderson, R.F., Snipes, M.B., Griffith, W.C., Mauderly, J.L., Cuddihy, R.G. & McClellan, R.O. (1987) Alterations in particle accumulation and clearance in lungs of rats chronically exposed to diesel exhaust. *Fundam. appl. Toxicol.*, *9*, 154–166

Wong, O., Morgan, R.W., Kheifets, L., Larson, S.R. & Whorton, M.D. (1985) Mortality among members of a heavy construction equipment operators union with potential exposure to diesel exhaust emissions. *Br. J. ind. Med.*, *42*, 435–448

Wong, D., Mitchell, C.E., Wolff, R.K., Mauderly, J.L. & Jeffrey, A.M. (1986) Identification of DNA damage as a result of exposure of rats to diesel engine exhaust. *Carcinogenesis*, *7*, 1595–1597

Woskie, S.R., Smith, T.J., Hammond, S.K., Schenker, M.B., Garshick, E. & Speizer, F.E. (1988a) Estimation of the diesel exhaust exposures of railroad workers: I. Current exposures. *Am. J. ind. Med.*, *13*, 381–394

Woskie, S.R., Smith, T.J., Hammond, S.K., Schenker, M.B., Garshick, E. & Speizer, F.E. (1988b) Estimation of the diesel exhaust exposures of railroad workers: II. National and historical exposures. *Am. J. ind. Med.*, *13*, 395–404

Wright, E.S. (1986) Effects of short-term exposure to diesel exhaust on lung cell proliferation and phospholipid metabolism. *Exp. Lung Res.*, *10*, 39–55

Wynder, E.L. & Hoffmann, D. (1962) A study of air pollution carcinogenesis. III. Carcinogenic activity of gasoline engine exhaust condensate. *Cancer*, *15*, 103–108

Wynder, E.L., Dieck, G.S., Hall, N.E.L. & Lahti, H. (1985) A case-control study of diesel exhaust exposure and bladder cancer. *Environ. Res.*, *37*, 475–489

Xu, G.B. & Yu, C.P. (1987) Deposition of diesel exhaust particles in mammalian lungs. A comparison between rodents and man. *Aerosol Sci. Technol.*, *7*, 117–123

Yamaki, N., Kohno, T., Ishiwata, S., Matsushita, H., Yoshihara, K., Iida, Y., Mizoguchi, T., Okuzawa, S., Sakamoto, K., Kachi, H., Goto, S., Sakamoto, T. & Daishima, S. (1986) The state of the art on the chemical characterization of diesel particulates in Japan. In: Ishinishi, N., Koizumi, A., McClellan, R.O. & Stöber, W., eds, *Carcinogenic and Mutagenic Effects of Diesel Engine Exhaust*, Amsterdam, Elsevier, pp. 17–40

Yoshimura, H. (1983) The influence of air pollution in the development of pulmonary cancer, with special reference to gasoline engines (Jpn.). *Nippon Eiseigaku Zasshi (Jpn. J. Hyg.)*, *37*, 848–865

Yu, C.P. & Xu, G.B. (1986) Predictive models for deposition of diesel exhaust particulates in human and rat lungs. *Aerosol Sci. Technol.*, *5*, 337–347

Yu, C.P. & Xu, G.B. (1987) Predicted disposition of diesel particles in young humans. *J. Aerosol Sci.*, *18*, 419–423

Zack, M., Cannon, S., Loyd, D., Heath, C.W., Jr, Falletta, J.M., Jones, B., Housworth, J. & Crowley, S. (1980) Cancer in children of parents exposed to hydrocarbon-related industries and occupations. *Am. J. Epidemiol.*, *111*, 329–336

Zaebst, D.D., Blade, L.M., Morris, J.A., Schuetzle, D. & Butler, J. (1988) Elemental carbon as a surrogate index of diesel exhaust exposure. In: *Proceedings of the American Industrial Hygiene Conference, 15–20 May 1988, San Francisco, CA*, Cincinnati, OH, National Institute for Occupational Safety and Health, Division of Surveillance, Hazard Evaluation and Field Studies

Zamora, P.O., Gregory, R.E. & Brooks, A.L. (1983) In vitro evaluation of the tumor-promoting potential of diesel-exhaust-particle extracts. *J. Toxicol. environ. Health, 11,* 187–197

Ziskind, R.A., Carlin, T.J. & Ballas, J. (1978) Evaluating toxic gas hazards inside heavy duty diesel truck cabs. In: *Proceedings of the 4th Joint Conference on Sensing Environmental Pollutants, New Orleans, 1977*, Washingon DC, American Chemical Society, pp. 377–383

Zweidinger, R.B. (1982) Emission factors from diesel and gasoline powered vehicles: correlation with the Ames test. In: Lewtas, J., ed., *Toxicological Effects of Emissions from Diesel Engines*, Amsterdam, Elsevier, pp. 83–96

# SOME NITROARENES

# 3,7-DINITROFLUORANTHENE

## 1. Chemical and Physical Data

### 1.1 Synonyms

*Chem. Abstr. Services Reg. No.*: 105735-71-5
*Chem. Abstr. Name*: Fluoranthene, 3,7-dinitro-
*IUPAC Systematic Name*: 3,7-Dinitrofluoranthene

### 1.2 Structural and molecular formulae and molecular weight

$C_{16}H_8N_2O_4$                                                                 Mol. wt: 292.3

### 1.3 Chemical and physical properties of the pure substance

From Nakagawa *et al.* (1987)
(*a*) *Description*: Yellow needles
(*b*) *Melting-point*: 203–204°C
(*c*) *Spectroscopy data*: Nuclear magnetic resonance and ultra-violet spectral data have been reported.

### 1.4 Technical products and impurities

No data were available to the Working Group.

## 2. Production, Use, Occurrence and Analysis

### 2.1 Production and use

No evidence was found that 3,7-dinitrofluoranthene has been produced in commercial quantities or used for other than laboratory applications.

### 2.2 Occurrence

3,7-Dinitrofluoranthene was detected at a concentration of 0.028 mg/kg in particles emitted from a diesel engine (Tokiwa *et al.*, 1986). Dinitrofluoranthenes have been found in incomplete combustion products of liquefied petroleum gas (Horikawa *et al.*, 1987).

Toners for use in photocopy machines have been produced in quantity since the late 1950s and have seen widespread use. 'Long-flow' furnace black was first used in photocopy toners in 1967; its manufacture involved an oxidation whereby some nitration also occurred. Subsequent changes in the production technique reduced the total extractable nitropyrene content from an uncontrolled level of 5–100 mg/kg to below 0.3 mg/kg (Rosenkranz *et al.*, 1980; Sanders, 1981; Butler *et al.*, 1983), and toners produced from that carbon black since 1980 have not been found to contain detectable levels of mutagenicity or, hence, nitropyrenes (Rosenkranz *et al.*, 1980; Butler *et al.*, 1983).

### 2.3 Analysis

See the monograph on 1-nitropyrene.

## 3. Biological Data Relevant to the Evaluation of Carcinogenic Risk to Humans

### 3.1 Carcinogenicity studies in animals[1]

*Subcutaneous administration*

*Rat*: A group of 21 male Fischer 344/DuCrj rats, six weeks old, received subcutaneous injections of 0.05 mg 3,7-dinitrofluoranthene (purity, 99.84%) dissolved in 0.2 ml dimethyl sulfoxide twice a week for ten weeks (total dose, 1 mg; Tokiwa *et al.*, 1987). A group of 21 males was injected similarly with 0.2 ml of the solvent. Animals were observed for 50 weeks; those with tumours at the site of injection were observed until moribund. The first subcutaneous tumour was observed in the treated group on day 155, and within 48 weeks after the beginning of treatment, all treated rats had developed tumours at the site of injection:

---

[1]The Working Group was aware of a study in progress in rats by single injection into the lung (IARC, 1988).

20 were described as malignant fibrous histiocytomas [a term used as a specific diagnosis for some subcutaneous and intraperitoneal sarcomas] and one as a rhabdomyosarcoma. Metastatic foci in the lungs were found in three animals. No subcutaneous tumour developed among the vehicle controls.

## 3.2 Other relevant data

*(a) Experimental systems*

(i) *Absorption, distribution, excretion and metabolism*

No data were available to the Working Group.

(ii) *Toxic effects*

No data were available to the Working Group.

(iii) *Genetic and related effects*

The genetic and related effects of nitroarenes and of their metabolites have been reviewed (Rosenkranz & Mermelstein, 1983; Beland *et al.*, 1985; Rosenkranz & Mermelstein, 1985; Tokiwa & Ohnishi, 1986).

3,7-Dinitrofluoranthene was mutagenic to *Salmonella typhimurium* TA1537, TA1538, TA97, TA98 and TA100 and preferentially inhibited the growth of DNA repair-deficient *Bacillus subtilis* (0.005—0.02 µg/disc; Tokiwa *et al.*, 1986; Nakagawa *et al.*, 1987).

As reported in an abstract, 3,7-dinitrofluoranthene induced mutations to 6-thioguanine resistance in Chinese hamster V79 cells and induced micronuclei in mouse erythrocytes (Horikawa *et al.*, 1987).

*(b) Humans*

No data were available to the Working Group.

## 3.3 Epidemiological studies and case reports of carcinogenicity in humans

No data were available to the Working Group.

# 4. Summary of Data Reported and Evaluation

## 4.1 Exposure data

3,7-Dinitrofluoranthene has been detected in the particulate fraction of the exhaust of a diesel engine.

## 4.2 Experimental data

3,7-Dinitrofluoranthene was tested for carcinogenicity in one experiment in rats by subcutaneous injection, producing sarcomas at the injection site.

## 4.3 Human data

No data were available to the Working Group.

## 4.4 Other relevant data

3,7-Dinitrofluoranthene induced DNA damage and mutation in bacteria.

## 4.5 Evaluation[1]

There is *limited evidence* for the carcinogenicity in experimental animals of 3,7-dinitrofluoranthene.

No data were available from studies in humans on the carcinogenicity of 3,7-dinitrofluoranthene.

### Overall evaluation

3,7-Dinitrofluoranthene *is not classifiable as to its carcinogenicity to humans (Group 3).*

# 5. References

Beland, F.A., Heflich, R.H., Howard, P.C. & Fu, P.P. (1985) The in vitro metabolic activation of nitro polycyclic aromatic hydrocarbons. In: Harvey, R.G., ed., *Polycyclic Hydrocarbons and Carcinogenesis (ACS Symposium Series, No. 283)*, Washington DC, American Chemical Society, pp. 371–396

Butler, M.A., Evans, D.L., Giammarise, A.T., Kiriazides, D.K., Marsh, D., McCoy, E.C., Mermelstein, R., Murphy, C.B. & Rosenkranz, H.S. (1983) Application of *Salmonella* assay to carbon blacks and toners. In: Cooke, M. & Dennis, A.J., eds, *Polynuclear Aromatic Hydrocarbons, 7th International Symposium, Formation, Metabolism and Measurement*, Columbus, OH, Battelle, pp. 225–241

Horikawa, K., Otofuji, T., Nakagawa, R., Sera, N., Kuroda, Y., Otsuka, H. & Tokiwa, H. (1987) Mutagenicity of dinitrofluoranthenes (DNFs) and their carcinogenicity in F344 rats (Abstract no. 11). *Mutat. Res., 182*, 360–361

IARC (1988) *Information Bulletin on the Survey of Chemicals Being Tested for Carcinogenicity*, No. 13, Lyon, p. 103

Nakagawa, R., Horikawa, K., Sera, N., Kodera, Y. & Tokiwa, H. (1987) Dinitrofluoranthene: induction, identification and gene mutation. *Mutat. Res., 191*, 85–91

---

[1]For definitions of the italicized terms, see Preamble, pp. 25–28.

## Summary table of genetic and related effects of 3,7-dinitrofluoranthene

| Nonmammalian systems | | | | | | | | | | | | Mammalian systems | | | | | | | | | | | | | | | | | |
|---|---|---|---|---|---|---|---|---|---|---|---|---|---|---|---|---|---|---|---|---|---|---|---|---|---|---|---|---|---|
| Proka-ryotes | | Lower eukaryotes | | | | | Plants | | | Insects | | In vitro | | | | | | | | | | | | In vivo | | | | | Humans |
| | | | | | | | | | | | | Animal cells | | | | | | | Human cells | | | | | | Animals | | | | |
| D | G | D | R | G | A | D | G | C | R | G | C | A | D | G | S | M | C | A | T | I | D | G | S | M | C | A | T | I | D | G | S | M | C | DL | A | D | S | M | C | A |
| + | +¹ | | | | | | | | | | | | | | | | | | | | | | | | | | | | | | | | | | | | | | | |

A, aneuploidy; C, chromosomal aberrations; D, DNA damage; DL, dominant lethal mutation; G, gene mutation; I, inhibition of intercellular communication; M, micronuclei; R, mitotic recombination and gene conversion; S, sister chromatid exchange; T, cell transformation

*In completing the table, the following symbols indicate the consensus of the Working Group with regard to the results for each endpoint:*
+ considered to be positive for the specific endpoint and level of biological complexity
+¹ considered to be positive, but only one valid study was available to the Working Group

Rosenkranz, H.S. & Mermelstein, R. (1983) Mutagenicity and genotoxicity of nitroarenes: all nitro-containing chemicals were not created equal. *Mutat. Res., 114*, 217–267

Rosenkranz, H.S. & Mermelstein, R. (1985) The genotoxicity, metabolism and carcinogenicity of nitrated polycyclic aromatic hydrocarbons. *J. environ. Sci. Health, C3*, 221–272

Rosenkranz, H.S., McCoy, E.C., Sanders, D.R., Butler, M., Kiriazides, D.K. & Mermelstein, R. (1980) Nitropyrenes: isolation, identification, and reduction of mutagenic impurities in carbon black and toners. *Science, 209*, 1039–1043

Sanders, D.R. (1981) Nitropyrenes: the isolation of trace mutagenic impurities from the toluene extract of an aftertreated carbon black. In: Cooke, M. & Dennis, A.J., eds, *Polynuclear Aromatic Hydrocarbons, 5th International Symposium, Chemical Analysis and Biological Fate*, Columbus, OH, Battelle, pp. 145–158

Tokiwa, H. & Ohnishi, Y. (1986) Mutagenicity and carcinogenicity of nitroarenes and their sources in the environment. *CRC crit. Rev. Toxicol., 17*, 23–60

Tokiwa, H., Otofuji, T., Nakagawa, R., Horikawa, K., Maeda, T., Sano, N., Izumi, K. & Otsuka, H. (1986) Dinitro derivatives of pyrene and fluoranthene in diesel emission particulates and their tumorigenicity in mice and rats. In: Ishinishi, N., Koizumi, A., McClellan, R.O. & Stöber, W., eds, *Carcinogenic and Mutagenic Effects of Diesel Engine Exhaust*, Amsterdam, Elsevier, pp. 253–270

Tokiwa, H., Otofuji, T., Horikawa, K., Sera, N., Nakagawa, R., Maeda, Y., Sano, N., Izumi, K. & Otsuka, H. (1987) Induction of subcutaneous tumors in rats by 3,7- and 3,9-dinitrofluoranthene. *Carcinogenesis, 8*, 1919–1922

# 3,9-DINITROFLUORANTHENE

## 1. Chemical and Physical Data

### 1.1 Synonyms

*Chem. Abstr. Services Reg. No.*: 22506-53-2
*Chem. Abstr. Name*: Fluoranthene, 3,9-dinitro-
*IUPAC Systematic Name*: 3,9-Dinitrofluoranthene

### 1.2 Structural and molecular formulae and molecular weight

$C_{16}H_8N_2O_4$   Mol. wt: 292.3

### 1.3 Chemical and physical properties of the pure substance

(a) *Description*: Yellow-orange crystals (Charlesworth & Lithown, 1969); yellow needles (Nakagawa *et al.*, 1987)

(b) *Melting-point*: 275–276°C (Charlesworth & Lithown, 1969); 222–224°C (Nakagawa *et al.*, 1987)

(c) *Spectroscopy data*: Nuclear magnetic resonance and ultra-violet spectral data have been reported (Nakagawa *et al.*, 1987).

### 1.4 Technical products and impurities

No data were available to the Working Group.

## 2. Production, Use, Occurrence and Analysis

### 2.1 Production and use

No evidence was found that 3,9-dinitrofluoranthene has been produced in commercial quantities or used for other than laboratory applications.

### 2.2 Occurrence

3,9-Dinitrofluoranthene was detected at a concentration of 0.013 mg/kg in particles emitted from a diesel engine (Tokiwa *et al.*, 1986). Dinitrofluoranthenes have been found in incomplete combustion products of liquefied petroleum gas (Horikawa *et al.*, 1987).

Toners for use in photocopy machines have been produced in quantity since the late 1950s and have seen widespread use. 'Long-flow' furnace black was first used in photocopy toners in 1967; its manufacture involved an oxidation whereby some nitration also occurred. Subsequent changes in the production technique reduced the total extractable nitropyrene content from an uncontrolled level of 5–100 mg/kg to below 0.3 mg/kg (Rosenkranz *et al.*, 1980; Sanders, 1981; Butler *et al.*, 1983), and toners produced from that carbon black since 1980 have not been found to contain detectable levels of mutagenicity or, hence, nitropyrenes (Rosenkranz *et al.*, 1980; Butler *et al.*, 1983).

### 2.3 Analysis

See the monograph on 1-nitropyrene.

## 3. Biological Data Relevant to the Evaluation of Carcinogenic Risk to Humans

### 3.1 Carcinogenicity studies in animals[1]

*Subcutaneous administration*

*Rat*: A group of 11 male Fischer 344/DuCrj rats, six weeks old, received subcutaneous injections of 0.05 mg 3,9-dinitrofluoranthene (purity, 99.9%) dissolved in 0.2 ml dimethyl sulfoxide twice a week for ten weeks (total dose, 1 mg; Tokiwa *et al.*, 1987). A group of 21 males was injected similarly with 0.2 ml of the solvent. Animals were observed for 50 weeks; those with tumours at the site of injection were observed until moribund. The first subcutaneous tumour was observed in the treated group on day 88, and 10/11 treated rats had developed tumours at the site of injection by 48 weeks after the beginning of treatment.

---

[1]The Working Group was aware of a study in progress in rats by single injection into the lung (IARC, 1988).

Seven were described as malignant fibrous histiocytomas [a term used as a specific diagnosis for some subcutaneous and intraperitoneal sarcomas] and three as rhabdomyosarcomas. No metastasis was found, and no subcutaneous tumour developed among the vehicle controls.

## 3.2 Other relevant data

(a) *Experimental systems*

(i) *Absorption, distribution, excretion and metabolism*

No data were available to the Working Group.

(ii) *Toxic effects*

No data were available to the Working Group.

(iii) *Genetic and related effects*

The genetic and related effects of nitroarenes and of their metabolites have been reviewed (Rosenkranz & Mermelstein, 1983; Beland *et al.*, 1985; Rosenkranz & Mermelstein, 1985; Tokiwa & Ohnishi, 1986).

3,9-Dinitrofluoranthene was mutagenic to *Salmonella typhimurium* TA1537, TA1538, TA97, TA98 and TA100 and preferentially inhibited the growth of DNA repair-deficient *Bacillus subtilis* (0.005–0.02 µg/disc; Tokiwa *et al.*, 1986; Nakagawa *et al.*, 1987).

As reported in an abstract, 3,9-dinitrofluoranthene induced mutations to 6-thioguanine resistance of Chinese hamster V79 cells and induced micronuclei in mouse erythrocytes (Horikawa *et al.*, 1987).

(b) *Humans*

No data were available to the Working Group.

## 3.3 Epidemiological studies and case reports of carcinogenicity in humans

No data were available to the Working Group.

# 4. Summary of Data Reported and Evaluation

## 4.1 Exposure data

3,9-Dinitrofluoranthene has been detected in the particulate fraction of the exhaust of a diesel engine.

## 4.2 Experimental data

3,9-Dinitrofluoranthene was tested for carcinogenicity in one experiment in rats by subcutaneous injection, producing sarcomas at the injection site.

## 4.3 Human data

No data were available to the Working Group.

## 4.4 Other relevant data

3,9-Dinitrofluoranthene induced DNA damage and mutation in bacteria.

## 4.5 Evaluation[1]

There is *limited evidence* for the carcinogenicity in experimental animals of 3,9-dinitrofluoranthene.

No data were available from studies in humans on the carcinogenicity of 3,9-dinitrofluoranthene.

### Overall evaluation

3,9-Dinitrofluoranthene *is not classifiable as to its carcinogenicity to humans (Group 3)*.

# 5. References

Beland, F.A., Heflich, R.H., Howard, P.C. & Fu, P.P. (1985) The in vitro metabolic activation of nitro polycyclic aromatic hydrocarbons. In: Harvey, R.G., ed., *Polycyclic Hydrocarbons and Carcinogenesis (ACS Symposium Series No. 283)*, Washington DC, American Chemical Society, pp. 371–396

Butler, M.A., Evans, D.L., Giammarise, A.T., Kiriazides, D.K., Marsh, D., McCoy, E.C., Mermelstein, R., Murphy, C.B. & Rosenkranz, H.S. (1983) Application of Salmonella assay to carbon blacks and toners. In: Cooke, M. & Dennis, A.J., eds, *Polynuclear Aromatic Hydrocarbons, 7th International Symposium, Formation, Metabolism and Measurement*, Columbus, OH, Battelle, pp. 225–241

Charlesworth, E.H. & Lithown, C.U. (1969) Fluoranthene studies. IV. Nitration of 2-nitro-, 3-nitro-, and 2-acetamido-fluoranthene. *Can. J. Chem.*, 47, 1595–1599

Horikawa, K., Otofuji, T., Nakagawa, R., Sera, N., Kuroda, Y., Otsuka, H. & Tokiwa, H. (1987) Mutagenicity of dinitrofluoranthenes (DNFs) and their carcinogenicity in F344 rats (Abstract No. 11). *Mutat. Res.*, 182, 360–361

---

[1]For definitions of the italicized terms, see Preamble, pp. 25–28.

## Summary table of genetic and related effects of 3,9-dinitrofluoranthene

| Nonmammalian systems | | | | | | | | | | | | Mammalian systems | | | | | | | | | | | | | | | | | | | | | |
|---|---|---|---|---|---|---|---|---|---|---|---|---|---|---|---|---|---|---|---|---|---|---|---|---|---|---|---|---|---|---|---|---|---|
| Proka-ryotes | | Lower eukaryotes | | | | Plants | | | | Insects | | In vitro | | | | | | | | | | | | | | | | | In vivo | | | | |
| | | | | | | | | | | | | Animal cells | | | | | | | Human cells | | | | | | | | | | Animals | | | | Humans |
| D | G | D | R | G | A | D | G | C | R | G | C | A | D | G | S | M | C | A | T | I | D | G | S | M | C | A | T | I | D | G | S | M | C | DL | A | D | S | M | C | A |
| + | +¹ | | | | | | | | | | | | | | | | | | | | | | | | | | | | | | | | |

A, aneuploidy; C, chromosomal aberrations; D, DNA damage; DL, dominant lethal mutation; G, gene mutation; I, inhibition of intercellular communication; M, micronuclei; R, mitotic recombination and gene conversion; S, sister chromatid exchange; T, cell transformation

*In completing the table, the following symbols indicate the consensus of the Working Group with regard to the results for each endpoint:*
+ considered to be positive for the specific endpoint and level of biological complexity
+¹ considered to be positive, but only one valid study was available to the Working Group

IARC (1988) *Information Bulletin on the Survey of Chemicals Being Tested for Carcinogenicity*, No. 13, Lyon, p. 103

Nakagawa, R., Horikawa, K., Sera, N., Kodera, Y. & Tokiwa, H. (1987) Dinitrofluoranthene: induction, identification and gene mutation. *Mutat. Res.*, *191*, 85–91

Rosenkranz, H.S. & Mermelstein, R. (1983) Mutagenicity and genotoxicity of nitroarenes: all nitro-containing chemicals were not created equal. *Mutat. Res.*, *114*, 217–267

Rosenkranz, H.S. & Mermelstein, R. (1985) The genotoxicity, metabolism and carcinogenicity of nitrated polycyclic aromatic hydrocarbons. *J. environ. Sci. Health*, *C3*, 221–272

Rosenkranz, H.S., McCoy, E.C., Sanders, D.R., Butler, M., Kiriazides, D.K. & Mermelstein, R. (1980) Nitropyrenes: isolation, identification and reduction of mutagenic impurities in carbon black and toners. *Science*, *209*, 1039–1043

Sanders, D.R. (1981) Nitropyrenes: the isolation of trace mutagenic impurities from the toluene extract of an aftertreated carbon black. In: Cooke, M. & Dennis, A.J., eds, *Polynuclear Aromatic Hydrocarbons, 5th International Symposium, Chemical Analysis and Biological Fate*, Columbus, OH, Battelle, pp. 145–158

Tokiwa, H. & Ohnishi, Y. (1986) Mutagenicity and carcinogenicity of nitroarenes and their sources in the environment. *CRC crit. Rev. Toxicol.*, *17*, 23–60

Tokiwa, H., Otofuji, T., Nakagawa, R., Horikawa, K., Maeda, T., Sano, N., Izumi, K. & Otsuka, H. (1986) Dinitro derivatives of pyrene and fluoranthene in diesel emission particulates and their tumorigenicity in mice and rats. In: Ishinishi, N., Koizumi, A., McClellan, R.O. & Stöber, W., eds, *Carcinogenic and Mutagenic Effects of Diesel Engine Exhaust*, Amsterdam, Elsevier, pp. 253–270

Tokiwa, H., Otofuji, T., Horikawa, K., Sera, N., Nakagawa, R., Maeda, T., Sano, N., Izumi, K. & Otsuka, H. (1987) Induction of subcutaneous tumors in rats by 3,7- and 3,9-dinitrofluoranthene. *Carcinogenesis*, *8*, 1919–1922

# 1,3-DINITROPYRENE

## 1. Chemical and Physical Data

### 1.1 Synonyms

*Chem. Abstr. Services Reg. No.*: 75321-20-9
*Chem. Abstr. Name*: Pyrene, 1,3-dinitro-
*IUPAC Systematic Name*: 1,3-Dinitropyrene

### 1.2 Structural and molecular formulae and molecular weight

$C_{16}H_8N_2O_4$                          Mol. wt: 292.3

### 1.3 Chemical and physical properties of the pure substance

(a) *Description*: Light-brown needles, recrystallized from benzene and methanol (Buckingham, 1985); orange crystalline solid (Chemsyn Science Laboratories, 1988)

(b) *Melting-point*: 274–276°C (Buckingham, 1985); 297–298°C (Chemsyn Science Laboratories, 1988)

(c) *Spectroscopy data*: Ultra-violet (Paputa-Peck *et al.*, 1983), infra-red (Hashimoto & Shudo, 1984), nuclear magnetic resonance (Kaplan, 1981; Paputa-Peck *et al.*, 1983; Hashimoto & Shudo, 1984) and mass (Schuetzle & Jensen, 1985) spectral data have been reported.

(d) *Solubility*: Moderately soluble in toluene (Chemsyn Science Laboratories, 1988)

### 1.4 Technical products and impurities

1,3-Dinitropyrene is available for research purposes at ⩾99% purity (Aldrich Chemical Co., 1988; Chemsyn Science Laboratories, 1988). It is also available in $^{14}$C- or $^{3}$H-labelled form at ⩾98% radiochemical purity (Chemsyn Science Laboratories, 1988).

## 2. Production, Use, Occurrence and Analysis

### 2.1 Production and use

Mixtures of 1,3-, 1,6- and 1,8-dinitropyrenes are produced by the nitration of pyrene, and 1,3-dinitropyrene has been isolated and purified from such preparations (Yoshikura et al., 1985). No evidence was found that it has been produced in commercial quantities or used for other than laboratory applications.

### 2.2 Occurrence

(a) *Engine exhaust*

Levels of 1,3-dinitropyrene in exhaust particulate emissions from mobile sources and in the extracts from these particles are given in Table 1.

Table 1. 1,3-Dinitropyrene levels in diesel exhaust particles and their extracts

| Sample[a] | Concentration (mg/kg particulate matter) | Reference |
| --- | --- | --- |
| HDD (mining), 100% load, 1200 rpm | 0.52 | Draper (1986) |
| HDD (mining), 75% load, 1800 rpm | 1.6 | Draper (1986) |
| Diesel emissions (LDD) | 0.3 | Salmeen et al. (1984) |
| Diesel emissions (LDD) | 0.6 | Nishioka et al. (1982) |
| Diesel emissions (LDD) | <0.5 | Schuetzle (1983) |
| Diesel emissions (LDD) | ⩽0.005 | Gibson (1983) |

[a]HDD, heavy-duty diesel; LDD, light-duty diesel

(b) *Other occurrence*

Small amounts of dinitropyrenes are generated by kerosene heaters, which are used extensively in Japan for heating residences and offices (Tokiwa et al., 1985). Such open, oil-burning space heaters were found to emit dinitropyrenes at a rate of 0.2 ng/h after only 1 h of operation; 1,3-dinitropyrene was found at 0.53 ± 0.59 mg/kg particulate extract, accounting for 2.9% of the mutagenicity of the fraction. Gas and liquefied petroleum gas

(LPG) burners, widely used for home heating and cooking, also produced detectable amounts of dinitropyrenes. A level of 0.6 mg/kg particulate extract of 1,3-dinitropyrene was found in emissions from one gas burner, representing 7.9% of the mutagenic activity. The authors suggested that dinitropyrenes result from the incomplete combustion of fuel in the presence of at least a few micrograms per cuber metre of nitrogen dioxide.

According to Takayama *et al.* (1985) and Pitts (1987), several dinitropyrenes have been detected in respirable particles from ambient atmospheric samples. Tanabe *et al.* (1986) measured 1,3-dinitropyrene at up to 4.7 pg/m$^3$ air and up to 56.2 ng/g particulate matter in the ambient atmosphere in Tokyo, Japan. Gibson (1986) found no 1,3-dinitropyrene in the ambient air at six sites in the USA, under various conditions; the detection limit was 0.001 μg/g particulate matter.

Toners for use in photocopy machines have been produced in quantity since the late 1950s and have seen widespread use. 'Long-flow' furnace black was first used in photocopy toners in 1967; its manufacture involved an oxidation whereby some nitration also occurred. Subsequent changes in the production technique reduced the total extractable nitropyrene content from an uncontrolled level of 5-100 mg/kg to below 0.3 mg/kg (Rosenkranz *et al.*, 1980; Sanders, 1981; Butler *et al.*, 1983), and toners produced from this carbon black since 1980 have not been found to contain detectable levels of mutagenicity or, hence, nitropyrenes (Rosenkranz *et al.*, 1980; Butler *et al.*, 1983).

A pre-1979 carbon black sample was reported to contain 6.3 mg/kg 1,3-dinitropyrene (Sanders, 1981); and a formerly available commercial carbon black was also found to contain this compound (Ramdahl & Urdal, 1982). A sample made in 1980 contained 0.07 mg/kg 1,3-dinitropyrene (Giammarise *et al.*, 1982).

## 2.3 Analysis

See the monograph on 1-nitropyrene.

# 3. Biological Data Relevant to the Evaluation of Carcinogenic Risk to Humans

### 3.1 Carcinogenicity studies in animals[1]

*(a) Oral administration*

*Rat*: A group of 36 female weanling CD rats received oral intubations of 10 μmol-[3 mg]/kg bw 1,3-dinitropyrene (purity, >99%) dissolved in dimethyl sulfoxide (DMSO; 1.7 μmol[0.5 mg]/ml DMSO) three times per week for four weeks (average total dose, 16 μmol[4.7 mg]/rat) and were observed for 76-78 weeks (King, 1988). A vehicle control group

---

[1]The Working Group was aware of a study in progress in mice by single subcutaneous injection (IARC, 1988).

of 36 animals received DMSO only. Average survival times of treated and control animals were 527 and 517 days, respectively. Three rats (9%) administered 1,3-dinitropyrene and none of the controls developed leukaemia. Mammary tumours (11 adenocarcinomas and 7 fibroadenomas) were found in 12/35 treated animals, but their incidence did not differ from that observed in vehicle controls (6 and 13 in 12/35). [The Working Group noted the short duration of both treatment and observation and that, in parallel studies, positive results were obtained with 1,6- and 1,8-dinitropyrene.]

*(b) Subcutaneous administration*

*Mouse*: A group of 20 male BALB/c mice, six weeks old, received subcutaneous injections of 0.05 mg 1,3-dinitropyrene (purity, >99.9%) dissolved in 0.2 ml DMSO once a week for 20 weeks (total dose, 1 mg; Otofuji *et al.*, 1987). A positive control group of 20 males received injections of 0.05 mg benzo[*a*]pyrene; a further 20 mice served as untreated controls. Animals were observed for 60 weeks or until moribund. The first subcutaneous tumour in the benzo[*a*]pyrene-treated group was seen in week 21, and all 16 mice surviving beyond this time developed tumours at the injection site which were diagnosed histologically as malignant fibrous histiocytomas [a term used as a specific diagnosis for some subcutaneous and intraperitoneal sarcomas]. No subcutaneous tumour was found in 1,3-dinitropyrene-treated or untreated controls up to 60 weeks. Some tumours developed in the lungs, liver and spleen of 1,3-dinitropyrene-treated animals, but the incidence was not statistically different from those in the positive or DMSO controls. [The Working Group noted the small number of animals used and the relatively short observation period.]

*Rat*: Ten male Fischer 344/DuCrj rats, six weeks old, received subcutaneous injections of 0.2 mg 1,3-dinitropyrene ([purity unspecified] impurities: 0.6% 1,6-dinitropyrene, <0.05% other nitropyrenes) dissolved in 0.2 ml DMSO twice a week for ten weeks (total dose, 4 mg; Ohgaki *et al.*, 1984). A control group of 20 rats received injections of 0.2 ml DMSO only. The animals were killed between days 169 and 347. Subcutaneous sarcomas developed at the site of injection in all treated rats between days 119 and 320. No 'tumorous' change was observed in other organs of the treated rats, and no tumour developed among control animals. [The Working Group noted the possible influence of the contamination with 1,6-dinitropyrene.]

A group of 43 female newborn CD rats received subcutaneous injections of 1,3-dinitropyrene (purity, >99%; total dose, 6.3 $\mu$mol [1.9 mg]) dissolved in DMSO (1.7 $\mu$mol[0.5 mg]/ml DMSO) into the suprascapular region once a week for eight weeks (King, 1988). A group of 40 animals injected with DMSO alone served as controls. The average length of survival was 468 days for treated animals and 495 days for controls. At the time of sacrifice, 67 weeks after the first treatment, 5/43 treated rats had developed malignant fibrous histiocytomas at the site of injection; no tumour of this type was found among vehicle controls ($p < 0.05$). Mammary tumours (six adenocarcinomas and three fibroadenomas) were observed in 9/43 treated animals and in 8/37 control animals (one adenocarcinoma, six fibroadenomas).

(c) *Intraperitoneal administration*

*Mouse*: Groups of 90 or 100 male and female newborn CD-1 mice received three intraperitoneal injections of 1,3-dinitropyrene (total dose, 200 nmol [58.5 µg]; purity, >99%) in 10, 20 and 40 µl DMSO on days 1, 8 and 15 after birth; a total dose of 560 nmol [140 µg] benzo[*a*]pyrene (purity, >99%); or three injections of DMSO only (Wislocki *et al.*, 1986). Treatment of a second vehicle control group was begun ten weeks after that of the other groups. At 25–27 days, when the mice were weaned, 30 males and 39 females in the treated group, 37 males and 27 females in the positive control group, and 28 and 31 males and 45 and 34 females in the two vehicle control groups were still alive. All remaining mice were killed after one year. In the group injected with 1,3-dinitropyrene, 6/30 male mice developed liver adenomas; this incidence was not significantly greater than that in the vehicle controls. No increase in the incidences of lung adenomas or malignant lymphomas was observed in males or females as compared to DMSO-treated animals. Benzo[*a*]pyrene induced liver tumours (adenomas and carcinomas) in 18/37 males and in 0/27 females, and the numbers of animals with lung adenomas (males, 13/37; females, 13/27) were significantly higher than those in DMSO controls. Malignant lymphomas were seen in 2/37 males and 4/27 females treated with benzo[*a*]pyrene. The numbers of animals with tumours in the two groups treated with DMSO only were 2/28 and 5/45 males with liver adenomas, 1/28 male with a lung adenoma and 4/45 with lung adenomas and carcinomas; only 2/34 females in the second vehicle control group had lung tumours. [The Working Group noted the short duration of the study.]

*Rat*: A group of 36 female weanling CD rats received intraperitoneal injections of 10 µmol[3 mg]/kg bw 1,3-dinitropyrene (purity, >99%) dissolved in DMSO (1.7 µmol[0.5 mg]/ml DMSO) three times per week for four weeks (total dose, 16 µmol[4.7 mg]/rat); 36 control animals were treated with DMSO only (King, 1988). Animals were sacrificed when moribund or after 76–78 weeks. At this time, malignant fibrous histiocytomas were found in the peritoneal cavity of two treated rats, and two animals had leukaemia. Neither malignancy developed in 31 surviving controls. Mammary tumours were observed in 19/36 treated rats (9 adenocarcinomas and 12 fibroadenomas) and in 7/31 controls (3 and 5, respectively); the difference in the total number of tumours was statistically significant ($p < 0.05$). [The Working Group noted the high and variable spontaneous incidence of mammary tumours seen in these studies.]

## 3.2 Other relevant data

(a) *Experimental systems*

(i) *Absorption, distribution, excretion and metabolism*

Under an argon atmosphere, rat and dog liver cytosol catalysed the reduction of 1,3-dinitropyrene to 1-amino-3-nitropyrene, 1-nitro-3-nitrosopyrene and 1,3-diaminopyrene. During this reduction, metabolites were formed that bound to exogenous DNA. When acetyl coenzyme A was added to the rat liver cytosolic incubations, 1-acetylamino-3-nitropyrene was also detected as a metabolite, and the extent of binding to DNA was increased 19-fold (Djurić et al., 1985). Subsequent studies showed that *Salmonella typhimurium* TA98 and rat liver microsomes obtained from a 105 000 g supernatant also reduced 1,3-dinitropyrene to 1-nitro-3-nitrosopyrene and 1-amino-3-nitropyrene (Djurić et al., 1986).

1-Amino-3-nitropyrene and 1,3-diaminopyrene were detected as metabolites in rat mammary gland cytosol incubated with 1,3-dinitropyrene under anaerobic conditions. When incubations were conducted in the presence of acetyl coenzyme A, binding to exogenous tRNA occurred. Metabolism was not detected in intact rat mammary gland cells (King et al., 1986; Imaida et al., 1988).

Hsieh et al. (1986) used $^{32}$P-postlabelling to detect a low level of DNA adduct formation (fewer than five adducts per $10^6$ nucleotides) in C3H 10T1/2 mouse embryo fibroblasts incubated with 1,3-dinitropyrene.

(ii) *Toxic effects*

Intraperitoneal administration of 1,3-dinitropyrene to young male Sprague-Dawley rats (three times at 2.5 mg/kg bw) resulted in a four-fold increase in 1-nitropyrene reductase activity in liver microsomes over that in controls (Chou et al., 1987).

(iii) *Genetic and related effects*

The genetic and related effects of nitroarenes and of their metabolites have been reviewed (Rosenkranz & Mermelstein, 1983; Beland et al., 1985; Rosenkranz & Mermelstein, 1985; Tokiwa & Ohnishi, 1986).

1,3-Dinitropyrene (0.0015 µg/ml) induced DNA damage in *Salmonella typhimurium* (Nakamura et al., 1987) and preferentially inhibited the growth of DNA repair-deficient *Bacillus subtilis* (Horikawa et al., 1986 (0.03–1.0 µg/disc); Tokiwa et al., 1986 (0.1 µg/disc)). It was mutagenic to *Escherichia coli* WP2 uvrA pKM101 (McCoy et al., 1985a) and to *S. typhimurium* TA96, TA97, TA98, TA100, TA102, TA104, TA1537 and TA1538 (Rosenkranz et al., 1980; Löfroth, 1981; Mermelstein et al., 1981; Pederson & Siak, 1981; Morotomi & Watanabe, 1984; McCoy et al., 1985b; Rosenkranz et al., 1985; Tokiwa et al., 1985).

1,3-Dinitropyrene (up to 500 µg/ml) did not induce gene conversion in the yeast *Saccharomyces cerevisiae* D4 (McCoy et al., 1983).

It induced marginal DNA damage in primary mouse hepatocytes, as measured by alkaline elution, at 5–20 µM (Møller & Thorgeirsson, 1985). It induced unscheduled DNA synthesis in rat and mouse hepatocytes at $1.1 \times 10^{-5} - 1.1 \times 10^{-2}$ mg/ml (Mori et al., 1987). 1,3-Dinitropyrene (0.5–2.0 µg/ml) induced the synthesis of polyoma virus DNA in polyoma virus-transformed rat fibroblasts (Lambert & Weinstein, 1987).

1,3-Dinitropyrene induced unscheduled DNA synthesis in cultured human hepatoma-derived HepG2 cells (Eddy et al., 1986). As reported in an abstract, it induced unscheduled DNA synthesis in human hepatocytes (Yoshimi et al., 1987).

1,3-Dinitropyrene (0.1–10 µg/ml) induced mutation to diphtheria toxin resistance in cultured Chinese hamster lung fibroblasts (Nakayasu et al., 1982) and to ouabain resistance in Chinese hamster V79 cells (1–10 µg/ml; Takayama et al., 1983; Katoh et al., 1984). It also marginally induced mutation to 6-thioguanine resistance in Chinese hamster CHO cells in the absence of an exogenous metabolic system (0.2–2 µg/ml) but was unequivocally active at 2 µg/ml in the presence of activation (Li & Dutcher, 1983).

1,3-Dinitropyrene induced mutations at the *hprt* locus of cultured human hepatoma-derived HepG2 cells (Eddy *et al.*, 1986).

As reported in an abstract, 1,3-dinitropyrene (2 µg/ml) induced chromosomal aberrations in cultured Chinese hamster lung fibroblasts in the absence of an exogenous metabolic system (Matsuoka *et al.*, 1987). As reported in an abstract, no transformation activity was observed when 1,3-dinitropyrene was tested at concentrations of up to 250 µg/ml in BALB/c 3T3 cells (Tu *et al.*, 1982).

(*b*) *Humans*

No data were available to the Working Group.

### 3.3 Epidemiological studies and case reports of carcinogenicity in humans

No data were available to the Working Group.

## 4. Summary of Data Reported and Evaluation

### 4.1 Exposure data

1,3-Dinitropyrene has been detected in some carbon blacks and in particulate emissions from diesel engines, kerosene heaters and gas burners. It has been found at low concentrations in ambient air.

### 4.2 Experimental data

1,3-Dinitropyrene was tested for carcinogenicity in single experiments in rats by oral administration, in mice, rats and newborn rats by subcutaneous injection and in newborn mice and in weanling rats by intraperitoneal injection. It was carcinogenic to rats, producing sarcomas at the site of its subcutaneous injection. The tests by oral and intraperitoneal routes in rats and by subcutaneous and intraperitoneal injection in mice were inadequate for evaluation.

### 4.3 Human data

No data were available to the Working Group.

### 4.4 Other relevant data

Metabolism of 1,3-dinitropyrene led to DNA binding *in vitro*. 1,3-Dinitropyrene caused DNA damage and mutation in cultured rodent and human cells and in bacteria. It did not cause gene conversion in yeast.

### 4.5 Evaluation[1]

There is *limited evidence* for the carcinogenicity in experimental animals of 1,3-dinitropyrene.

No data were available from studies in humans on the carcinogenicity of 1,3-dinitropyrene.

**Overall evaluation**

1,3-Dinitropyrene *is not classifiable as to its carcinogenicity to humans (Group 3).*

## 5. References

Aldrich Chemical Co. (1988) *Aldrich Catalog/Handbook of Fine Chemicals 1988–1989*, Milwaukee, WI, p. 633

Beland, F.A., Heflich, R.H., Howard, P.C. & Fu, P.P. (1985) The in vitro metabolic activation of nitro polycyclic aromatic hydrocarbons. In: Harvey, R.G., ed., *Polycyclic Hydrocarbons and Carcinogenesis (ACS Symposium Series No. 283)*, Washington DC, American Chemical Society, pp. 371–396

Buckingham, J., ed. (1985) *Dictionary of Organic Compounds*, 5th ed., 3rd Supplement, New York, Chapman & Hall, p. 182 (D-30522)

Butler, M.A., Evans, D.L., Giammarise, A.T., Kiriazides, D.K., Marsh, D., McCoy, E.C., Mermelstein, R., Murphy, C.B. & Rosenkranz, H.S. (1983) Application of *Salmonella* assay to carbon blacks and toners. In: Cooke, M. & Dennis, A.J., eds, *Polynuclear Aromatic Hydrocarbons, 7th International Symposium, Formation, Metabolism and Measurement*, Columbus, OH, Battelle, pp. 225–241

Chemsyn Science Laboratories (1988) *1,3-Dinitropyrene (Product Code U1037)*, Lenexa, KS, pp. 66–68

Chou, M.W., Wang, B., Von Tungeln, L.S., Beland, F.A. & Fu, P.P. (1987) Induction of rat hepatic cytochromes P-450 by environmental nitropolycyclic aromatic hydrocarbons. *Biochem. Pharmacol.*, 36, 2449–2454

Djurić, Z., Fifer, E.K. & Beland, F.A. (1985) Acetyl coenzyme A-dependent binding of carcinogenic and mutagenic dinitropyrenes to DNA. *Carcinogenesis*, 6, 941–944

---

[1] For definitions of the italicized terms, see Preamble, pp. 25–28.

## Summary table of genetic and related effects of 1,3-dinitropyrene

| Nonmammalian systems | | | | | | | | | | | | | | | | | Mammalian systems | | | | | | | | | | | | | | | | | | | |
|---|---|---|---|---|---|---|---|---|---|---|---|---|---|---|---|---|---|---|---|---|---|---|---|---|---|---|---|---|---|---|---|---|---|---|---|
| Proka-ryotes | | | | Lower eukaryotes | | | | Plants | | | | Insects | | | | In vitro | | | | | | | | | | | | In vivo | | | | | | | |
| | | | | | | | | | | | | | | | | Animal cells | | | | | | | Human cells | | | | | Animals | | | | | | Humans | | |
| D | G | D | R | G | A | E | D | G | C | R | G | C | A | D | G | S | M | C | A | T | I | D | G | S | M | C | A | T | I | D | G | S | M | C | DL | A | D | S | M | C | A |
| + | + | | −¹ | | | | | | | | | | | | + | + | | | | | | | | +¹ | +¹ | | | | | | | | | | | | | | | | |

A, aneuploidy; C, chromosomal aberrations; D, DNA damage; DL, dominant lethal mutation; G, gene mutation; I, inhibition of intercellular communication; M, micronuclei; R, mitotic recombination and gene conversion; S, sister chromatid exchange; T, cell transformation

*In completing the table, the following symbols indicate the consensus of the Working Group with regard to the results for each endpoint:*

\+ considered to be positive for the specific endpoint and level of biological complexity
+¹ considered to be positive, but only one valid study was available to the Working Group
−¹ considered to be negative, but only one valid study was available to the Working Group

Djurić, Z., Potter, D.W., Heflich, R.H. & Beland, F.A. (1986) Aerobic and anaerobic reduction of nitrated pyrenes in vitro. *Chem.-biol. Interactions*, *59*, 309–324

Draper, W.M. (1986) Quantitation of nitro- and dinitropolycyclic aromatic hydrocarbons in diesel exhaust particulate matter. *Chemosphere*, *15*, 437–447

Eddy, E.P., McCoy, E.C., Rosenkranz, H.S. & Mermelstein, R. (1986) Dichotomy in the mutagenicity and genotoxicity of nitropyrenes: apparent effect of the number of electrons involved in nitroreduction. *Mutat. Res.*, *161*, 109–111

Giammarise, A.T., Evans, D.L., Butler, M.A., Murphy, C.B., Kiriazides, D.K., Marsh, D. & Mermelstein, R. (1982) Improved methodology for carbon black extraction. In: Cooke, M., Dennis, A.J. & Fisher, G.L., eds, *Polynuclear Aromatic Hydrocarbons, 6th International Symposium, Physical and Biological Chemistry*, Columbus, OH, Battelle, pp. 325–334

Gibson, T.L. (1983) Sources of direct-acting nitroarene mutagens in airborne particulate matter. *Mutat. Res.*, *122*, 115–121

Gibson, T.L. (1986) Sources of nitroaromatic mutagens in atmospheric polycyclic organic matter. *J. Air Pollut. Control Assoc.*, *36*, 1022–1025

Hashimoto, Y. & Shudo, K. (1984) Preparation of pure isomers of dinitropyrenes. *Chem. pharm. Bull.*, *32*, 1992–1994

Horikawa, K., Sera, N., Tokiwa, H. & Kada, T. (1986) Results of the *rec*-assay of nitropyrenes in the *Bacillus subtilis* test system. *Mutat. Res.*, *174*, 89–92

Hsieh, L.L., Wong, D., Heisig, V., Santella, R.M., Mauderly, J.L., Mitchell, C.E., Wolff, R.K. & Jeffrey, A.M. (1986) Analysis of genotoxic components in diesel engine emissions. In: Ishinishi, N., Koizumi, A., McClellan, R.O. & Stöber, W., eds, *Carcinogenic and Mutagenic Effects of Diesel Engine Exhaust*, Amsterdam, Elsevier, pp. 223–232

IARC (1988) *Information Bulletin on the Survey of Chemicals Being Tested for Carcinogenicity*, No. 13, Lyon, p. 13

Imaida, K., Tay, L.K., Lee, M.-S., Wang, C.Y., Ito, N. & King, C.M. (1988) Tumor induction by nitropyrenes in the female CD rat. In: King, C.M., Romano, L.J. & Schuetzle, D., eds, *Carcinogenic and Mutagenic Responses to Aromatic Amines and Nitroarenes*, Amsterdam, Elsevier, pp. 187–197

Kaplan, S. (1981) Carbon-13 chemical shift assignments of the nitration products of pyrene. *Org. magn. Resonance*, *15*, 197–199

Katoh, Y., Takayama, S. & Shudo, K. (1984) Inhibition by hemin of dinitropyrene-induced mutagenesis in Chinese hamster V79 cells. *Gann*, *75*, 574–577

King, C.M. (1988) *Metabolism and Biological Effects of Nitropyrene and Related Compounds (Research Report No. 16)*, Cambridge, MA, Health Effects Institute

King, C.M., Tay, L.K., Lee, M.-S., Imaida, K. & Wang, C.Y. (1986) Mechanisms of tumor induction by dinitropyrenes in the female CD rat. In: Ishinishi, N., Koizumi, A., McClellan, R.O. & Stöber, W., eds, *Carcinogenic and Mutagenic Effects of Diesel Engine Exhaust*, Amsterdam, Elsevier, pp. 279–290

Lambert, M.E. & Weinstein, I.B. (1987) Nitropyrenes are inducers of polyoma viral DNA synthesis. *Mutat. Res.*, *183*, 203–211

Li, A.P. & Dutcher, J.S. (1983) Mutagenicity of mono-, di- and tri-nitropyrenes in Chinese hamster ovary cells. *Mutat. Res.*, *119*, 387–392

Löfroth, G. (1981) Comparison of the mutagenic activity in carbon particulate matter and in diesel and gasoline engine exhaust. In: Waters, M.D., Sandhu, S.S., Lewtas Huisingh, J., Claxton, L. & Nesnow, S., eds, *Short-term Bioassays in the Analysis of Complex Environmental Mixtures, II*, New York, Plenum, pp. 319–336

Matsuoka, A., Sofuni, T., Sato, S., Miyata, N. & Ishidate, M., Jr (1987) In vitro clastogenicity of nitropyrenes and nitrofluorenes (Abstract No. 25). *Mutat. Res., 182*, 366–367

McCoy, E.C., Anders, M., Rosenkranz, H.S. & Mermelstein, R. (1983) Apparent absence of recombinogenic activity of nitropyrenes for yeast. *Mutat. Res., 116*, 119–127

McCoy, E.C., Anders, M., Rosenkranz, H.S. & Mermelstein, R. (1985a) Mutagenicity of nitropyrenes for *Escherichia coli*: requirement for increased cellular permeability. *Mutat. Res., 142*, 163–167

McCoy, E.C., Holloway, M., Frierson, M., Klopman, G., Mermelstein, R. & Rosenkranz, H.S. (1985b) Genetic and quantum chemical basis of the mutagenicity of nitroarenes for adenine-thymine base pairs. *Mutat. Res., 149*, 311–319

Mermelstein, R., Kiriazides, D.K., Butler, M., McCoy, E.C. & Rosenkranz, H.S. (1981) The extraordinary mutagenicity of nitropyrenes in bacteria. *Mutat. Res., 89*, 187–196

Møller, M.E. & Thorgeirsson, S.S. (1985) DNA damage induced by nitropyrenes in primary mouse hepatocytes and in rat H4-II-E hepatoma cells. *Mutat. Res., 151*, 137–146

Mori, H., Sugie, S., Yoshimi, N., Kinouchi, T. & Ohnishi, Y. (1987) Genotoxicity of a variety of nitroarenes and other nitro compounds in DNA-repair tests with rat and mouse hepatocytes. *Mutat. Res., 190*, 159–167

Morotomi, M. & Watanabe, T. (1984) Metabolism of exogenous compounds by the intestinal microflora (Jpn). *Tikoshikoroji Foramu (Toxicol. Forum), 7*, 395–408

Nakamura, S.-I., Oda, Y., Shimada, T., Oki, I. & Sugimoto, K. (1987) SOS-inducing activity of chemical carcinogens and mutagens in *Salmonella typhimurium* TA1535/pSK 1002: examination with 151 chemicals. *Mutat. Res., 192*, 239–246

Nakayasu, M., Sakamoto, H., Wakabayashi, K., Terada, M., Sugimura, T. & Rosenkranz, H.S. (1982) Potent mutagenic activity of nitropyrenes on Chinese hamster lung cells with diphtheria toxin resistance as a selective marker. *Carcinogenesis, 3*, 917–922

Nishioka, M.G., Petersen, B.A. & Lewtas, J. (1982) Comparison of nitro-aromatic content and direct-acting mutagenicity of diesel emissions. In: Cooke, M., Dennis, A.J. & Fisher, G.L., eds, *Polynuclear Aromatic Hydrocarbons, 6th International Symposium, Physical and Biological Chemistry*, Columbus, OH, Battelle, pp. 603–613

Ohgaki, H., Negishi, C., Wakabayashi, K., Kusama, K., Sato, S. & Sugimura, T. (1984) Induction of sarcomas in rats by subcutaneous injection of dinitropyrenes. *Carcinogenesis, 5*, 583–585

Otofuji, T., Horikawa, K., Maeda, T., Sano, N., Izumi, K., Otsuka, H. & Tokiwa, H. (1987) Tumorigenicity test of 1,3- and 1,8-dinitropyrene in BALB/c mice. *J. natl Cancer Inst., 79*, 185–188

Paputa-Peck, M.C., Marano, R.S., Schuetzle, D., Riley, T.L., Hampton, C.V., Prater, T.J., Skewes, L.M. & Jensen, T.E. (1983) Determination of nitrated polynuclear aromatic hydrocarbons in particulate extracts by capillary column gas chromatography with nitrogen selective detection. *Anal. Chem., 55*, 1946–1954

Pederson, T.C. & Siak, J.-C. (1981) The role of nitroaromatic compounds in the direct-acting mutagenicity of diesel particle extracts. *J. Appl. Toxicol., 1*, 54–60

Pitts, J.N., Jr (1987) Nitration of gaseous polycyclic aromatic hydrocarbons in simulated and ambient urban atmospheres: a source of mutagenic nitroarenes. *Atmos. Environ., 21*, 2531–2547

Ramdahl, T. & Urdal, K. (1982) Determination of nitrated polycyclic aromatic hydrocarbons by fused silica capillary gas chromatography/negative ion chemical ionization mass spectrometry. *Anal. Chem., 54*, 2256–2260

Rosenkranz, H.S. & Mermelstein, R. (1983) Mutagenicity and genotoxicity of nitroarenes: all nitro-containing chemicals were not created equal. *Mutat. Res., 114*, 217–267

Rosenkranz, H.S. & Mermelstein, R. (1985) The genotoxicity, metabolism and carcinogenicity of nitrated polycyclic aromatic hydrocarbons. *J. environ. Sci. Health, C3*, 221–272

Rosenkranz, H.S., McCoy, E.C., Sanders, D.R., Butler, M., Kiriazides, D.K. & Mermelstein, R. (1980) Nitropyrenes: isolation, identification and reduction of mutagenic impurities in carbon black and toners. *Science, 209*, 1039–1043

Rosenkranz, H.S., McCoy, E.C., Frierson, M. & Klopman, G. (1985) The role of DNA sequence and structure of the electrophile on the mutagenicity of nitroarenes and arylamine derivatives. *Environ. Mutagenesis, 7*, 645–653

Salmeen, I.T., Pero, A.M., Zator, R., Schuetzle, D. & Riley, T.L. (1984) Ames assay chromatograms and the identification of mutagens in diesel particle extracts. *Environ. Sci. Technol., 18*, 375–382

Sanders, D.R. (1981) Nitropyrenes: the isolation of trace mutagenic impurities from the toluene extract of an aftertreated carbon black. In: Cooke, M. & Dennis, A.J., eds, *Polynuclear Aromatic Hydrocarbons, 5th International Symposium, Chemical Analysis and Biological Fate*, Columbus, OH, Battelle, pp. 145–158

Schuetzle, D. (1983) Sampling of vehicle emissions for chemical analysis and biological testing. *Environ. Health Perspect., 47*, 65–80

Schuetzle, D. & Jensen, T.E. (1985) Analysis of nitrated polycyclic aromatic hydrocarbons (nitro-PAH) by mass spectrometry. In: White, C.M., ed., *Nitrated Polycyclic Aromatic Hydrocarbons*, Heidelberg, A. Hüthig Verlag, pp. 121–167

Takayama, S., Tanaka, M., Katoh, Y., Terada, M. & Sugimura, T. (1983) Mutagenicity of nitropyrenes in Chinese hamster V79 cells. *Gann, 74*, 338–341

Takayama, S., Ishikawa, T., Nakajima, H. & Sato, S. (1985) Lung carcinoma induction in Syrian golden hamsters by intratracheal instillation of 1,6-dinitropyrene. *Jpn. J. Cancer Res. (Gann), 76*, 457–461

Tanabe, K., Matsushita, H., Kuo, C.-T. & Imamiya, S. (1986) Determination of carcinogenic nitroarenes in airborne particulates by high performance liquid chromatography (Jpn.). *Taiki Osen Gakkaishi (J. Jpn. Soc. Air Pollut.), 21*, 535–544

Tokiwa, H. & Ohnishi, Y. (1986) Mutagenicity and carcinogenicity of nitroarenes and their sources in the environment. *CRC crit. Rev. Toxicol., 17*, 23–69

Tokiwa, H., Nakagawa, R. & Horikawa, K. (1985) Mutagenic/carcinogenic agents in indoor pollutants; the dinitropyrenes generated by kerosene heaters and fuel gas and liquefied petroleum gas burners. *Mutat. Res., 157*, 39–47

Tokiwa, H., Otofuji, T., Nakagawa, R., Horikawa, K., Maeda, T., Sano, N., Izumi, K. & Otsuka, H. (1986) Dinitro derivatives of pyrene and fluoranthene in diesel emission particulates and their tumorigenicity in mice and rats. In: Ishinishi, N., Koizumi, A., McClellan, R.O. & Stöber, eds, *Carcinogenic and Mutagenic Effects of Diesel Engine Exhaust*, Amsterdam, Elsevier, pp. 253–270

Tu, A.S., Sivak, A. & Mermelstein, R. (1982) Evaluation of in vitro transforming activity of nitropyrenes (Abstract). In: *Proceedings of the Fifth CIIT Conference on Toxicology: Toxicity of Nitroaromatic Compounds*, Raleigh, NC, Chemical Industry Institute of Toxicology, p. 8

Wislocki, P.G., Bagan, E.S., Lu, A.Y.H., Dooley, K.L., Fu, P.P., Han-Hsu, H., Beland, F.A. & Kadlubar, F.F. (1986) Tumorigenicity of nitrated derivatives of pyrene, benz[*a*]anthracene, chrysene and benzo[*a*]pyrene in the newborn mouse assay. *Carcinogenesis*, 7, 1317–1322

Yoshikura, T., Kuroda, K., Kamiura, T., Masumoto, K., Fukushima, M., Yamamoto, T. & Torii, M. (1985) Synthesis of 1,3-, 1,6- and 1,8-dinitropyrenes and evaluation of their mutagenicities. *Annu. Rep. Osaka City Inst. public Health environ. Sci.*, 47, 31–35 [*Chem. Abstr.*, 106, 49745t]

Yoshimi, N., Sugie, S., Mori, H., Kinouchi, T. & Ohnishi, Y. (1987) Genotoxicity of various nitroarenes in DNA repair tests with human hepatocytes (Abstract No. 73). *Mutat. Res.*, 182, 384

# 1,6-DINITROPYRENE

## 1. Chemical and Physical Data

### 1.1 Synonyms

*Chem. Abstr. Services Reg. No.*: 42397-64-8
*Chem. Abstr. Name*: Pyrene, 1,6-dinitro-
*IUPAC Systematic Name*: 1,6-Dinitropyrene

### 1.2 Structural and molecular formulae and molecular weight

$C_{16}H_8N_2O_4$                      Mol. wt: 292.3

### 1.3 Chemical and physical properties of the pure substance

(a) *Description*: Light-brown needles, recrystallized from benzene and methanol (Buckingham, 1985); yellow crystalline solid (Chemsyn Science Laboratories, 1988)

(b) *Melting-point*: >300°C (Buckingham, 1985); 310°C (Chemsyn Science Laboratories, 1988)

(c) *Spectroscopy data*: Ultra-violet (Paputa-Peck *et al.*, 1983), infra-red (Hashimoto & Shudo, 1984), nuclear magnetic resonance (Kaplan, 1981; Paputa-Peck *et al.*, 1983; Hashimoto & Shudo, 1984) and mass (Schuetzle & Jensen, 1985) spectral data have been reported.

(d) *Solubility*: Moderately soluble in toluene (Chemsyn Science Laboratories, 1988)

### 1.4 Technical products and impurities

1,6-Dinitropyrene is available for research purposes at 98% (Aldrich Chemical Co., 1988) or ⩾99% purity (Chemsyn Science Laboratories, 1988). It is also available in $^{14}$C- or $^3$H-labelled form at ⩾98% radiochemical purity (Chemsyn Science Laboratories, 1988).

## 2. Production, Use, Occurrence and Analysis

### 2.1 Production and use

*(a) Production*

Mixtures of 1,3-, 1,6- and 1,8-dinitropyrenes are produced by the nitration of pyrene, and 1,6-dinitropyrene has been isolated and purified from such preparations (Yoshikura *et al.*, 1985). The Katsura Chemical Co., Tokyo, Japan, synthesized >99.9% pure 1,6-dinitropyrene for Takayama *et al.* (1985), according to the method of Hashimoto and Shudo (1984).

*(b) Use*

No evidence was found that 1,6-dinitropyrene has been used for other than laboratory applications.

### 2.2 Occurrence

*(a) Engine exhaust*

1,6-Dinitropyrene has been found at levels of 0.81 mg/kg (Manabe *et al.*, 1985) and 1.2 mg/kg (Nakagawa *et al.*, 1983) in extracts of particles from the exhaust of heavy-duty diesel engines, and at $0.4 \pm 0.2$ mg/kg extract (Salmeen *et al.*, 1984), 0.6 mg/kg extract (Nishioka *et al.*, 1982) and 0.033–0.034 mg/kg particles (Gibson, 1983) from the exhaust of light-duty diesel engines.

*(b) Other occurrence*

Small amounts of dinitropyrenes are generated by kerosene heaters, which are used extensively in Japan for heating residences and offices (Tokiwa *et al.*, 1985). Such open, oil-burning space heaters were found to emit dinitropyrenes at a rate of 0.2 ng/h after only 1 h of operation; a mixture of 1,6- and 1,8-dinitropyrenes was found at $3.25 \pm 0.63$ mg/kg particulate extract, accounting for 13% of the mutagenic activity of the sample. Gas and liquefied petroleum gas (LPG) burners, widely used for home heating and cooking, also produced detectable amounts of dinitropyrenes: 1.88 mg/kg extract (36.8% of mutagenicity) and 0.88 mg/kg extract (25.2% of mutagenicity), respectively. The authors suggested that dinitropyrenes result from the incomplete combustion of fuel in the presence of at least a few micrograms per cubic metre of nitrogen dioxide.

According to Takayama *et al.* (1985) and Pitts (1987), several dinitropyrenes have been detected in respirable particles from ambient atmospheric samples. Gibson (1986) reported higher amounts in heavy industrialized areas than in nonindustrialized urban and suburban sites. Levels of 1,6-dinitropyrene in samples of airborne particulates are given in Table 1.

Table 1. 1,6-Dinitropyrene levels in atmospheric particulates

| Sample source | Concentration | | Reference |
|---|---|---|---|
| | Particulate extract (mg/kg) | Atmosphere (pg/m³) | |
| Tokyo, Japan | 0.0047–0.105 | 0.33–8.74 | Tanabe *et al.* (1986) |
| Bermuda (remote) | | | Gibson (1986) |
|   Summer | 0.0081 | 0.15[a] | |
|   Winter | 0.0083 | 0.12[a] | |
| Delaware, USA (rural) | | | Gibson (1986) |
|   Summer | 0.0049 | 0.12[a] | |
| Warren, MI, USA (suburban) | | | Gibson (1986) |
|   Winter | <0.006 | 0.15[a] | |
|   Summer | 0.0046 | 0.30[a] | |
| Detroit, MI, USA (urban) | 0.0036 | 0.48[a] | Gibson (1986) |
|   Summer | | | |
| River Rouge, MI, USA (industrial) | | | Gibson (1986) |
|   Summer | 0.046 | 4.44[a] | |
| Dearborn, MI, USA (industrial) | | | Gibson (1986) |
|   Summer | 0.041 | 7.50[a] | |
| Southeast, MI, USA | | | Siak *et al.* (1985) |
|   Summer | 0.31 (mean) | 0.026 (mean) | |
| Santiago, Chile (urban) | 0.2 | – | Tokiwa *et al.* (1983) |

[a]Calculated by the Working Group

Toners for use in photocopy machines have been produced in quantity since the late 1950s and have seen widespread use. 'Long-flow' furnace black was first used in photocopy toners in 1967; its manufacture involved an oxidation whereby some nitration also occurred. Subsequent changes in the production technique reduced the total extractable nitropyrene content from an uncontrolled level of 5–100 mg/kg to below 0.3 mg/kg (Rosenkranz *et al.*, 1980; Sanders, 1981; Butler *et al.*, 1983), and toners produced from this carbon black since 1980 have not been found to contain detectable levels of mutagenicity or, hence, nitropyrenes (Rosenkranz *et al.*, 1980; Butler *et al.*, 1983).

Some carbon black samples have also been found to contain 1,6-dinitropyrene: 21 mg/kg in a pre-1979 aftertreated carbon black (Sanders, 1981) and in a commercial sample (Ramdahl & Urdal, 1982). A sample made in 1980 was found to contain 0.13 mg/kg 1,6-dinitropyrene (Giammarise et al., 1982).

## 2.3 Analysis

See the monograph on 1-nitropyrene.

# 3. Biological Data Relevant to the Evaluation of Carcinogenic Risk to Humans

## 3.1 Carcinogenicity studies in animals[1]

### (a) Oral administration

*Rat*: A group of 36 female weanling CD rats received oral intubations of 10 μmol-[3 mg]/kg bw 1,6-dinitropyrene (purity, >99%) dissolved in dimethyl sulfoxide (DMSO; 1.7 μmol[0.5 mg]/ml DMSO) three times per week for four weeks (average total dose, 16 μmol[4.7 mg]/rat) and were observed for 76–78 weeks (King, 1988). A vehicle control group of 36 animals received DMSO only. Two rats treated with 1,6-dinitropyrene and none of the controls developed leukaemia. Mammary tumours were found in 17/36 treated (19 adenocarcinomas and 11 fibroadenomas) and in 12/35 control rats (6 adenocarcinomas and 13 fibroadenomas); the difference between the groups was not statistically significant. [The Working Group noted the short duration of both treatment and observation.]

### (b) Intratracheal instillation

*Hamster*: A group of ten male and ten female Syrian golden hamsters, ten weeks old, received intratracheal instillations of 0.5 mg 1,6-nitropyrene (purity, >99.9%) suspended in 0.2 ml saline once a week for 26 weeks (total dose, 13 mg; Takayama et al., 1985). A group of ten males and ten females received instillations of saline only and served as controls. The experiment was terminated at 11 months. Lung adenocarcinomas developed in ten males and nine females treated with 1,6-nitropyrene in weeks 20–48; 65% had multiple tumour nodules. In addition, myeloid leukaemia developed in six males and six females. No such tumour was detected among controls.

### (c) Intrapulmonary administration

*Rat*: A group of 28 male Fischer 344/DuCrj rats, 10–11 weeks old, received a single injection of 0.05 ml beeswax-tricaprylin containing 0.15 mg 1,6-dinitropyrene (purity,

---

[1]The Working Group was aware of studies in progress in rats by single intrapleural instillation and in mice by single subcutaneous injection (IARC, 1988).

>99.9%) directly into the lower third of the left lung after left lateral thoracotomy (Maeda et al., 1986). A group of 19 rats received a single injection of 0.05 ml beeswax-tricaprylin containing 0.5 mg 3-methylcholanthrene [purity unspecified], and another group of 31 rats received an injection of beeswax-tricaprylin only. Animals were observed for 72 weeks after treatment, at which time the experiment was terminated. Of the 1,6-dinitropyrene-treated rats, 21/28 (75%) developed squamous-cell carcinomas and 2/28 developed undifferentiated carcinomas. Squamous-cell carcinomas were induced in all 19 rats treated with 3-methylcholanthrene earlier than in 1,6-dinitropyrene-treated rats. No squamous-cell carcinoma was observed in the control group ($p < 0.005$). Distant metastases of induced tumours were observed in four 1,6-dinitropyrene-treated and one 3-methylcholanthrene-treated rats. The incidence of Leydig-cell tumours of the testis was significantly lower in 1,6-dinitropyrene- and 3-methylcholanthrene-treated rats than in the controls ($p < 0.05$). The incidences of other tumours did not differ among the groups.

(d) *Subcutaneous administration*

*Mouse*: A group of 20 male BALB/c mice, six weeks old, received subcutaneous injections of 0.1 mg 1,6-dinitropyrene (purity, >99.9%) dissolved in 0.2 ml DMSO once a week for 20 weeks (total dose, 2 mg; Tokiwa et al., 1984). A further group of 20 mice treated with 0.2 ml DMSO only served as vehicle controls. Animals were observed for 60 weeks or, for mice with tumours at the site of injection, until moribund. The first tumour in the 1,6-dinitropyrene-treated group was seen on day 112; 45 weeks after the first treatment, 10/20 mice had developed tumours at the injection site which were diagnosed histologically as malignant fibrous histiocytomas [a term used as a specific diagnosis for some subcutaneous and intraperitoneal sarcomas]. No subcutaneous tumour was detected in vehicle controls ($p < 0.002$). Lung tumours were found in 6/20 treated and 7/20 control mice.

*Rat*: Ten male Fischer 344/DuCrj rats, six weeks old, received subcutaneous injections of 0.2 mg 1,6-dinitropyrene ([purity unspecified] impurities: <0.05% each of 1,3-dinitropyrene, 1,8-dinitropyrene, 1,3,6-trinitropyrene and 1,3,6,8-tetranitropyrene) dissolved in 0.2 ml DMSO twice a week for ten weeks (total dose, 4 mg; Ohgaki et al., 1985). A control group of 20 rats received injections of 0.2 ml DMSO only. Treated animals were killed on day 320 and control rats on day 650. Sarcomas developed at the site of injection in all treated rats between days 103 and 123. No tumour developed at the injection site among control animals, although 16 interstitial-cell tumours of the testis, two C-cell adenomas of the thyroid gland, two pancreatic islet-cell adenomas and one phaeochromocytoma were seen.

A group of 46 female newborn CD rats received subcutaneous injections of 1,6-dinitropyrene (purity, >99%) dissolved in DMSO (1.7 $\mu$mol[0.5 mg]/ml DMSO) into the suprascapular region once a week for eight weeks (total dose, 6.3 $\mu$mol[1.8 mg]; King, 1988). A group of 40 animals injected with DMSO alone served as controls. The average survival time was 149 days for treated rats and 495 days for controls. Malignant fibrous histiocytomas developed rapidly at the site of injection among treated rats; the first tumour was seen 15 weeks after the initial treatment, and by 18 weeks all rats had developed this tumour. In addition, nine rats had leukaemia. Vehicle controls developed neither malignancy ($p < 0.0001$ and $p < 0.005$). Mammary tumours (mainly adenocarcinomas) were seen in 5/46 treated rats; 8/40 controls had mammary tumours (mainly fibroadenomas).

*(e) Intraperitoneal administration*

*Mouse*: Groups of 90 or 100 male and female newborn CD-1 mice received three intraperitoneal injections of 1,6-dinitropyrene (purity, >99%; total dose, 200 nmol [58.7 μg] in 10, 20 and 40 μl DMSO on days 1, 8 and 15 after birth; a total dose of 560 nmol [140 μg] benzo[a]pyrene (purity, >99%) as three injections; or three injections of DMSO only (Wislocki *et al.*, 1986). Treatment of a second vehicle control group was begun ten weeks after that of the other groups. At 25–27 days, when the mice were weaned, 25 males and 29 females in the treated group, 37 males and 37 females in the positive control group, and 28 and 31 males and 45 and 34 females in the two vehicle control groups were still alive. All remaining mice were killed after one year. In the group injected with 1,6-dinitropyrene, 8/25 male mice developed liver tumours (three with adenomas, five with carcinomas); this incidence was significantly greater than that in the vehicle controls ($p < 0.025$). No increase in the incidences of lung tumours or malignant lymphomas was observed in males or females as compared to DMSO-treated animals. Benzo[a]pyrene induced liver tumours in 18/37 males and 0/27 females and lung adenomas in 13/37 males and 13/27 females; the latter incidences were significantly higher than those in DMSO controls ($p < 0.005$). Malignant lymphomas were seen in 2/37 males and 4/27 females treated with benzo[a]pyrene. In the two DMSO-treated groups, 2/28 and 5/45 males had liver adenomas and 1/28 and 4/45 had lung tumours, and 0/31 and 0/34 females had liver tumours and 0/31 and 2/34 had lung tumours.

*Rat*: A group of 36 female weanling CD rats received intraperitoneal injections of 10 μmol[3 mg]/kg bw 1,6-dinitropyrene (purity, >99%) dissolved in DMSO (1.7 μmol[0.5 mg]/ml DMSO) three times per week for four weeks (average total dose, 16 μmol[4.7 mg]/rat); 36 control animals were treated with DMSO only (King, 1988). Treatment with 1,6-dinitropyrene resulted in some early deaths 12–15 weeks after the initial treatment. Tumours were first identified in a rat autopsied 17 weeks after the first injection. All 23 1,6-dinitropyrene-treated animals that survived longer than 21 weeks had developed malignant fibrous histiocytomas in the peritoneal cavity, but none of the vehicle controls, observed for 76–78 weeks, developed these tumours ($p < 0.0001$). Mammary tumours developed in both groups at approximately the same incidence.

## 3.2 Other relevant data

*(a) Experimental systems*

(i) *Absorption, distribution, excretion and metabolism*

In preweanling male CD mice treated with a single intraperitoneal dose of 115 nmol [33.6 μg] [$^3$H]1,6-dinitropyrene, analysis of lung and liver DNA 24 h later indicated the presence of one major adduct, *N*-(deoxyguanosin-8-yl)-1-amino-6-nitropyrene (Delclos *et al.*, 1987). In male Sprague-Dawley rats treated with an intraperitoneal dose of 200 µg/kg bw [$^3$H]1,6-dinitropyrene, DNA binding was detected in the mammary epithelium, liver, lung, kidney and urinary bladder; *N*-(deoxyguanosin-8-yl)-1-amino-6-nitropyrene was detected in the urinary bladder, liver, kidney and mammary epithelium. Pretreatment of these animals with 1-nitropyrene, which induced nitroreductase, did not affect DNA binding, except in the kidney where it was increased 1.6-fold (Djurić *et al.*, 1988).

Under an argon atmosphere, rat and dog liver cytosol catalysed the reduction of 1,6-dinitropyrene to 1-amino-6-nitropyrene, 1-nitro-6-nitrosopyrene and 1,6-diaminopyrene. During this reduction, metabolites were formed that bound to exogenous DNA. When acetyl coenzyme A was added to the rat liver cytosolic incubations, 1-acetylamino-6-nitropyrene was also detected as a metabolite, and the extent of binding was increased 24-fold (Djurić *et al.*, 1985). Subsequent studies showed that *Salmonella typhimurium* TA98, rat liver microsomes obtained from a 105 000 *g* supernatant and human liver cytosol also reduced 1,6-dinitropyrene to 1-nitro-6-nitrosopyrene and 1-amino-6-nitropyrene (Djurić *et al.*, 1986, 1988).

1-Nitro-6-nitrosopyrene, 1-amino-6-nitropyrene and 1,6-diaminopyrene were detected as metabolites in rat mammary gland cytosol incubated with 1,6-dinitropyrene under anaerobic conditions. When incubations were conducted in the presence of acetyl coenzyme A, binding to exogenous tRNA occurred. Incubation with intact rat mammary gland cells resulted in the formation of 1-amino-6-nitropyrene (King *et al.*, 1986; Imaida *et al.*, 1988).

A low level of DNA adduct formation (fewer than five adducts per $10^6$ nucleotides) was detected by $^{32}$P-postlabelling in C3H 10T1/2 mouse embryo fibroblasts incubated with 1,6-dinitropyrene (Hsieh *et al.*, 1986).

A Fischer 2408 rat fibroblast cell line, H3, transformed by a temperature-sensitive mutant of polyoma virus, metabolized 1,6-dinitropyrene to several polar products; one major and several minor DNA adducts were formed at the same time (Lambert & Weinstein, 1987).

Incubation of 1,6-dinitropyrene with purified nitroreductases from the anaerobic bacterium, *Bacteroides fragilis*, in the presence of various polynucleotides resulted in preferential binding to the deoxyguanine moiety of poly(dG) nucleic acids, binding to the deoxy adenine moiety poly(dA) being about 75% lower (Kinouchi & Ohnishi, 1986).

(ii) *Toxic effects*

A group of 28 male Fischer 344 rats was given a single injection of 0.15 mg 1,6-dinitropyrene directly into the lower third of the left lung after left lateral thoracotomy. Squamous metaplasia of the lung was seen in two animals and granulomatous lesions containing foreign-body giant cells in three (Maeda *et al.*, 1986).

Intraperitoneal administration of 1,6-dinitropyrene to young male Sprague Dawley rats (three times at 2.5 mg/kg bw) resulted in a 2.5-fold increase in 1-nitropyrene reductase activity in liver microsomes over that in controls (Chou *et al.*, 1987).

(iii) *Genetic and related effects*

The genetic and related effects of nitroarenes and of their metabolites have been reviewed (Rosenkranz & Mermelstein, 1983; Beland *et al.*, 1985; Rosenkranz & Mermelstein, 1985; Tokiwa & Ohnishi, 1986).

1,6-Dinitropyrene (0.005 µg/ml) induced DNA damage in *S. typhimurium* (Nakamura *et al.*, 1987) and preferentially inhibited the growth of DNA repair-deficient *Bacillus subtilis* (Horikawa *et al.*, 1986 (0.02–0.06 µg/disc); Tokiwa *et al.*, 1986 (0.04 µg/disc)). It was mutagenic to *Escherichia coli* WP2 *uvrA* pkM101 (Tokiwa *et al.*, 1984; McCoy *et al.*, 1985a) and to *S. typhimurium* TA96, TA97, TA98, TA100, TA102, TA104, TA1537 and TA1538 (Rosenkranz *et al.*, 1980; Löfroth, 1981; Mermelstein *et al.*, 1981; Tokiwa *et al.*, 1981; Nakayasu *et al.*, 1982; Ashby *et al.*, 1983; Morotomi & Watanabe, 1984; Tokiwa *et al.*, 1984; McCoy *et al.*, 1985b; Rosenkranz *et al.*, 1985; Tokiwa *et al.*, 1985; El-Bayoumy & Hecht, 1986; Fifer *et al.*, 1986; Fu *et al.*, 1986).

Conflicting results have been reported concerning the induction by 1,6-dinitropyrene of gene conversion in the yeast, *Saccharomyces cerevisiae*: positive results were reported in strain JDI (Wilcox & Parry, 1981 (1.6–25 µg/ml); Wilcox *et al.*, 1982 (2.9–4.4 ng/ml)) and negative results in strain D4 (McCoy *et al.*, 1983 (up to 500 µg/ml)). It has been suggested that these differences reflect intracellular oxygen levels (Rosenkranz & Mermelstein, 1983).

As determined by alkaline elution, 1,6-dinitropyrene induced a marginal effect on the formation of single-strand DNA breaks in primary mouse hepatocytes at 5–20 µM (Møller & Thorgeirsson, 1985) and in Chinese hamster V79 cells at the only concentration tested, 15 µM (Saito *et al.*, 1984), but not in cultured rat hepatoma cells at up to 10 µM (Møller & Thorgeirsson, 1985). 1,6-Dinitropyrene (15 µM) did not induce DNA-protein cross-links in cultured rat hepatoma cells (Møller & Thorgeirsson, 1985). When tested at 0.5–2 µg/ml, it induced the synthesis of viral DNA in polyoma virus-transformed rat fibroblasts (Lambert & Weinstein, 1987).

1,6-Dinitropyrene induced unscheduled DNA synthesis in mouse (Mori *et al.*, 1987 (1.0 $\times 10^{-5}$–1.0 $\times 10^{-2}$ mg/ml)), rat (Butterworth *et al.*, 1983 (0.00005–0.005 mM); Mori *et al.*, 1987 (1.0 $\times 10^{-5}$–1.0 $\times 10^{-2}$ mg/ml)) and human (Butterworth *et al.*, 1983 (0.00005–0.005 mM); Yoshimi *et al.*, 1987)) hepatocytes, and in rat (Doolittle & Butterworth, 1984 (0.05–0.5 µM)) and human (Sugimura & Takayama, 1983 ($10^{-4}$M); Doolittle *et al.*, 1985 (0.5–5.0 µM)) cultured tracheal or bronchial epithelial cells. It induced unscheduled DNA synthesis in rabbit lung Clara and alveolar type II cells (Haugen *et al.*, 1986 (0.63–10 ng/ml)), but not in human hepatoma-derived HepG2 cells (Eddy *et al.*, 1985, 1986 (up to 2 µg/ml)) or in isolated rat spermatocytes (Working & Butterworth, 1984 (0.05–5 µM)).

1,6-Dinitropyrene (0.05–5 µg/ml) induced mutations at the *hprt* locus of cultured Chinese hamster CHO cells (Li & Dutcher, 1983 (0.2–2 µg/ml); Edgar & Brooker, 1985) and was weakly active at 5–20 µM (Fifer *et al.*, 1986); it did not induce this mutation in human hepatoma-derived HepG2 cells at up to 2 µg/ml (Eddy *et al.*, 1985, 1986). It induced mutation to ouabain resistance (only one dose tested, 0.1 µg/ml) in Chinese hamster V79 cells (Katoh *et al.*, 1984) and to diphtheria toxin resistance (0.1–10 µg/ml; Nakayasu *et al.*, 1982) in cultured Chinese hamster lung fibroblasts.

1,6-Dinitropyrene (0.05–5 µg/ml) induced sister chromatid exchange and chromosomal aberrations in cultured Chinese hamster CHO cells (Edgar & Brooker, 1985). It induced chromosomal aberrations, primarily of the chromatid type, in cultured rat (Wilcox *et al.*, 1982; Danford *et al.*, 1982 (0.01–2.5 µg/ml)) and Chinese hamster liver epithelial cells (Danford *et al.*, 1983 (2 mg/ml)) and in human fibroblasts (Wilcox *et al.*, 1982 (0.02–5.0 µg/ml)). As reported in an abstract, 1,6-dinitropyrene (0.1 µg/ml) induced chromosomal aberrations in cultured Chinese hamster lung fibroblasts (Matsuoka *et al.*, 1987).

Oral administration of 1,6-dinitropyrene to rats (50 mg/kg bw) did not result in the induction of unscheduled DNA synthesis in either hepatocytes (Butterworth *et al.*, 1983) or spermatocytes (Working & Butterworth, 1984).

1,6-Dinitropyrene-induced rat fibrosarcomas contained activated H-*ras* and N-*ras* oncogenes (Ishizaka *et al.*, 1987).

*(b) Humans*

No data were available to the Working Group.

## 3.3 Epidemiological studies and case reports of carcinogenicity in humans

No data were available to the Working Group.

# 4. Summary of Data Reported and Evaluation

## 4.1 Exposure data

1,6-Dinitropyrene has been detected in some carbon blacks and in particulate emissions from diesel engines, kerosene heaters and gas burners. It has also been found at low concentrations in ambient air.

## 4.2 Experimental data

1,6-Dinitropyrene was tested for carcinogenicity by intratracheal instillation in hamsters, by intrapulmonary injection in rats, by subcutaneous injection in mice and rats and by intraperitoneal injection in newborn mice and weanling rats. After intratracheal instillation, it induced adenocarcinomas of the lung and leukaemia. After intrapulmonary injection, it induced a high incidence of squamous-cell carcinomas of the lung. After subcutaneous injection, it induced a high incidence of sarcomas at the injection site in weanling and newborn rats and in mice and leukaemia in newborn rats. After intraperitoneal injection, it increased the incidence of liver-cell tumours in male mice and induced sarcomas of the peritoneal cavity in rats. A study by oral administration in rats was inadequate for evaluation.

## 4.3 Human data

No data were available to the Working Group.

## 4.4 Other relevant data

Metabolism of 1,6-dinitropyrene led to DNA adduct formation *in vivo* and *in vitro*. 1,6-Dinitropyrene induced DNA damage and chromosomal aberrations but not mutations in cultured human cells. It induced DNA damage, mutation, sister chromatid exchange and chromosomal aberrations in cultured rodent cells, and DNA damage and mutation in bacteria.

## 4.5 Evaluation[1]

There is *sufficient evidence* for the carcinogenicity in experimental animals of 1,6-dinitropyrene.

No data were available from studies in humans on the carcinogenicity of 1,6-dinitropyrene.

### Overall evaluation

1,6-Dinitropyrene *is possibly carcinogenic to humans (Group 2B)*.

# 5. References

Aldrich Chemical Co. (1988) *Aldrich Catalog/Handbook of Fine Chemicals 1988*–1989, Milwaukee, WI, p. 633

Ashby, J., Paton, D., Wilcox, P. & Parry, J.M. (1983) Synthesis of 1,6-diaminopyrene from 1,6-dinitropyrene and its S9 dependent mutagenicity to *S. typhimurium*. *Carcinogenesis*, 4, 787–789

Beland, F.A., Heflich, R.H., Howard, P.C. & Fu, P.P. (1985) The in vitro metabolic activation of nitro polycyclic aromatic hydrocarbons. In: Harvey, R.G., ed., *Polycyclic Hydrocarbons and Carcinogenesis (ACS Symposium Series No. 283)*, Washington DC, American Chemical Society, pp. 371–396

Buckingham, J., ed. (1985) *Dictionary of Organic Compounds*, 5th ed., 3rd Supplement, New York, Chapman & Hall, p. 182 (D-30522)

Butler, M.A., Evans, D.L., Giammarise, A.T., Kiriazides, D.K., Marsh, D., McCoy, E.C., Mermelstein, R., Murphy, C.B. & Rosenkranz, H.S. (1983) Application of *Salmonella* assay to carbon blacks and toners. In: Cooke, M. & Dennis, A.J., eds, *Polynuclear Aromatic Hydrocarbons, 7th International Symposium, Formation, Metabolism and Measurement*, Columbus, OH, Battelle, pp. 225–241

---

[1] For definitions of the italicized terms, see Preamble, pp. 25–28.

# Summary table of genetic and related effects of 1,6-dinitropyrene

| Nonmammalian systems | | | | | Mammalian systems | | | |
|---|---|---|---|---|---|---|---|---|
| Proka-ryotes | Lower eukaryotes | Plants | Insects | | In vitro | | In vivo | |
| | | | | | Animal cells | Human cells | Animals | Humans |
| D G | D R G C A D G | A D G C R | G C A | | D G S M C A T | D G S M C A T I | D G S M C DL A | D S M C A |
| + + | ? | | | | + + +¹ + | + −¹ +¹ | + | |

A, aneuploidy; C, chromosomal aberrations; D, DNA damage; DL, dominant lethal mutation; G, gene mutation; I, inhibition of intercellular communication; M, micronuclei; R, mitotic recombination and gene conversion; S, sister chromatid exchange; T, cell transformation

*In completing the table, the following symbols indicate the consensus of the Working Group with regard to the results for each endpoint:*

+ considered to be positive for the specific endpoint and level of biological complexity
+¹ considered to be positive, but only one valid study was available to the Working Group
−¹ considered to be negative, but only one valid study was available to the Working Group
? considered to be equivocal or inconclusive (e.g., there were contradictory results from different laboratories; there were confounding exposures; the results were equivocal)

Butterworth, B.E., Earle, L.L., Strom, D., Jirtle, R. & Michalopoulos, G. (1983) Induction of DNA repair in human and rat hepatocytes by 1,6-dinitropyrene. *Mutat. Res., 122*, 73–80

Chemsyn Science Laboratories (1988) *1,6-Dinitropyrene (Product Code U1036)*, Lenexa, KS, pp. 69–71

Chou, M.W., Wang, B., Von Tungeln, L.S., Beland, F.A. & Fu, P.P. (1987) Induction of rat hepatic cytochromes P-450 by environmental nitropolycyclic aromatic hydrocarbons. *Biochem. Pharmacol., 36*, 2449–2454

Danford, N., Wilcox, P. & Parry, J.M. (1982) The clastogenic activity of dinitropyrenes in a rat-liver epithelial cell line. *Mutat. Res., 105*, 349–355

Danford, N., Hogan, L. & Parry, J.M. (1983) A modified hypotonic treatment to measure mitotic aneuploidy in a Chinese hamster primary cell line (Abstract). *Environ. Mutagenesis, 5*, 948

Delclos, K.B., Walker, R.P., Dooley, K.L., Fu, P.P. & Kadlubar, F.F. (1987) Carcinogen-DNA adduct formation in the lungs and livers of preweanling CD-1 male mice following administration of [$^3$H]-6-nitrochrysene, [$^3$H]-6-aminochrysene, and [$^3$H]-1,6-dinitropyrene. *Cancer Res., 47*, 6272–6277

Djurić, Z., Fifer, E.K. & Beland, F.A. (1985) Acetyl coenzyme A-dependent binding of carcinogenic and mutagenic dinitropyrenes to DNA. *Carcinogenesis, 6*, 941–944

Djurić, Z., Potter, D.W., Heflich, R.H. & Beland, F.A. (1986) Aerobic and anaerobic reduction of nitrated pyrenes *in vitro*. *Chem.-biol. Interactions, 59*, 309–324

Djurić, Z., Fifer, E.K., Yamazoe, Y. & Beland, F.A. (1988) DNA binding by 1-nitropyrene and 1,6-dinitropyrene *in vitro* and *in vivo*: effects of nitroreductase induction. *Carcinogenesis, 9*, 357–364

Doolittle, D.J. & Butterworth, B.E. (1984) Assessment of chemically-induced DNA repair in rat tracheal epithelial cells. *Carcinogenesis, 5*, 773–779

Doolittle, D.J., Furlong, J.W. & Butterworth, B.E. (1985) Assessment of chemically induced DNA repair in primary cultures of human bronchial epithelial cells. *Toxicol. appl. Pharmacol., 79*, 28–38

Eddy, E.P., Howard, P.C. & Rosenkranz, H.S. (1985) Metabolism, DNA repair and mutagenicity of 1-nitropyrene in the human hepatoma cell line HepG2 (Abstract No. 378). *Proc. Am. Assoc. Cancer Res., 26*, 96

Eddy, E.P., McCoy, E.C., Rosenkranz, H.S. & Mermelstein, R. (1986) Dichotomy in the mutagenicity and genotoxicity of nitropyrenes: apparent effect of the number of electrons involved in nitroreduction. *Mutat. Res., 161*, 109–111

Edgar, D.H. & Brooker, P.C. (1985) Induction of 6-thioguanine resistance, chromosome aberrations and SCE by dinitropyrenes in Chinese hamster ovary cells *in vitro*. *Mutat. Res., 158*, 209–215

El-Bayoumy, K. & Hecht, S.S. (1986) Mutagenicity of K-region derivatives of 1-nitropyrene; remarkable activity of 1- and 3-nitro-5*H*-phenanthro[4,5-*bcd*]pyran-5-one. *Mutat. Res., 170*, 31–40

Fifer, E.K., Heflich, R.H., Djurić, Z., Howard, P.C. & Beland, F.A. (1986) Synthesis and mutagenicity of 1-nitro-6-nitrosopyrene and 1-nitro-8-nitrosopyrene, potential intermediates in the metabolic activation of 1,6- and 1,8-dinitropyrene. *Carcinogenesis, 7*, 65–70

Fu, P.P., Heflich, R.H., Von Tungeln, L.S., Yang, D.T.C., Fifer, E.K. & Beland, F.A. (1986) Effect of the nitro group conformation on the rat liver microsomal metabolism and bacterial mutagenicity of 2- and 9-nitroanthracene. *Carcinogenesis, 7*, 1819–1827

Giammarise, A.T., Evans, D.L., Butler, M.A., Murphy, C.B., Kiriazides, D.K., Marsh, D. & Mermelstein, R. (1982) Improved methodology for carbon black extraction. In: Cooke, M., Dennis, A.J. & Fisher, G.L., eds, *Polynuclear Aromatic Hydrocarbons, 6th International Symposium, Physical and Biological Chemistry*, Columbus, OH, Battelle Press, pp. 325–334

Gibson, T.L. (1983) Sources of direct-acting nitroarene mutagens in airborne particulate matter. *Mutat. Res.*, *122*, 115–121

Gibson, T.L. (1986) Sources of nitroaromatic mutagens in atmospheric polycyclic organic matter. *J. Air Pollut. Control Assoc.*, *36*, 1022–1025

Hashimoto, Y. & Shudo, K. (1984) Preparation of pure isomers of dinitropyrenes. *Chem. pharm. Bull.*, *32*, 1992–1994

Haugen, A., Aune, T. & Deilhaug, T. (1986) Nitropyrene-induced DNA repair in Clara cells and alveolar type-II cells isolated from rabbit lung. *Mutat. Res.*, *175*, 259–262

Horikawa, K., Sera, N., Tokiwa, H. & Kada, T. (1986) Results of the *rec*-assay of nitropyrenes in the *Bacillus subtilis* test system. *Mutat. Res.*, *174*, 89–92

Hsieh, L.L., Wong, D., Heisig, V., Santella, R.M., Mauderly, J.L., Mitchell, C.E., Wolff, R.K. & Jeffrey, A.M. (1986) Analysis of genotoxic components in diesel engine emissions. In: Ishinishi, N., Koizumi, A., McClellan, R.O. & Stöber, W., eds, *Carcinogenic and Mutagenic Effects of Diesel Engine Exhaust*, Amsterdam, Elsevier, pp. 223–232

IARC (1988) *Information Bulletin on the Survey of Chemicals Being Tested for Carcinogenicity*, No. 13, Lyon, pp. 13, 103

Imaida, K., Tay, L.K., Lee, M.-S., Wang, C.Y., Ito, N. & King, C.M. (1988) Tumor induction by nitropyrenes in the female CD rat. In: King, C.M., Romano, L.J. & Schuetzle, D., eds, *Carcinogenic and Mutagenic Responses to Aromatic Amines and Nitroarenes*, Amsterdam, Elsevier, pp. 187–197

Ishizaka, Y., Ochiai, M., Ohgaki, H., Ishikawa, F., Sato, S., Miura, Y., Nagao, M. & Sugimura, T. (1987) Active H-*ras* and N-*ras* in rat fibrosarcomas induced by 1,6-dinitropyrene. *Cancer Lett.*, *34*, 317–324

Kaplan, S. (1981) Carbon-13 chemical shift assignments of the nitration products of pyrene. *Org. magn. Resonance*, *15*, 197–199

Katoh, Y., Takayama, S. & Shudo, K. (1984) Inhibition by hemin of dinitropyrene-induced mutagenesis in Chinese hamster V79 cells. *Gann*, *75*, 574–577

King, C.M. (1988) *Metabolism and Biological Effects of Nitropyrene and Related Compounds (Research Report No. 16)*, Cambridge, MA, Health Effects Institute

King, C.M., Tay, L.K., Lee, M.-S., Imaida, K. & Wang, C.Y. (1986) Mechanisms of tumor induction by dinitropyrenes in the female CD rat. In: Ishinishi, N., Koizumi, A., McClellan, R.O. & Stöber, W., eds, *Carcinogenic and Mutagenic Effects of Diesel Engine Exhaust*, Amsterdam, Elsevier, pp. 279–290

Kinouchi, T. & Ohnishi, Y. (1986) Metabolic activation of 1-nitropyrene and 1,6-dinitropyrene by nitroreductases from *Bacteroides fragilis* and distribution of nitroreductase activity in rats. *Microbiol. Immunol.*, *30*, 979–992

Lambert, M.E. & Weinstein, I.B. (1987) Nitropyrenes are inducers of polyoma viral DNA synthesis. *Mutat. Res.*, *183*, 203–211

Li, A.P. & Dutcher, J.S. (1983) Mutagenicity of mono-, di- and tri-nitropyrenes in Chinese hamster ovary cells. *Mutat. Res.*, *119*, 387–392

Löfroth, G. (1981) Comparison of the mutagenic activity in carbon particulate matter and in diesel and gasoline engine exhaust. In: Waters, M.D., Sandhu, S.S., Lewtas Huisingh, J., Claxton, L. & Nesnow, S., eds, *Application of Short-term Bioassays in the Analysis of Complex Environmental Mixtures, II*, New York, Plenum, pp. 319-336

Maeda, T., Izumi, K., Otsuka, H., Manabe, Y., Kinouchi, T. & Ohnishi, Y. (1986) Induction of squamous cell carcinoma in the rat lung by 1,6-dinitropyrene. *J. natl Cancer Inst.*, *76*, 693-701

Manabe, Y., Kinouchi, T. & Ohnishi, Y. (1985) Identification and quantification of highly mutagenic nitroacetoxypyrenes and nitrohydroxypyrenes in diesel-exhaust particles. *Mutat. Res.*, *158*, 3-18

Matsuoka, A., Sofuni, T., Sato, S., Miyata, N. & Ishidate, M., Jr (1987) In vitro clastogenicity of nitropyrenes and nitrofluorenes (Abstract No. 25). *Mutat. Res.*, *182*, 366-367

McCoy, E.C., Anders, M., Rosenkranz, H.S. & Mermelstein, R. (1983) Apparent absence of recombinogenic activity of nitropyrenes for yeast. *Mutat. Res.*, *116*, 119-127

McCoy, E.C., Anders, M., Rosenkranz, H.S. & Mermelstein, R. (1985a) Mutagenicity of nitropyrenes for *Escherichia coli*: requirement for increased cellular permeability. *Mutat. Res.*, *142*, 163-167

McCoy, E.C., Holloway, M., Frierson, M., Klopman, G., Mermelstein, R. & Rosenkranz, H.S. (1985b) Genetic and quantum chemical basis of the mutagenicity of nitroarenes for adenine-thymine base pairs. *Mutat. Res.*, *149*, 311-319

Mermelstein, R., Kiriazides, D.K., Butler, M., McCoy, E.C. & Rosenkranz, H.S. (1981) The extraordinary mutagenicity of nitropyrenes in bacteria. *Mutat. Res.*, *89*, 187-196

Møller, M.E. & Thorgeirsson, S.S. (1985) DNA damage induced by nitropyrenes in primary mouse hepatocytes and in rat H4-II-E hepatoma cells. *Mutat. Res.*, *151*, 137-146

Mori, H., Sugie, S., Yoshimi, N., Kinouchi, T. & Ohnishi, Y. (1987) Genotoxicity of a variety of nitroarenes and other nitro compounds in DNA-repair tests with rat and mouse hepatocytes. *Mutat. Res.*, *190*, 159-167

Morotomi, M. & Watanabe, T. (1984) Metabolism of exogenous compounds by the intestinal microflora (Jpn.). *Tikoshikoroji Foramu* [*Toxicol. Forum*], *7*, 395-408

Nakagawa, R., Kitamori, S., Horikawa, K., Nakashima, K. & Tokiwa, H. (1983) Identification of dinitropyrenes in diesel-exhaust particles. Their probable presence as the major mutagens. *Mutat. Res.*, *124*, 201-211

Nakamura, S.-I., Oda, Y., Shimada, T., Oki, I. & Sugimoto, K. (1987) SOS-inducing activity of chemical carcinogens and mutagens in *Salmonella typhimurium* TA1535/pSK1002: examination with 151 chemicals. *Mutat. Res.*, *192*, 239-246

Nakayasu, M., Sakamoto, H., Wakabayashi, K., Terada, M., Sugimura, T. & Rosenkranz, H.S. (1982) Potent mutagenic activity of nitropyrenes on Chinese hamster lung cells with diphtheria toxin resistance as a selective marker. *Carcinogenesis*, *3*, 917-922

Nishioka, M.G., Petersen, B.A. & Lewtas, J. (1982) Comparison of nitro-aromatic content and direct-acting mutagenicity of diesel emissions. In: Cooke, M., Dennis, A.J. & Fisher, G.L., eds, *Polynuclear Aromatic Hydrocarbons, 6th International Symposium, Physical and Biological Chemistry*, Columbus, OH, Battelle, pp. 603-613

Ohgaki, H., Hasegawa, H., Kato, T., Negishi, C., Sato, S. & Sugimura, T. (1985) Absence of carcinogenicity of 1-nitropyrene, correction of previous results, and new demonstration of carcinogenicity of 1,6-dinitropyrene in rats. *Cancer Lett.*, *25*, 239-245

Paputa-Peck, M.C., Marano, R.S., Schuetzle, D., Riley, T.L., Hampton, C.V., Prater, T.J., Skewes, L.M., Jensen, T.E., Ruehle, P.H., Bosch, L.C. & Duncan, W.P. (1983) Determination of nitrated polynuclear aromatic hydrocarbons in particulate extracts by capillary column gas chromatography with nitrogen selective detection. *Anal. Chem.*, 55, 1946–1954

Pitts, J.N., Jr (1987) Nitration of gaseous polycyclic aromatic hydrocarbons in simulated and ambient urban atmospheres: a source of mutagenic nitroarenes. *Atmos. Environ.*, 21, 2531–2547

Ramdahl, T. & Urdal, K. (1982) Determination of nitrated polycyclic aromatic hydrocarbons by fused silica capillary gas chromatography/negative ion chemical ionization mass spectrometry. *Anal. Chem.*, 54, 2256–2260

Rosenkranz, H.S. & Mermelstein, R. (1983) Mutagenicity and genotoxicity of nitroarenes: all nitro-containing chemicals were not created equal. *Mutat. Res.*, 114, 217–267

Rosenkranz, H.S. & Mermelstein, R. (1985) The genotoxicity, metabolism and carcinogenicity of nitrated polycyclic aromatic hydrocarbons. *J. environ. Sci. Health*, C3, 221–272

Rosenkranz, H.S., McCoy, E.C., Sanders, D.R., Butler, M., Kiriazides, D.K. & Mermelstein, R. (1980) Nitropyrenes: isolation, identification, and reduction of mutagenic impurities in carbon black and toners. *Science*, 209, 1039–1043

Rosenkranz, H.S., McCoy, E.C., Frierson, M. & Klopman, G. (1985) The role of DNA sequence and structure of the electrophile on the mutagenicity of nitroarenes and arylamine derivatives. *Environ. Mutagenesis*, 7, 645–653

Saito, K., Mita, S., Kamataki, T. & Kato, R. (1984) DNA single-strand breaks by nitropyrenes and related compounds in Chinese hamster V79 cells. *Cancer Lett.*, 24, 121–127

Salmeen, I.T., Pero, A.M., Zator, R., Schuetzle, D. & Riley, T.L. (1984) Ames assay chromatograms and the identification of mutagens in diesel particle extracts. *Environ. Sci. Technol.*, 18, 375–382

Sanders, D.R. (1981) Nitropyrenes: the isolation of trace mutagenic impurities from the toluene extract of an aftertreated carbon black. In: Cooke, M. & Dennis, A.J., eds, *Polynuclear Aromatic Hydrocarbons, 5th International Symposium, Chemical Analysis and Biological Fate*, Columbus, OH, Battelle, pp. 145–158

Schuetzle, D. & Jensen, T.E. (1985) Analysis of nitrated polycyclic aromatic hydrocarbons (nitro-PAH) by mass spectrometry. In: White, C.M., ed., *Nitrated Polycyclic Aromatic Hydrocarbons*, Heidelberg, A. Hüthig Verlag, pp. 121–167

Siak, J., Chan, T.L., Gibson, T.L. & Wolff, G.T. (1985) Contribution to bacterial mutagenicity from nitro-PAH compounds in ambient aerosols. *Atmos. Environ.*, 19, 369–376

Sugimura, T. & Takayama, S. (1983) Biological actions of nitroarenes in short-term tests on *Salmonella*, cultured mammalian cells and cultured human tracheal tissues: possible basis for regulatory control. *Environ. Health Perspect.*, 47, 171–176

Takayama, S., Ishikawa, T., Nakajima, H. & Sato, S. (1985) Lung carcinoma induction in Syrian golden hamsters by intratracheal instillation of 1,6-dinitropyrene. *Jpn. J. Cancer Res. (Gann)*, 76, 457–461

Tanabe, K., Matsushita, H., Kuo, C.-T. & Imamiya, S. (1986) Determination of carcinogenic nitroarenes in airborne particulates by high performance liquid chromatography (Jpn.). *Taiki Osen Gakkaishi (J. Jpn. Soc. Air Pollut.)*, 21, 535–544

Tokiwa, H. & Ohnishi, Y. (1986) Mutagenicity and carcinogenicity of nitroarenes and their sources in the environment. *CRC crit. Rev. Toxicol.*, 17, 23–60

Tokiwa, H., Nakagawa, R. & Ohnishi, Y. (1981) Mutagenic assay of aromatic nitro compounds with *Salmonella typhimurium*. *Mutat. Res.*, *91*, 321—325

Tokiwa, H., Kitamori, S., Nakagawa, R., Horikawa, K. & Matamala, L. (1983) Demonstration of a powerful mutagenic dinitropyrene in airborne particulate matter. *Mutat. Res.*, *121*, 107—116

Tokiwa, H., Otofuji, T., Horikawa, K., Kitamori, S., Otsuka, H., Manabe, Y., Kinouchi, T. & Ohnishi, Y. (1984) 1,6-Dinitropyrene: mutagenicity in *Salmonella* and carcinogenicity in BALB/c mice. *J. natl Cancer Inst.*, *73*, 1359—1363

Tokiwa, H., Nakagawa, R. & Horikawa, K. (1985) Mutagenic/carcinogenic agents in indoor pollutants; the dinitropyrenes generated by kerosene heaters and fuel gas and liquefied petroleum gas burners. *Mutat. Res.*, *157*, 39—47

Tokiwa, H., Otofuji, T., Nakagawa, R., Horikawa, K., Maeda, T., Sano, N., Izumi, K. & Otsuka, H. (1986) Dinitro derivatives of pyrene and fluoranthene in diesel emission particulates and their tumorigenicity in mice and rats. In: Ishinishi, N., Koizumi, A., McClellan, R.O. & Stöber, W., eds, *Carcinogenic and Mutagenic Effects of Diesel Engine Exhaust*, Amsterdam, Elsevier, pp. 253—270

Wilcox, P. & Parry, J.M. (1981) The genetic activity of dinitropyrenes in yeast: unusual dose response curves for induced mitotic gene conversion. *Carcinogenesis*, *2*, 1201—1205

Wilcox, P., Danford, N. & Parry, J.M. (1982) The genetic activity and metabolism of dinitropyrenes in eucaryotic cells. In: Sorsa, M. & Vainio, H., eds, *Mutagens in Our Environment*, New York, Alan R. Liss, pp. 249—258

Wislocki, P.G., Bagan, E.S., Lu, A.Y.H., Dooley, K.L., Fu, P.P., Han-Hsu, H., Beland, F.A. & Kadlubar, F.F. (1986) Tumorigenicity of nitrated derivatives of pyrene, benz[a]anthracene, chrysene and benzo[a]pyrene in the newborn mouse assay. *Carcinogenesis*, *7*, 1317—1322

Working, P.K. & Butterworth, B.E. (1984) An assay to detect chemically induced DNA repair in rat spermatocytes. *Environ. Mutagenesis*, *6*, 273—286

Yoshikura, T., Kuroda, K., Kamiura, T., Masumoto, K., Fukushima, M., Yamamoto, T. & Torii, M. (1985) Synthesis of 1,3-, 1,6- and 1,8-dinitropyrenes and evaluation of their mutagenicities. *Annu. Rep. Osaka City Inst. public Health environ. Sci.*, *47*, 31—35 [*Chem. Abstr.*, *106*, 49745t]

Yoshimi, N., Sugie, S., Mori, H., Kinouchi, T. & Ohnishi, Y. (1987) Genotoxicity of various nitroarenes in DNA repair tests with human hepatocytes (Abstract No. 73). *Mutat. Res.*, *182*, 384

# 1,8-DINITROPYRENE

This substance was considered by a previous Working Group, in June 1983 (IARC, 1984). Since that time, new data have become available and these have been incorporated into the monograph and taken into consideration in the present evaluation.

## 1. Chemical and Physical Data

### 1.1 Synonyms

*Chem. Abstr. Services Reg. No.*: 42397-65-9
*Chem. Abstr. Name*: Pyrene, 1,8-dinitro-
*IUPAC Systematic Name*: 1,8-Dinitropyrene

### 1.2 Structural and molecular formulae and molecular weight

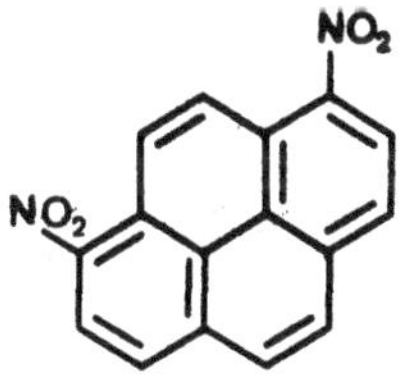

$C_{16}H_8N_2O_4$ 

Mol. wt: 292.3

### 1.3 Chemical and physical properties of the pure substance

(a) *Description*: Light-brown needles, recrystallized from benzene and methanol (Buckingham, 1985); yellow, fluffy, crystalline solid (Chemsyn Science Laboratories, 1988)

(b) *Melting-point*: >300°C (Buckingham, 1985); 300°C (Chemsyn Science Laboratories, 1988)

(c) *Spectroscopy data*: Ultra-violet, infra-red, nuclear magnetic resonance (Kaplan, 1981; Paputa-Peck *et al.*, 1983; Hashimoto & Shudo, 1984) and mass (Schuetzle & Jensen, 1985) spectral data have been reported.

### 1.4 Technical products and impurities

1,8-Dinitropyrene is available for research purposes at 98% (Aldrich Chemical Co., 1988) and ⩾99% purity (Chemsyn Science Laboratories, 1988). It is also available in $^{14}$C- or $^{3}$H-labelled form in ⩾98% radiochemical purity (Chemsyn Science Laboratories, 1988).

## 2. Production, Use, Occurrence and Analysis

### 2.1 Production and use

*(a) Production*

Mixtures of 1,3-, 1,6- and 1,8-dinitropyrenes are produced by the nitration of pyrene, and 1,8-dinitropyrene has been isolated and purified from such preparations (Yoshikura *et al.*, 1985).

*(b) Use*

1,8-Dinitropyrene has been reported to be a photosensitizer, increasing the spectral activity of bis-azide compounds with light (Tsunoda *et al.*, 1973). However, no evidence was found that 1,8-dinitropyrene is currently used commercially for this or other applications.

### 2.2 Occurrence

*(a) Engine exhaust*

1,8-Dinitropyrene has been found at a level of 3.4 mg/kg extract of particles from the exhaust of a heavy-duty diesel engine (Nakagawa *et al.*, 1983), and at $0.5 \pm 0.3 - 0.7 \pm 0.2$ mg/kg extract (Salmeen *et al.*, 1984), 0.4 mg/kg extract (Nishioka *et al.*, 1982) and 0.013-0.025 mg/kg particles (Gibson, 1983) from the exhausts of light-duty diesel engines.

*(b) Other occurrence*

Toners for use in photocopy machines have been produced in quantity since the late 1950s and have seen widespread use. 'Long-flow' furnace black was first used in photocopy toners in 1967; its manufacture involved an oxidation whereby some nitration also occurred. Subsequent changes in the production technique reduced the total extractable nitropyrene content from an uncontrolled level of 5-100 mg/kg to below 0.3 mg/kg (Rosenkranz *et al.*, 1980; Sanders, 1981; Butler *et al.*, 1983), and toners produced from this carbon black since 1980 have not been found to contain detectable levels of mutagenicity or, hence, nitropyrenes (Rosenkranz *et al.*, 1980; Butler *et al.*, 1983).

1,8-Dinitropyrene was found in an extract of a pre-1979 sample of furnace black that had been after-treated by an oxidation-nitration process, at a level of 23.4 mg/kg (Sanders, 1981). One lot of this grade made in 1980 was found to contain 0.16 mg/kg (Giammarise *et al.*, 1982). An undetermined level of 1,8-dinitropyrene was detected in an extract of a formerly available commercial furnace black produced before 1980 (Ramdahl & Urdal, 1982).

Small amounts of dinitropyrenes are generated by kerosene heaters, which are used extensively in Japan for heating residences and offices (Tokiwa *et al.*, 1985). Such open, oil-burning space heaters were found to emit dinitropyrenes at a rate of 0.2 ng/h after only 1 h of operation; a mixture of 1,8- and 1,6-dinitropyrenes was found at $3.25 \pm 0.63$ mg/kg particulate extract, accounting for 27% of the mutagenic activity of the sample. Gas and liquified petroleum gas (LPG) burners, widely used for home heating and cooking, also produced detectable amounts of dinitropyrenes: 0.68 mg/kg extract (28% of mutagenicity) and 0.96 mg/kg extract (58% of mutagenicity), respectively. The authors suggested that dinitropyrenes result from the incomplete combustion of fuel in the presence of at least a few micrograms per cubic metre of nitrogen dioxide.

According to Takayama *et al.* (1985) and Pitts (1987), several dinitropyrenes have been detected in respirable particulates from ambient atmospheric samples. Gibson (1986) reported higher amounts in heavy industrialized areas than in nonindustrialized urban and suburban sites. Levels of 1,8-dinitropyrene in samples of airborne particulates are given in Table 1.

### 2.3 Analysis

See the monograph on 1-nitropyrene.

## 3. Biological Data Relevant to the Evaluation of Carcinogenic Risk to Humans

### 3.1 Carcinogenicity studies in animals[1]

*(a) Oral administration*

*Rat*: A group of 36 female weanling CD rats received oral intubations of 10 μmol-[3 mg]/kg bw 1,8-dinitropyrene (purity, >99%) dissolved in dimethyl sulfoxide (DMSO; 1.7 μmol[0.5 mg]/ml DMSO) three times per week for four weeks (average total dose, 16 μmol[4.7 mg]/rat) and were observed for 76-78 weeks (King, 1988). A vehicle control group of 36 animals received DMSO only. The number of animals with mammary tumours was significantly increased in treated animals (22/36) as compared to controls (12/35; $p < 0.05$).

*(b) Subcutaneous administration*

*Mouse*: A group of 20 male BALB/c mice, six weeks old, received subcutaneous injections of 0.05 mg 1,8-dinitropyrene (purity, >99.9%) dissolved in 0.2 ml DMSO once a

---

[1]The Working Group was aware of a study in progress by single subcutaneous injection in mice (IARC, 1988).

## Table 1. 1,8-Dinitropyrene levels in atmospheric particulates

| Sample | 1,8-Dinitropyrene concentration | | Reference |
|---|---|---|---|
| | Particulate extract (mg/kg) | Atmosphere (pg/m³) | |
| Tokyo, Japan | | 0.658 | Tanabe et al. (1986) |
| Bermuda (remote) | | | Gibson (1986) |
| Summer | 0.0035 | 0.07[a] | |
| Winter | 0.0044 | 0.06[a] | |
| Delaware, USA (rural) | | | Gibson (1986) |
| Summer | 0.0024 | 0.06[a] | |
| Warren, MI, USA (suburban) | | | Gibson (1986) |
| Winter | <0.004 | <0.10[a] | |
| Summer | 0.0021 | 0.13[a] | |
| Detroit, MI, USA (urban) | | | Gibson (1986) |
| Summer | 0.0025 | 0.34[a] | |
| River Rouge, MI, USA (industrial) | | | Gibson (1986) |
| Summer | 0.0131 | 1.26[a] | |
| Dearborn, MI, USA (industrial) | | | Gibson (1986) |
| Summer | 0.02 | 3.80[a] | |
| Southeast, MI, USA | | | Siak et al. (1985) |
| Summer | 0.46 | 0.04 | |
| Santiago, Chile (urban) | 0.2 | – | Tokiwa et al. (1983) |

[a]Calculated by the Working Group

week for 20 weeks (Otofuji et al., 1987). A positive control group of 20 males received of 0.05 mg benzo[a]pyrene, and a further 20 mice were untreated. Animals were observed for 60 weeks or until moribund. The first subcutaneous tumour in the benzo[a]pyrene-treated group was seen in week 21; all 16 mice surviving beyond this time developed sarcomas at the injection site. After 60 weeks, 6/15 mice injected with 1,8-dinitropyrene had developed subcutaneous tumours; no such tumour was found in untreated controls ($p < 0.05$). All of the subcutaneous tumours were diagnosed histologically as malignant fibrous histiocytomas [a term used as a specific diagnosis for some subcutaneous and intraperitoneal sarcomas]. Some animals in the 1,8-dinitropyrene-treated group developed tumours in the lung and liver.

*Rat*: Ten male Fischer 344/DuCrj rats, six weeks old, received subcutaneous injections of 0.2 mg 1,8-dinitropyrene ([purity unspecified] impurities: 0.4% 1,3-dinitropyrene, <0.05% other nitropyrenes) dissolved in 0.2 ml DMSO twice a week for ten weeks (total dose, 4 mg; Ohgaki et al., 1984). A control group of 20 rats received injections of 0.2 ml

DMSO only. The animals were killed between days 140 and 169. Sarcomas developed at the site of injection in all treated rats between days 113 and 127. No 'tumorous' change was observed in other organs of the treated rats, and no local tumour developed among control animals.

Two groups of ten male Fischer 344/DuCrj rats, six weeks old, received subcutaneous injections of 0.002 or 0.02 mg 1,8-dinitropyrene ([purity unspecified] impurities: 0.4% 1,3-dinitropyrene) dissolved in 0.2 ml DMSO twice a week for ten weeks (total doses, 0.04 or 0.4 mg; Ohgaki et al., 1985). A control group of 20 rats received injections of 0.2 ml DMSO only. All treated animals were killed on day 320 and control rats on day 650. Sarcomas developed at the site of injection between days 123 and 156 in all rats treated with 0.4 mg 1,8-dinitropyrene and between days 213 and 320 in 9/10 rats treated with 0.04 mg 1,8-dinitropyrene. No tumour was observed in other organs of the treated rats or at the injection site in control animals.

A group of 37 female newborn CD rats received subcutaneous injections of 1,8-dinitropyrene (purity, >99%; total dose, 6.3 $\mu$mol [1.8 mg]) dissolved in DMSO (1.7 $\mu$mol[0.5 mg]/ml DMSO) into the suprascapular region once a week for eight weeks (King, 1988). A group of 40 or more animals injected with DMSO alone served as controls. Average survival was 163 days for treated animals and 495 days for controls. Malignant fibrous histiocytomas developed rapidly at the injection site in treated rats; the first tumour was seen 122 days after the initial injection, and by 20 weeks all treated rats had developed this tumour. In addition, eight rats (22%) in this group had leukaemia. Controls developed neither malignancy ($p < 0.0001$ and $p < 0.005$).

*(d) Intraperitoneal administration*

*Mouse*: Groups of 90 or 100 male and female newborn CD-1 mice received three intraperitoneal injections of 1,8-dinitropyrene (total dose, 200 nmol [58.7 $\mu$g]; purity, >99%) in 10, 20 and 40 $\mu$l DMSO on days 1, 8 and 15 after birth; a total dose of 560 nmol [140 $\mu$g] benzo[a]pyrene (purity, >99%) as three injections; or three injections of DMSO only (Wislocki et al., 1986). Treatment of a second vehicle control group was begun ten weeks after that of the other groups. At 25–27 days, when the mice were weaned, 31 males and 33 females in the treated group, 37 males and 27 females in the positive control group and 28 and 31 males and 45 and 34 females in the two vehicle control groups were still alive. All remaining mice were killed after one year. In the group injected with 1,8-dinitropyrene, 5/31 male mice developed liver tumours (four with adenomas, one with a carcinoma). No increase in the incidences of lung tumours or malignant lymphomas was observed in males or females as compared to DMSO-treated animals. Benzo[a]pyrene induced liver tumours in 18/37 males and in 0/27 females and lung adenomas in 13/37 males and 13/27 females; the latter incidences were significantly higher than those in DMSO controls ($p < 0.005$). In the two DMSO control groups, 2/28 and 5/45 males had liver adenomas and 1/28 and 4/45 lung tumours, and 0/31 and 0/34 females had liver tumours and 0/31 and 2/34 lung tumours. [The Working Group noted the small number of animals per group and the short observation period.]

*Rat*: A group of 36 female weanling CD rats received intraperitoneal injections of 10 μmol[3 mg]/kg bw 1,8-dinitropyrene (purity, >99%) dissolved in DMSO (1.7 μmol [0.5 mg]/ml DMSO) three times per week for four weeks (total dose, 16 μmol[4.7 mg]/rat); 36 control animals were treated with DMSO only (King, 1988). Treatment with 1,8-dinitropyrene resulted in early deaths 12–15 weeks after the initial treatment. The first intraperitoneal tumour was detected at week 17; after 44 weeks, 29/33 of the treated rats had developed malignant fibrous histiocytomas in the peritoneal cavity ($p < 0.0001$), and a significantly increased incidence of myelocytic leukaemia (7/33) was observed in this group ($p < 0.01$). Neither malignancy developed among 31 vehicle controls after an observation period of 76–78 weeks.

## 3.2 Other relevant data

(a) *Experimental systems*

(i) *Absorption, distribution, excretion and metabolism*

$N,N'$-Diacetyl-1,8-diaminopyrene, 1,8-diaminopyrene, 1-acetylamino-8-nitro-pyrene, 1-amino-8-nitropyrene and unidentified polar metabolites were detected in the faeces of conventional male CD rats treated orally with 1.0 μmol [0.3 mg] 1,8-dinitropyrene. In germ-free rats treated similarly, only 1-amino-8-nitropyrene and the polar metabolites were found. In both groups of animals, $N$-(deoxyguanosin-8-yl)-1-amino-8-nitropyrene was detected as the major DNA adduct in both liver and mammary gland; however, the extent of binding was considerably lower in the germ-free rats (Heflich *et al.*, 1986a).

Under an argon atmosphere, rat and dog liver cytosol catalysed the reduction of 1,8-dinitropyrene to 1-amino-8-nitropyrene, 1-nitro-8-nitrosopyrene and 1,8-diaminopyrene. During this reduction, metabolites were formed that bound to exogenous DNA. When acetyl coenzyme A was added to the rat liver cytosolic incubations, 1-acetylamino-8-nitropyrene was also detected as a metabolite, and the extent of binding was increased 39-fold (Djurić *et al.*, 1985). Subsequent studies showed that *Salmonella typhimurium* TA98, rat liver microsomes obtained from a 105 000 $g$ supernatant, human liver cytosol and Chinese hamster ovary cell cytosol also reduced 1,8-dinitropyrene to 1-nitro-8-nitrosopyrene and 1-amino-8-nitropyrene (Djurić *et al.*, 1986; Heflich *et al.*, 1986b).

1-Nitro-8-nitrosopyrene, 1-amino-8-nitropyrene and 1,8-diaminopyrene were detected as metabolites in rat mammary gland cytosol incubated with 1,8-dinitropyrene under anaerobic conditions. When incubations were conducted in the presence of acetyl coenzyme A, binding to exogenous tRNA occurred. Incubation with intact rat mammary gland cells resulted in the formation of 1-amino-8-nitropyrene and 1-acetylamino-8-nitropyrene (King *et al.*, 1986; Imaida *et al.*, 1988).

A low level of DNA adduct formation (fewer than five adducts per $10^6$ nucleotides) was detected by $^{32}$P-postlabelling in C3H 10T1/2 mouse embryo fibroblasts incubated with 1,8-dinitropyrene (Hsieh *et al.*, 1986). Several DNA adducts were detected when similar incubations were conducted with [$^3$H]1,8-dinitropyrene. Incubation of Chinese hamster ovary cells with 1,8-dinitropyrene resulted in the formation of 1-amino-8-nitropyrene and a DNA adduct identified as *N*-(deoxyguanosin-8-yl)-1-amino-8-nitropyrene (Heflich *et al.*, 1986b).

As reported in an abstract, the major DNA adduct in rabbit tracheal epithelial cells incubated with 1,8-dinitropyrene and its partially reduced derivative, 1-nitroso-8-nitropyrene, was *N*-(deoxyguanosin-8-yl)-1-amino-8-nitropyrene (Norman *et al.*, 1988). Anaerobic bacterial suspensions from human faeces and intestinal contents of rhesus monkeys and rats were reported to reduce 1,8-dinitropyrene to 1-amino-8-nitropyrene and 1,8-diaminopyrene (Cerniglia *et al.*, 1986).

1,8-Dinitropyrene is metabolized to 1-amino-8-nitropyrene, 1,8-diaminopyrene, 1-*N*-acetylamino-8-nitropyrene and *N*,*N'*-diacetyl-1,8-diaminopyrene by several strains of *S. typhimurium* (Bryant *et al.*, 1984; Heflich *et al.*, 1985; Orr *et al.*, 1985). *N*-(Deoxyguanosin-8-yl)-1-amino-8-nitropyrene has been detected in DNA of *S. typhimurium* cells (Helflich *et al.*, 1985; Andrews *et al.*, 1986). In *S. typhimurium* TA1538, the concentration of this adduct was correlated with the induction of frameshift mutations (Heflich *et al.*, 1985).

(ii) *Toxic effects*

Intraperitoneal administration of 1,8-dinitropyrene to young male Sprague-Dawley rats (three times at 2.5 mg/kg bw) resulted in increases in the activities of aryl hydrocarbon hydroxylase, 7-ethoxycoumarin-*O*-deethylase, aminopyrine-*N*-demethylase and 1-nitropyrene reductase in liver microsomes over that in controls (Chou *et al.*, 1987).

(iii) *Genetic and related effects*

The genetic and related effects of nitroarenes and of their metabolites have been reviewed (Rosenkranz & Mermelstein, 1983; Beland *et al.*, 1985; Rosenkranz & Mermelstein, 1985; Tokiwa & Ohnishi, 1986).

1,8-Dinitropyrene (0.0003 $\mu$g/ml) induced DNA damage in *S. typhimurium* TA1535 (Nakamura *et al.*, 1987) and preferentially inhibited the growth of DNA repair-deficient *Bacillus subtilis* (Horikawa *et al.*, 1986 (0.01–0.04 $\mu$g/disc); Tokiwa *et al.*, 1986 (0.02 $\mu$g/disc)). It was mutagenic to *Escherichia coli* WP2 *uvrA* pKM101 (McCoy *et al.*, 1985a) and to *S. typhimurium* TA96, TA97, TA98, TA100, TA102, TA104, TA1537 and TA1538 (Rosenkranz *et al.*, 1980; Löfroth, 1981; Mermelstein *et al.*, 1981; Pederson & Siak, 1981; Tokiwa *et al.*, 1981; Nakayasu *et al.*, 1982; Morotomi & Watanabe, 1984; Pitts *et al.*, 1984; Heflich *et al.*, 1985; McCoy *et al.*, 1985b; Rosenkranz *et al.*, 1985; Tokiwa *et al.*, 1985; Fifer *et al.*, 1986; Holloway *et al.*, 1987; Zielinska *et al.*, 1987).

Conflicting results have been reported concerning the induction by 1,8-dinitropyrene of gene conversion in the yeast, *Saccharomyces cerevisiae*: positive results were reported in strain JDI (1.6–25 $\mu$g/ml) (Wilcox & Parry, 1981; Wilcox *et al.*, 1982) and negative results in strain D4 at up to 500 $\mu$g/ml (McCoy *et al.*, 1983). It has been suggested that these differences reflect intracellular oxygen levels (Rosenkranz & Mermelstein, 1983).

As determined by alkaline elution, 1,8-dinitropyrene induced a marginal effect on the formation of single-strand DNA breaks in primary mouse hepatocytes at 5–20 $\mu$M (Møller

& Thorgeirsson, 1985) and in cultured Chinese hamster V79 cells at the only dose tested, 15 µM (Saito et al., 1984); it also caused single-strand DNA breaks in cultured rat hepatoma cells (3–10 µM), but it did not induce DNA-protein cross-links at 15 µM (Møller & Thorgeirsson, 1985). It activated the synthesis of viral DNA in polyoma virus-transformed rat fibroblasts at 0.5–2.0 µg/ml (Lambert & Weinstein, 1987).

1,8-Dinitropyrene induced unscheduled DNA synthesis in mouse and rat hepatocytes (Mori et al., 1987 ($1.0 \times 10^{-5} – 1.0 \times 10^{-2}$ mg/ml)), in rabbit lung Clara and alveolar type II cells (Haugen et al., 1986 (0.63–10.0 ng/ml)) and, as reported in an abstract, in human hepatocytes (Yoshimi et al., 1987); however, the combined results from Eddy et al. (1985, 1986) suggest that unscheduled DNA synthesis was not induced in human hepatoma-derived HepG2 cells at up to 2 µg/ml. 1,8-Dinitropyrene (2.5 µg/ml) did not exhibit preferential toxicity for DNA repair-deficient human xeroderma pigmentosum fibroblasts (Arlett, 1984).

1,8-Dinitropyrene (0.025–2.5 µg/ml) induced mutations to thioguanine, methotrexate, ouabain and arabinofuranosyl cytosine resistance in cultured mouse lymphoma L5178Y cells (Cole et al., 1982; Arlett, 1984) and at the thymidine kinase locus (0.1–5 µg/ml; Edgar, 1985). It induced mutations at the *hprt* locus of cultured Chinese hamster CHO cells (Li & Dutcher, 1983 (0.2–2 µg/ml); Edgar & Brooker, 1985 (0.05–5 µg/ml); Heflich et al., 1986b (2–20 µM)). It also induced mutation to diphtheria toxin resistance (Nakayasu et al., 1982 (0.03–8 µg/ml)) in cultured Chinese hamster lung fibroblasts and to ouabain resistance in V79 cells (Takayama et al., 1983 (0.01–0.1 µg/ml); Katoh et al., 1984 (0.1 µg/ml)). It was reported in an abstract that 1,8-dinitropyrene (100–500 ng/ml) induced mutation to ouabain resistance in human diploid lymphoblasts (Sanders et al., 1983). At up to 2 µg/ml, it did not induce mutation at the *hprt* locus of human hepatoma-derived HepG2 cells (Eddy et al., 1985, 1986) or of normal and xeroderma pigmentosum human fibroblasts [probably at 2.5 µg/ml] (Arlett, 1984).

1,8-Dinitropyrene induced sister chromatid exchange in cultured Chinese hamster CHO cells (Nachtman & Wolff, 1982 (1.6 µM); Edgar & Brooker, 1985 (0.05–5 µg/ml), but did not induce micronuclei in cultured normal and xeroderma pigmentosum human fibroblasts (Arlett, 1984; 2.5 µg/ml). It induced chromosomal aberrations in cultured Chinese hamster CHO cells (Edgar & Brooker, 1985 (0.05–5 µg/ml)) and, to some extent, in human fibroblasts (Wilcox et al., 1982 (0.02–5.0 µg/ml)). It induced chromosomal aberrations, primarily of the chromatid type, in rat epithelial cells (Danford et al., 1982 (0.01–2.5 µg/ml); Wilcox et al., 1982). As reported in an abstract, 1,8-dinitropyrene at 0.025 µg/ml induced chromosomal aberrations in cultured Chinese hamster lung fibroblasts (Matsuoka et al., 1987).

1,8-Dinitropyrene at 1.7–17 µM induced morphological transformation in Syrian hamster embryo cells (DiPaolo et al., 1983). It was reported in an abstract that no transformation activity was observed when 1,8-dinitropyrene was tested at concentrations of up to 250 µg/ml in BALB/c 3T3 cells (Tu et al., 1982).

Rat sarcomas induced by this chemical contained activated c-Ki-*ras* oncogenes (Ochiai et al., 1985; Tahira et al., 1986).

(b) *Humans*

No data were available to the Working Group.

### 3.3 Epidemiological studies and case reports of carcinogenicity in humans

No data were available to the Working Group.

## 4. Summary of Data Reported and Evaluation

### 4.1 Exposure data

1,8-Dinitropyrene has been detected in some carbon blacks and in particulate emissions from diesel engines, kerosene heaters and gas burners. It has also been found at low concentrations in ambient air.

### 4.2 Experimental data

1,8-Dinitropyrene was tested for carcinogenicity by oral administration in rats, by subcutaneous injection in mice and in young and newborn rats and by intraperitoneal injection in newborn mice and rats. After oral administration, it increased the incidence of mammary tumours. After subcutaneous injection, it produced sarcomas at the site of injection in mice and rats and an increased incidence of leukaemia in newborn rats. After intraperitoneal injection, it induced injection-site sarcomas and leukaemia in rats and liver tumours in male mice.

### 4.3 Human data

No data were available to the Working Group.

### 4.4 Other relevant data

Metabolism of 1,8-dinitropyrene led to DNA adduct formation *in vivo* and *in vitro*. It induced chromosomal aberrations but not DNA damage, mutation or micronuclei in cultured human cells. It induced DNA damage, sister chromatid exchange, chromosomal aberrations, mutation and morphological transformation in cultured rodent cells and DNA damage and mutation in bacteria.

### 4.5 Evaluation[1]

There is *sufficient evidence* for the carcinogenicity in experimental animals of 1,8-dinitropyrene.

---

[1]For definitions of the italicized terms, see Preamble, pp. 25–28.

## Summary table of genetic and related effects of 1,8-dinitropyrene

| Nonmammalian systems | | | | Mammalian systems | | | | | |
|---|---|---|---|---|---|---|---|---|---|
| Prokaryotes | Lower eukaryotes | Plants | Insects | In vitro | | | | In vivo | |
| | | | | Animal cells | | Human cells | | Animals | Humans |
| D G R | D G R | A D G C R | G C A | D G S M C A T I | | D G S M C A T I | | D G S M C DL A | D S M C A |
| + + ? | | | | + + + + + ±  | | − − − ± | | ± | |

A, aneuploidy; C, chromosomal aberrations; D, DNA damage; DL, dominant lethal mutation; G, gene mutation; I, inhibition of intercellular communication; M, micronuclei; R, mitotic recombination and gene conversion; S, sister chromatid exchange; T, cell transformation

*In completing the table, the following symbols indicate the consensus of the Working Group with regard to the results for each endpoint:*

+  considered to be positive for the specific endpoint and level of biological complexity
± considered to be positive, but only one valid study was available to the Working Group
−  considered to be negative
∓ considered to be negative, but only one valid study was available to the Working Group
?  considered to be equivocal or inconclusive (e.g., there were contradictory results from different laboratories; there were confounding exposures; the results were equivocal)

No data were available from studies in humans on the carcinogenicity of 1,8-dinitropyrene.

**Overall evaluation**

1,8-Dinitropyrene *is possibly carcinogenic to humans (Group 2B).*

## 5. References

Aldrich Chemical Co. (1988) *Aldrich Catalog/ Handbook of Fine Chemicals 1988*–1989, Milwaukee, WI, p. 633

Andrews, P.J., Quilliam, M.A., McCarry, B.E., Bryant, D.W. & McCalla, D.R. (1986) Identification of the DNA adduct formed by metabolism of 1,8-dinitropyrene in *Salmonella typhimurium. Carcinogenesis*, 7, 105–110

Arlett, C.F. (1984) Mutagenicity of 1,8-dinitropyrene in cultured mammalian cells. In: Rickert, D.E., ed., *Toxicity of Nitroaromatic Compounds*, Washington DC, Hemisphere, pp. 185–194

Beland, F.A., Heflich, R.H., Howard, P.C. & Fu, P.P. (1985) The in vitro metabolic activation of nitro polycyclic aromatic hydrocarbons. In: Harvey, R.G., ed., *Polycyclic Hydrocarbons and Carcinogenesis (ACS Symposium Series No. 283)*, Washington DC, American Chemical Society, pp. 371–396

Bryant, D.W., McCalla, D.R., Lultschik, P., Quilliam, M.A. & McCarry, B.E. (1984) Metabolism of 1,8-dinitropyrene by *Salmonella typhimurium. Chem.-biol. Interactions*, 49, 351–368

Buckingham, J., ed. (1985) *Dictionary of Organic Compounds*, 5th ed., 3rd Suppl., New York, Chapman & Hall, p. 183 (D-30524)

Butler, M.A., Evans, D.L., Giammarise, A.T., Kiriazides, D.K., Marsh, D., McCoy, E.C., Mermelstein, R., Murphy, C.B. & Rosenkranz, H.S. (1983) Application of Salmonella assay to carbon blacks and toners. In: Cooke, M. & Dennis, A.J., eds, *Polynuclear Aromatic Hydrocarbons, 7th International Symposium, Formation, Metabolism and Measurement*, Columbus, OH, Battelle, pp. 225–241

Cerniglia, C.E., Lambert, K.J., White, G.L., Heflich, R.H., Fifer, E.K. & Beland, F.A. (1986) Reductive metabolism and detoxification of 1,8-dinitropyrene by human, rhesus monkey and rat intestinal microflora (Abstract 449). *Proc. Am. Assoc. Cancer Res.*, 27, 114

Chemsyn Science Laboratories (1988) *1,8-Dinitropyrene (Product Code U1033)*, Lenexa, KS, pp. 72–74

Chou, M.W., Wang, B., Von Tungeln, L.S., Beland, F.A. & Fu, P.P. (1987) Induction of rat hepatic cytochromes P-450 by environmental nitropolycyclic aromatic hydrocarbons. *Biochem. Pharmacol.*, 36, 2449–2454

Cole, J., Arlett, C.F., Lowe, J. & Bridges, B.A. (1982) The mutagenic potency of 1,8-dinitropyrene in cultured mouse lymphoma cells. *Mutat. Res.*, 93, 213–220

Danford, N., Wilcox, P. & Parry, J.M. (1982) The clastogenic activity of dinitropyrenes in a rat-liver epithelial cell line. *Mutat. Res.*, 105, 349–355

DiPaolo, J.A., DeMarinis, A.J., Chow, F.L., Garner, R.C., Martin, C.N. & Doniger, J. (1983) Nitration of carcinogenic and non-carcinogenic polycyclic aromatic hydrocarbons results in products able to induce transformation of Syrian hamster cells. *Carcinogenesis*, 4, 357–359

Djurić, Z., Fifer, E.K. & Beland, F.A. (1985) Acetyl coenzyme A-dependent binding of carcinogenic and mutagenic dinitropyrenes to DNA. *Carcinogenesis*, 6, 941–944

Djurić, Z., Potter, D.W., Heflich, R.H. & Beland, F.A. (1986) Aerobic and anaerobic reduction of nitrated pyrenes *in vitro*. *Chem.-biol. Interactions*, 59, 309–324

Eddy, E.P., Howard, P.C. & Rosenkranz, H.S. (1985) Metabolism, DNA repair and mutagenicity of 1-nitropyrene in the human hepatoma cell line HepG2 (Abstract No. 378). *Proc. Am. Assoc. Cancer Res.*, 26, 96

Eddy, E.P., McCoy, E.C., Rosenkranz, H.S. & Mermelstein, R. (1986) Dichotomy in the mutagenicity and genotoxicity of nitropyrenes: apparent effect of the number of electrons involved in nitroreduction. *Mutat. Res.*, 161, 109–111

Edgar, D.H. (1985) The mutagenic potency of 4 agents at the thymidine kinase locus in mouse lymphoma L5178Y cells *in vitro*: effects of exposure time. *Mutat. Res.*, 157, 199–204

Edgar, D.H. & Brooker, P.C. (1985) Induction of 6-thioguanine resistance, chromosome aberrations and SCE by dinitropyrenes in Chinese hamster ovary cells *in vitro*. *Mutat. Res.*, 209–215

Fifer, E.K., Heflich, R.H., Djurić, Z., Howard, P.C. & Beland, F.A. (1986) Synthesis and mutagenicity of 1-nitro-6-nitrosopyrene and 1-nitro-8-nitrosopyrene, potential intermediates in the metabolic activation of 1,6- and 1,8-dinitropyrene. *Carcinogenesis*, 7, 65–70

Giammarise, A.T., Evans, D.L., Butler, M.A., Murphy, C.B., Kiriazides, D.K., Marsh, D. & Mermelstein, R. (1982) Improved methodology for carbon black extraction. In: Cooke, M., Dennis, A.J. & Fisher, G.L., eds, *Polynuclear Aromatic Hydrocarbons, 6th International Symposium, Physical and Biological Chemistry*, Columbus, OH, Battelle Press, pp. 325–334

Gibson, T.L. (1983) Sources of direct-acting nitroarene mutagens in airborne particulate matter. *Mutat. Res.*, 122, 115–121

Gibson, T.L. (1986) Sources of nitroaromatic mutagens in atmospheric polycyclic organic matter. *J. Air Pollut. Control Assoc.*, 36, 1022–1025

Hashimoto, Y. & Shudo, K. (1984) Preparation of pure isomers of dinitropyrenes. *Chem. pharm. Bull.*, 32, 1992–1994

Haugen, A., Aune, T. & Deilhaug, T. (1986) Nitropyrene-induced DNA repair in Clara cells and alveolar type-II cells isolated from rabbit lung. *Mutat. Res.*, 175, 259–262

Heflich, R.H., Fifer, E.K., Djurić, Z. & Beland, F.A. (1985) DNA adduct formation and mutation induction by nitropyrenes in *Salmonella* and Chinese hamster ovary cells: relationships with nitroreduction and acetylation. *Environ. Health Perspect.*, 62, 135–143

Heflich, R.H., Djurić, Z., Fifer, E.K., Cerniglia, C.E. & Beland, F.A. (1986a) Metabolism of dinitropyrenes to DNA-binding derivatives *in vitro* and *in vivo*. In: Ishinishi, N., Koizumi, A., McClellan, R.O. & Stöber, W., eds, *Carcinogenic and Mutagenic Effects of Diesel Engine Exhaust*, Amsterdam, Elsevier, pp. 185–197

Heflich, R.H., Fifer, E.K., Djurić, Z. & Beland, F.A. (1986b) Mutation induction and DNA adduct formation by 1,8-dinitropyrene in Chinese hamster ovary cells. In: Ramel, C., Lambert, B. & Monson, J., eds, *Genetic Toxicology of Environmental Chemicals, Part A: Basic Principles and Mechanisms of Action*, New York, Alan R. Liss, pp. 265–273

Holloway, M.P., Biaglow, M.C., McCoy, E.C., Anders, M., Rosenkranz, H.S. & Howard, P.C. (1987) Photochemical instability of 1-nitropyrene, 3-nitrofluoranthene, 1,8-dinitropyrene and their parent polycyclic aromatic hydrocarbons. *Mutat. Res.*, *187*, 199—207

Horikawa, K., Sera, N., Tokiwa, H. & Kada, T. (1986) Results of the rec-assay of nitropyrenes in the *Bacillus subtilis* test system. *Mutat. Res.*, *174*, 89—92

Hsieh, L.L., Wong, D., Heisig, V., Santella, R.M., Mauderly, J.L., Mitchell, C.E., Wolff, R.K. & Jeffrey, A.M. (1986) Analysis of genotoxic components in diesel engine emissions. In: Ishinishi, N., Koizumi, A., McClellan, R.O. & Stöber, W., eds, *Carcinogenic and Mutagenic Effects of Diesel Engine Exhaust*, Amsterdam, Elsevier, pp. 223—232

IARC (1984) *IARC Monographs on the Evaluation of the Carcinogenic Risk of Chemicals to Humans*, Vol. 33, *Polynuclear Aromatic Compounds, Part 2, Carbon Blacks, Mineral Oils and Some Nitroarenes*, Lyon, pp. 171—178

IARC (1988) *Information Bulletin on the Survey of Chemicals Being Tested for Carcinogenicity*, No. 13, Lyon, p. 13

Imaida, K., Tay, L.K., Lee, M.-S., Wang, C.Y., Ito, N. & King, C.M. (1988) Tumor induction by nitropyrenes in the female CD rat. In: King, C.M., Romano, L.J. & Schuetzle, D., eds, *Carcinogenic and Mutagenic Responses to Aromatic Amines and Nitroarenes*, Amsterdam, Elsevier, pp. 187—197

Kaplan, S. (1981) Carbon-13 chemical shift assignments of the nitration products of pyrene. *Org. magn. Resonance*, *15*, 197—199

Katoh, Y., Takayama, S. & Shudo, K. (1984) Inhibition by hemin of dinitropyrene-induced mutagenesis in Chinese hamster V79 cells. *Gann*, *75*, 574—577

King, C.M. (1988) *Metabolism and Biological Effects of Nitropyrene and Related Compounds (Research Report No. 16)*, Cambridge, MA, Health Effects Institute

King, C.M., Tay, L.K., Lee, M.-S., Imaida, K. & Wang, C.Y. (1986) Mechanisms of tumor induction by dinitropyrenes in the female CD rat. In: Ishinishi, N., Koizumi, A., McClellan, R.O. & Stöber, W., eds, *Carcinogenic and Mutagenic Effects of Diesel Engine Exhaust*, Amsterdam, Elsevier, pp. 279—290

Lambert, M.E. & Weinstein, I.B. (1987) Nitropyrenes are inducers of polyoma viral DNA synthesis. *Mutat. Res.*, *183*, 203—211

Li, A.P. & Dutcher, J.S. (1983) Mutagenicity of mono-, di- and tri-nitropyrenes in Chinese hamster ovary cells. *Mutat. Res.*, *119*, 387—392

Löfroth, G. (1981) Comparison of the mutagenic activity in carbon particulate matter and in diesel and gasoline engine exhaust. In: Waters, M.D., Sandhu, S.S., Lewtas Huisingh, J., Claxton, L. & Nesnow, S., eds, *Application of Short-term Bioassays in the Analysis of Complex Environmental Mixtures, II*, New York, Plenum, pp. 319—336

Matsuoka, A., Sofuni, T., Sato, S., Miyata, N. & Ishidate, M., Jr (1987) In vitro clastogenicity of nitropyrenes and nitrofluorenes (Abstract No. 25). *Mutat. Res.*, *182*, 366—367

McCoy, E.C., Anders, M., Rosenkranz, H.S. & Mermelstein, R. (1983) Apparent absence of recombinogenic activity of nitropyrenes for yeast. *Mutat. Res.*, *116*, 119—127

McCoy, E.C., Anders, M., Rosenkranz, H.S. & Mermelstein, R. (1985a) Mutagenicity of nitropyrenes for *Escherichia coli*: requirement for increased cell permeability. *Mutat. Res.*, *142*, 163—167

McCoy, E.C., Holloway, M., Frierson, M., Klopman, G., Mermelstein, R. & Rosenkranz, H.S. (1985b) Genetic and quantum chemical basis of the mutagenicity of nitroarenes for adenine-thymine base pairs. *Mutat. Res.*, *149*, 311–319

Mermelstein, R., Kiriazides, D.K., Butler, M., McCoy, E.C. & Rosenkranz, H.S. (1981) The extraordinary mutagenicity of nitropyrenes in bacteria. *Mutat. Res.*, *89*, 187–196

Møller, M.E. & Thorgeirsson, S.S. (1985) DNA damage induced by nitropyrenes in primary mouse hepatocytes and in rat H4-II-E hepatoma cells. *Mutat. Res.*, *151*, 137–146

Mori, H., Sugie, S., Yoshimi, N., Kinouchi, T. & Ohnishi, Y. (1987) Genotoxicity of a variety of nitroarenes and other nitro compounds in DNA-repair tests with rat and mouse hepatocytes. *Mutat. Res.*, *190*, 159–167

Morotomi, M. & Watanabe, T. (1984) Metabolism of exogenous compounds by the intestinal microflora (Jpn.). *Tikoshikoroji Foramu* [*Toxicol. Forum*], *7*, 395–408

Nachtman, J.P. & Wolff, S. (1982) Activity of nitro-polynuclear aromatic hydrocarbons in the sister chromatid exchange assay with and without metabolic activation. *Environ. Mutagenesis*, *4*, 1–5

Nakagawa, R., Kitamori, S., Horikawa, K., Nakashima, K. & Tokiwa, H. (1983) Identification of dinitropyrenes in diesel-exhaust particles. Their probable presence as the major mutagens. *Mutat. Res.*, *124*, 201–211

Nakamura, S.-I., Oda, Y., Shimada, T., Oki, I. & Sugimoto, K. (1987) SOS-inducing activity of chemical carcinogens and mutagens in *Salmonella typhimurium* TA1535/pSK 1002: examination with 151 chemicals. *Mutat. Res.*, *192*, 239–246

Nakayasu, M., Sakamoto, H., Wakabayashi, K., Terada, M., Sugimara, T. & Rosenkranz, H.S. (1982) Potent mutagenic activity of nitropyrenes on Chinese hamster lung cells with diphtheria toxin resistance as a selective marker. *Carcinogenesis*, *3*, 917–922

Nishioka, M.G., Petersen, B.A. & Lewtas, J. (1982) Comparison of nitro-aromatic content and direct-acting mutagenicity of diesel emissions. In: Cooke, A., Dennis, A.J. & Fisher, G.L., eds, *Polynuclear Aromatic Hydrocarbons, 6th International Symposium, Physical and Biological Chemistry*, Columbus, OH, Battelle, pp. 603–613

Norman, C.A., Davison, L.M., Lambert, I.B., Bryant, D.W. & McCalla, D.R. (1988) P-32 postlabelling analysis of DNA adducts formed in primary rabbit tracheal epithelial cells following treatment with 1,8-dinitropyrene and its partially reduced derivative, 1-nitroso-8-nitropyrene (Abstract No. 189). *Environ. mol. Mutagenesis*, *11*, 78

Ochiai, M., Nagao, M., Tahira, T., Ishikawa, F., Hayashi, K., Ohgaki, H., Terada, M., Tsuchida, N. & Sugimura, T. (1985) Activation of K-*ras* and oncogenes other than *ras* family in rat fibrosarcomas induced by 1,8-dinitropyrene. *Cancer Lett.*, *29*, 119–125

Ohgaki, H., Negishi, C., Wakabayashi, K., Kusama, K., Sato, S. & Sugimura, T. (1984) Induction of sarcomas in rats by subcutaneous injection of dinitropyrenes. *Carcinogenesis*, *5*, 583–585

Ohgaki, H., Hasegawa, H., Kato, T., Negishi, C., Sato, S. & Sugimura, T. (1985) Absence of carcinogenicity of 1-nitropyrene, correction of previous results, and new demonstration of carcinogenicity of 1,6-dinitropyrene in rats. *Cancer Lett.*, *25*, 239–245

Orr, J.C., Bryant, D.W., McCalla, D.R. & Quilliam, M.A. (1985) Dinitropyrene-resistant *Salmonella typhimurium* are deficient in an acetyl-CoA acetyltransferase. *Chem.-biol. Interactions*, *54*, 281–288

Otofuji, T., Horikawa, K., Maeda, T., Sano, N., Izumi, K., Otsuka, H. & Tokiwa, H. (1987) Tumorigenicity test of 1,3- and 1,8-dinitropyrene in BALB/c mice. *J. natl Cancer Inst.*, *79*, 185–188

Paputa-Peck, M.C., Marano, R.S., Schuetzle, D., Riley, T.L., Hampton, C.V., Prater, T.J., Skewes, L.M. & Jensen, T.E. (1983) Determination of nitrated polynuclear aromatic hydrocarbons in particulate extracts by capillary column gas chromatography with nitrogen selective detection. *Anal. Chem.*, *55*, 1946-1954

Pederson, T.C. & Siak, J.C. (1981) The role of nitroaromatic compounds in the direct-acting mutagenicity of diesel particle extracts. *J. appl. Toxicol.*, *1*, 54-60

Pitts, J.N., Jr (1987) Nitration of gaseous polycyclic aromatic hydrocarbons in simulated and ambient urban atmospheres: a source of mutagenic nitroarenes. *Atmos. Environ.*, *21*, 2531-2547

Pitts, J.N., Jr, Zielinska, B. & Harger, W.P. (1984) Isomeric mononitrobenzo[*a*]pyrenes: synthesis, identification and mutagenic activities. *Mutat. Res.*, *140*, 81-85

Ramdahl, T. & Urdal, K. (1982) Determination of nitrated polycyclic aromatic hydrocarbons by fused silica capillary gas chromatography/negative ion chemical ionization mass spectrometry. *Anal. Chem.*, *54*, 2256-2260

Rosenkranz, H.S. & Mermelstein, R. (1983) Mutagenicity and genotoxicity of nitroarenes: all nitro-containing chemicals were not created equal. *Mutat. Res.*, *114*, 217-267

Rosenkranz, H.S. & Mermelstein, R. (1985) The genotoxicity, metabolism and carcinogenicity of nitrated polycyclic aromatic hydrocarbons. *J. environ. Sci. Health*, *C3*, 221-272

Rosenkranz, H.S., McCoy, E.C., Sanders, D.R., Butler, M., Kiriazides, D.K. & Mermelstein, R. (1980) Nitropyrenes: isolation, identification, and reduction of mutagenic impurities in carbon black and toners. *Science*, *209*, 1039-1043

Rosenkranz, H.S., McCoy, E.C., Frierson, M. & Klopman, G. (1985) The role of DNA sequence and structure of the electrophile on the mutagenicity of nitroarenes and arylamine derivatives. *Environ. Mutagenesis*, *7*, 645-653

Saito, K., Mita, S., Kamataki, T. & Kato, R. (1984) DNA single-strand breaks by nitropyrenes and related compounds in Chinese hamster V79 cells. *Cancer Lett.*, *24*, 121-127

Salmeen, I.T., Pero, A.M., Zator, R., Schuetzle, D. & Riley, T.L. (1984) Ames assay chromatograms and the identification of mutagens in diesel particle extracts. *Environ. Sci. Technol.*, *18*, 375-382

Sanders, D.R. (1981) Nitropyrenes: the isolation of trace mutagenic impurities from the toluene extract of an aftertreated carbon black. In: Cooke, M. & Dennis, A.J., eds, *Polynuclear Aromatic Hydrocarbons, 5th International Symposium, Chemical Analysis and Biological Fate*, Columbus, OH, Battelle, pp. 145-158

Sanders, D.R., Temcharoen, P. & Thilly, W.G. (1983) 1,8-Dinitropyrene mutagenicity in bacteria and human cells (Abstract No. EC-6). *Environ. Mutagenesis*, *5*, 457

Schuetzle, D. & Jensen, T.E. (1985) Analysis of nitrated polycyclic aromatic hydrocarbons (nitro-PAH) by mass spectrometry. In: White, C.M., ed., *Nitrated Polycyclic Aromatic Hydrocarbons*, Heidelberg, A. Hüthig Verlag, pp. 121-167

Siak, J., Chan, T.L., Gibson, T.L. & Wolff, G.T. (1985) Contribution to bacterial mutagenicity from nitro-PAH compounds in ambient aerosols. *Atmos. Environ.*, *19*, 369-376

Tahira, T., Hayashi, K., Ochiai, M., Tsuchida, N., Nagao, M. & Sugimura, T. (1986) Structure of the c-Ki-*ras* gene in rat fibrosarcoma induced by 1,8-dinitropyrene. *Mol. cell. Biol.*, *6*, 1349-1351

Takayama, S., Tanaka, M., Katoh, Y., Terada, M. & Sugimura, T. (1983) Mutagenicity of nitropyrenes in Chinese hamster V79 cells. *Gann*, *74*, 338-341

Takayama, S., Ishikawa, T., Nakajima, H. & Sato, S. (1985) Lung carcinoma induction in Syrian golden hamsters by intratracheal instillation of 1,6-dinitropyrene. *Jpn. J. Cancer Res. (Gann)*, *76*, 457–461

Tanabe, K., Matsushita, H., Kuo, C.T. & Imamiya, S. (1986) Determination of carcinogen nitroarenes in airborne particulates by high performance liquid chromatography. *Taiki Osen Gakkaishi*, *21*, 535–544

Tokiwa, H. & Ohnishi, Y. (1986) Mutagenicity and carcinogenicity of nitroarenes and their sources in the environment. *CRC crit. Rev. Toxicol.*, *17*, 23–60

Tokiwa, H., Nakagawa, R. & Ohnishi, Y. (1981) Mutagenic assay of aromatic nitro compounds with *Salmonella typhimurium*. *Mutat. Res.*, *91*, 321–325

Tokiwa, H., Kitamori, S., Nakagawa, R., Horikawa, K. & Matamala, L. (1983) Demonstration of a powerful mutagenic dinitropyrene in airborne particulate matter. *Mutat. Res.*, *121*, 107–116

Tokiwa, H., Nakagawa, R. & Horikawa, K. (1985) Mutagenic/carcinogenic agents in indoor pollutants: the dinitropyrenes generated by kerosene heaters and fuel gas and liquified petroleum gas burners. *Mutat. Res.*, *157*, 39–47

Tokiwa, H., Otofuji, T., Nakagawa, R., Horikawa, K., Maeda, T., Sano, N., Izumi, E. & Otsuka, H. (1986) Dinitro derivatives of pyrene and fluoranthene in diesel emission particulates and their tumorigenicity in mice and rats. In: Ishinishi, N., Koizumi, A., McClellan, R.O. & Stöber, W., eds, *Carcinogenic and Mutagenic Effects of Diesel Engine Exhaust*, Amsterdam, Elsevier, pp. 253–270

Tsunoda, T., Yamaoka, T. & Nagamatsu, G. (1973) Spectral sensitization of bisazide compounds. *Photogr. Sci. Eng.*, *17*, 390–393

Tu, A.S., Sivak, A. & Mermelstein, R. (1982) Evaluation of in vitro transforming ability of nitropyrenes (Abstract). In: *Proceedings of the Fifth CIIT Conference on Toxicology: Toxicity of Nitroaromatic Compounds*, Raleigh, NC, Chemical Industry Institute of Toxicology, p. 8

Wilcox, P. & Parry, J.M. (1981) The genetic activity of dinitropyrenes in yeast: unusual dose response curves for induced mitotic gene conversion. *Carcinogenesis*, *2*, 1201–1205

Wilcox, P., Danford, N. & Parry, J.M. (1982) The genetic activity and metabolism of dinitropyrenes in eucaryotic cells. In: Sorsa, M. & Vainio, H., eds, *Mutagens in Our Environment*, New York, Alan R. Liss, pp. 249–258

Wislocki, P.G., Bagan, E.S., Lu, A.Y.H., Dooley, K.L., Fu, P.P., Han-Hsu, H., Beland, F.A. & Kadlubar, F.F. (1986) Tumorigenicity of nitrated derivatives of pyrene, benz[a]anthracene, chrysene and benzo[a]pyrene in the newborn mouse assay. *Carcinogenesis*, *7*, 1317–1322

Yoshikura, T., Kuroda, K., Kamiura, T., Masumoto, K., Fukushima, M., Yamamoto, T. & Torii, M. (1985) Synthesis of 1,3- 1,6- and 1,8-dinitropyrenes and evaluation of their mutagenicities. *Annu. Rep. Osaka City Inst. public Health environ. Sci.*, *47*, 31–35 [*Chem. Abstr.*, *106*, 49745t]

Yoshimi, N., Sugie, S., Mori, H., Kinouchi, T. & Ohnishi, Y. (1987) Genotoxicity of various nitroarenes in DNA repair tests with human hepatocytes (Abstract No. 73). *Mutat. Res.*, *182*, 384

Zielinska, B., Harger, W.P., Arey, J., Winer, A.M., Haas, R.A. & Hanson, C.V. (1987) The mutagenicity of 2-nitrofluoranthene and its in vitro hepatic metabolites. *Mutat. Res.*, *190*, 259–266

# 7-NITROBENZ[a]ANTHRACENE

## 1. Chemical and Physical Data

### 1.1 Synonyms

*Chem. Abstr. Services Reg. No.*: 20268-51-3
*Chem. Abstr. Name*: Benz[a]anthracene, 7-nitro-
*IUPAC Systematic Name*: 7-Nitrobenz[a]anthracene

### 1.2 Structural and molecular formulae and molecular weight

$C_{18}H_{11}NO_2$            Mol. wt: 273.3

### 1.3 Chemical and physical properties of the pure substance

(a) *Description*: Yellow crystals (Newman & Lilje, 1979; Chemsyn Science Laboratories, 1988)

(b) *Melting-point*: 159–161°C (Newman & Lilje, 1979); 160–163°C (Buckingham, 1987)

(c) *Spectroscopy data*: Infra-red, nuclear magnetic resonance (Iversen et al., 1985) and mass (Schuetzle & Jensen, 1985) spectral data have been reported.

(d) *Solubility*: Limited solubility in toluene and benzene (Chemsyn Science Laboratories, 1988)

### 1.4 Technical products and impurities

7-Nitrobenz[a]anthracene is available for research purposes in ⩾99% purity (Chemsyn Science Laboratories, 1988).

## 2. Production, Use, Occurrence and Analysis

### 2.1 Production and use

*(a) Production*

7-Nitrobenz[*a*]anthracene is the main product of the nitration of benz[*a*]anthracene (Buckingham, 1987). No evidence was found that this compound has been produced in commercial quantities.

*(b) Use*

No evidence was found that 7-nitrobenz[*a*]anthracene has been used for commercial applications.

### 2.2 Occurrence

7-Nitrobenz[*a*]anthracene was not detected in an extract of the exhaust of a light-duty diesel vehicle (detection limit, ~0.3 mg/kg; Paputa-Peck *et al.*, 1983).

Toners for use in photocopy machines have been produced in quantity since the late 1950s and have seen widespread use. 'Long-flow' furnace black was first used in photocopy toners in 1967; its manufacture involved an oxidation whereby some nitration also occurred. Subsequent changes in the production technique reduced the total extractable nitropyrene content from an uncontrolled level of 5–100 mg/kg to below 0.3 mg/kg (Rosenkranz *et al.*, 1980; Sanders, 1981; Butler *et al.*, 1983), and toners produced from this carbon black since 1980 have not been found to contain detectable levels of mutagenicity or, hence, nitropyrenes (Rosenkranz *et al.*, 1980; Butler *et al.*, 1983).

### 2.3 Analysis

See the monograph on 1-nitropyrene.

## 3. Biological Data Relevant to the Evaluation of Carcinogenic Risk to Humans

### 3.1 Carcinogenicity studies in animals

*Intraperitoneal administration*

*Mouse*: Groups of 90 or 100 male and female newborn CD-1 mice received three intraperitoneal injections of 7-nitrobenz[*a*]anthracene (total dose, 2800 nmol [0.8 mg]; purity, >99%) in 10, 20 and 40 µl dimethyl sulfoxide (DMSO) on days 1, 8 and 15 after birth; a total dose of 560 nmol [0.14 mg] benzo[*a*]pyrene (purity, >99%) as three injections; or three injections of DMSO only (Wislocki et al., 1986). Treatment of a second vehicle control group was begun ten weeks after that of the other groups. At 25-27 days, when the mice were weaned, 25 males and 33 females in the treated group, 37 males and 27 females in the positive control group and 28 and 31 males and 45 and 34 females in the two vehicle control groups were still alive. All remaining mice were killed after one year. Liver tumours occurred in 7/25 7-nitrobenz[a]anthracene-treated males (six adenomas and one carcinoma; $p < 0.05$ compared with DMSO controls), 0/33 7-nitrobenz[a]anthracene-treated females, 18/37 benzo[a]pyrene-treated males, 0/27 benzo[a]pyrene-treated females, 2/28 and 5/45 DMSO-treated males, and 0/31 and 0/34 DMSO-treated females. Lung adenomas occurred in significantly more benzo[a]pyrene-treated males (13/37) and females (13/27) than in controls ($p < 0.005$), but no significant increase occurred among 7-nitrobenz[a]anthracene-treated males (2/25) or females (3/33). The incidences of lung tumours in the DMSO groups were 1/28 and 4/45 in males and 0/31 and 2/34 in females. [The Working Group noted the short duration of the experiment.]

## 3.2 Other relevant data

### (a) Experimental systems

#### Absorption, distribution, excretion and metabolism

Liver microsomes from male Sprague-Dawley rats pretreated with 3-methylcholanthrene catalysed the conversion of 7-nitrobenz[a]anthracene to 7-nitrobenz[a]anthracene *trans*-3,4-dihydrodiol and 7-nitrobenz[a]anthracene *trans*-8,9-dihydrodiol (Fu & Yang, 1989).

Rat liver microsomes and xanthine oxidase, a mammalian nitroreductase, catalysed the binding of 7-nitrobenz[a]anthracene to exogenous DNA (Colvert & Fu, 1986; Colvert et al., 1989).

#### Toxic effects

No data were available to the Working Group.

#### Genetic and related effects

The genetic and related effects of nitroarenes and of their metabolites have been reviewed (Rosenkranz & Mermelstein, 1983; Beland et al., 1985; Rosenkranz & Mermelstein, 1985; Tokiwa & Ohnishi, 1986).

7-Nitrobenz[a]anthracene did not induce mutation in *Salmonella typhimurium* TA98 or TA100 in the presence or absence of an exogenous metabolic system from Aroclor 1254-induced rat liver (Greibrokk et al., 1984; Fu et al., 1985; White et al., 1985 (10 µg/plate)).

### (b) Humans

No data were available to the Working Group.

## 3.3 Epidemiological studies and case reports of carcinogenicity in humans

No data were available to the Working Group.

# 4. Summary of Data Reported and Evaluation

## 4.1 Exposure data

No data were available to the Working Group.

## 4.2 Experimental data

7-Nitrobenz[a]anthracene was tested for carcinogenicity in one experiment by intraperitoneal injection into newborn mice, resulting in an increased incidence of liver-cell tumours in males.

## 4.3 Human data

No data were available to the Working Group.

## 4.4 Other relevant data

Metabolism of 7-nitrobenz[a]anthracene led to binding to exogenous DNA. It was not mutagenic to bacteria.

## 4.5 Evaluation[1]

There is *limited evidence* for the carcinogenicity in experimental animals of 7-nitrobenz[a]anthracene.

No data were available from studies in humans on the carcinogenicity of 7-nitrobenz[a]anthracene.

### Overall evaluation

7-Nitrobenz[a]anthracene *is not classifiable as to its carcinogenicity to humans (Group 3)*.

---

[1]For definitions of the italicized terms, see Preamble, pp. 25–28.

## Summary table of genetic and related effects of 7-nitrobenz[a]anthracene

| Nonmammalian systems | | | | | | | | | | | | | Mammalian systems | | | | | | | | | | | | | | | | | | | | | |
|---|---|---|---|---|---|---|---|---|---|---|---|---|---|---|---|---|---|---|---|---|---|---|---|---|---|---|---|---|---|---|---|---|---|---|
| Proka-ryotes | | | | Lower eukaryotes | | | | Plants | | | | Insects | In vitro | | | | | | | | | | | | | | | | | In vivo | | | | |
| | | | | | | | | | | | | | Animal cells | | | | | | | Human cells | | | | | | | | | | Animals | | | | | Humans |
| D | G | D | R | G | A | D | G | C | R | G | C | A | D | G | S | M | C | A | T | I | D | G | S | M | C | A | T | I | D | G | S | M | C | DL | A | D | S | M | C | A |
| − | | | | | | | | | | | | | | | | | | | | | | | | | | | | | | | | | | | | | | | | |

A, aneuploidy; C, chromosomal aberrations; D, DNA damage; DL, dominant lethal mutation; G, gene mutation; I, inhibition of intercellular communication; M, micronuclei; R, mitotic recombination and gene conversion, S, sister chromatid exchange; T, cell transformation
−, considered to be negative for the specific end point and level of biological complexity

## 5. References

Beland, F.A., Heflich, R.H., Howard, P.C. & Fu, P.P. (1985) The in vitro metabolic activation of nitro polycyclic aromatic hydrocarbons. In: Harvey, R.G., ed., *Polycyclic Hydrocarbons and Carcinogenesis (ACS Symposium Series, No. 283)*, Washington DC, American Chemical Society, pp. 371–396

Buckingham, J., ed. (1987) *Dictionary of Organic Compounds*, 5th ed., 5th Suppl., New York, Chapman & Hall, p. 476 (N-50107)

Butler, M.A., Evans, D.L., Giammarise, A.T., Kiriazides, D.K., Marsh, D., McCoy, E.C., Mermelstein, R., Murphy, C.B. & Rosenkranz, H.S. (1983) Application of *Salmonella* assay to carbon blacks and toners. In: Cooke, M. & Dennis, A.J., eds, *Polynuclear Aromatic Hydrocarbons, 7th International Symposium, Formation, Metabolism and Measurement*, Columbus, OH, Battelle, pp. 225–241

Chemsyn Science Laboratories (1988) *7-Nitrobenz[a]anthracene (Product Code U1028)*, Lenexa, KS, p. 78

Colvert, K.K. & Fu, P.P. (1986) Xanthine oxidase-catalyzed DNA binding of dihydrodiol derivatives of nitro-polycyclic aromatic hydrocarbons. *Biochem. biophys. Res. Commun.*, 141, 245–250

Colvert, K.K., Chou, M.W., Von Tungeln, L.S. & Fu, P.P. (1989) In vitro binding of nitro-polycyclic aromatic hydrocarbons and their oxidative metabolites to macromolecules. In: *Polynuclear Aromatic Hydrocarbons, 11th International Symposium*, Columbus, OH, Battelle (in press)

Fu, P.P. & Yang, S.K. (1983) Stereoselective metabolism of 7-nitrobenz[*a*]-anthracene to 3,4- and 8,9-*trans*-dihydrodiols. *Biochem. biophys. Res. Commun.*, 115, 123–129

Fu, P.P., Chou, M.W., Miller, D.W., White, G.L., Heflich, R.H. & Beland, F.A. (1985) The orientation of the nitro substituent predicts the direct-acting bacterial mutagenicity of nitrated polycyclic aromatic hydrocarbons. *Mutat. Res.*, 143, 173–181

Greibrokk, T., Löfroth, G., Nilsson, L., Toftgård, R., Carlstedt-Duke, J. & Gustafsson, J.-Å. (1984) Nitroarenes: mutagenicity in the Ames *Salmonella*/microsome assay and affinity to the TCDD-receptor protein. In: Rickert, D.E., ed., *Toxicity of Nitroaromatic Compounds*, Washington DC, Hemisphere, pp. 167–183

Iversen, B., Sydnes, L.K. & Greibrokk, T. (1985) Characterization of nitrobenzanthracenes and nitrodibenzanthracenes. *Acta chem. scand.*, B39, 837–847

Newman, M.S. & Lilje, K.C. (1979) Synthesis of 7-fluorobenz[a]anthracene. *J. org. Chem.*, 44, 1347–1348

Paputa-Peck, M.C., Marano, R.S., Schuetzle, D., Riley, T.L., Hampton, C.V., Prater, T.J., Skewes, L.M. & Jensen, T.E. (1983) Determination of nitrated polynuclear aromatic hydrocarbons in particulate extracts by capillary column gas chromatography with nitrogen selective detection. *Anal. Chem.*, 55, 1946–1954

Rosenkranz, H.S. & Mermelstein, R. (1983) Mutagenicity and genotoxicity of nitroarenes: all nitro-containing chemicals were not created equal. *Mutat. Res.*, 114, 217–267

Rosenkranz, H.S. & Mermelstein, R. (1985) The genoxotoxicity, metabolism and carcinogenicity of nitrated polycyclic aromatic hydrocarbons. *J. environ. Sci. Health*, C3, 221–272

Rosenkranz, H.S., McCoy, E.C., Sanders, D.R., Butler, M., Kiriazides, D.K. & Mermelstein, R. (1980) Nitropyrenes: isolation, identification and reduction of mutagenic impurities in carbon black and toners. *Science*, 209, 1039–1043

Sanders, D.R. (1981) Nitropyrenes: the isolation of trace mutagenic impurities from the toluene extract of an aftertreated carbon black. In: Cooke, M. & Dennis, A.J., eds, *Polynuclear Aromatic Hydrocarbons, 5th International Symposium, Chemical Analysis and Biological Fate*, Columbus, OH, Battelle, pp. 145–158

Schuetzle, D. & Jensen, T.E. (1985) Analysis of nitrated polycyclic aromatic hydrocarbons (nitro-PAH) by mass spectrometry. In: White, C.M., ed., *Nitrated Polycyclic Aromatic Hydrocarbons*, Heidelberg, A. Hüthig Verlag, pp. 121–167

Tokiwa, H. & Ohnishi, Y. (1986) Mutagenicity and carcinogenicity of nitroarenes and their sources in the environment. *CRC crit. Rev. Toxicol.*, *17*, 23–69

White, G.L., Fu, P.P. & Heflich, R.H. (1985) Effect of nitro substitution on the light-mediated mutagenicity of polycyclic aromatic hydrocarbons in *Salmonella typhimurium* TA98. *Mutat. Res.*, *144*, 1–7

Wislocki, P.G., Bagan, E.S., Lu, A.Y.H., Dooley, K.L., Fu, P.P., Han-Hsu, H., Beland, F.A. & Kadlubar, F.F. (1986) Tumorigenicity of nitrated derivatives of pyrene, benz[*a*]anthracene, chrysene and benzo[*a*]pyrene in the newborn mouse assay. *Carcinogenesis*, *7*, 1317–1322

# 6-NITROBENZO[*a*]PYRENE

This substance was considered by a previous Working Group, in June 1983 (IARC, 1984). Since that time, new data have become available and these have been incorporated into the monograph and taken into consideration in the present evaluation.

## 1. Chemical and Physical Data

### 1.1 Synonyms

*Chem. Abstr. Services Reg. No.*: 63041-90-7
*Chem. Abstr. Name*: Benzo[*a*]pyrene, 6-nitro-
*IUPAC Systematic Name*: 6-Nitrobenzo[*a*]pyrene

### 1.2 Structural and molecular formulae and molecular weight

$C_{20}H_{11}NO_2$     Mol. wt: 297.3

### 1.3 Chemical and physical properties of the pure substance

(*a*) *Description*: Orange-yellow needles, recrystallized from benzene (Boit, 1965); yellow crystalline solid (Chemsyn Science Laboratories, 1988); orange crystals (Buckingham, 1985)

(*b*) *Melting-point*: 250.5–251°C (Boit, 1965); 255–256°C (Buckingham, 1985)

(*c*) *Spectroscopy data*: Ultra-violet, nuclear magnetic resonance and mass spectral data have been reported (Dewar *et al.*, 1956; Fu *et al.*, 1982a; Chou *et al.*, 1984; Johansen *et al.*, 1984; Schuetzle & Jensen, 1985).

(d) *Solubility*: Limited solubility in toluene and benzene (Chemsyn Science Laboratories, 1988)

(e) *Reactivity*: Reacts with chromic acid in acetic acid to form 7-oxo-7H-benz[de]-anthracene dicarboxylic acid-3,4-anhydride (Boit, 1965)

### 1.4 Technical products and impurities

6-Nitrobenzo[a]pyrene is available at a certified purity of 99.75% (Belliardo et al., 1988). It is also available at ⩾99% purity and at ⩾98% radiochemical purity as the $^3$H-labelled compound (Chemsyn Science Laboratories, 1988).

## 2. Production, Use, Occurrence and Analysis

### 2.1 Production and use

(a) *Production*

6-Nitrobenzo[a]pyrene was first synthesized by Windaus and Rennhak in 1937 by treating benzo[a]pyrene with aqueous nitric acid in either acetic acid or benzene and acetic acid (Boit, 1965). It has been reported to be formed under simulated environmental atmospheric conditions by reacting benzo[a]pyrene with nitrogen oxide and traces of nitric acid (Pitts et al., 1978). No evidence was found that 6-nitrobenzo[a]pyrene has been produced in commercial quantities.

(b) *Use*

No evidence was found that 6-nitrobenzo[a]pyrene has been used for other than laboratory applications.

### 2.2 Occurrence

(a) *Engine exhaust*

Pitts et al. (1982) and Gibson (1982, 1983) have reported the occurrence of 6-nitrobenzo[a]pyrene in diesel emissions.

Illustrative values for levels of 6-nitrobenzo[a]pyrene found in engine emissions are given in Table 1. Pitts et al. (1982) reported finding 50 mg/kg in an extract and 5 mg/kg in particulate matter from the exhaust of a six-cylinder diesel-powered car. The rates of emission of 6-nitrobenz[a]pyrene in automobile exhaust have been reported to be 1.46 ± 0.74 µg/mile [0.9 ± 0.5 µg/km] for a gasoline-powered car with a precatalyst engine running on leaded fuel, 0.45 ± 0.22 µg/mile [0.28 ± 0.14 µg/km] for an engine with the catalyst removed running on unleaded fuel and 0.012 µg/mile [0.008 µg/km] for a gasoline-powered engine with a catalytic converter. A production model diesel engine emitted <0.15 µg/mile [<0.09 µg/km] and a diesel trap model, 0.01 µg/mile [0.006 µg/km] (Gibson, 1982).

### Table 1. 6-Nitrobenzo[a]pyrene levels in exhaust particles[a]

| Sample | 6-Nitrobenzo[a]pyrene concentration (mg/kg particulate matter) |
|---|---|
| Gasoline-powered cars | |
| 1974 engine (precatalyst), leaded fuel | 32.8 ± 16.2 |
| 1980 engine (catalyst removed), unleaded fuel | 17.3 ± 8.5 |
| 1981 engine with catalyst | 0.21 ± 0.1 |
| Diesel-powered cars | |
| trap model | 0.1 |
| 1980 engine | <0.4 |

[a]From Gibson (1982)

*(b) Other occurrence*

Toners for use in photocopy machines have been produced in quantity since the late 1950s and have seen widespread use. 'Long-flow' furnace black was first used in photocopy toners in 1967; its manufacture involved an oxidation whereby some nitration also occurred. Subsequent changes in the production technique reduced the total extractable nitropyrene content from an uncontrolled level of 5–100 mg/kg to below 0.3 mg/kg (Rosenkranz *et al.*, 1980; Sanders, 1981; Butler *et al.*, 1983), and toners produced from this carbon black since 1980 have not been found to contain detectable levels of mutagenicity or, hence, nitropyrenes (Rosenkranz *et al.*, 1980; Butler *et al.*, 1983).

6-Nitrobenzo[a]pyrene has been detected in airborne particles in Prague, Czechoslovakia (Jäger, 1978). Ambient particles collected in the area of Detroit, MI, USA, during the spring and summer of 1981 contained levels of 0.9–2.5 mg/kg, corresponding to airborne concentrations of 0.04–0.28 ng/m$^3$ (Gibson, 1982). Nielsen *et al.* (1984) detected 6-nitrobenzo[a]pyrene in airborne particles in rural Denmark during the late winter and early spring of 1982, but the levels were one to two orders of magnitude lower than those of most common polyciclic aromatic hydrocarbons such as benzo[a]pyrene. The authors suggested that formation may have occurred during sampling.

Other reported sources of emissions of 6-nitrobenzo[a]pyrene include stack gases from aluminium smelters (Oehme *et al.*, 1982). A fireplace in which red oak was burned yielded diluted emissions of 0.11 and 0.12 mg/kg particles (Gibson, 1982).

## 2.3 Analysis

See the monograph on 1-nitropyrene.

## 3. Biological Data Relevant to the Evaluation of Carcinogenic Risk to Humans

### 3.1 Carcinogenicity studies in animals[1]

*(a) Skin application*

*Mouse*: In a study of initiating activity, two groups of 20 female CD-1 Charles River mice, aged 50–55 days, received ten applications of 5 μg 6-nitrobenzo[a]pyrene or benzo[a]pyrene (purity, >99%) in 0.1 ml acetone onto shaved back skin every other day for 20 days (total dose, 0.05 mg; El-Bayoumy *et al.*, 1982). A group of 20 female mice receiving acetone alone served as controls. Starting ten days after initiation had been completed, all animals received applications of 2.5 μg 12-*O*-tetradecanoylphorbol 13-acetate in 0.1 ml acetone three times per week for 25 weeks. At the end of this time, 5/20 animals treated with 6-nitrobenzo[a]pyrene, 18/20 benzo[a]pyrene-treated animals and 1/20 control animals had developed skin tumours (mainly papillomas). The incidence of papillomas in 6-nitrobenzo[a]pyrene-treated animals was not statistically significant from that in untreated controls [$p = 0.09$]. [The Working Group noted the small number of animals tested.]

*(b) Intraperitoneal administration*

*Mouse*: Groups of 90 or 100 male and female newborn CD-1 mice received three intraperitoneal injections of 6-nitrobenzo[a]pyrene (total dose, 560 nmol [0.17 mg]; purity, >99%) in 10, 20 and 40 μl dimethyl sulfoxide (DMSO) on days 1, 8 and 15 after birth; a total dose of 560 nmol [0.14 mg] benzo[a]pyrene (purity, 99%); or three injections of DMSO only (Wislocki *et al.*, 1986). Treatment of a second vehicle control group was begun ten weeks after that of the other groups. At 25–27 days, when the mice were weaned, 29 males and 44 females in the treated group, 37 males and 27 females in the positive control group, and 28 and 31 males and 45 and 34 females in the two vehicle control groups were still alive. All remaining mice were killed after one year. Liver tumours occurred in 8/29 6-nitrobenzo[a]pyrene-treated males (five adenomas, three carcinomas; $p < 0.05$), 0/44 6-nitrobenzo[a]pyrene-treated females, 18/37 benzo[a]pyrene-treated males, 0/27 benzo[a]pyrene-treated females, 2/28 and 5/45 DMSO-treated males and 0/31 and 0/34 DMSO-treated females. Lung adenomas occurred in significantly more benzo[a]pyrene-treated males (13/37) and females (13/27) than in controls ($p < 0.005$), but no significant increase occurred among 6-nitrobenzo[a]pyrene-treated males (4/29) or females (1/44). The incidences of lung tumours in the DMSO groups were 1/28 and 4/45 in males and 0/31 and 2/34 in females. [The Working Group noted the short duration of the experiment.]

---

[1]The Working Group was aware of studies in progress in mice by single subcutaneous injection and by intraperitoneal injection (IARC, 1988).

## 3.2 Other relevant data

(a) *Experimental systems*

(i) *Absorption, distribution, excretion and metabolism*

Among female F344 rats administered 1 nmol [297 ng] [$^{14}$C]6-nitrobenzo[a]pyrene by intratracheal instillation, the majority of the material (86%) was cleared from the lungs with a half-life of 0.2 h, while the remaining 14% had a half-life of 36 h (Bond *et al.*, 1985).

In-vitro incubation of 6-nitrobenzo[a]pyrene with rat liver microsomes, 9000 g supernatant of rat liver or lung, rat lung microsomes or 9000 g supernatant of mouse liver has been reported to give rise to benzo[a]pyrene, 6-nitrobenzo[a]pyrene-7,8- and 9,10-dihydrodiols, 6-hydroxybenzo[a]pyrene, 1- and 3-hydroxy-6-nitrobenzo[a]pyrenes, 1,9-and 3,9-dihydroxy-6-nitrobenz[a]pyrenes, benzo[a]pyrene-1,6-, -3,6- and -6,12-quinones, 6-acetoxybenzo[a]pyrene, and mono- and diacetoxy-6-nitrobenzo[a]pyrenes (Fu *et al.*, 1982a,b; Chou *et al.*, 1983; Raha *et al.*, 1984, 1986a,b, 1987a,b). Similar incubation with 9000 g supernatant of liver from rats pretreated with 3-methylcholanthrene led to binding to exogenous DNA (Kaneko & Nagata, 1983).

Anaerobic bacterial suspensions from human faeces and intestinal contents, rat faeces and intestinal contents and pure cultures of anaerobic bacteria reduced 6-nitrobenzo[a]pyrene to 6-aminobenzo[a]pyrene (Cerniglia *et al.*, 1984; Richardson *et al.*, 1988).

6-Nitrobenzo[a]pyrene was reduced to metabolites soluble in organic solvents (predominant presence of dihydrodiols) and in water by hamster embryo fibroblasts. The metabolism was accompanied by binding to RNA, DNA and nuclear protein (Selkirk *et al.*, 1981; Tong & Selkirk, 1983).

Incubation of explants of human colon and bronchus with 6-nitrobenzo[a]pyrene resulted in the formation of one major metabolite, 3-hydroxy-6-nitrobenzo[a]pyrene, which bound to the DNA of both tissues. Two adducts were identified in bronchial DNA, one of which had a retention time in high-performance liquid chromatograms similar to that of the major adduct found in lung and liver DNA of Sprague-Dawley rats treated with an intraperitoneal dose of 2 mg/kg bw 6-nitrobenzo[a]pyrene. By comparison, three adducts were detected in the DNA of *Salmonella typhimurium* TA98 that had been incubated with 6-nitrobenzo[a]pyrene in the presence of an exogenous metabolic system from rat liver. One of these adducts appeared to have a similar retention time to the major adduct detected in rat lung and liver (Garner *et al.*, 1985).

(ii) *Toxic effects*

Intraperitoneal administration of 6-nitrobenzo[a]pyrene to young male Sprague-Dawley rats (three times at 5 mg/kg bw) resulted in a 1.6-fold increase in aryl hydrocarbon hydroxylase activity over that in controls (Chou *et al.*, 1987).

(iii) *Genetic and related effects*

The genetic and related effects of nitroarenes and of their metabolites have been reviewed (Rosenkranz & Mermelstein, 1983; Beland *et al.*, 1985; Rosenkranz & Mermelstein, 1985; Tokiwa & Ohnishi, 1986).

6-Nitrobenzo[a]pyrene (1–5 nmol/plate) was mutagenic to *S. typhimurium* TA98 and TA100, generally only in the presence of an exogenous metabolic system from rat liver (Wang *et al.*, 1978; Tokiwa *et al.*, 1981; Fu *et al.*, 1982a,b; Pitts *et al.*, 1982; Chou *et al.*, 1984; Greibrokk *et al.*, 1984; Fu *et al.*, 1985; White *et al.*, 1985; Hass *et al.*, 1986a; Löfroth *et al.*, 1984; Anderson *et al.*, 1987).

Early studies indicated that 6-nitrobenzo[a]pyrene was mutagenic to the *hprt* locus of cultured Chinese hamster CHO cells in the absence of an exogenous metabolic system (1–3 $\mu$g/ml; Chou *et al.*, 1984), but subsequent reports indicated positive results in the presence (one dose only, 5 $\mu$g/ml) and negative results in the absence (up to 10 $\mu$g/ml) of metabolic activation (Hass *et al.*, 1986b).

6-Nitrobenzo[a]pyrene induced morphological transformation in cultured Syrian hamster embryo cells (DiPaolo *et al.*, 1983 (6.6–34 $\mu$M); Sala *et al.*, 1987 (marginally active at 2–8 $\mu$M)) and transformation (induction of growth in soft agar and invasiveness in chicken embryo skin culture) in human diploid fibroblasts when oxygen tension was reduced (Howard *et al.*, 1983 (4–67 $\mu$M)) and in mouse BALB/c 3T3 cells (Sala *et al.*, 1987 (4–32 $\mu$M)). It did not induce transformation of mouse C3H 10T1/2 cells (at up to 8 $\mu$M), nor did it act as an initiator in these cells (Sala *et al.*, 1987).

*(b) Humans*

No data were available to the Working Group.

## 3.3 Epidemiological studies and case reports of carcinogenicity in humans

No data were available to the Working Group.

# 4. Summary of Data Reported and Evaluation

## 4.1 Exposure data

6-Nitrobenzo[a]pyrene has been detected in stack gases from aluminium smelters and in particulate emissions from diesel and gasoline engines. It has also been measured at low concentrations in ambient air.

## 4.2 Experimental data

6-Nitrobenzo[a]pyrene was tested for carcinogenicity in a two-stage initiation-promotion study in mouse skin and by intraperitoneal injection into newborn mice. The study by skin application was inadequate for evaluation. An increased incidence of liver-cell tumours was observed in male mice after intraperitoneal injection.

## 4.3 Human data

No data were available to the Working Group.

## 4.4 Other relevant data

Metabolism of 6-nitrobenzo[a]pyrene led to DNA adduct formation in bacteria, explanted human tissues and animals. 6-Nitrobenzo[a]pyrene caused transformation of animal and human cultured cells and was mutagenic to cultured animal cells. It induced mutations in bacteria in the presence of an exogenous metabolic system.

## 4.5 Evaluation[1]

There is *limited evidence* for the carcinogenicity in experimental animals of 6-nitrobenzo[a]pyrene.

No data were available from studies in humans on the carcinogenicity of 6-nitrobenzo[a]pyrene.

### Overall evaluation

6-Nitrobenzo[a]pyrene *is not classifiable as to its carcinogenicity to humans (Group 3).*

# 5. References

Anderson, J.G., McCalla, D.R., Bryant, D.W., McCarry, B.E. & Bromke, A.M. (1987) Metabolic activation of 3-nitroperylene in the *Salmonella*/S9 assay. *Mutagenesis, 2,* 279–285

Beland, F.A., Heflich, R.H., Howard, P.C. & Fu, P.P. (1985) The in vitro metabolic activation of nitro polycyclic aromatic hydrocarbons. In: Harvey, R.G., ed., *Polycyclic Hydrocarbons and Carcinogenesis (ACS Symposium Series No. 283)*, Washington DC, American Chemical Society, pp. 371–396

Belliardo, J.J., Jacob, J. & Lindsey, A.S. (1988) *The Certification of the Purity of Seven Nitropolycyclic Aromatic Compounds, CRM Nos 305, 306, 307, 308, 310, 311, 312, BCR Information, Reference Materials (EUR 11254 EN)*, Brussels, Commission of the European Communities, p. III

Boit, H.-G., ed. (1965) *Beilsteins Handbuch der Organischen Chemie*, Vol. 5, 4th ed., 3rd Suppl., Syst. No. 490, Berlin (West), Springer-Verlag, p. 2520

Bond, J.A., Baker, S.M. & Bechtold, W.E. (1985) Correlation of the octanol/water partition coefficient with clearance halftimes of intratracheally instilled aromatic hydrocarbons in rats. *Toxicology, 36,* 285–295

Buckingham, J., ed. (1985) *Dictionary of Organic Compounds*, 5th ed., 3rd Suppl., New York, Chapman & Hall, p. 323 (N-30046)

---

[1]For definitions of the italicized terms, see Preamble, pp. 25–28.

## Summary table of genetic and related effects of 6-nitrobenzo[a]pyrene

| Nonmammalian systems | | | | | | | | | | | | | | | Mammalian systems | | | | | | | | | | | | | | | | | | | | | | |
|---|---|---|---|---|---|---|---|---|---|---|---|---|---|---|---|---|---|---|---|---|---|---|---|---|---|---|---|---|---|---|---|---|---|---|---|---|
| Proka-ryotes | | | | Lower eukaryotes | | | | | | Plants | | | | Insects | | In vitro | | | | | | | | | | | | | | | In vivo | | | | | | |
| | | | | | | | | | | | | | | | | Animal cells | | | | | | | Human cells | | | | | | | | Animals | | | | Humans | | |
| D | G | D | R | G | A | D | G | C | R | G | C | A | C | R | G | C | A | D | G | S | M | C | A | T | I | D | G | S | M | C | A | T | I | D | G | S | M | C | DL | A | D | S | M | C | A |
| ±  | + | | | | | | | | | | | | | | | | | + | | | | | | | | ± | | | | + | | ± | | ±  | | | | | | | | | | | |

A, aneuploidy; C, chromosomal aberrations; D, DNA damage; DL, dominant lethal mutation; G, gene mutation; I, inhibition of intercellular communication; M, micronuclei; R, mitotic recombination and gene conversion; S, sister chromatid exchange; T, cell transformation

*In completing the table, the following symbols indicate the consensus of the Working Group with regard to the results for each endpoint:*
+ considered to be positive for the specific endpoint and level of biological complexity
± considered to be positive, but only one valid study was available to the Working Group

Butler, M.A., Evans, D.L., Giammarise, A.T., Kiriazides, D.K., Marsh, D., McCoy, E.C., Mermelstein, R., Murphy, C.B. & Rosenkranz, H.S. (1983) Application of *Salmonella* assay to carbon blacks and toners. In: Cooke, M. & Dennis, A.J., eds, *Polynuclear Aromatic Hydrocarbons, 7th International Symposium, Formation, Metabolism and Measurement*, Columbus, OH, Battelle, pp. 225—241

Cerniglia, C.E., Howard, P.C., Fu, P.P. & Franklin, W. (1984) Metabolism of nitropolycyclic aromatic hydrocarbons by human intestinal microflora. *Biochem. biophys. Res. Commun.*, *123*, 262—270

Chemsyn Science Laboratories (1988) *6-Nitrobenzo[a]pyrene (Product Code U1027)*, Lenexa, KS, pp. 79—80

Chou, M.W., Evans, F.E., Yang, S.K. & Fu, P.P. (1983) Evidence for a 2,3-epoxide as an intermediate in the microsomal metabolism of 6-nitrobenzo[*a*]pyrene. *Carcinogenesis*, *4*, 699—702

Chou, M.W., Heflich, R.H., Casciano, D.A., Miller, D.W., Freeman, J.P., Evans, F.E. & Fu, P.P. (1984) Synthesis, spectral analysis, and mutagenicity of 1-, 3- and 6-nitrobenzo[*a*]pyrene. *J. med. Chem.*, *27*, 1156—1161

Chou, M.W., Wang, B., Von Tungeln, L.S., Beland, F.A. & Fu, P.P. (1987) Induction of rat hepatic cytochromes P-450 by environmental nitropolycyclic aromatic hydrocarbons. *Biochem. Pharmacol.*, *36*, 2449—2454

Dewar, M.J.S., Mole, T., Urch, D.S. & Warford, E.W.T. (1956) Electrophilic substitution. Part IV. The nitration of diphenyl, chrysene, benzo[*a*]pyrene, and anthanthrene. *J. chem. Soc.*, 3572—3575

DiPaolo, J.A., DeMarinis, A.J., Chow, F.L., Garner, R.C., Martin, C.N. & Doniger, J. (1983) Nitration of carcinogenic and non-carcinogenic polycyclic aromatic hydrocarbons results in products able to induce transformation of Syrian hamster cells. *Carcinogenesis*, *4*, 357—359

El-Bayoumy, K., Hecht, S.S. & Hoffmann, D. (1982) Comparative tumor initiating activity on mouse skin of 6-nitrobenzo[*a*]pyrene, 6-nitrochrysene, 3-nitroperylene, 1-nitropyrene and their parent hydrocarbons. *Cancer Lett.*, *16*, 333—337

Fu, P.P., Chou, M.W., Yang, S.K., Beland, F.A., Kadlubar, F.F., Casciano, D.A., Heflich, R.H. & Evans, F.E. (1982a) Metabolism of the mutagenic environmental pollutant, 6-nitrobenzo[*a*]pyrene: metabolic activation via ring oxidation. *Biochem. biophys. Res. Commun.*, *105*, 1037—1043

Fu, P.P., Chou, M.W., Yang, S.K., Unruh, L.E., Beland, F.A., Kadlubar, F.F., Casciano, D.A., Heflich, R.H. & Evans, F.E. (1982b) In vitro metabolism of 6-nitrobenzo[a]pyrene: identification and mutagenicity of its metabolites. In: *Polynuclear Aromatic Hydrocarbons, Sixth International Symposium, Physical and Biochemical Chemistry*, Columbus, OH, Battelle, pp. 287—295

Fu, P.P., Chou, M.W., Miller, D.W., White, G.L., Heflich, R.H. & Beland, F.A. (1985) The orientation of the nitro substituent predicts the direct-acting bacterial mutagenicity of nitrated polycyclic aromatic hydrocarbons. *Mutat. Res.*, *143*, 173—181

Garner, R.C., Stanton, C.A., Martin, C.N., Harris, C.C. & Grafstrom, R.C. (1985) Rat and human explant metabolism, binding studies, and DNA adduct analysis of benzo(*a*)pyrene and its 6-nitro derivative. *Cancer Res.*, *45*, 6225—6231

Gibson, T.L. (1982) Nitro derivatives of polynuclear aromatic hydrocarbons in airborne and source particulate matter. *Atmos. Environ.*, *16*, 2037—2040

Gibson, T.L. (1983) Sources of direct-acting nitroarene mutagens in airborne particulate matter. *Mutat. Res.*, *122*, 115–121

Greibrokk, T., Löfroth, G., Nilsson, L., Toftgård, R., Carlstedt-Duke, J. & Gustafsson, J.-Å. (1984) Nitroarenes: mutagenicity in the Ames *Salmonella*/microsome assay and affinity in the TCDD-receptor protein. In: Rickert, D.E., ed., *Toxicity of Nitroaromatic Compounds*, Washington DC, Hemisphere, pp. 167–183

Hass, B.S., Heflich, R.H., Chou, M.W., White, G.L., Fu, P.P. & Casciano, D.A. (1986a) Hepatocyte-mediated mutagenicity of mononitrobenzo[a]pyrenes in *Salmonella typhimurium* strains. *Mutat. Res.*, *171*, 123–129

Hass, B.S., Heflich, R.H., Schol, H.M., Chou, M.W., Fu, P.P. & Casciano, D.A. (1986b) Mutagenicity of the mononitrobenzo[a]pyrenes in Chinese hamster ovary cells mediated by rat hepatocytes of liver S9. *Carcinogenesis*, *7*, 681–684

Howard, P.C., Gerrard, J.A., Milo, G.E., Fu, P.P., Beland, F.A. & Kadlubar, F.F. (1983) Transformation of normal human skin fibroblasts by 1-nitropyrene and 6-nitrobenzo(a)pyrene. *Carcinogenesis*, *4*, 353–355

IARC (1984) *IARC Monographs on the Evaluation of the Carcinogenic Risk of Chemicals to Humans*, Vol. 33, *Polynuclear Aromatic Compounds, Part 2, Carbon Blacks, Mineral Oils and Some Nitroarenes*, Lyon, pp. 187–194

IARC (1988) *Information Bulletin on the Survey of Chemicals Being Tested for Carcinogenicity*, No. 13, Lyon, pp. 19, 171

Jäger, J. (1978) Detection and characterization of nitro derivatives of some polycyclic aromatic hydrocarbons by fluorescence quenching after thin-layer chromatography: application to air pollution analysis. *J. Chromatogr.*, *152*, 575–578

Johansen, E., Sydnes, L.K. & Greibrokk, T. (1984) Separation and characterization of mononitro derivatives of benzo[a]pyrene, benzo[e]pyrene and benzo[ghi]perylene. *Acta chem. scand.*, *B38*, 309–318

Kaneko, M. & Nagata, C. (1983) Covalent binding of 6-nitrobenzo[a]pyrene metabolites to DNA *in vitro*. *Gann*, *74*, 5–7

Löfroth, G., Toftgård, R., Nilsson, L., Agurell, E. & Gustafsson, J.-Å. (1984) Short-term bioassays of nitro derivatives of benzo[a]pyrene and perylene. *Carcinogenesis*, *5*, 925–930

Nielsen, T., Seitz, B. & Ramdahl, T. (1984) Occurrence of nitro-PAH in the atmosphere in a rural area. *Atmos. Environ.*, *18*, 2159–2165

Oehme, M., Manø, S. & Stray, H. (1982) Determination of nitrated polycyclic hydrocarbons in aerosols using capillary gas chromatography combined with different electron capture detection methods. *J. High Resolut. Chromatogr. Chromatogr. Commun.*, *5*, 417–423

Pitts, J.N., Jr, Van Cauwenberghe, K.A., Grosjean, D., Schmid, J.P., Fitz, D.R., Belser, W.L., Jr, Knudson, G.B. & Hynds, P.M. (1978) Atmospheric reactions of polycyclic aromatic hydrocarbons: facile formation of mutagenic nitro derivatives. *Science*, *202*, 515–519

Pitts, J.N., Jr, Lokensgard, D.M., Harger, W., Fisher, T.S., Mejia, V., Schuler, J.J., Scorziell, G.M. & Katzenstein, Y.A. (1982) Mutagens in diesel exhaust particulate: identification and direct activities of 6-nitrobenzo[a]pyrene, 9-nitroanthracene, 1-nitropyrene and 5$H$-phenanthro[4,5-bcd]pyran-5-one. *Mutat. Res.*, *103*, 241–249

Raha, C., Hines, R. & Bresnick, E. (1984) Demonstration of microsomal oxygenation of the benzo ring of 6-nitrobenzo[a]pyrene by thin-layer chromatography. *J. Chromatogr.*, *291*, 231–239

Raha, C., Hart-Anstey, M., Cheung, M.-S. & Bresnick, E. (1986a) 6-Nitrobenzo[*a*]pyrene can be denitrated during mammalian metabolism. *J. Toxicol. environ. Health*, *19*, 55–64

Raha, C., Hart-Anstey, M. & Bresnick, E. (1986b) High-pressure liquid chromatographic separation of 6-acetoxybenzo(a)pyrene from *in vitro* incubation of 6-nitrobenzo(a)pyrene. *J. Liquid Chromatogr.*, *9*, 2945–2953

Raha, C.R., Cheung, M.-S. & Bresnick, E. (1987a) Metabolism of 6-nitrobenzo[*a*]pyrene in rat lung preparations. *Toxicol. Lett.*, *37*, 229–233

Raha, C., Williamson, D., Hart-Anstey, M., Maiefski, T., Stohs, S.J. & Bresnick, E. (1987b) Ring oxidation of 6-nitrobenzo(a)pyrene by female mouse liver. *Res. Commun. chem. Pathol. Pharmacol.*, *58*, 63–74

Richardson, K.E., Fu, P.P. & Cerniglia, C.E. (1988) Metabolism of 1-, 3-and 6-nitrobenzo[*a*]pyrene by intestinal microflora. *J. Toxicol. environ. Health*, *23*, 527–537

Rosenkranz, H.S. & Mermelstein, R. (1983) Mutagenicity and genotoxicity of nitroarenes: all nitro-containing chemicals were not created equal. *Mutat. Res.*, *114*, 217–267

Rosenkranz, H.S. & Mermelstein, R. (1985) The genotoxicity, metabolism and carcinogenicity of nitrated polycyclic aromatic hydrocarbons. *J. environ. Sci. Health*, *C3*, 221–272

Rosenkranz, H.S., McCoy, E.C., Sanders, D.R., Butler, M., Kiriazides, D.K. & Mermelstein, R. (1980) Nitropyrenes: isolation, identification and reduction of mutagenic impurities in carbon black and toners. *Science*, *209*, 1039–1043

Sala, M., Lasne, C., Lu, Y.P. & Chouroulinkov, I. (1987) Morphological transformation in three mammalian cell systems following treatment with 6-nitrochrysene and 6-nitrobenzo[*a*]pyrene. *Carcinogenesis*, *8*, 503–507

Sanders, D.R. (1981) Nitropyrenes: the isolation of trace mutagenic impurities from the toluene extract of an aftertreated carbon black. In: Cooke, M. & Dennis, A.J., eds, *Polynuclear Aromatic Hydrocarbons, 5th International Symposium, Chemical Analysis and Biological Fate*, Columbus, OH, Battelle, pp. 145–158

Schuetzle, D. & Jensen, T.E. (1985) Analysis of nitrated polycyclic aromatic hydrocarbons (nitro-PAH) by mass spectrometry. In: White, C.M., ed., *Nitrated Polycyclic Aromatic Hydrocarbons*, Heidelberg, A. Hüthig Verlag, pp. 121–167

Selkirk, J.K., Tong, S., Stoner, G.D., Nikbakht, A. & Mansfield, B.K. (1981) Benzo[*a*]pyrene and 6-nitrobenzo[*a*]pyrene metabolism in human and rodent microsomes and tissue culture. *Environ. Sci. Res.*, *31*, 429–446

Tokiwa, H. & Ohnishi, Y. (1986) Mutagenicity and carcinogenicity of nitroarenes and their sources in the environment. *CRC crit. Rev. Toxicol.*, *17*, 23–69

Tokiwa, H., Nakagawa, R. & Ohnishi, Y. (1981) Mutagenic assay of aromatic nitro compounds with *Salmonella typhimurium*. *Mutat. Res.*, *91*, 321–325

Tong, S. & Selkirk, J.K. (1983) Metabolism of 6-nitrobenzo[*a*]pyrene by hamster embryonic fibroblasts and its interaction with nuclear macromolecules. *J. Toxicol. environ. Health*, *11*, 381–393

Wang, Y.Y., Rappaport, S.M., Sawyer, R.F., Talcott, R.E. & Wei, E.T. (1978) Direct-acting mutagens in automobile exhaust. *Cancer Lett.*, *5*, 39–47

White, G.L., Fu, P.P. & Heflich, R.H. (1985) Effect of nitro substitution on the light-mediated mutagenicity of polycyclic aromatic hydrocarbons in *Salmonella typhimurium* TA98. *Mutat. Res.*, *144*, 1–7

Wislocki, P.G., Bagan, E.S., Lu, A.Y.H., Dooley, K.L., Fu, P.P., Han-Hsu, H., Beland, F.A. & Kadlubar, F.F. (1986) Tumorigenicity of nitrated derivatives of pyrene, benz[a]anthracene, chrysene and benzo[a]pyrene in the newborn mouse assay. *Carcinogenesis*, 7, 1317–1322

# 6-NITROCHRYSENE

This substance was considered by a previous Working Group, in June 1983 (IARC, 1984). Since that time, new data have become available, and these have been incorporated into the monograph and taken into consideration in the present evaluation.

## 1. Chemical and Physical Data

### 1.1 Synonyms

*Chem. Abstr. Services Reg. No.*: 7496-02-8
*Chem. Abstr. Name*: Chrysene, 6-nitro
*IUPAC Systematic Name*: 6-Nitrochrysene

### 1.2 Structural and molecular formulae and molecular weight

$C_{18}H_{11}NO_2$                                        Mol. wt: 273.3

### 1.3 Chemical and physical properties of the pure substance

(*a*) *Description*: Chrome-red, thick prismatic crystals (Prager & Jacobson, 1922); orange-yellow needles (Boit, 1965); light-yellow needles (Chemsyn Science Laboratories, 1988)

(*b*) *Boiling-point*: Sublimes without decomposition (Prager & Jacobson, 1922)

(*c*) *Melting-point*: 209°C (Boit, 1965)

(d) *Spectroscopy data*: Mass spectral data have been reported (Schuetzle & Jensen, 1985).

(e) *Solubility*: Slightly soluble in cold ethanol, diethyl ether and carbon disulfide; somewhat more soluble in benzene and acetic acid; soluble in hot nitrobenzene (Prager & Jacobson, 1922)

(f) *Reactivity*: Forms 6-aminochrysene upon heating with tin and concentrated hydrochloric acid in acetic acid at 100°C. Reacts with bromine to form 12-bromo-6-nitrochrysene, and reacts with fuming nitric acid to form 6,12-dinitrochrysene (Boit, 1965)

### 1.4 Technical products and impurities

6-Nitrochrysene is offered for sale in research quantities at ≥98% purity (Chemsyn Science Laboratories, 1988) and is also available at a certified purity of 98.9% as a reference material (Belliardo *et al.*, 1988).

## 2. Production, Use, Occurrence and Analysis

### 2.1 Production and use

(a) *Production*

6-Nitrochrysene was first synthesized in 1890 by heating chrysene with aqueous nitric acid in acetic acid (Prager & Jacobson, 1922). It can also be synthesized by briefly heating chrysene with nitric acid and concentrated sulfuric acid in acetic acid at 40°C (Boit, 1965).

(b) *Use*

No evidence was found that 6-nitrochrysene has been used in commercial applications. It is used as an internal standard in the chemical analysis of nitroarenes (see monograph on 1-nitropyrene).

### 2.2 Occurrence

Toners for use in photocopy machines have been produced in quantity since the late 1950s and have seen widespread use. 'Long-flow' furnace black was first used in photocopy toners in 1967; its manufacture involved an oxidation whereby some nitration also occurred. Subsequent changes in the production technique reduced the total extractable nitropyrene content from an uncontrolled level of 5–100 mg/kg to below 0.3 mg/kg (Rosenkranz *et al.*, 1980; Sanders, 1981; Butler *et al.*, 1983), and toners produced from this carbon black since 1980 have not been found to contain detectable levels of mutagenicity or, hence, nitropyrenes (Rosenkranz *et al.*, 1980; Butler *et al.*, 1983).

Garner *et al.* (1986) identified 6-nitrochrysene at a level of ~1 ng/m$^3$ in ambient air in Upper Frankonia, Federal Republic of Germany. Atmospheric transformation of chrysene to mononitrochrysene is reported to occur in the presence of 19 mg/m$^3$ nitrogen dioxide (Tokiwa & Ohnishi, 1986).

### 2.3 Analysis

See the monograph on 1-nitropyrene.

## 3. Biological Data Relevant to the Evaluation of Carcinogenic Risk to Humans

### 3.1 Carcinogenicity studies in animals[1]

*(a) Skin application*

*Mouse*: In a study of initiating activity, a group of 20 female CD-1 Charles River mice, aged 50—55 days, received ten applications of 0.1 mg 6-nitrochrysene (purity, >99%) in 0.1 ml acetone onto shaved back skin every other day for 20 days (total dose, 1 mg; El-Bayoumy *et al.*, 1982). Another group of 20 female mice receiving acetone alone served as controls. Starting ten days after the initiation treatment had been completed, all animals received applications of 2.5 µg 12-*O*-tetradecanoylphorbol 13-acetate in 0.1 ml acetone three times per week for 25 weeks. At the end of this time, 12/20 of the treated animals had developed skin tumours (mainly papillomas; 2.1 tumours/animal) compared with 1/20 controls ($p < 0.01$).

*(b) Intraperitoneal administration*

*Mouse*: A group of 22 male and 29 female newborn Swiss-Webster BLU-Ha mice received three intraperitoneal injections of 6-nitrochrysene (total dose, 38.5 µg/mouse [purity unspecified] in 5, 10 and 20 µl dimethyl sulfoxide (DMSO) on days 1, 8 and 15 after birth (Busby *et al.*, 1985). Another group of 23 male and 21 female newborn mice received three injections to give a total dose of 189 µg 6-nitrochrysene. A further group of 22 males and 15 females received injections of DMSO only and served as controls. Animals were killed and necropsied at 26 weeks of age. All mice injected with 6-nitrochrysene developed multiple lung tumours, the incidence of which was significantly different from that in controls (three males and one female with lung tumours; $p < 0.0001$); 70% of treated animals had adenocarcinomas. Control mice with tumours of the lung did not develop more than two adenomas per mouse, but the average number of lung tumours was increased by 150

---

[1]The Working Group was aware of a study in progress in mice by single subcutaneous injection (IARC, 1988). Subsequent to the meeting, the Secretariat became aware of a study in newborn mice by intraperitoneal injection in which lung tumours were induced in animals of each sex and liver tumours were induced in males (El-Bayoumy *et al.*, 1989).

and 250 fold in the two treated groups, respectively. Female mice in both treatment groups developed ~40% more lung tumours than males, although this difference was not statistically significant. A few lymphomas and nodular hyperplasia of the liver were observed in treated but not in control animals.

Groups of 90 or 100 male and female newborn CD-1 mice received three intraperitoneal injections of 6-nitrochrysene (total dose, 2800 nmol [0.77 mg]; purity, >99%) in 10, 20 and 40 µl DMSO on days 1, 8 and 15 after birth; a total dose of 700 nmol [0.2 mg] 6-nitrochrysene; a total dose of 560 nmol [0.14 mg] benzo[a]pyrene (purity, >99%); or three injections of DMSO only (Wislocki et al., 1986). Treatment of a second vehicle control group and of the group administered 700 nmol 6-nitrochrysene was begun ten weeks after that of the other groups. At 25–27 days, when the mice were weaned, nine males and 11 females in the group that received 2800 nmol 6-nitrochrysene, 33 males and 40 females in the group that received 700 nmol 6-nitrochrysene, 37 males and 27 females in the positive control group, and 28 and 31 males and 45 and 34 females in the vehicle control groups were still alive. All remaining mice were killed after one year. Liver-cell tumours occurred in 3/9 males given 2800 nmol (carcinomas; $p < 0.05$), in 3/11 females given 2800 nmol (two adenomas, one carcinoma; $p < 0.05$); in 25/33 males given 700 nmol (one adenoma, 24 carcinomas; $p < 0.05$); in 9/40 females given 700 nmol (five adenomas, four carcinomas; $p < 0.005$); in 2/28 and 5/45 DMSO-treated males and in 0/31 and 0/34 DMSO-treated females. Treatment with 700 nmol 6-nitrochrysene increased the multiplicity of hepatic nodules per tumour-bearing mouse. Lung tumours occurred in 7/9 males given 2800 nmol, 9/11 females given 2800 nmol, 28/33 males given 700 nmol (11 adenomas, 17 carcinomas) and 36/40 females given 700 nmol (19 adenomas, 17 carcinomas); all of these incidences were statistically significantly different ($p < 0.005$) from those in DMSO controls (1/28 and 4/45 in males and 0/31 and 2/34 in females). The numbers of mice with malignant lymphomas were substantially increased in both groups administered 6-nitrochrysene ($p < 0.005$ for the 700 nmol group). In the group given benzo[a]pyrene, 18/37 males had hepatic tumours and 13/37 had lung adenomas, and 13/27 females had lung adenomas; no significant increase in the incidence of malignant lymphomas was observed.

### 3.2 Other relevant data

(a) *Experimental systems*

(i) *Absorption, distribution, excretion and metabolism*

Incubation of 6-nitrochrysene with an exogenous metabolic system from rat liver has been reported to result in the formation of *trans*-1,2-dihydro-1,2-dihydroxy-6-nitrochrysene and 6-aminochrysene (El-Bayoumy & Hecht, 1984). Anaerobic bacteria from human faeces metabolized 6-nitrochrysene to 6-nitrosochrysene, 6-aminochrysene, *N*-formyl-6-aminochrysene and 6-acetyl aminochrysene. Mixed cultures of rat and mouse intestinal bacteria and pure cultures of anaerobic bacteria reduced 6-nitrochrysene to 6-aminochrysene (Manning et al., 1988).

Incubation of primary cultures of rat liver hepatocytes with 6-nitrochrysene resulted in the formation of two DNA adducts, $N$-(deoxyguanosin-8-yl)-6-aminochrysene and $N$-(deoxyinosin-8-yl)-6-aminochrysene. The latter adduct was suggested to arise from the deamination of $N$-(deoxyadenosin-8-yl)-6-aminochrysene. The same two adducts plus 5-(deoxyguanosin-$N^2$-yl)-6-aminochrysene were formed by reacting $N$-hydroxy-6-aminochrysene with DNA (Delclos et al., 1987a).

After preweanling male CD mice were given one or three intraperitoneal doses of 6-nitrochrysene, analysis of lung and liver DNA indicated a single major adduct that corresponded to the adduct detected after the microsomal incubation of 6-aminochrysene trans-1,2-dihydrodiol with calf thymus DNA (Delclos et al., 1988). The same adduct was found at lower levels in mice treated with 6-aminochrysene (Delclos et al., 1987b).

As reported in an abstract, 6-nitrochrysene was incubated with liver microsomes from preweanling BLU:Ha mice, from 3-methylcholanthrene-pretreated Sprague-Dawley rats and from Aroclor-pretreated Fischer rats, and with human lung explants and lung and liver microsomes. 6-Nitrochrysene trans-1,2-dihydrodiol and 6-nitrochrysene trans-9,10-dihydrodiol were found as metabolites. The metabolic profile detected with the human lung explants and in preweanling mice was similar to that observed in the microsomal incubations. A DNA adduct was detected in the human lung explants that appeared to be identical to that previously found in mouse liver DNA (Delclos et al., 1987c).

(ii) *Toxic effects*

Intraperitoneal administration of a total dose of 2800 nmol 6-nitrochrysene to newborn CD mice increased mortality at weaning by two fold (Wislocki et al., 1986).

Two intraperitoneal administrations of 5 mg/kg bw 6-nitrochrysene to young male Sprague-Dawley rats resulted in an eight-fold increase in aryl hydrocarbon hydroxylase activity over that in controls; two injections of 2.5 mg/kg bw resulted in a 4.5-fold increase. Three-fold increases in the activities of 7-ethoxycoumarin-$O$-deethylase and 1-nitropyrene reductase were seen at the lower dose (Chou et al., 1987).

(iii) *Genetic and related effects*

The genetic and related effects of nitroarenes and of their metabolites have been reviewed (Rosenkranz & Mermelstein, 1983; Beland et al., 1985; Rosenkranz & Mermelstein, 1985; Tokiwa & Ohnishi, 1986).

6-Nitrochrysene (0.5 µg/disc) preferentially inhibited the growth of DNA repair-deficient *Bacillus subtilis* (Tokiwa et al., 1987) and was mutagenic to *Salmonella typhimurium* TA98 and TA100 (2 µg/plate; Pederson & Siak, 1981; Tokiwa et al., 1981a,b; Sugimura & Takayama, 1983; El Bayoumy & Hecht, 1984; Greibrokk et al., 1984).

6-Nitrochrysene induced morphological transformation in cultured Syrian hamster embryo cells (DiPaolo et al., 1983 (3.7–73 µM); Sala et al., 1987 (3.6–10.8 µg/ml)). It did not induce transformation in murine BALB/c 3T3 (at up to 40 µM) or C3H 10T1/2 cells (at up to 55 µM; Sala et al., 1987).

(b) *Humans*

No data were available to the Working Group.

## 3.3 Epidemiological studies and case reports of carcinogenicity in humans

No data were available to the Working Group.

# 4. Summary of Data Reported and Evaluation

## 4.1 Exposure data

6-Nitrochrysene was found in ambient air at a low concentration in one study.

## 4.2 Experimental data

6-Nitrochrysene was tested for initiating activity on mouse skin and was found to be active. It was also tested for carcinogenicity in two experiments by intraperitoneal injection into newborn mice, producing increased incidences of lung and liver-cell tumours and of malignant lymphomas.

## 4.3 Human data

No data were available to the Working Group.

## 4.4 Other relevant data

Intraperitoneal injection of 6-nitrochrysene caused a substantial increase in aryl hydrocarbon hydroxylase activity in rat liver. Metabolism of 6-nitrochrysene led to DNA adduct formation in cultured mammalian cells and in animals. 6-Nitrochrysene caused transformation in cultured animal cells. It was mutagenic to and induced DNA damage in bacteria.

## 4.5 Evaluation[1]

There is *sufficient evidence* for the carcinogenicity in experimental animals of 6-nitrochrysene.

No data were available from studies in humans on the carcinogenicity of 6-nitrochrysene.

---

[1]For definitions of the italicized terms, see Preamble, pp. 25–28.

## Summary table of genetic and related effects of 6-nitrochrysene

| Nonmammalian systems | | | | Mammalian systems | | | |
|---|---|---|---|---|---|---|---|
| Proka-ryotes | Lower eukaryotes | Plants | Insects | In vitro | | | In vivo |
| | | | | Animal cells | Human cells | | Animals | Humans |
| D G D R G A D G C R G C A D | | | | D G S M C A T I | D G S M C A T I | | D G S M C DL A D S M C A |
| +¹ + | | | | +¹ | + | | +¹ |

A, aneuploidy; C, chromosomal aberrations; D, DNA damage; DL, dominant lethal mutation; G, gene mutation; I, inhibition of intercellular communication; M, micronuclei; R, mitotic recombination and gene conversion; S, sister chromatid exchange; T, cell transformation

*In completing the table, the following symbols indicate the consensus of the Working Group with regard to the results for each endpoint:*
+ considered to be positive for the specific endpoint and level of biological complexity
+¹ considered to be positive, but only one valid study was available to the Working Group

**Overall evaluation**

6-Nitrochrysene *is possibly carcinogenic to humans (Group 2B).*

## 5. References

Beland, F.A., Heflich, R.H., Howard, P.C. & Fu, P.P. (1985) The in vitro metabolic activation of nitro polycyclic aromatic hydrocarbons. In: Harvey, R.G., ed., *Polycyclic Hydrocarbons and Carcinogenesis (ACS Symposium Series No. 283)*, Washington DC, American Chemical Society, pp. 371–396

Belliardo, J.J., Jacob, J. & Lindsey, A.S. (1988) *The Certification of the Purity of Seven Nitropolycyclic Aromatic Compounds, CRM Nos 305, 306, 307, 308, 310, 311, 312, BCR Information, Reference Materials (Addendum to EUR 11254 EN), CRM No. 309 6-Nitrochrysene*, Brussels, Commission of the European Communities

Boit, H.-G., ed. (1965) *Beilsteins Handbuch der Organischen Chemie*, Vol. 5, 4th ed., 3rd Suppl., Syst. No. 490, Berlin (West), Springer-Verlag, p. 2583

Busby, W.F., Jr, Garner, R.C., Chow, F.L., Martin, C.N., Stevens, E.K., Newberne, P.M. & Wogan, G.N. (1985) 6-Nitrochrysene is a potent tumorigen in newborn mice. *Carcinogenesis, 6*, 801–803

Butler, M.A., Evans, D.L., Giammarise, A.T., Kiriazides, D.K., Marsh, D., McCoy, E.C., Mermelstein, R., Murphy, C.B. & Rosenkranz, H.S. (1983) Application of *Salmonella* assay to carbon blacks and toners. In: Cooke, M. & Dennis, A.J., eds, *Polynuclear Aromatic Hydrocarbons, 7th International Symposium, Formation, Metabolism and Measurement*, Colombus, OH, Battelle, pp. 225–241

Chemsyn Science Laboratories (1988) *6-Nitrochrysene (Product Code U1010)*, Lenexa, KS, p. 85

Chou, M.W., Wang, B., Von Tungeln, L.S., Beland, F.A. & Fu, P.P. (1987) Induction of rat hepatic cytochromes P-450 by environmental nitropolycyclic aromatic hydrocarbons. *Biochem. Pharmacol., 36*, 2449–2454

Delclos, K.B., Miller, D.W., Lay, J.O., Jr, Casciano, D.A., Walker, R.P., Fu, P.P. & Kadlubar, F.F. (1987a) Identification of C8-modified deoxyinosine and $N^2$- and C8-modified deoxyguanosine as major products of the in vitro reaction of N-hydroxy-6-aminochrysene with DNA and the formation of these adducts in isolated rat hepatocytes treated with 6-nitrochrysene and 6-aminochrysene. *Carcinogenesis, 8*, 1703–1709

Delclos, K.B., Walker, R.P., Dooley, K.L., Fu, P.P. & Kadlubar, F.F. (1987b) Carcinogen-DNA adduct formation in the lungs and livers of preweanling CD-1 male mice following administration of [$^3$H]-6-nitrochrysene, [$^3$H]-6-aminochrysene, and [$^3$H]-1,6-dinitropyrene. *Cancer Res., 47*, 6272–6277

Delclos, K.B., El-Bayoumy, K., Hecht, S.S., Shivapurkar, N., Stoner, G.D., Walker, R. & Kadlubar, F.F. (1987c) Microsomal metabolism of 6-nitrochrysene (NC) by mouse, rat and human lung and liver: its relation to DNA adduct formation (Abstract No. 502). *Proc. Am. Assoc. Cancer Res., 28*, 126

Delclos, K.B., El-Bayoumy, K., Hecht, S.S., Walker, R.P. & Kadlubar, F.F. (1988) Metabolic activation of 6-aminochrysene and 6-nitrochrysene: a diol-epoxide of 6-aminochrysene as a probable ultimate carcinogen in preweanling mice. In: King, C.M., Romano, L.J. & Schuetzle, D., eds, *Carcinogenic and Mutagenic Responses to Aromatic Amines and Nitroarenes*, New York, Elsevier, pp. 103–106

DiPaolo, J.A., DeMarinis, A.J., Chow, F.L., Garner, R.C., Martin, C.N. & Doniger, J. (1983) Nitration of carcinogenic and non-carcinogenic polycyclic aromatic hydrocarbons results in products able to induce transformation of Syrian hamster cells. *Carcinogenesis*, 4, 357–359

El-Bayoumy, K. & Hecht, S.S. (1984) Identification of *trans*-1,2-dihydro-1,2-dihydroxy-6-nitrochrysene as a major mutagenic metabolite of 6-nitrochrysene. *Cancer Res.*, 44, 3408–3413

El-Bayoumy, K., Hecht, S.S. & Hoffmann, D. (1982) Comparative tumor initiating activity on mouse skin of 6-nitrobenzo[*a*]pyrene, 6-nitrochrysene, 3-nitroperylene, 1-nitropyrene and their parent hydrocarbons. *Cancer Lett.*, 16, 333–337

El-Bayoumy, K., Shive, G.-H. & Hecht, S.S. (1989) Comparative tumorigenicity of 6-nitrochrysene and its metabolites in newborn mice. *Carcinogenesis*, 10, 369–372

Garner, R.C., Stanton, C.A., Martin, C.N., Chow, F.L., Thomas, W., Hubner, D. & Herrmann, R. (1986) Bacterial mutagenicity and chemical analysis of polycyclic aromatic hydrocarbons and some nitroderivatives in environmental samples collected in West Germany. *Environ. Mutagenesis*, 8, 109–117

Greibrokk, T., Lofröth, G., Nilsson, L., Toftgård, R., Carlstedt-Duke, J. & Gustafsson, J.-Å. (1984) Nitroarenes: mutagenicity in the Ames *Salmonella*/microsome assay and affinity in the TCDD-receptor protein. In: Rickert, D.E., ed., *Toxicity of Nitroaromatic Compounds*, Washington DC, Hemisphere, pp. 167–183

IARC (1984) *IARC Monographs on the Evaluation of the Carcinogenic Risk of Chemicals to Humans*, Vol. 33, *Polynuclear Aromatic Compounds, Part 2, Carbon Blacks, Mineral Oils and Some Nitroarenes*, Lyon, pp. 195–200

IARC (1988) *Information Bulletin on the Survey of Chemicals Being Tested for Carcinogenicity*, No. 13, Lyon, pp. 19, 283–284

Manning, B.W., Campbell, W.L., Frankin, W., Delclos, K.B. & Cerniglia, C.E. (1988) Metabolism of 6-nitrochrysene by intestinal microflora. *Appl. environ. Microbiol.*, 54, 197–203

Pederson, T.C. & Siak, J.-C. (1981) The role of nitroaromatic compounds in the direct-acting mutagenicity of diesel particles extracts. *J. appl. Toxicol.*, 1, 54–60

Prager, B. & Jacobson, P., eds (1922) *Beilsteins Handbuch der Organischen Chemie*, Vol. 5, 4th ed., Syst. No. 488, Berlin (West), Springer-Verlag, pp. 719–720

Rosenkranz, H.S. & Mermelstein, R. (1983) Mutagenicity and genotoxicity of nitroarenes: all nitro-containing chemicals were not created equal. *Mutat. Res.*, 114, 217–267

Rosenkranz, H.S. & Mermelstein, R. (1985) The genotoxicity, metabolism and carcinogenicity of nitrated polycyclic aromatic hydrocarbons. *J. environ. Sci. Health*, C3, 221–272

Rosenkranz, H.S., McCoy, E.C., Sanders, D.R., Butler, M., Kiriazides, D.K. & Mermelstein, R. (1980) Nitropyrenes: isolation, identification and reduction of mutagenic impurities in carbon black and toners. *Science*, 209, 1039–1043

Sala, M., Lasne, C., Lu, Y.P. & Chouroulinkov, I. (1987) Morphological transformation in three mammalian cell systems following treatment with 6-nitrochrysene and 6-nitrobenzo[*a*]pyrene. *Carcinogenesis*, 8, 503–507

Sanders, D.R. (1981) Nitropyrenes: the isolation of trace mutagenic impurities from the toluene extract of an aftertreated carbon black. In: Cooke, M. & Dennis, A.J., eds, *Polynuclear Aromatic Hydrocarbons, 5th International Symposium, Chemical Analysis and Biological Fate*, Columbus, OH, Battelle, pp. 145–158

Schuetzle, D. & Jensen, T.E. (1985) Analysis of nitrated polycyclic aromatic hydrocarbons (nitro-PAH) by mass spectrometry. In: White, C.M., ed., *Nitrated Polycyclic Aromatic Hydrocarbons*, Heidelberg, A. Hüthig Verlag, pp. 121–167

Sugimura, T. & Takayama, S. (1983) Biological actions of nitroarenes in short-term tests on *Salmonella*, cultured mammalian cells and cultured human tracheal tissues: possible basis for regulatory control. *Environ. Health Perspect.*, 47, 171–176

Tokiwa, H. & Ohnishi, Y. (1986) Mutagenicity and carcinogenicity of nitroarenes and their sources in the environment. *CRC crit. Rev. Toxicol.*, 17, 23–69

Tokiwa, H., Nakagawa, R., Morita, K. & Ohnishi, Y. (1981a) Mutagenicity of nitro derivatives induced by exposure of aromatic compounds to nitrogen dioxide. *Mutat. Res.*, 85, 195–205

Tokiwa, H., Nakagawa, R. & Ohnishi, Y. (1981b) Mutagenic assay of aromatic nitro compounds with *Salmonella typhimurium*. *Mutat. Res.*, 91, 321–325

Tokiwa, H., Nakagawa, R., Horikawa, K. & Ohkubo, A. (1987) The nature of the mutagenicity and carcinogenicity of nitrated, aromatic compounds in the environment. *Environ. Health Perspect.*, 73, 191–199

Wislocki, P.G., Bagan, E.S., Lu, A.Y.H., Dooley, K.L., Fu, P.P., Han-Hsu, H., Beland, F.A. & Kadlubar, F.F. (1986) Tumorigenicity of nitrated derivatives of pyrene, benz[a]anthracene, chrysene and benzo[a]pyrene in the newborn mouse assay. *Carcinogenesis*, 7, 1317–1322

# 2-NITROFLUORENE

## 1. Chemical and Physical Data

### 1.1 Synonyms

*Chem. Abstr. Services Reg. No.*: 607-57-8
*Chem. Abstr. Name*: 9*H*-Fluorene, 2-nitro-
*IUPAC Systematic Names*: 2-Nitro-9*H*-fluorene; 2-nitrofluorene

### 1.2 Structural and molecular formulae and molecular weight

$C_{13}H_9NO_2$            Mol. wt: 211.2

### 1.3 Chemical and physical properties of the pure substance

(*a*) *Description*: Needles, recrystallized from 50% acetic acid or acetone (Weast, 1985); light-yellow, fluffy solid (Chemsyn Science Laboratories, 1988)

(*b*) *Melting-point*: 156°C (Buckingham, 1982)

(*c*) *Spectroscopy data*: Ultra-violet (Sawicki, 1954) and mass (Schuetzle & Jensen, 1985) spectral data have been reported.

(*d*) *Solubility*: Sparingly soluble in water (Beije & Möller, 1988); soluble in acetone, benzene (Weast, 1985), tetrahydrofluorenone and toluene (Chemsyn Science Laboratories, 1988)

### 1.4 Technical products and impurities

2-Nitrofluorene is available for research purposes at 95% (Pfaltz & Bauer, Inc. 1988), 98% (Aldrich Chemical Co., 1988) or ⩾99% purity and in radiolabelled form at ⩾98% [$^{14}$C] or ⩾99% [$^{3}$H] purity (Chemsyn Science Laboratories, 1988).

## 2. Production, Use, Occurrence and Analysis

### 2.1 Production and use

#### (a) Production

No evidence was found that 2-nitrofluorene is currently produced other than for laboratory use. It is reported on the 1985 *Toxic Substances Control Act Chemical Substance Inventory* (US Environmental Protection Agency, 1986).

#### (b) Use

No evidence was found that 2-nitrofluorene has been used for commercial applications.

### 2.2 Occurrence

#### (a) Engine exhaust

2-Nitrofluorene has been identified in diesel emissions. Levels of two isomers of nitrofluorene in exhausts from light-duty diesel passenger cars were 71–186 mg/kg of particulates (Schuetzle, 1983). Emission levels from 1980–85 model engines running on an urban Federal Test Procedure cycle were 90 μg/mile (56 μg/km) for the gas phase and 97 μg/mile (61 μg/km) for the particulate phase (Schuetzle & Frazier, 1986). Concentrations of 0.63 mg/kg in particulates were reported for a heavy-duty mining diesel engine run at 100% load and 1200 revolutions/min and 8.8 mg/kg in particulates for the same engine at 75% load and 1800 revolutions/min (Draper, 1986).

#### (b) Other occurrence

Toners for use in photocopy machines have been produced in quantity since the late 1950s and have seen widespread use. 'Long-flow' furnace black was first used in photocopy toners in 1967; its manufacture involved an oxidation whereby some nitration also occurred. Subsequent changes in the production technique reduced the total extractable nitropyrene content from an uncontrolled level of 5–100 mg/kg to below 0.3 mg/kg (Rosenkranz *et al.*, 1980; Sanders, 1981; Butler *et al.*, 1983), and toners produced from this carbon black since 1980 have not been found to contain detectable levels of mutagenicity or, hence, nitropyrenes (Rosenkranz *et al.*, 1980; Butler *et al.*, 1983).

2-Nitrofluorene has been detected in airborne particulates in Tokyo, Japan, at concentrations of 0–21.8 mg/kg and in air at concentrations of 0–27.2 pg/m$^3$ (Tanabe *et al.*,

1986) and 24–71 pg/m³, in China at 36–700 pg/m³ and in the Federal Republic of Germany at 170–5200 pg/m³ (Möller, 1988; Beije & Möller, 1988).

2-Nitrofluorene was identified in particulate extracts of emissions from kerosene heaters, gas burners and liquefied petroleum gas burners (Tokiwa et al., 1985). In the exhaust from an open, oil-burning space heater, of the type used extensively in Japan in urban and rural residential and public office spaces, a concentration of 568 ng/m³ 2-nitrofluorene was reported (Möller, 1988).

2-Nitrofluorene was found in a river sediment at 1.5 µg/kg (Möller, 1988).

## 2.3 Analysis

See the monograph on 1-nitropyrene.

# 3. Biological Data Relevant to the Evaluation of Carcinogenic Risk to Humans

### 3.1 Carcinogenicity studies in animals[1]

*(a) Oral administration*

*Rat*: A group of six male and three female Minnesota strain [albino] rats [age unspecified] was fed a basal diet containing 2.37 mmol[500 mg]/kg diet 2-nitrofluorene ([purity unspecified] melting-point, 157°C) for 23 weeks (average estimated total dose, 756 mg per rat), after which time animals were placed on basal control diet until they developed gross tumours or became moribund (Morris et al., 1950). Average survival time was 308 days for tumour-bearing animals and 310 days for animals without tumours. Three males and three females fed basal diet alone served as controls (average survival time, 280 days). At the end of the experiment, two females in the treated group had one adenocarcinoma of the mammary gland and one squamous-cell carcinoma of the ear duct; no tumour was observed in controls. [The Working Group noted the small number of animals used.]

Nine male and nine female Holtzman [albino] rats weighing 190–210 g [age unspecified] were fed a basal grain diet containing 1.62 mmol[342 mg]/kg diet 2-nitrofluorene ([purity unspecified] melting-point, 155–157°C) for eight months (Miller et al., 1955). A group of 26 males and 27 females receiving a diet containing 1.62 mmol[361 mg]/kg diet 2-acetylaminofluorene (a metabolite of 2-nitrofluorene) served as positive controls. After eight months, both groups were maintained on grain diet alone for two months. A group of 18 male and 20 female rats received basal grain diet alone for ten months, at which time the experiment was terminated. 2-Acetylaminofluorene induced high incidences of liver-cell tumours in males (24/26) and of mammary gland tumours, described as adenocarcinomas,

---

[1]The Working Group was aware of a study in progress in mice by single subcutaneous injection (IARC, 1988).

in females (22/25) and caused moderate incidences of carcinomas of the ear duct (11/26 in males, 19/27 in females) and adenocarcinomas of the small intestinal epithelium (13/26 in males, 6/27 in females). Four mammary gland tumours were seen in 2-nitrofluorene-treated females and only one fibroadenoma in an untreated female. Most rats given 2-nitrofluorene developed multiple papillomas or squamous-cell carcinomas in the forestomach (5/7 males and 2/2 females examined). To confirm this observation, a group of 20 male rats was fed 1.62 mmol[342 mg]/kg diet 2-nitrofluorene for 12 months, during which time a further ten males were maintained on basal diet. Of these rats, 17/18 that survived for 10–12 months had squamous-cell carcinomas of the forestomach. In addition, 13 rats in this group had developed tumours of the liver, four had tumours of the ear duct, two had tumours of the small intestinal epithelium, and one had a tumour of the mammary gland by 12 months. No tumour was found in the control group.

(b) *Initiation-promotion study*

In a initiation-promotion model, Möller *et al.* (1989) gave weanling male Wistar rats 20, 100 or 200 mg/kg bw 2-nitrofluorene intraperitoneally 16 h after a two-thirds hepatectomy. Two weeks later, the animals were fed a diet supplemented with 0.02% 2-acetylaminofluorene for two weeks, 2 ml/kg bw carbon tetrachloride intragastrically when the rats had been on this diet for one week, and then a basic diet for a further four weeks. In a second experiment, weanling male Wistar rats received an intraperitoneal injection of 200 mg/kg bw *N*-nitrosodiethylamine. Two weeks later, they were given 30 or 120 mg/kg bw 2-nitrofluorene intragastrically in six equal doses: four doses were given on consecutive days followed by a two-thirds hepatectomy, followed by two additional doses of 2-nitrofluorene. Seven weeks after initiation, the rats were killed, and γ-glutamyl transferase-positive liver foci were identified microscopically and quantitified using morphometric techniques. A statistically significant increase ($p < 0.001$) in the number of foci was observed in the first experiment. A dose-response effect was seen in the second study, the highest response being approximately three times the background.

## 3.2 Other relevant data

(a) *Experimental systems*

(i) *Absorption, distribution, excretion and metabolism*

The metabolism of 2-nitrofluorene *in vivo* has been reviewed by Möller (1988).

After male albino rabbits were administered 2-nitrofluorene orally at 100 mg/kg bw per day for two days, 2-aminofluorene, 2-acetylaminofluorene and 2-formylaminofluorene were found in urine collected for three days after dosing. The same metabolites were found in the faeces but not in urine of male Wistar rats treated similarly. 2-Formylaminofluorene was also detected in in-vitro incubations of rabbit, rat, mouse, guinea-pig and hamster cytosol supplemented with *N*-formyl-L-kynurenine and 2-aminofluorene (Tatsumi & Amano, 1987). [The Working Group noted that 2-aminofluorene and 2-acetylaminofluorene are carcinogenic in a variety of experimental animal species. See for example, Garner et al. (1984).]

In an eight-day period after Sprague-Dawley rats were given a single oral dose of 5 mg [$^{14}$C]2-nitrofluorene, approximately 60% was excreted in the urine and 30% was found in the faeces; *N*-, 1-, 3-, 5-, 7-, 8- and 9-hydroxy-2-acetylaminofluorenes were identified as metabolites. The major products were 5- and 7-hydroxy-2-acetylaminofluorenes (Möller et al., 1985, 1987a). [The Working Group noted that *N*-hydroxy-2-acetylaminofluorene is carcinogenic in a variety of experimental species and 9-hydroxy-2-acetylaminofluorene in rats. See for example, Garner et al., 1984]. After intratracheal instillation in rats, 2-nitrofluorene was rapidly excreted into the perfusate (Möller et al., 1987b). Intestinal microflora appeared to reduce the excretion of mutagenic metabolites of 2-nitrofluorene (Möller et al., 1988).

As reported in an abstract, covalent binding to haemoglobin was detected in male Sprague-Dawley rats treated orally with 0.5 mmol[106 mg]/kg bw 2-nitrofluorene, although the level was lower than that found with 2-aminofluorene (Suzuki et al., 1987).

Under anaerobic conditions, rat liver microsomes and rabbit liver microsomes and cytosol catalysed the reduction of 2-nitrofluorene to *N*-hydroxy-2-aminofluorene and 2-aminofluorene (Uehleke & Nestel, 1967; Sternson, 1975; Kitamura et al., 1983; Tatsumi et al., 1986). [The Working Group noted that *N*-hydroxy-2-aminofluorene is carcinogenic to rats. See, for example, Garner et al., 1984).]

Incubation of 2-nitrofluorene with postmitochondrial supernatants from the livers of Wistar rats pretreated with sodium phenobarbital, 3-methylcholanthrene or Kenechlor-500 resulted in a time-dependent loss of substrate. The rate of metabolism was faster with homogenates from animals pretreated with 3-methylcholanthrene or Kanechlor-500 than with those from animals given phenobarbital (Ohe, 1985).

The major metabolites in isolated perfused lungs from male Sprague-Dawley rats were 9-hydroxy-2-nitrofluroene and an unidentified hydroxylated nitrofluorene. The same metabolites were detected in perfused livers from Wistar rats following treatment with β-glucuronidase (Möller et al., 1987b).

(ii) *Toxic effects*

No data were available to the Working Group.

(iii) *Genetic and related effects*

The genetic and related effects of nitroarenes and of their metabolites have been reviewed (Rosenkranz & Mermelstein, 1983; Beland et al., 1985; Rosenkranz & Mermelstein, 1985; Tokiwa & Ohnishi, 1986).

2-Nitrofluorene induced DNA damage in *Salmonella typhimurium* (Nakamura et al., 1987; lowest effective dose, 31 μg/ml) and in *Escherichia coli* (Ohta et al., 1984 (50–200 μg/ml); Quillardet et al., 1985; Mamber et al., 1986; Marzin et al., 1986 (lowest effective dose, 100 nM/ml)). Treatment of *E. coli* with 2-nitrofluorene induced binding of cellular DNA to the bacterial envelope (Kubinski et al., 1981). Conflicting results have been reported regarding the ability of 2-nitrofluorene to induce prophage in *E. coli* (Ho & Ho,

1981; Mamber et al., 1984). 2-Nitrofluorene (only dose tested, 10 μg/ml) preferentially inhibited the growth of DNA repair-deficient *E. coli* (Rosenkranz & Poirier, 1979; Doudney et al., 1981; McCarroll et al., 1981a; Mamber et al., 1983) and *Bacillus subtilis* (McCarroll et al., 1981b; Suter & Jaeger, 1982).

Conflicting results have been reported regarding the mutagenicity of 2-nitrofluorene to *E. coli* (Sakamoto et al., 1980; Dunkel et al., 1984; Mitchell & Gilbert, 1984, 1985). Over 200 independent reports are available on the mutagenicity of 2-nitrofluorene in *S. typhimurium*, as the compound is often used as a positive reference compound. These studies gave generally positive results: e.g., mutagenic to *S. typhimurium* TA97, TA98, TA100, TA1538, TA1978 (Purchase et al., 1978; Rosenkranz & Poirier, 1979; Sakamoto et al., 1980; Wang et al., 1980; McCoy et al., 1981; Pederson & Siak, 1981; Tokiwa et al., 1981; Pitts et al., 1982; Rosenkranz & Mermelstein, 1983; Dunkel et al., 1984; Xu et al., 1984; Vance et al., 1987) and BA9 (Ruiz-Rubio et al., 1984; Hera & Pueyo, 1986) but not to strain SV50 (Xu et al., 1984). 2-Nitrofluorene (0.7 μg/ml) was also mutagenic to *Photobacterium leiognathi* (Ulitzur, 1982).

2-Nitrofluorene (5%) induced recombination in the yeast *Saccharomyces cerevisiae* D3 (Simmon, 1979) but not strain D4 (at up to 100 μg/ml; Mitchell, 1980). It was not mutagenic to *Aspergillus nidulans* at up to 2000 μg/ml (Bignami et al., 1982). 2-Nitrofluorene has been reported to be mutagenic to the *Tradescantia* stamen hair (Schairer & Sautkulis, 1982).

In the mouse host-mediated assay, 2-nitrofluorene (at 125–1600 mg/kg) induced mutation in *S. typhimurium* but not recombination in *S. cerevisiae* D3 (Simmon et al., 1979). The urine of rats administered 2-nitrofluorene was mutagenic to *S. typhimurium* (Beije & Möller, 1988).

2-Nitrofluorene caused inhibition of DNA synthesis in HeLa cells (Painter & Howard, 1982). At a dose of $10^{-4}$–$10^{-1}$ mg/ml, it induced unscheduled DNA synthesis in mouse hepatocytes (Mori et al., 1987), but conflicting results were obtained with rat hepatocytes: negative at 1000 nmol/ml (Probst et al., 1981) but active at $10^{-4}$–$10^{-1}$ mg/ml (Mori et al., 1987). It induced sister chromatid exchange in Chinese hamster CHO cells (at 30 μM) in the presence of an exogenous metabolic system (Nachtman & Wolff, 1982) and mutation in mouse lymphoma L5178Y $TK^{+/-}$ cells (Amacher et al., 1979; Oberly et al., 1984).

2-Nitrofluorene induced morphological transformation of Syrian hamster embryo cells in the presence of hamster hepatocytes (Poiley et al., 1979; Pienta, 1980).

Oral administration of 2-nitrofluorene (125–500 mg/kg) to Chinese hamsters resulted in an increased incidence of sister chromatid exchange in bone-marrow cells; no such effect was observed after intraperitoneal administration of 50–200 mg/kg (Neal & Probst, 1983).

(b) *Humans*

No data were available to the Working Group.

### 3.3 Epidemiological studies and case reports of carcinogenicity in humans

No data were available to the Working Group.

## 4. Summary of Data Reported and Evaluation

### 4.1 Exposure data

2-Nitrofluorene has been detected in particulate emissions from diesel engines, kerosene heaters and gas burners. It has also been found at low concentrations in ambient air.

### 4.2 Experimental data

2-Nitrofluorene was tested for carcinogenicity in rats by oral administration, producing tumours of the mammary gland, forestomach, liver and ear duct. In a liver initiation-promotion model, it was shown to be an initiator of preneoplastic foci.

### 4.3 Human data

No data were available to the Working Group.

### 4.4 Other relevant data

2-Nitrofluorene induced sister chromatid exchange in Chinese hamsters *in vivo*. It induced DNA damage, sister chromatid exchange, mutation and morphological transformation in cultured animal cells. It was recombinogenic but not mutagenic to fungi and induced DNA damage and mutation in bacteria.

2-Aminofluorene, 2-acetylaminofluorene, *N*-hydroxy-2-amino-fluorene and *N*-hydroxy-2-acetylaminofluorene, which are model carcinogens, have been detected as metabolites of 2-nitrofluorene.

### 4.5 Evaluation[1]

There is *sufficient evidence* for the carcinogenicity in experimental animals of 2-nitrofluorene.

No data were available from studies in humans on the carcinogenicity of 2-nitrofluorene.

#### Overall evaluation

2-Nitrofluorene is *possibly carcinogenic to humans (Group 2B)*.

---

[1]For definitions of the italicized terms, see Preamble, pp. 25–28.

## Summary table of genetic and related effects of 2-nitrofluorene

| Nonmammalian systems | | | | | | | | | | | | Mammalian systems | | | | | | | | | | | | | | | | | | | | |
|---|---|---|---|---|---|---|---|---|---|---|---|---|---|---|---|---|---|---|---|---|---|---|---|---|---|---|---|---|---|---|---|---|
| Proka-ryotes | | | Lower eukaryotes | | | | Plants | | | Insects | | In vitro | | | | | | | | | | | | | | | In vivo | | | | | |
| | | | | | | | | | | | | Animal cells | | | | | | Human cells | | | | | | | | | Animals | | | | | Humans |
| D | G | R | D | G | R | G | C | A | D | G | C | A | D | G | S | M | C | A | T | I | D | G | S | M | C | A | T | I | D | G | S | M | C | DL | A | D | S | M | C | A |
| + | + |   | + | -¹ |   |   |   |   |   |   |   |   | + | + | ±¹ |   |   |   |   |   |   |   |   |   |   | ±¹ |   |   |   |   | +¹ |   |   |   |   |   |   |   |   |   |

A, aneuploidy; C, chromosomal aberrations; D, DNA damage; DL, dominant lethal mutation; G, gene mutation; I, inhibition of intercellular communication; M, micronuclei; R, mitotic recombination and gene conversion; S, sister chromatid exchange; T, cell transformation

*In completing the table, the following symbols indicate the consensus of the Working Group with regard to the results for each endpoint:*
+ considered to be positive for the specific endpoint and level of biological complexity
+¹ considered to be positive, but only one valid study was available to the Working Group
−¹ considered to be negative, but only one valid study was available to the Working Group

## 5. References

Aldrich Chemical Co. (1988) *Aldrich Catalog/Handbook of Fine Chemicals 1988*–1989, Milwaukee, WI, p. 1114

Amacher, D.E., Paillet, S.C. & Turner, G.N. (1979) Utility of the mouse lymphoma L5178Y/TK assay for the detection of chemical mutagens. In: Hsie, A.W., O'Neill, J.P. & McElheny, V.K., eds, *Mammalian Cell Mutagenesis, The Maturation of Test Systems* (*Banbury Report No. 2*), Cold Spring Harbor, NY, CSH Press, pp. 277–289

Beije, B. & Möller, L. (1988) Correlation between induction of unscheduled DNA synthesis in the liver and excretion of mutagenic metabolites in the urine of rats exposed to the carcinogenic air pollutant 2-nitrofluorene. *Carcinogenesis, 9*, 1465–1470

Beland, F.A., Heflich, R.H., Howard, P.C. & Fu, P.P. (1985) The in vitro metabolic activation of nitro polycyclic aromatic hydrocarbons. In: Harvey, R.G., ed., *Polycyclic Hydrocarbons and Carcinogenesis* (*ACS Symposium Series No. 283*), Washington DC, American Chemical Society, pp. 371–396

Bignami, M., Carere, A., Conti, L., Crebelli, R. & Fabrizi, M. (1982) Evaluation of two different genetic markers for the detection of frameshift and missense mutagens in *A. nidulans*. *Mutat. Res., 97*, 293–302

Buckingham, J., ed. (1982) *Dictionary of Organic Compounds*, 5th ed., New York, Chapman & Hall, p. 4247 (N-00938)

Butler, M.A., Evans, D.L., Giammarise, A.T., Kiriazides, D.K., Marsh, D., McCoy, E.C., Mermelstein, R., Murphy, C.B. & Rosenkranz, H.S. (1983) Application of *Salmonella* assay to carbon blacks and toners. In: Cooke, M. & Dennis, A.J., eds, *Polynuclear Aromatic Hydrocarbons, 7th International Symposium, Formation, Metabolism and Measurement*, Columbus, OH, Battelle, pp. 225–241

Chemsyn Science Laboratories (1988) *2-Nitrofluroene (Product Code U1046)*, Lenexa, KS, pp. 111–113

Doudney, C.O., Franke, M.A. & Rinaldi, C.N. (1981) The DNA damage activity (DDA) assay and its application to river waters and diesel exhausts. *Environ. int., 5*, 293–297

Draper, W.M. (1986) Quantitation of nitro- and dinitropolycyclic aromatic hydrocarbons in diesel exhaust particulate matter. *Chemosphere, 15*, 437–447

Dunkel, V.C., Zeiger, E., Brusick, D., McCoy, E., McGregor, D., Mortelmans, K., Rosenkranz, H.S. & Simmon, V.F. (1984) Reproducibility of microbial mutagenicity assays: I. Tests with *Salmonella typhimurium* and *Escherichia coli* using a standardized protocol. *Environ. Mutagenesis, 6*, Suppl. 2, 1–254

Garner, R.C., Martin, C.N. & Clayson, D.B. (1984) Carcinogenic aromatic amines and related compounds. In: Searle, C.F., ed., *Chemical Carcinogens*, 2nd ed., Vol. 1 (*ACS Monograph 182*), Washington DC, American Chemical Society, pp. 175–276

Hera, C. & Pueyo, C. (1986) Conditions for the optimal use of the L-arabinose-resistance mutagenesis test with *Salmonella typhimurium*. *Mutagenesis, 1*, 267–273

Ho, Y.L. & Ho, S.K. (1981) Screening of carcinogens with the prophage λcIts857 induction test. *Cancer Res., 41*, 532–536

IARC (1988) *Information Bulletin on the Survey of Chemicals Being Tested for Carcinogenicity*, No. 13, Lyon, p. 20

Kitamura, S., Narai, N., Hayashi, M. & Tatsumi, K. (1983) Rabbit liver enzymes responsible for reduction of nitropolycyclic aromatic hydrocarbons. *Chem. pharm. Bull.*, *31*, 776-779

Kubinski, H., Gutzke, G.E. & Kubinski, Z.O. (1981) DNA-cell-binding (DCB) assay for suspected carcinogens and mutagens. *Mutat. Res.*, *89*, 95-136

Mamber, S.W., Bryson, V. & Katz, S.E. (1983) The *Escherichia coli* WP2/WP100 rec assay for detection of potential chemical carcinogens. *Mutat. Res.*, *119*, 135-144

Mamber, S.W., Bryson, V. & Katz, S.E. (1984) Evaluation of the *Escherichia coli* K12 inductest for detection of potential chemical carcinogens. *Mutat. Res.*, *130*, 141-151

Mamber, S.W., Okasinski, W.G., Pinter, C.D. & Tunac, J.B. (1986) The *Escherichia coli* K-12 SOS chromotest agar spot test for simple, rapid detection of genotoxic agents. *Mutat. Res.*, *171*, 83-90

Marzin, D.R., Olivier, P. & Vophi, H. (1986) Kinetic determination of enzymatic activity and modification of the metabolic activation system in the SOS chromotest. *Mutat. Res.*, *164*, 353-359

McCarroll, N.E., Piper, C.E. & Keech, B.H. (1981a) An *E. coli* microsuspension assay for the detection of DNA damage induced by direct-acting agents and promutagens. *Environ. Mutagenesis*, *3*, 429-444

McCarroll, N.E., Keech, B.H. & Piper, C.E. (1981b) A microsuspension adaptation of the *Bacillus subtilis* 'rec' assay. *Environ. Mutagenesis*, *3*, 607-616

McCoy, E.C., Rosenkranz, E.J., Rosenkranz, H.S. & Mermelstein, R. (1981) Nitrated fluorene derivatives are potent frameshift mutagens. *Mutat. Res.*, *90*, 11-20

Miller, J.A., Sandin, R.B., Miller, E.C. & Rusch, H.P. (1955) The carcinogenicity of compounds related to 2-acetylaminofluorene. II. Variations in the bridges and the 2-substituent. *Cancer Res.*, *15*, 188-199

Mitchell, I. deG. (1980) Forward mutation in *Escherichia coli* and gene conversion in *Saccharomyces cerevisiae* compared quantitatively with reversion in *Salmonella typhimurium*. *Agents Actions*, *10*, 287-295

Mitchell, I. deG. & Gilbert, P.J. (1984) The effect of pretreatment of *Escherichia coli* CM891 with ethylenediaminetetraacetate on sensitivity to a variety of standard mutagens. *Mutat. Res.*, *140*, 13-19

Mitchell, I. deG. & Gilbert, P.J. (1985) An assessment of the importance of error-prone repair and point mutations to forward mutation to L-azetidine-2-carboxylic acid resistance in *Escherichia coli*. *Mutat. Res.*, *149*, 303-310

Möller, L. (1988) *2-Nitrofluorene, in vivo Metabolism and Assessment of Cancer Risk of an Air Pollutant*, Stockholm, Karolinska Institute

Möller, L., Nilsson, L., Gustafsson, J.-Å. & Rafter, J. (1985) Formation of mutagenic metabolites from 2-nitrofluorene in the rat. *Environ. int.*, *11*, 363-368

Möller, L., Rafter, J. & Gustafsson, J.-Å. (1987a) Metabolism of the carcinogenic air pollutant 2-nitrofluorene in the rat. *Carcinogenesis*, *8*, 637-645

Möller, L., Törnquist, S., Beije, B., Rafter, J., Toftgård, R. & Gustafsson, J.-Å. (1987b) Metabolism of the carcinogenic air pollutant 2-nitrofluorene in the isolated perfused rat lung and liver. *Carcinogenesis*, *8*, 1847-1852

Möller, L., Corrie, M., Midtvedt, T., Rafter, J. & Gustafsson, J.-Å. (1988) The role of the intestinal microflora in the formation of mutagenic metabolites from the carcinogenic air pollutant 2-nitrofluorene. *Carcinogenesis*, 9, 823–830

Möller, L., Torndal, U.B., Eriksson, L.C. & Gustafsson, J.-Å. (1989) The air pollutant 2-nitrofluorene as initiator and promotor in a liver model for chemical carcinogenesis. *Carcinogenesis* (in press)

Mori, H., Sugie, S., Yoshimi, N., Kinouchi, T. & Ohnishi, Y. (1987) Genotoxicity of a variety of nitroarenes and other nitro compounds in DNA-repair tests with rat and mouse hepatocytes. *Mutat. Res.*, 190, 159–167

Morris, H.P., Dubnik, C.S. & Johnson, J.M. (1950) Studies of the carcinogenic action in the rat of 2-nitro-, 2-amino-, 2-acetylamino-, and 2-diacetylaminofluorene after ingestion and after painting. *J. natl Cancer Inst.*, 10, 2101–1213

Nachtman, J.P. & Wolff, S. (1982) Activity of nitro-polynuclear aromatic hydrocarbons in the sister chromatid exchange assay with and without metabolic activation. *Environ. Mutagenesis*, 4, 1–5

Nakamura, S.-I., Oda, Y., Shimada, T., Oki, I. & Sugimoto, K. (1987) SOS-inducing activity of chemical carcinogens and mutagens in *Salmonella typhimurium* TA1535/pSK1002: examination with 151 chemicals. *Mutat. Res.*, 192, 239–246

Neal, S.B. & Probst, G.S. (1983) Chemically-induced sister-chromatid exchange *in vivo* in bone marrow of Chinese hamsters. *Mutat. Res.*, 113, 33–43

Oberly, T.J., Bewsey, B.J. & Probst, G.S. (1984) An evaluation of the L5178Y TK$^{+/-}$ mouse lymphoma forward mutation assay using 42 chemicals. *Mutat. Res.*, 125, 291–306

Ohe, T. (1985) Studies on comparative decomposition rate by rat liver homogenate and on micronucleus test of nitrated polycyclic aromatic hydrocarbons. *Bull. environ. Contam. Toxicol.*, 34, 715–721

Ohta, T., Nakamura, N., Moriya, M., Shirasu, Y. & Kada, T. (1984) The SOS-function-inducing activity of chemical mutagens in *Escherichia coli*. *Mutat. Res.*, 131, 101–109

Painter, R.B. & Howard, R. (1982) The HeLa DNA synthesis test as a rapid screen for mutagenic carcinogens. *Mutat. Res.*, 92, 427–437

Pederson, T.C. & Siak, J.C. (1981) The role of nitroaromatic compounds in the direct-acting mutagenicity of diesel particle extracts. *J. Appl. Toxicol.*, 1, 54–60

Pfaltz & Bauer, Inc. (1988) *Organic and Inorganic Chemicals for Research*, 11th ed., Waterbury, CT, p. 291

Pienta, R.J. (1980) Evaluation and relevance of the Syrian hamster embryo cell system. In: Williams, G.M., Kroes, R., Waaijers, H.W. & van de Poll, K.W., eds, *The Predictive Value of Short-term Screening Tests in Carcinogenicity Evaluation*, Amsterdam, Elsevier, pp. 149–169

Pitts, J.N., Jr, Lokensgard, D.M., Harger, W., Fisher, T.S., Mejia, V., Schuler, J.J., Scorziell, G.M. & Katzenstein, Y.A. (1982) Mutagens in diesel exhaust particulate: identification and direct activities of 6-nitrobenzo[*a*]pyrene, 9-nitroanthracene, 1-nitropyrene and 5*H*-phenanthro[4,5-*bcd*]pyran-5-one. *Mutat. Res.*, 103, 241–249

Poiley, J.A., Raineri, R. & Pienta, R.J. (1979) Use of hamster hepatocytes to metabolize carcinogens in an in vitro bioassay. *J. natl Cancer Institute*, 63, 519–524

Probst, G.S., McMahon, R.E., Hill, L.E., Thompson, C.Z., Epp, J.K. & Neal, S.B. (1981) Chemically-induced unscheduled DNA synthesis in primary rat hepatocyte cultures: a comparison with bacterial mutagenicity using 218 compounds. *Environ. Mutagenesis*, 3, 11–32

Purchase, L.F.H., Longstaff, E., Ashby, J., Styles, J.A., Anderson, D., Lefevre, P.A. & Westwood, F.R. (1978) An evaluation of six short-term tests for detecting organic chemical carcinogens. *Br. J. Cancer, 37*, 873–959

Quillardet, P., de Bellecombe, C. & Hofnung, M. (1985) The SOS chromotest, a colorimetric bacterial assay for genotoxins: validation study with 83 compounds. *Mutat. Res., 147*, 79–95

Rosenkranz, H.S. & Mermelstein, R. (1983) Mutagenicity and genotoxicity of nitroarenes: all nitro-containing chemicals were not created equal. *Mutat. Res., 114*, 217–267

Rosenkranz, H.S. & Mermelstein, R. (1985) The genotoxicity, metabolism and carcinogenicity of nitrated polycyclic aromatic hydrocarbons. *J. environ. Sci. Health, C3*, 221–272

Rosenkranz, H.S. & Poirier, L.A. (1979) An evaluation of the mutagenicity and DNA-modifying activity of carcinogens and noncarcinogens in microbial systems. *J. natl Cancer Inst., 62*, 873–892

Rosenkranz, H.S., McCoy, E.C., Sanders, D.R., Butler, M., Kiriazides, D.K. & Mermelstein, R. (1980) Nitropyrenes: isolation, identification and reduction of mutagenic impurities in carbon black and toners. *Science, 209*, 1039–1043

Ruiz-Rubio, M., Hera, C. & Pueyo, C. (1984) Comparison of a forward and a reverse mutation assay in *Salmonella typhimurium* measuring L-arabinose resistance and histidine prototrophy. *EMBO J., 3*, 1435–1440

Sakamoto, Y., Yamamoto, K. & Kikuchi, Y. (1980) Difference in sensitivity against various mutagens in variants with *E. coli* repair ability (Jpn.). *Environ. Mutagen. Res. Commun., 2*, 10–12

Sanders, D.R. (1981) Nitropyrenes: the isolation of trace mutagenic impurities from the toluene extract of an aftertreated carbon black. In: Cooke, M. & Dennis, A.J., eds, *Polynuclear Aromatic Hydrocarbons, 5th International Symposium, Chemical Analysis and Biological Fate*, Columbus, OH, Battelle, pp. 145–158

Sawicki, E. (1954) 7-Alkyl derivatives of 2-aminofluorene. *J. Am. chem. Soc., 76*, 2269–2271

Schairer, L.A. & Sautkulis, R.C. (1982) Detection of ambient levels of mutagenic atmospheric pollutants with the higher plant *Tradescantia*. In: Klekowski, E.J., Jr, ed., *Environmental Mutagenesis, Carcinogenesis and Plant Biology*, Vol. 2, New York, Praeger, pp. 154–194

Schuetzle, D. (1983) Sampling of vehicle emissions for chemical analysis and biological testing. *Environ. Health Perspect., 47*, 65–80

Schuetzle, D. & Jensen, T.E. (1985) Analysis of nitrated polycyclic aromatic hydrocarbons (nitro-PAH) by mass spectrometry. In: White, C.M., ed., *Nitrated Polycyclic Aromatic Hydrocarbons*, Heidelberg, A. Hüthig Verlag, pp. 121–167

Schuetzle, D. & Frazier, J.A. (1986) Factors influencing the emission of vapor and particulate phase components from diesel engines. In: Ishinishi, N., Koizumi, A., McClellan, R.O. & Stöber, W., eds, *Carcinogenic and Mutagenic Effects of Diesel Engine Exhaust*, Amsterdam, Elsevier, pp. 41–63

Simmon, V.F. (1979) In vitro assays for recombinogenic activity of chemical carcinogens and related compounds with *Saccharomyces cerevisiae* D3. *J. natl Cancer Inst., 62*, 901–909

Simmon, V.F., Rosenkranz, H.S., Zeiger, E. & Poirier, L.A. (1979) Mutagenic activity of chemical carcinogens and related compounds in the intraperitoneal host-mediated assay. *J. natl Cancer Inst., 62*, 911–918

Sternson, L.A. (1975) Detection of arylhydroxylamines as intermediates in the metabolic reduction of nitro compounds. *Experientia, 31*, 268–270

Suter, W. & Jaeger, I. (1982) Comparative evaluation of different pairs of DNA repair-deficient and DNA repair-proficient bacterial tester strains for rapid detection of chemical mutagens and carcinogens. *Mutat. Res., 97*, 1–18

Suzuki, J., Meguro, S. & Suzuki, S. (1987) Comparison of in vivo binding of aromatic nitro and amino compounds to rat hemoglobin (Abstract F 06-Y-13). *J. pharm. Sci., 76*, S126

Tanabe, K., Matsushita, H., Kuo, C.-T. & Imamiya, S. (1986) Determination of carcinogenic nitroarenes in airborne particulates by high performance liquid chromatography (Jpn.). *Taiki Osen Gakkaishi (J. Jpn. Soc. Air Pollut.), 21*, 535–544

Tatsumi, K. & Amano, H. (1987) Biotransformation of 1-nitropyrene and 2-nitrofluorene to novel metabolites, the corresponding formylamino compounds, in animal bodies. *Biochem. biophys. Res. Commun., 142*, 376–382

Tatsumi, K., Kitamura, S. & Narai, N. (1986) Reductive metabolism of aromatic nitro compounds including carcinogens by rabbit liver preparations. *Cancer Res., 46*, 1089–1093

Tokiwa, H. & Ohnishi, Y. (1986) Mutagenicity and carcinogenicity of nitroarenes and their sources in the environment. *CRC crit. Rev. Toxicol., 17*, 23–69

Tokiwa, H., Nakagawa, R. & Ohnishi, Y. (1981) Mutagenic assay of aromatic nitro compounds with *Salmonella typhimurium*. *Mutat. Res., 91*, 321–325

Tokiwa, H., Nakagawa, R. & Horikawa, K. (1985) Mutagenic/carcinogenic agents in indoor pollutants: the dinitropyrenes generated by kerosene heaters and fuel gas and liquified petroleum gas burners. *Mutat. Res., 157*, 39–47

Uehleke, H. & Nestel, K. (1967) Hydroxylamino- and nitrosobiphenyl: biological oxidation products of 4-aminobiphenyl and reduction metabolites of 4-nitrobiphenyl (Ger.). *Naunyn-Schmiedebergs Arch. Pharmacol. exp. Pathol., 257*, 151–171

Ulitzur, S. (1982) A bioluminescence test for genetoxic agents. *Trends anal. Chem., 1*, 329–333

US Environmental Protection Agency (1986) *Toxic Substances Control Act Chemical Substance Inventory*, 1985 ed., Vol. III, *Substance Name Index (EPA-560/7-85-002c)*, Washington DC, Office of Toxic Substances

Vance, W.A., Wang, Y.Y. & Okamoto, H.S. (1987) Disubstituted amino-, nitroso-, and nitro-fluorenes: a physicochemical basis for structure-activity relationships in *Salmonella typhimurium*. *Environ. Mutagenesis, 9*, 123–141

Wang, C.Y., Lee, M.-S., King, C.M. & Warner, P.O. (1980) Evidence for nitroaromatics as direct-acting mutagens of airborne particulates. *Chemosphere, 9*, 83–87

Weast, R.C., ed. (1985) *CRC Handbook of Chemistry and Physics*, 66th ed., Boca Raton, FL, CRC Press, p. C-277

Xu, J., Whong, W.-Z. & Ong, T.M. (1984) Validation of the *Salmonella* (SV50)/arabinose-resistant forward mutation assay system with 26 compounds. *Mutat. Res., 130*, 79–86

# 1-NITRONAPHTHALENE

## 1. Chemical and Physical Data

### 1.1 Synonyms

*Chem. Abstr. Services Reg. No.*: 86-57-7
*Chem. Abstr. Name*: Naphthalene, 1-nitro-
*IUPAC Systematic Name*: 1-Nitronaphthalene
*Synonyms*: α-Nitronaphthalene; nitrol

### 1.2 Structural and molecular formulae and molecular weight

$C_{10}H_7NO_2$                                    Mol. wt: 173.2

### 1.3 Chemical and physical properties of the pure substance

(a) *Description*: Yellow needles, recrystallized from ethanol (Weast, 1985)

(b) *Boiling-point*: 304°C (Windholz, 1983)

(c) *Melting-point*: 61.5°C (Weast, 1985)

(d) *Spectroscopy data*: Ultra-violet (National Cancer Institute, 1978), proton and nuclear magnetic resonance (Lucchini & Wells, 1976; Kitching *et al.*, 1977) and mass (Schuetzle & Jensen, 1985) spectral data have been reported.

(e) *Relative density*: 1.331 relative to water at 4°C (Buckingham, 1982)

(f) *Solubility*: Insoluble in water; soluble in ethanol, diethyl ether, chloroform, carbon disulfide (Windholz, 1983), benzene and pyrene (Weast, 1985)

(g) *Flash-point*: 164°C (Sax & Lewis, 1987)

### 1.4 Technical products and impurities

1-Nitronaphthalene is available for research purposes at 99% purity (Aldrich Chemical Co., 1988). It is also available in a certified purity of 99.61% as a reference material (Belliardo *et al.*, 1988).

## 2. Production, Use, Occurrence and Analysis

### 2.1 Production and use

(a) *Production*

1-Nitronaphthalene is synthesized by the action of a mixture of nitric and sulfuric acids on finely ground naphthalene (Sax & Lewis, 1987). Reaction of naphthalene with nitric acid and sulfuric acid in dichloromethane (or another suitable inert solvent) was reported to give a 80% yield of 99.2% purity (Kameo & Hirashima, 1986).

There is one producer of this substance in the USA. 1-Nitronaphthalene is reported on the 1985 *Toxic Substances Control Act Chemical Substance Inventory* (US Environmental Protection Agency, 1986).

(b) *Use*

The uses of 1-nitronaphthalene include a chemical intermediate in the manufacture of dyes [drugs, perfumes, rubber chemicals, tanning agents and pesticides]; a fluorescence quencher for mineral oils (Sax & Lewis, 1987); a 'debloomer' for petroleum oils (Windholz, 1983); a vapour-phase corrosion inhibitor (Foley & Brown, 1979); a wood preservative; and a fungicide (Kasperczak & Lutomski, 1973; Dominik, 1978). A Chinese patent was issued in which [a compound presumed to be] 1-nitronaphthalene was proposed as a component at 1–2% in sulfur-free, fragrant fireworks powder (Ying *et al.*, 1986).

### 2.2 Occurrence

(a) *Engine exhaust*

1-Nitronaphthalene concentrations of 0.77 mg/kg of particulates were reported in the emissions of a heavy-duty diesel engine run at 100% load and 1200 revolutions/min; at 75% load and 1800 revolutions/min, the same engine produced concentrations of 0.47 mg/kg of particulates (Draper, 1986). Nishioka *et al.* (1982) detected 1-nitronaphthalene in the exhaust emissions of light-duty diesel engines (0.3-0.7 mg/kg), and Liberti *et al.* (1984) found this compound in the gas phase of diesel engine exhaust.

*(b) Other occurrence*

Toners for use in photocopy machines have been produced in quantity since the late 1950s and have seen widespread use. 'Long-flow' furnace black was first used in photocopy toners in 1967; its manufacture involved an oxidation whereby some nitration also occurred. Subsequent changes in the production technique reduced the total extractable nitropyrene content from an uncontrolled level of 5–100 mg/kg to below 0.3 mg/kg (Rosenkranz *et al.*, 1980; Sanders, 1981; Butler *et al.*, 1983), and toners produced from this carbon black since 1980 have not been found to contain detectable levels of mutagenicity or, hence, nitropyrenes (Rosenkranz *et al.*, 1980; Butler *et al.*, 1983). 1-Nitronaphthalene has been detected in formerly available commercial carbon blacks (Fitch *et al.*, 1978; Ramdahl & Urdal, 1982).

1-Nitronaphthalene was detected in urban ambient airborne particulates in St Louis, MO, USA (Ramdahl & Urdal, 1982; Ramdahl *et al.*, 1982), and trace quantities were identified in urban air particulates in Göteborg, Sweden (Brorström-Lundén & Lindskog, 1985). In a laboratory experiment, 1-nitronaphthalene was formed by a gas-phase naphthalene nitration reaction at room temperature and atmospheric pressure with a yield of 18% (Pitts *et al.*, 1985). It was postulated that significant amounts of 1-nitronaphthalene result from the night-time gas-phase reaction of naphthalene with nitrogen pentoxide (Pitts, 1987).

1-Nitronaphthalene was found at 3.5 mg/kg particulate matter in a hexane/benzene fraction and at 3.1 mg/kg particulate matter in a polycyclic aromatic hydrocarbon fraction of suburban/industrial ambient air in north-west Philadelphia, PA, USA. It was not found in polar I and II fractions (Wise *et al.*, 1985). A level of 2.3 ng/m$^3$ was found in a night-time sample of ambient air in Torrance, CA, USA, calculated as the sum of the concentrations on the filter and three polyurethane foam plugs. A day-time sample contained 3.0 ng/m$^3$ in approximately equal amounts of 1- and 2-nitronaphthalene; however, this was considered to be a lower limit, since the adsorption capacity of the three polyurethane foam plugs was exceeded (Arey *et al.*, 1987).

## 2.3 Analysis

See the monograph on 1-nitropyrene.

# 3. Biological Data Relevant to the Evaluation of Carcinogenic Risk to Humans

## 3.1 Carcinogenicity studies in animals[1]

*Oral administration*

*Mouse*: Two groups of 50 male and 50 female B6C3F1 mice, approximately six weeks old, were fed a basal diet containing 0.06% or 0.12% 1-nitronaphthalene ([purity and impurities unspecified] melting-point, 50–53°C) for 78 weeks and observed for a further 18–20 weeks (National Cancer Institute, 1978). Two untreated groups of 50 males and 50 females served as controls. Statistical analyses were based on animals that survived at least 52 weeks; more than 80% of the mice survived to 80 weeks. At the end of the experiment, tumours were observed in the respiratory, digestive and endocrine systems in both treated and control animals; the incidences did not differ significantly among the four groups. [The Working Group noted that the dose administered was not the maximal tolerated dose.]

*Rat*: Two groups of 50 male and 50 female Fischer 344 rats, approximately six weeks old, were fed a basal diet containing 0.05% then 0.06% or 0.18% 1-nitronaphthalene ([purity and impurities unspecified] melting-point, 50–53°C) for 78 weeks and observed for a further 29–31 weeks (National Cancer Institute, 1978). Two untreated groups of 25 females and 25 males and 50 males and 50 females served as controls for the high- and low-dose groups, respectively. Statistical analyses were based on animals that survived at least 52 weeks; more than 80% of the rats survived to 80 weeks. At the end of the experiment, tumours were observed in the respiratory, digestive and endocrine systems in both treated and control animals; the incidences did not differ significantly among the four groups. [The Working Group noted that the dose administered was not the maximal tolerated dose and that it was changed during treatment of the low-dose group.]

## 3.2 Other relevant data

(*a*) *Experimental systems*

(i) *Absorption, distribution, excretion and metabolism*

1-Naphthylamine (see IARC, 1987) was detected in the urine of male Sprague-Dawley rats administered single intraperitoneal doses of 100 mg/kg bw 1-nitronaphthalene (Johnson & Cornish, 1978).

Incubation of 1-nitronaphthalene under anaerobic conditions with a postmitochondrial supernatant from the livers of male Fischer rats resulted in the stoichiometric formation of 1-naphthylamine (Poirier & Weisburger, 1974). Under aerobic conditions, a rat liver

---

[1]The Working Group was aware of a study in progress in mice by single subcutaneous injection (IARC, 1988).

metabolic system converted 1-nitronaphthalene into dihydrodiol and phenol metabolites (El-Bayoumy & Hecht, 1982).

Under anaerobic conditions, rabbit liver microsomes catalysed the reduction of 1-nitronaphthalene to N-hydroxy-1-naphthylamine and 1-naphthylamine (Sternson, 1975; Tatsumi *et al.*, 1986). [The Working Group noted that N-hydroxy-1-naphthylamine is carcinogenic to experimental animals. See, for example, Garner *et al.* (1984).]

Lung and liver microsomes from male Swiss-Webster mice metabolized 1-nitronaphthalene to products that bound microsomal macromolecules. The binding was NADPH- and oxygen-dependent and was inhibited by carbon monoxide, nitrogen and SKF-525A. Little binding was detected with kidney microsomes. Pretreatment of the mice with β-naphthoflavone enhanced the binding to lung microsomal macromolecules; phenobarbital pretreatment increased the binding to liver microcomes. Incubations were also conducted with lung slices and isolated lung cells. Autoradiographs of the lung slices showed that most of the binding occurred in the epithelial cells of the bronchioles and smaller airways. With the isolated lung cells, there was preferential binding of 1-nitronaphthalene to cell populations enriched in Clara cells. β-Naphthoflavone pretreatment increased the binding of 1-nitronaphthalene in both the lung slices and isolated lung cells (Rasmussen, 1986).

(ii) *Toxic effects*

A single intraperitoneal injection of 1-nitronaphthalene (25–200 mg/kg bw) to male Sprague-Dawley rats resulted in respiratory distress, which generally developed within 24 h ($ED_{50}$, 60 mg/kg bw). At necropsy at 24 h, there was diffuse, irregular red mottling on the pleural surface of the lungs and necrosis of nonciliated bronchiolar epithelial cells (Clara cells). Hepatotoxicity was also observed after intraperitoneal injection of 100 mg/kg bw, increasing in severity over 72 h after injection (Johnson *et al.*, 1984).

No toxic effect was observed in mice administered 1-nitronaphthalene for 78 weeks at doses up to 0.12% or in rats at doses up to 0.18% in the diet (National Cancer Institute, 1978).

(iii) *Genetic and related effects*

The genetic and related effects of nitroarenes and of their metabolites have been reviewed (Rosenkranz & Mermelstein, 1983; Beland *et al.*, 1985; Rosenkranz & Mermelstein, 1985; Tokiwa & Ohnishi, 1986).

1-Nitronaphthalene (100 µg/disc) preferentially inhibited the growth of DNA repair-deficient *Bacillus subtilis* (Tokiwa *et al.*, 1987) and induced DNA damage in *Salmonella typhimurium* (lowest effective dose, 19 µg/ml; Nakamura *et al.*, 1987).

1-Nitronaphthalene was mutagenic to *S. typhimurium*, TA1535, TA1538, TA98 and TA100 (Scribner *et al.*, 1979; El-Bayoumy *et al.*, 1981; Matsuda, 1981; McCoy *et al.*, 1981; Tokiwa *et al.*, 1981; Löfroth *et al.*, 1984; Vance & Levin, 1984; Dunkel *et al.*, 1985; Mortelmans *et al.*, 1986). It was not mutagenic to TA97 or TA1537 (McCoy *et al.*, 1981;

Dunkel et al., 1985; Rosenkranz et al., 1985; Mortelmans et al., 1986) or to *Escherichia coli* WP2 *uvr*A (Dunkel et al., 1985).

This compound did not induce sex-linked recessive lethal mutation in *Drosophila melanogaster* when administered orally or by injection (Valencia et al., 1985).

1-Nitronaphthalene has been reported [data not given] to induce chromosomal aberrations but not sister chromatid exchange [in Chinese hamster CHO cells] (Shelby & Stasiewicz, 1984).

*(b) Humans*

No data were available to the Working Group.

### 3.3 Epidemiological studies and case reports of carcinogenicity in humans

No data were available to the Working Group.

## 4. Summary of Data Reported and Evaluation

### 4.1 Exposure data

1-Nitronaphthalene is used as an intermediate in chemical synthesis. It has been detected in some carbon blacks and in particulate exhaust of diesel engines and has been found at low concentrations in ambient air.

### 4.2 Experimental data

1-Nitronaphthalene was tested for carcinogenicity in mice and rats by oral administration. No carcinogenic effect was observed, but the dose used did not induce toxic effects.

### 4.3 Human data

No data were available to the Working Group.

### 4.4 Other relevant data

*N*-Hydroxy-1-naphthylamine (which has been shown to induce tumours in experimental animals) has been detected as a metabolite of 1-nitronaphthalene *in vitro*. A single intraperitoneal injection of 1-nitronaphthalene to rats caused hepatotoxicity and necrosis of Clara cells of the lung. 1-Nitronaphthalene induced DNA damage and mutation in bacteria but was not mutagenic to *Drosophila melanogaster*.

## Summary table of genetic and related effects of 1-nitronaphthalene

| Nonmammalian systems | | | | | | | | | | | | Mammalian systems | | | | | | | | | | | | | | | | | | | |
|---|---|---|---|---|---|---|---|---|---|---|---|---|---|---|---|---|---|---|---|---|---|---|---|---|---|---|---|---|---|---|---|
| Proka-ryotes | | | Lower eukaryotes | | | | Plants | | | Insects | | In vitro | | | | | | | | | | | | | | In vivo | | | | | |
| | | | | | | | | | | | | Animal cells | | | | | | | Human cells | | | | | | | Animals | | | | | Humans | |
| D | G | D | R | G | A | D | G | C | R | G | C | A | D | G | S | M | C | A | T | I | D | G | S | M | C | A | T | I | D | G | S | M | C | DL | A | D | S | M | C | A |
| + | + | | | | | | | | | –¹ | | | | | | | | | | | | | | | | | | | | | | | | | | | | | | |

A, aneuploidy; C, chromosomal aberrations; D, DNA damage; DL, dominant lethal mutation; G, gene mutation; I, inhibition of intercellular communication; M, micronuclei; R, mitotic recombination and gene conversion; S, sister chromatid exchange; T, cell transformation

*In completing the table, the following symbols indicate the consensus of the Working Group with regard to the results for each endpoint:*

+ considered to be positive for the specific endpoint and level of biological complexity
–¹ considered to be negative, but only one valid study was available to the Working Group

## 4.5 Evaluation[1]

There is *inadequate evidence* for the carcinogenicity in experimental animals of 1-nitronaphthalene.

No data were available from studies in humans on the carcinogenicity of 1-nitronaphthalene.

**Overall evaluation**

1-Nitronaphthalene *is not classifiable as to its carcinogenicity to humans (Group 3).*

# 5. References

Aldrich Chemical Co. (1988) *Aldrich Catalog/ Handbook of Fine Chemicals 1988*–1989, Milwaukee, WI, p. 1118

Arey, J., Zielinska, B., Atkinson, R. & Winer, A.M. (1987) Polycyclic aromatic hydrocarbon and nitroarene concentrations in ambient air during a wintertime high-$NO_x$ episode in the Los Angeles basin. *Atmos. Environ.*, *21*, 1437–1444

Beland, F.A., Heflich, R.H., Howard, P.C. & Fu, P.P. (1985) The in vitro metabolic activation of nitro polycyclic aromatic hydrocarbons. In: Harvey, R.G., ed., *Polycyclic Hydrocarbons and Carcinogenesis (ACS Symposium Series No. 283)*, Washington DC, American Chemical Society, pp. 371–396

Belliardo, J.J., Jacob, J. & Lindsey, A.S. (1988) *The Certification of the Purity of Seven Nitropolycyclic Aromatic Compounds, CRM Nos 305, 306, 307, 308, 310, 311, 312, BCR Information Reference Materials (EUR 11254 EN)*, Brussels, Commission of the European Communities, p. III

Brorström-Lundén, E. & Lindskog, A. (1985) Characterization of organic compounds on airborne particles. *Environ. int.*, *11*, 183–188

Buckingham, J., ed. (1982) *Dictionary of Organic Compounds*, 5th ed., New York, Chapman & Hall, p. 4257 (N-01040)

Butler, M.A., Evans, D.L., Giammarise, A.T., Kiriazides, D.K., Marsh, D., McCoy, E.C., Mermelstein, R., Murphy, C.B. & Rosenkranz, H.S. (1983) Application of *Salmonella* assay to carbon blacks and toners. In: Cooke, M. & Dennis, A.J., eds, *Polynuclear Aromatic Hydrocarbons, 7th International Symposium, Formation, Metabolism and Measurement*, Columbus, OH, Battelle, pp. 225–241

Dominik, J. (1978) Studies of the stability of insecticidal activity of some oily wood preservations 15 years after their application (Pol.). *Zesz. Probl. Postepow Nauk Roln.*, *209*, 135–141

Draper, W.M. (1986) Quantitation of nitro- and dinitropolycyclic aromatic hydrocarbons in diesel exhaust particulate matter. *Chemosphere*, *15*, 437–447

---

[1]For definitions of the italicized terms, see Preamble, pp. 25–28.

Dunkel, V.C., Zeiger, E., Brusick, D., McCoy, E., McGregor, D., Mortelmans, K., Rosenkranz, H.S. & Simmon, V.F. (1985) Reproducibility of microbial mutagenicity assays: II. Testing of carcinogens and noncarcinogens in *Salmonella typhimurium* and *Escherichia coli*. *Environ. Mutagenesis*, 7, Suppl. 5, 1–248

El-Bayoumy, K. & Hecht, S.S. (1982) Comparative metabolism in vitro of 5-nitroacenaphthene and 1-nitronaphthalene. In: Cooke, W.M., Dennis, A.J. & Fisher, G.L., eds, *Polynuclear Aromatic Hydrocarbons, Sixth International Symposium, Physical and Biological Chemistry*, Columbus, OH, Battelle, pp. 263–273

El-Bayoumy, K., Lavoie, E.J., Hecht, S.S., Fow, E.A. & Hoffmann, D. (1981) The influence of methyl substitution on the mutagenicity of nitronaphthalenes and nitrobiphenyls. *Mutat. Res.*, 81, 143–153

Fitch, W.L., Everhart, E.T. & Smith, D.H. (1978) Characterization of carbon black adsorbates and artifacts formed during extraction. *Anal. Chem.*, 50, 2122–2126

Foley, R.T. & Brown, B.F. (1979) Corrosion and corrosion inhibitors. In: Mark, H.F., Othmer, D.F., Overberger, C.G., Seaborg, G.T. & Grayson, M., eds, *Kirk-Othmer Encyclopedia of Chemical Technology*, 3rd ed., Vol. 11, New York, John Wiley & Sons, pp. 113–142

Garner, R.C., Martin, C.N. & Clayson, D.B. (1984) Carcinogenic aromatic amines and related compounds. In: Searle, C.E., ed, *Chemical Carcinogens*, 2nd ed., Vol. 1 (*ACS Monograph 182*), Washington DC, American Chemical Society, pp. 175–276

IARC (1987) *IARC Monographs on the Evaluation of Carcinogenic Risks to Humans, Supplement 7, Overall Evaluations of Carcinogenicity: An Updating of IARC Monographs Volumes 1 to 42*, Lyon, pp. 260–261

IARC (1988) *Information Bulletin on the Survey of Chemicals Being Tested for Carcinogenicity*, No. 13, Lyon, p. 20

Johnson, D.E. & Cornish, H.H. (1978) Metabolic conversion of 1- and 2-nitronaphthalene to 1- and 2-naphthylamine in the rat. *Toxicol. appl. Pharmacol.*, 46, 549–553

Johnson, D.E., Riley, M.G.I. & Cornish, H.H. (1984) Acute target organ toxicity of 1-nitronaphthalene in the rat. *J. appl. Toxicol.*, 4, 253–257

Kameo, T. & Hirashima, T. (1986) Mononitration of naphthalene with nitric acid in inert solvents (Jpn.). *Chem. Express*, 1, 371–374 [*Chem. Abstr.*, 106, 119419r]

Kasperczak, B. & Lutomski, K. (1973) Fungicidal properties of by-products formed during the production of dinitrophenol and α-nitronaphthalene (Pol.). *Rocz. Akad. Roln. Poznaniu*, 62, 87–100

Kitching, W., Bullpitt, M., Gartshore, D., Adcock, W., Khor, T.O., Doddrell, D. & Rae, I.D. (1977) Carbon-13 nuclear magnetic resonance examination of naphthalene derivatives. Assignments and analysis of substituent chemical shifts. *J. org. Chem.*, 42, 2411–2418

Liberti, A., Ciccioli, P., Cecinato, A., Brancaleoni, E. & Di Palo, C. (1984) Determination of nitrated-polyaromatic hydrocarbons (nitro-PAHs) in environmental samples by high resolution chromatographic techniques. *J. high Resolut. Chromatogr. Chromatogr. Commun.*, 7, 389–397

Löfroth, G., Toftgård, R., Nilsson, L., Agurell, E. & Gustafsson, J.-Å. (1984) Short-term bioassays of nitro derivatives of benzo[a]pyrene and perylene. *Carcinogenesis*, 5, 925–930

Lucchini, V. & Wells, P.R. (1976) Proton magnetic resonance spectra of monosubstituted naphthalenes. *Org. magn. Resonance*, 8, 137–140

Matsuda, A. (1981) Studies on the mutagenicity of nitro-aromatic compounds in the environment (Jpn.). *Gifu Daigaku Igakuba Kiyo*, 29, 278–296

McCoy, E.C., Rosenkranz, E.J., Petrullo, L.A., Rosenkranz, H.S. & Mermelstein, R. (1981) Structural basis of the mutagenicity in bacteria of nitrated naphthalene and derivatives. *Environ. Mutagenesis*, *3*, 499–511

Mortelmans, K., Haworth, S., Lawlor, T., Speck, W., Tainer, B. & Zeiger, E. (1986) *Salmonella* mutagenicity tests: II. Results from the testing of 270 chemicals. *Environ. Mutagenesis*, *8*, Suppl. 7, 1–119

Nakamura, S.-I., Oda, Y., Shimada, T., Oki, I. & Sugimoto, K. (1987) SOS-inducing activity of chemical carcinogens and mutagens in *Salmonella typhimurium* TA1535/pSK1002: examination with 151 chemicals. *Mutat. Res.*, *192*, 239–246

National Cancer Institute (1978) *Bioassay of 1-Nitronaphthalene for Possible Carcinogenicity* (*NCI-CG-TR-64*) (*DHEW Publication No. NIH 78-1314*), Bethesda, MD, US Department of Health, Education, and Welfare

Nishioka, M.G., Petersen, B.A. & Lewtas, J. (1982) Comparison of nitro-aromatic content and direct-acting mutagenicity of diesel emissions. In: Cooke, M., Dennis, A.J. & Fisher, G.L., *Polynuclear Aromatic Hydrocarbons, Sixth International Symposium, Physical and Biological Chemistry*, Columbus, OH, Battelle, pp. 603–613

Pitts, J.N., Jr (1987) Nitration of gaseous polycyclic aromatic hydrocarbons in simulated and ambient urban atmospheres: a source of mutagenic nitroarenes. *Atmos. Environ.*, *21*, 2531–2547

Pitts, J.N., Jr, Atkinson, R., Sweetman, J.A. & Zielinska, B. (1985) The gas-phase reactions of naphthalene with $N_2O_5$ to form nitronaphthalenes. *Atmos. Environ.*, *19*, 701–705

Poirier, L.A. & Weisburger, J.H. (1974) Enzymic reduction of carcinogenic aromatic nitro compounds by rat and mouse liver fractions. *Biochem. Pharmacol.*, *23*, 661–669

Ramdahl, T. & Urdal, K. (1982) Determination of nitrated polycyclic aromatic hydrocarbons by fused silica capillary gas chromatography/negative ion chemical ionization mass spectrometry. *Anal. Chem.*, *54*, 2256–2260

Ramdahl, T., Becher, G. & Bjørseth, A. (1982) Nitrated polycyclic aromatic hydrocarbons in urban air particulates. *Environ. Sci. Technol.*, *16*, 861–865

Rasmussen, R.E. (1986) Metabolism and macromolecular binding of 1-nitronaphthalene in the mouse. *Toxicology*, *41*, 233–247

Rosenkranz, H.S. & Mermelstein, R. (1983) Mutagenicity and genotoxicity of nitroarenes: all nitro-containing chemicals were not created equal. *Mutat. Res.*, *114*, 217–267

Rosenkranz, H.S. & Mermelstein, R. (1985) The genotoxicity, metabolism and carcinogenicity of nitrated polycyclic aromatic hydrocarbons. *J. environ. Sci. Health*, *C3*, 221–272

Rosenkranz, H.S., McCoy, E.C., Sanders, D.R., Butler, M., Kiriazides, D.K. & Mermelstein, R. (1980) Nitropyrenes: isolation, identification and reduction of mutagenic impurities in carbon black and toners. *Science*, *209*, 1039–1043

Rosenkranz, H.S., McCoy, E.C., Frierson, M. & Klopman, G. (1985) The role of DNA sequence and structure of the electrophile on the mutagenicity of nitroarenes and arylamine derivatives. *Environ. Mutagenesis*, *7*, 645–653

Sanders, D.R. (1981) Nitropyrenes: the isolation of trace mutagenic impurities from the toluene extract of an aftertreated carbon black. In: Cooke, M. & Dennis, A.J., eds, *Polynuclear Aromatic Hydrocarbons, 5th International Symposium, Chemical Analysis and Biological Fate*, Columbus, OH, Battelle, pp. 145–158

Sax, N.I. & Lewis, R.J., eds (1987) *Hawley's Condensed Chemical Dictionary*, 11th ed., New York, Van Nostrand Reinhold, p. 735

Schuetzle, D. & Jensen, T.E. (1985) Analysis of nitrated polycyclic aromatic hydrocarbons (nitro-PAH) by mass spectrometry. In: White, C.M., ed., *Nitrated Polycyclic Aromatic Hydrocarbons*, Heidelberg, A., Hüthig Verlag, pp. 121–167

Scribner, J.D., Fisk, S.R. & Scribner, N.K. (1979) Mechanisms of action of carcinogenic aromatic amines: an investigation using mutagenesis in bacteria. *Chem.-biol. Interactions*, 26, 11–25

Shelby, M.D. & Stasiewicz, S. (1984) Chemicals showing no evidence of carcinogenicity in long-term, two-species rodent studies: the need for short-term test data. *Environ. Mutagenesis*, 6, 871–878

Sternson, L.A. (1975) Detection of arylhydroxylamines as intermediates in the metabolic reduction of nitro compounds. *Experientia*, 31, 268–270

Tatsumi, K., Kitamura, S. & Narai, N. (1986) Reductive metabolism of aromatic nitro compounds including carcinogens by rabbit liver preparations. *Cancer Res.*, 46, 1089–1093

Tokiwa, H. & Ohnishi, Y. (1986) Mutagenicity and carcinogenicity of nitroarenes and their sources in the environment. *CRC crit. Rev. Toxicol.*, 17, 23–69

Tokiwa, H., Nakagawa, R. & Ohnishi, Y. (1981) Mutagenic assay of aromatic nitro compounds with *Salmonella typhimurium*. *Mutat. Res.*, 91, 321–325

Tokiwa, H., Nakagawa, R., Horikawa, K. & Ohkubo, A. (1987) The nature of the mutagenicity and carcinogenicity of nitrated, aromatic compounds in the environment. *Environ. Health Perspect.*, 73, 191–199

US Environmental Protection Agency (1986) *Toxic Substances Control Act Chemical Substance Inventory*, 1985 ed., Vol. III, *Substance Name Index (EPA-560/7-85-002c)*, Washington DC, Office of Toxic Substances

Valencia, R., Mason, J.M., Woodruff, R.C. & Zimmering, S. (1985) Chemical mutagenesis testing in *Drosophila*. III. Results of 48 coded compounds tested for the National Toxicology Program. *Environ. Mutagenesis*, 7, 325–348

Vance, W.A. & Levin, D.E. (1984) Structural features of nitroaromatics that determine mutagenic activity in *Salmonella typhimurium*. *Environ. Mutagenesis*, 6, 797–811

Weast, R.C. (1985) *CRC Handbook of Chemistry and Physics*, 66th ed., Boca Raton, FL, CRC Press, p. C-361

Windholz, M., ed. (1983) *The Merck Index*, 10th ed., Rahway, NJ, Merck & Co., p. 949

Wise, S.A., Chesler, S.N., Hilpert, L.R., May, W.E., Rebbert, R.E., Vogt, C.R., Nishioka, M.G., Austin, A. & Lewtas, J. (1985) Quantification of polycyclic aromatic hydrocarbons and nitro-substituted polycyclic aromatic hydrocarbons and mutagenicity testing for the characterization of ambient air particulate matter. *Environ. int.*, 11, 147–160

Ying, B., Zhong, Z., Liu, J., Li, J. & Xian, P. (1986) *Sulfur-free Fragrant Fireworks Powder*. Patent issued 10 April 1986, CN 85,101,596 (F42B4/04) [*Chem. Abstr.*, 106, 122513x]

# 2-NITRONAPHTHALENE

## 1. Chemical and Physical Data

### 1.1 Synonyms

*Chem. Abstr. Services Reg. No.*: 581-89-5
*Chem. Abstr. Name*: Naphthalene, 2-nitro-
*IUPAC Systematic Name*: 2-Nitronaphthalene
*Synonym*: β-Nitronaphthalene

### 1.2 Structural and molecular formulae and molecular weight

$C_{10}H_7NO_2$                                                       Mol. wt: 173.2

### 1.3 Chemical and physical properties of the pure substance

(a) *Description*: Yellow needles or plates from ethanol (Weast, 1985)

(b) *Boiling-point*: 165°C at 15°C (Weast, 1985)

(c) *Melting-point*: 79°C (Weast, 1985)

(d) *Spectroscopy data*: Proton and nuclear magnetic resonance and mass spectral data have been reported (Lucchini & Wells, 1976; Kitching *et al.*, 1977; Schuetzle & Jensen, 1985).

(e) *Solubility*: Soluble in ethanol and diethyl ether (Weast, 1985)

### 1.4 Technical products and impurities

2-Nitronaphthalene is available for research purposes (Aldrich Chemical Co., 1988). It is also available at a purity of 99.7% as a reference material (Belliardo *et al.*, 1988).

## 2. Production, Use, Occurrence and Analysis

### 2.1 Production and use

*(a) Production*

2-Nitronaphthalene is a by-product (2–3%) from the commercial preparation of 1-nitronaphthalene by direct nitration of naphthalene (Verschueren, 1983). It can be produced by the Bucherer reaction, starting with 2-naphthalenol (2-naphthol), and by other indirect methods; however, the Bucherer method, which yields 2-naphthylamine (see IARC, 1987), is seldom used (Gaydos, 1981).

*(b) Use*

No evidence was found that 2-nitronaphthalene has been used for commercial applications.

### 2.2 Occurrence

*(a) Engine exhaust*

Emissions from a heavy-duty diesel engine contained 2-nitronaphthalene at concentrations of 0.94 mg/kg in particulates when the engine was run at 100% load and 1200 revolutions/min and 0.87 mg/kg in particulates when the same engine was run at 75% load and 1800 revolutions/min (Draper, 1986).

*(b) Other occurrence*

Toners for use in photocopy machines have been produced in quantity since the late 1950s and have seen widespread use. 'Long-flow' furnace black was first used in photocopy toners in 1967; its manufacture involved an oxidation whereby some nitration also occurred. Subsequent changes in the production technique reduced the total extractable nitropyrene content from an uncontrolled level of 5–100 mg/kg to below 0.3 mg/kg (Rosenkranz *et al.*, 1980; Sanders, 1981; Butler *et al.*, 1983), and toners produced from this carbon black since 1980 have not been found to contain detectable levels of mutagenicity or, hence, nitropyrenes (Rosenkranz *et al.*, 1980; Butler *et al.*, 1983). One sample of a formerly available commercial carbon black was reported to contain detectable concentrations of unspecified nitronaphthalene (Ramdahl & Urdal, 1982).

2-Nitronaphthalene was detected in urban ambient airborne particulates in St Louis, MO, USA (Ramdahl & Urdal, 1982; Ramdahl *et al.*, 1982). In a laboratory experiment, 2-nitronaphthalene was formed by a gas-phase napthhalene nitration reaction at room temperature and atmospheric pressure with a yield of about 8% (Pitts *et al.*, 1985). It was postulated that significant amounts of 2-nitronaphthalene result from the night-time gas-phase reaction of naphthalene with nitrogen pentoxide (Pitts, 1987). Approximately equal amounts of 1- and 2-nitronaphthalene were found in day-time samples of ambient air in Torrance, CA, USA. 2-Nitronaphthalene concentrations were 1.1 ng/m$^3$ of sample during night-time sampling and 2.9 ng/m$^3$ of sample during day-time sampling (Arey *et al.*, 1987).

### 2.3 Analysis

See the monograph on 1-nitropyrene.

## 3. Biological Data Relevant to the Evaluation of Carcinogenic Risk to Humans

### 3.1 Carcinogenicity studies in animals[1]

*(a) Oral administration*

*Monkey*: One female rhesus monkey (*Macaca mulatta*) that had been infected with a laboratory strain of *Plasmodium cynomolgi* and cured with chloroquine at least 12 weeks before the beginning of the experiment received a daily dose of 242 mg/kg bw 2-nitronaphthalene ['purified' but purity not given] administered orally in hard gelatin capsules on six days per week for 54 months. The monkey was then killed (terminal weight, 5.7 kg) and necropsied, three papillomas were found in the urinary bladder; no tumour was found in other organs (Conzelman *et al.*, 1970). [The Working Group noted that results were available for only one animal.]

*(b) Bladder implantation*

*Mouse*: Three groups of 41, 76 and 80 mice [strain and age unspecified] received a surgical implant of a cholesterol pellet containing 2-nitronaphthalene [dose and purity unspecified] into the urinary bladder (Bryan *et al.*, 1964). Three groups of 72, 82 and 140 controls received implants of cholesterol only. In a further group of 38 mice, a sham operation was performed which consisted of incising the bladder, momentarily inserting a pellet of pure cholesterol, removing the pellet, closing the bladder and suturing the abdomen. Animals were observed for up to 490 days, and only animals surviving longer than 175 days were evaluated. At the end of the experiment, the incidences of carcinomas and benign tumours of the bladder did not differ significantly between the various groups: 2/41, 2/76 and 7/80 in the treated groups; 4/72, 1/82 and 2/140 in the cholesterol controls and none in the sham-operated animals.

---

[1]The Working Group was aware of studies in progress by single subcutaneous injection in mice (IARC, 1988).

## 3.2 Other relevant data

*(a) Experimental systems*

(i) *Absorption, distribution, excretion and metabolism*

2-Naphthylamine (see IARC, 1987) was detected in the urine of male Sprague-Dawley rats administered single intraperitoneal doses of 100 mg/kg bw 2-nitronaphthalene (Johnson & Cornish, 1978).

After male Wistar rats had been administered 2 mmol[350 mg]/kg bw 2-nitronaphthalene orally, the following metabolites (either free or conjugated) were excreted in the urine over the subsequent 32 h: 2-amino-1-naphthyl sulfate, 2-amino-1-naphthol and N-hydroxy-2-naphthylamine. All of these products were detected in the urine of rats treated similarly with 2-naphthylamine (Kadlubar *et al.*, 1981). [The Working Group noted that N-hydroxy-2-naphthylamine is tumorigenic to experimental animals. See, for example, Garner *et al.* (1984).] The urine of monkeys given oral doses of 2-nitronaphthalene was found to contain 2-amino-1-naphthyl sulfate and 2-acetamido-6-naphthyl glucuronide (Conzelman *et al.*, 1970).

As reported in an abstract, in male Sprague-Dawley rats treated orally with 0.5 mmol[87 mg]/kg bw 2-nitronaphthalene, covalent binding to haemoglobin was detected, although the level was lower than that found with 2-naphthylamine (Suzuki *et al.*, 1987).

Under anaerobic conditions, liver postmitochondrial supernatants and cytosol from male Fischer rats and female Swiss mice catalysed the stoichiometric conversion of 2-nitronaphthalene to 2-naphthylamine (Poirier & Weisburger, 1974).

Incubation of 2-nitronaphthalene with liver postmitochondrial supernatants from Wistar rats pretreated with sodium phenobarbital, 3-methylcholanthrene or Kanechlor-500 resulted in a time-dependent loss of substrate. The rate of metabolism was faster with homogenates from animals pretreated with 3-methylcholanthrene or Kanechlor-500 than with those from animals given phenobarbital (Ohe, 1985).

(ii) *Toxic effects*

A single intraperitoneal injection of 2-nitronaphthalene (100 mg/kg bw) to male Sprague-Dawley rats did not cause respiratory distress or lung or liver toxicity, in contrast to observations made with 1-nitronaphthalene (see monograph on 1-nitronaphthalene; Johnson *et al.*, 1984).

(iii) *Genetic and related effects*

The genetic and related effects of nitroarenes and of their metabolites have been reviewed (Rosenkranz & Mermelstein, 1983; Beland *et al.*, 1985; Rosenkranz & Mermelstein, 1985; Tokiwa & Ohnishi, 1986).

2-Nitronaphthalene preferentially inhibited the growth of DNA repair-deficient *Escherichia coli* (Rosenkranz & Poirier, 1979; DeFlora *et al.*, 1984) and *Bacillus subtilis* (at 100 μg/disc; Tokiwa *et al.*, 1987) and induced DNA damage in *Salmonella typhimurium* (lowest effective dose, 6 μg/ml; Nakamura *et al.*, 1987).

2-Nitronaphthalene was mutagenic to *S. typhimurium* strains TA1535, TA1537, TA1538, TA98 and TA100 (McCann *et al.*, 1975; Wang *et al.*, 1978; De Flora, 1979; Rosenkranz & Poirier, 1979; Scribner *et al.*, 1979; Simmon, 1979a; Wang *et al.*, 1980; De Flora, 1981; El-Bayoumy *et al.*, 1981; Ho *et al.*, 1981; Löfroth, 1981; McCoy *et al.*, 1981; De Flora *et al.*, 1984; Morotomi & Watanabe, 1984) but not to strain TA97 (Rosenkranz *et al.*, 1985).

This compound induced recombination in the yeast, *Saccharomyces cerevisiae* D3 (Simmon, 1979b).

In a host-mediated assay in mice, 2-nitronaphthalene (at 125–1300 mg/kg) induced mutation in *S. typhimurium* TA1530 and TA1538 but not recombination in *S. cerevisiae* D3 (Simmon *et al.*, 1979).

2-Nitronaphthalene did not induce unscheduled DNA synthesis in cultured rat or mouse hepatocytes (Mori *et al.*, 1987) but did induce morphological transformation of Syrian hamster embryo cells (Pienta, 1980).

*(b) Humans*

No data were available to the Working Group.

### 3.3 Epidemiological studies and case reports of carcinogenicity in humans

No data were available to the Working Group.

## 4. Summary of Data Reported and Evaluation

### 4.1 Exposure data

2-Nitronaphthalene has been detected in particulate emissions from diesel engines. It has also been found at low concentrations in ambient air.

### 4.2 Experimental data

2-Nitronaphthalene was tested for carcinogenicity by prolonged oral administration in one monkey, producing papillomas in the urinary bladder. Implantation of cholesterol pellets containing 2-nitronaphthalene into the bladder of mice did not increase the incidence of urinary bladder tumours.

### 4.3 Human data

No data were available to the Working Group.

### 4.4 Other relevant data

*N*-Hydroxy-2-naphthylamine (which has been shown to induce tumours in experimental animals) and 2-naphthylamine (which is causally associated with cancer in humans) have been detected as metabolites of 2-nitronaphthalene in the urine of rats.

2-Nitronaphthalene induced morphological transformation in cultured animal cells but did not induce DNA damage in cultured rodent hepatocytes. It induced DNA damage and mutation in bacteria and recombination in yeast.

### 4.5 Evaluation[1]

There is *inadequate evidence* for the carcinogenicity in experimental animals of 2-nitronaphthalene.

No data were available from studies in humans on the carcinogenicity of 2-nitronaphthalene.

**Overall evaluation**

2-Nitronaphthalene *is not classifiable as to its carcinogenicity to humans (Group 3)*.

## 5. References

Aldrich Chemical Co. (1988) *Aldrich Catalog/Handbook of Fine Chemicals 1988-1989*, Milwaukee, WI, p. 1118

Arey, J., Zielinska, B., Atkinson, R. & Winer, A.M. (1987) Polycyclic aromatic hydrocarbon and nitroarene concentrations in ambient air during a wintertime high-$NO_x$ episode in the Los Angeles basin. *Atmos. Environ.*, 21, 1437–1444

Beland, F.A., Heflich, R.H., Howard, P.C. & Fu, P.P. (1985) The in vitro metabolic activation of nitro polycyclic aromatic hydrocarbons. In: Harvey, R.G., ed., *Polycyclic Hydrocarbons and Carcinogenesis (ACS Symposium Series No. 283)*, Washington DC, American Chemical Society, pp. 371–396

Belliardo, J.J., Jacob, J. & Lindsey, A.S. (1988) *The Certification of the Purity of Seven Nitropolycyclic Aromatic Compounds, CRM Nos 305, 306, 307, 308, 310, 311, 312, Reference Materials, BCR Information (EUR 11254 EN)*, Brussels, Commission of the European Communities, p. III

Bryan, G.T., Brown, R.R. & Price, J.M. (1964) Mouse bladder carcinogenicity of certain tryptophan metabolites and other aromatic nitrogen compounds suspended in cholesterol. *Cancer Res.*, 24, 596–602

---

[1] For definitions of the italicized terms, see Preamble, pp. 25–28.

## Summary table of genetic and related effects of 2-nitronaphthalene

| Nonmammalian systems | | | | | | | | | | | | | | Mammalian systems | | | | | | | | | | | | | | | | | | | | |
|---|---|---|---|---|---|---|---|---|---|---|---|---|---|---|---|---|---|---|---|---|---|---|---|---|---|---|---|---|---|---|---|---|---|---|
| Proka-ryotes | Lower eukaryotes | | | Plants | | | | Insects | | | | | | In vitro | | | | | | | | | | | | | | | In vivo | | | | | |
| | | | | | | | | | | | | | | Animal cells | | | | | | | | | Human cells | | | | | | Animals | | | | | Humans |
| D | D | G | R | A | D | G | C | R | G | C | A | D | G | S | M | C | A | T | I | D | G | S | M | C | A | T | I | D | G | S | M | C | DL | A | D | S | M | C | A |
| + | +¹ | | | | | | | | | | | – | | | | | | | +¹ | | | | | | | | | | | | | | | | | | | | |

A, aneuploidy; C, chromosomal aberrations; D, DNA damage; DL, dominant lethal mutation; G, gene mutation; I, inhibition of intercellular communication; M, micronuclei; R, mitotic recombination and gene conversion; S, sister chromatid exchange; T, cell transformation

*In completing the table, the following symbols indicate the consensus of the Working Group with regard to the results for each endpoint:*
+ considered to be positive for the specific endpoint and level of biological complexity
+¹ considered to be positive, but only one valid study was available to the Working Group
– considered to be negative

Butler, M.A., Evans, D.L., Giammarise, A.T., Kiriazides, D.K., Marsh, D., McCoy, E.C., Mermelstein, R., Murphy, C.B. & Rosenkranz, H.S. (1983) Application of *Salmonella* assay to carbon blacks and toners. In: Cooke, M. & Dennis, A.J., eds, *Polynuclear Aromatic Hydrocarbons, 7th International Symposium, Formation, Metabolism and Measurement*, Columbus, OH, Battelle, pp. 225–241

Conzelman, G.M., Jr, Moulton, J.E. & Flanders, L.E., III (1970) Tumors in the urinary bladder of a monkey: induction with 2-nitronaphthalene. *Gann, 61*, 79–80

DeFlora, S. (1979) Metabolic activation and deactivation of mutagens and carcinogens. *Ital. J. Biochem., 28*, 81–103

De Flora, S. (1981) Study of 106 organic and inorganic compounds in the *Salmonella*/microsome test. *Carcinogenesis, 2*, 283–298

De Flora, S., Zanacchi, P., Camoirano, A., Bennicelli, C. & Badolati, G.S. (1984) Genotoxic activity and potency of 135 compounds in the Ames reversion test and in a bacterial DNA-repair test. *Mutat. Res., 133*, 161–198

Draper, W.M. (1986) Quantitation of nitro- and dinitropolycyclic aromatic hydrocarbons in diesel exhaust particulate matter. *Chemosphere, 15*, 437–447

El-Bayoumy, K., Lavoie, E.J., Hecht, S.S., Fow, E.A. & Hoffmann, D. (1981) The influence of methyl substitution on the mutagenicity of nitronaphthalenes and nitrobiphenyls. *Mutat. Res., 81*, 143–153

Garner, R.C., Martin, C.N. & Clayson, D.B. (1984) Carcinogenic aromatic amines and related compounds. In: Searle, C.E., ed, *Chemical Carcinogens*, 2nd ed., Vol. 1 (*ACS Monograph 182*), Washington DC, American Chemical Society, pp. 175–276

Gaydos, R.M. (1981) Naphthalene. In: Mark, H.F., Othmer, D.F., Overberger, C.G., Seaborg, G.T. & Grayson, M., eds, *Kirk-Othmer Encyclopedia of Chemical Technology*, 3rd ed., Vol. 15, New York, John Wiley & Sons, pp. 698–719

Ho, C.H., Clark, B.R., Guerin, M.R., Barkenbus, B.D., Rao, T.K. & Epler, J.L. (1981) Analytical and biological analyses of test materials from the synthetic fuel technologies. IV. Studies of chemical structure-mutagenic activity relationships of aromatic nitrogen compounds relevant to synfuels. *Mutat. Res., 85*, 335–345

IARC (1987) *IARC Monographs on the Evaluation of Carcinogenic Risks to Humans*, Suppl. 7, *Overall Evaluations of Carcinogenicity: An Updating of IARC Monographs Volumes 1 to 42*, Lyon, pp. 261–263

IARC (1988) *Information Bulletin on the Survey of Chemicals Being Tested for Carcinogenicity*, No. 13, Lyon, p. 20

Johnson, D.E. & Cornish, H.H. (1978) Metabolic conversion of 1- and 2-nitronaphthalene to 1- and 2-naphthylamine in the rat. *Toxicol. appl. Pharmacol., 46*, 549–553

Johnson, D.E., Riley, M.G.I. & Cornish, H.H. (1984) Acute target organ toxicity of 1-nitronaphthalene in the rat. *J. appl. Toxicol., 4*, 253–257

Kadlubar, F.F., Unruh, L.E., Flammang, T.J., Sparks, D., Mitchum, R.K. & Mulder, G.J. (1981) Alteration of urinary levels of the carcinogen, $N$-hydroxy-2-naphthylamine, and its $N$-glucuronide in the rat by control of urinary pH, inhibition of metabolic sulfation, and changes in biliary excretion. *Chem.-biol. Interactions, 33*, 129–147

Kitching, W., Bullpitt, M., Gartshore, D., Adcock, W., Khor, T.C., Doddrell, D. & Rae, I.D. (1977) Carbon-13 nuclear magnetic resonance examination of naphthalene derivatives. Assignments and analysis of substituent chemical shifts. *J. org. Chem., 42*, 2411–2418

Löfroth, G. (1981) Comparison of the mutagenic activity in carbon particulate matter and in diesel and gasoline engine exhaust. In: Waters, M.D., Sandhu, S., Lewtas Huisingh, J., Claxton, L. & Nesnow, S., eds, *Application of Short-term Bioassays in the Analysis of Complex Environmental Mixtures, II*, New York, Plenum, pp. 319–336

Lucchini, V. & Wells, P.R. (1976) Proton magnetic resonance spectra of monosubstituted naphthalenes. *Org. magn. Resonance*, 8, 137–140

McCann, J., Choi, E., Yamasaki, E. & Ames, B.N. (1975) Detection of carcinogens as mutagens in the *Salmonella*/microsome test: assay of 300 chemicals. *Proc. natl Acad. Sci. USA*, 72, 5135–5139

McCoy, E.C., Rosenkranz, E.J., Petrullo, L.A., Rosenkranz, H.S. & Mermelstein, R. (1981) Structural basis of the mutagenicity in bacteria of nitrated naphthalene and derivatives. *Environ. Mutagenesis*, 3, 499–511

Mori, H., Sugie, S., Yoshimi, N., Kinouchi, T. & Ohnishi, Y. (1987) Genotoxicity of a variety of nitroarenes and other nitro compounds in DNA-repair tests with rat and mouse hepatocytes. *Mutat. Res.*, 190, 159–167

Morotomi, M. & Watanabe, T. (1984) Metabolism of exogenous compounds by the intestinal microflora (Jpn.). *Tikoshikoroji Foramu* [*Toxicol. Forum*], 7, 395–408

Nakamura, S., Oda, Y., Shimada, T., Oki, I. & Sugimoto, K. (1987) SOS-inducing activity of chemical carcinogens and mutagens in *Salmonella typhimurium* TA1535/pSK1002: examination with 151 chemicals. *Mutat. Res.*, 192, 239–246

Ohe, T. (1985) Studies on comparative decomposition rate by rat liver homogenate and on micronucleus test of nitrated polycyclic aromatic hydrocarbons. *Bull. environ. Contam. Toxicol.*, 34, 715–721

Pienta, R.J. (1980) Transformation of Syrian hamster embryo cells by diverse chemicals and correlation with their reported carcinogenic and mutagenic activities. In: de Serres, F.J. & Hollaender, A., eds, *Chemical Mutagens, Principles and Methods for Their Detection*, Vol. 6, New York, Plenum, pp. 175–202

Pitts, J.N., Jr (1987) Nitration of gaseous polycyclic aromatic hydrocarbons in simulated and ambient urban atmospheres: a source of mutagenic nitroarenes. *Atmos. Environ.*, 21, 2531–2547

Pitts, J.N., Jr, Atkinson, R., Sweetman, J.A. & Zielinska, B. (1985) The gas-phase reactions of naphthalene with $N_2O_5$ to form nitronaphthalenes. *Atmos. Environ.*, 19, 701–705

Poirier, L.A. & Weisburger, J.H. (1974) Enzymic reduction of carcinogenic aromatic nitro compounds by rat and mouse liver fractions. *Biochem. Pharmacol.*, 23, 661–669

Ramdahl, T. & Urdal, K. (1982) Determination of nitrated polycyclic aromatic hydrocarbons by fused silica capillary gas chromatography/negative ion chemical ionization mass spectrometry. *Anal. Chem.*, 54, 2256–2260

Ramdahl, T., Becher, G. & Bjørseth, A. (1982) Nitrated polycyclic aromatic hydrocarbons in urban air particles. *Environ. Sci. Technol.*, 16, 861–865

Rosenkranz, H.S. & Mermelstein, R. (1983) Mutagenicity and genotoxicity of nitroarenes: all nitro-containing chemicals were not created equal. *Mutat. Res.*, 114, 217–267

Rosenkranz, H.S. & Mermelstein, R. (1985) The genotoxicity, metabolism and carcinogenicity of nitrated polycyclic aromatic hydrocarbons. *J. environ. Sci. Health*, C3, 221–272

Rosenkranz, H.S. & Poirier, L.A. (1979) Evaluation of the mutagenicity and DNA-modifying activity of carcinogens and non-carcinogens in microbial systems. *J. natl Cancer Inst.*, 62, 873–892

Rosenkranz, H.S., McCoy, E.C., Sanders, D.R., Butler, M., Kiriazides, D.K. & Mermelstein, R. (1980) Nitropyrenes: isolation, identification and reduction of mutagenic impurities in carbon black and toners. *Science*, 209, 1039—1043

Rosenkranz, H.S., McCoy, E.C., Frierson, M. & Klopman, G. (1985) The role of DNA sequence and structure of the electrophile on the mutagenicity of nitroarenes and arylamine derivatives. *Environ. Mutagenesis*, 7, 645—653

Sanders, D.R. (1981) Nitropyrenes: the isolation of trace mutagenic impurities from the toluene extract of an aftertreated carbon black. In: Cooke, M. & Dennis, A.J., eds, *Polynuclear Aromatic Hydrocarbons, 5th International Symposium, Chemical Analysis and Biological Fate*, Columbus, OH, Battelle, pp. 145—158

Schuetzle, D. & Jensen, T.E. (1985) Analysis of nitrated polycyclic aromatic hydrocarbons (nitro-PAH) by mass spectrometry. In: White, C.M., ed., *Nitrated Polycyclic Aromatic Hydrocarbons*, Heidelberg, A. Hüthig Verlag, pp. 121—167

Scribner, J.D., Fisk, S.R. & Scribner, N.K. (1979) Mechanisms of action of carcinogenic aromatic amines: an investigation using mutagenesis in bacteria. *Chem.-biol. Interactions*, 26, 11—25

Simmon, V.F. (1979a) In vitro mutagenicity assays of chemical carcinogens and related compounds with *Salmonella typhimurium*. *J. natl Cancer Inst.*, 62, 893—899

Simmon, V.F. (1979b) In vitro assays for recombinogenic activity of chemical carcinogens and related compounds with *Saccharomyces cerevisiae* D3. *J. natl Cancer Inst.*, 62, 901—909

Simmon, V.F., Rosenkranz, H.S., Zeiger, E. & Poirier, L.A. (1979) Mutagenic activity of chemical carcinogens and related compounds in the intraperitoneal host-mediated assay. *J. natl Cancer Inst.*, 62, 911—918

Suzuki, J., Meguro, S. & Suzuki, S. (1987) Comparison of in vivo binding of aromatic nitro and amino compounds to rat hemoglobin (Abstract F 06-Y-13). *J. pharm. Sci.*, 76, S126

Tokiwa, H. & Ohnishi, Y. (1986) Mutagenicity and carcinogenicity of nitroarenes and their sources in the environment. *CRC crit. Rev. Toxicol.*, 17, 23—69

Tokiwa, H., Nakagawa, R., Horikawa, K. & Ohkubo, A. (1987) The nature of the mutagenicity and carcinogenicity of nitrated, aromatic compounds in the environment. *Environ. Health Perspect.*, 73, 191—199

Verschueren, K. (1983) *Handbook of Environmental Data on Organic Chemicals*, 2nd ed., New York, Van Nostrand Reinhold, p. 917

Wang, Y.Y., Rappaport, S.M., Sawyer, R.F., Talcott, R.E. & Wei, E.T. (1978) Direct-acting mutagens in automobile exhaust. *Cancer Lett.*, 5, 39—47

Wang, C.Y., Lee, M.-S., King, C.M. & Warner, P.O. (1980) Evidence for nitroaromatics as direct-acting mutagens of airborne particulates. *Chemosphere*, 9, 83—87

Weast, R.C. (1985) *CRC Handbook of Chemistry and Physics*, 66th ed., Boca Raton, FL, CRC Press, p. C-361

# 3-NITROPERYLENE

## 1. Chemical and Physical Data

### 1.1 Synonyms

*Chem. Abstr. Services Reg. No.*: 20589-63-3
*Chem. Abstr. Name*: Perylene, 3-nitro-
*IUPAC Systematic Name*: 3-Nitroperylene

### 1.2 Structural and molecular formulae and molecular weight

$C_{20}H_{11}NO_2$                      Mol. wt: 297.3

### 1.3 Chemical and physical properties of the pure substance

(a) *Description*: Brick-red crystals from benzene (Buckingham, 1984)

(b) *Melting-point*: 210–212°C (Buckingham, 1984)

(c) *Spectroscopy data*: Nuclear magnetic resonance and mass spectral data have been reported (Looker, 1972; Eberson & Radner, 1985; Schuetzle & Jensen, 1985).

### 1.4 Technical products and impurities

No data were available to the Working Group.

## 2. Production, Use, Occurrence and Analysis

### 2.1 Production and use

No evidence was found that 3-nitroperylene has been produced in commercial quantities or used for commercial applications.

### 2.2 Occurrence

Toners for use in photocopy machines have been produced in quantity since the late 1950s and have seen widespread use. 'Long-flow' furnace black was first used in photocopy toners in 1967; its manufacture involved an oxidation whereby some nitration also occurred. Subsequent changes in the production technique reduced the total extractable nitropyrene content from an uncontrolled level of 5–100 mg/kg to below 0.3 mg/kg (Rosenkranz *et al.*, 1980; Sanders, 1981; Butler *et al.*, 1983), and toners produced from this carbon black since 1980 have not been found to contain detectable levels of mutagenicity or, hence, nitropyrenes (Rosenkranz *et al.*, 1980; Butler *et al.*, 1983).

3-Nitroperylene was formed when perylene, deposited on high-volume filters, was exposed to simulated atmospheres with 0.5 ppm (1 mg/m$^3$) nitrogen dioxide and 0.35 ppm (0.9 mg/m$^3$) gaseous nitric acid, or 0.3–5 ppm (0.6–0.5 mg/m$^3$) nitrogen dioxide, 0.1 ppm (0.3 mg/m$^3$) nitric acid, 1.5 ppm (6.6 mg/m$^3$) nitrogen pentoxide and traces of NO$_3$ radicals (Pitts *et al.*, 1985). A compound with a mass number of 297 detected in an extract of diesel particulates was characterized tentatively as 3-nitroperylene (Paputa-Peck *et al.*, 1983).

### 2.3 Analysis

See the monograph on 1-nitropyrene.

## 3. Biological Data Relevant to the Evaluation of Carcinogenic Risk to Humans

### 3.1 Carcinogenicity studies in animals[1]

*Skin application*

*Mouse*: In a study of initiating activity, a group of 20 female CD-1 Charles River mice, aged 50–55 days, received ten applications of 0.1 mg 3-nitroperylene (purity, >99%) in 0.1 ml acetone onto shaved back skin every other day for 20 days (total dose, 1.0 mg; El-Bayoumy *et al.*, 1982). A further group received a total dose of 0.05 mg benzo[*a*]pyrene

---

[1]The Working Group was aware of a study in progress in mice by single subcutaneous injection (IARC, 1988).

(purity, >99%), and a group of 20 females receiving acetone alone served as vehicle controls. Starting ten days after initiation had been completed, the animals received applications of 2.5 µg 12-O-tetradecanoylphorbol 13-acetate in 0.1 ml acetone three times per week for 25 weeks. At the end of this time, skin tumours (mainly squamous-cell papillomas) were observed in 8/20 3-nitroperylene-treated, in 1/20 vehicle controls and in 18/20 benzo[a]-pyrene-treated animals. The tumour incidence in the 3-nitroperylene-treated group was significantly greater than that in vehicle controls ($p < 0.01$).

### 3.2 Other relevant data

*(a) Experimental systems*

*Absorption, distribution, excretion and metabolism*

Incubation of *Salmonella typhimurium* TA98 with [$^3$H]3-nitroperylene in the presence of a rat liver postmitochondrial supernatant gave rise to a number of polar metabolites (Andrews *et al.*, 1983). Similar results were obtained with liver microsomes from Sprague-Dawley rats pretreated with Aroclor 1254 (Anderson *et al.*, 1987).

*Toxic effects*

No data were available to the Working Group.

*Genetic and related effects*

The genetic and related effects of nitroarenes and of their metabolites have been reviewed (Rosenkranz & Mermelstein, 1983; Beland *et al.*, 1985; Rosenkranz & Mermelstein, 1985; Tokiwa & Ohnishi, 1986).

3-Nitroperylene induced mutation in *Salmonella typhimurium* TA100 and TA98 in the presence of an exogenous metabolic system from rat liver (Ho *et al.*, 1981; Pitts, 1983; Greibrokk *et al.*, 1984; Löfroth *et al.*, 1984; Anderson *et al.*, 1987).

*(b) Humans*

No data were available to the Working Group.

### 3.3 Epidemiological studies and case reports of carcinogenicity to humans

No data were available to the Working Group.

## 4. Summary of Data Reported and Evaluation

### 4.1 Exposure data

No data were available to the Working Group.

## 4.2 Experimental carcinogenicity data

3-Nitroperylene was tested for carcinogenicity in an initiation-promotion experiment on mouse skin and was active as an initiator.

## 4.3 Human carcinogenicity data

No data were available to the Working Group.

## 4.4 Other relevant data

3-Nitroperylene was mutagenic to bacteria in the presence of an exogenous metabolic system.

## 4.5 Evaluation[1]

There is *inadequate evidence* for the carcinogenicity in experimental animals of 3-nitroperylene.

No data were available from studies in humans on the carcinogenicity of 3-nitroperylene in humans.

### Overall evaluation

3-Nitroperylene *is not classifiable as to its carcinogenicity to humans (Group 3)*.

# 5. References

Anderson, J.G., McCalla, D.R., Bryant, D.W., McCarry, B.E. & Bromke, A.M. (1987) Metabolic activation of 3-nitroperylene in the *Salmonella*/S9 assay. *Mutagenesis*, 2, 279–285

Andrews, P.A., Bryant, D., Vitakunas, S., Gouin, M., Anderson, G., McCarry, B.E., Quilliam, M.A. & McCalla, D.R. (1983) Metabolism of nitrated polycyclic aromatic hydrocarbons and formation of DNA-adducts in *Salmonella* typhimurium. In: Cooke, M. & Dennis, A.J., eds, *Polycyclic Aromatic Hydrocarbons, 7th International Symposium, Formation, Metabolism and Measurement*, Columbus, OH, Battelle, pp. 89–98

Beland, F.A., Heflich, R.H., Howard, P.C. & Fu, P.P. (1985) The in vitro metabolic activation of nitro polycyclic aromatic hydrocarbons. In: Harvey, R.G., ed., *Polycyclic Hydrocarbons and Carcinogenesis (ACS Symposium Series No. 283)*, Washington DC, American Chemical Society, pp. 371–396

Buckingham, J., ed. (1984) *Dictionary of Organic Compounds*, 4th ed., 2nd Suppl., New York, Chapman & Hall, pp. 340–341 (N-20063)

---

[1]For definitions of the italicized terms, see Preamble, pp. 25–28.

## Summary table of genetic and related effects of 3-nitroperylene

| Nonmammalian systems | | | | | | | | | | | | | Mammalian systems | | | | | | | | | | | | | | | | | | | | | |
|---|---|---|---|---|---|---|---|---|---|---|---|---|---|---|---|---|---|---|---|---|---|---|---|---|---|---|---|---|---|---|---|---|---|---|
| Proka-ryotes | | | | Lower eukaryotes | | | | Plants | | | | Insects | In vitro | | | | | | | | | | | | | | | In vivo | | | | | | |
| | | | | | | | | | | | | | Animal cells | | | | | | | | Human cells | | | | | | | | Animals | | | | | Humans | |
| D | G | D | R | G | A | D | G | C | R | G | C | A | D | G | S | M | C | A | T | I | D | G | S | M | C | A | T | I | D | G | S | M | C | DL | A | D | S | M | C | A |
| + | | | | | | | | | | | | | | | | | | | | | | | | | | | | | | | | | | | | | | | | |

A, aneuploidy; C, chromosomal aberrations; D, DNA damage; DL, dominant lethal mutation; G, gene mutation; I, inhibition of intercellular communication; M, micronuclei; R, mitotic recombination and gene conversion; S, sister chromatid exchange; T, cell transformation

+, considered to be positive for the specific endpoint and level of biological complexity

Butler, M.A., Evans, D.L., Giammarise, A.T., Kiriazides, D.K., Marsh, D., McCoy, E.C., Mermelstein, R., Murphy, C.B. & Rosenkranz, H.S. (1983) Application of *Salmonella* assay to carbon blacks and toners. In: Cooke, M. & Dennis, A.J., eds, *Polynuclear Aromatic Hydrocarbons, 7th International Symposium, Formation, Metabolism and Measurement*, Columbus, OH, Battelle, pp. 225–241

Eberson, L. & Radner, F. (1985) Nitration of aromatics via electron transfer. IV. On the reaction between perylene radical cation and nitrogen dioxide or nitrite ion. *Acta chem. scand. Ser. B, 39*, 357–374

El-Bayoumy, K., Hecht, S.S. & Hoffmann, D. (1982) Comparative tumor intiating activity on mouse skin of 6-nitrobenzo[*a*]pyrene, 6-nitrochrysene, 3-nitroperylene, 1-nitropyrene and their parent hydrocarbons. *Cancer Lett., 16*, 333–337

Greibrokk, T., Löfroth, G., Nilsson, L., Toftgård, R., Carlstedt-Duke, J. & Gustafsson, J.-Å. (1984) Nitroarenes: mutagenicity in the Ames *Salmonella*/microsome assay and affinity to the TCDD-receptor protein. In: Rickert, D.E., ed., *Toxicity of Nitroaromatic Compounds*, Washington DC, Hemisphere, pp. 167–183

Ho, C.-H., Clark, B.R., Guerin, M.R., Barkenbus, B.D., Rao, T.K. & Epler, J.L. (1981) Analytical and biological analyses of test materials from the synthetic fuel technologies. IV. Studies of chemical structure-mutagenic activity relationships of aromatic nitrogen compounds relevant to synfuels. *Mutat. Res., 85*, 335–345

IARC (1988) *Information Bulletin on the Survey of Chemicals Being Tested for Carcinogenicity*, No. 13, Lyon, p. 21

Löfroth, G., Toftgård, R., Nilsson, L., Agurell, E. & Gustafsson, J.-Å. (1984) Short-term bioassays of nitro derivatives of benzo[*a*]pyrene and perylene. *Carcinogenesis, 5*, 925–930

Looker, J.J. (1972) Mononitration of perylene. Preparation and structure proof of the 1 and 3 isomers. *J. org. Chem., 37*, 3379–3381

Paputa-Peck, M.C., Marano, R.S., Schuetzle, D., Riley, T.L., Hampton, C.V., Prater, T.J., Skewes, L.M., Jensen, T.E., Ruehle, P.H., Bosch, L.C. & Duncan, W.P. (1983) Determination of nitrated polynuclear aromatic hydrocarbons in particulate extracts by capillary column gas chromatography with nitrogen selective detection. *Anal. Chem., 55*, 1946–1954

Pitts, J.N., Jr (1983) Formation and fate of gaseous and particulate mutagens and carcinogens in real and simulated atmospheres. *Environ. Health Perspect., 47*, 115–140

Pitts, J.N., Jr, Zielinska, B., Sweetman, J.A., Atkinson, R. & Winer, A.M. (1985) Reaction of adsorbed pyrene and perylene with gaseous $N_2O_5$ under simulated atmospheric conditions. *Atmos. Environ., 19*, 911–915

Rosenkranz, H.S. & Mermelstein, R. (1983) Mutagenicity and genotoxicity of nitroarenes: all nitro-containing chemicals were not created equal. *Mutat. Res., 114*, 217–267

Rosenkranz, H.S. & Mermelstein, R. (1985) The genotoxicity, metabolism and carcinogenicity of nitrated polycyclic aromatic hydrocarbons. *J. environ. Sci. Health, C3*, 221–272

Rosenkranz, H.S., McCoy, E.C., Sanders, D.R., Butler, M., Kiriazides, D.K. & Mermelstein, R. (1980) Nitropyrenes: isolation, identification and reduction of mutagenic impurities in carbon black and toners. *Science, 209*, 1039–1043

Sanders, D.R. (1981) Nitropyrenes: the isolation of trace mutagenic impurities from the toluene extract of an aftertreated carbon black. In: Cooke, M. & Dennis, A.J., eds, *Polynuclear Aromatic Hydrocarbons, 5th International Symposium, Chemical Analysis and Biological Fate*, Columbus, OH, Battelle, pp. 145–158

Schuetzle, D. & Jensen, T.E. (1985) Analysis of nitrated polycyclic aromatic hydrocarbons (nitro-PAH) by mass spectrometry. In: White, C.M., ed., *Nitrated Polycyclic Aromatic Hydrocarbons*, Heidelberg, A. Hüthig Verlag, pp. 121–167

Tokiwa, H. & Ohnishi, Y. (1986) Mutagenicity and carcinogenicity of nitroarenes and their sources in the environment. *CRC crit. Rev. Toxicol.*, *17*, 23–69

# 1-NITROPYRENE

This substance was considered by a previous Working Group, in June 1983 (IARC, 1984). Since that time, new data have become available, and these have been incorporated into the monograph and taken into consideration in the present evaluation.

## 1. Chemical and Physical Data

### 1.1 Synonyms

*Chem. Abstr. Services Reg. No.*: 5522-43-0
*Chem. Abstr. Name*: Pyrene, 1-nitro-
*IUPAC Systematic Name*: 1-Nitropyrene
*Synonym*: 3-Nitropyrene

### 1.2 Structural and molecular formulae and molecular weight

$C_{16}H_9NO_2$  Mol. wt: 247.3

### 1.3 Chemical and physical properties of the pure substance

(a) *Description*: Yellow needles or prisms from ethanol (Prager & Jacobson, 1922)

(b) *Melting-point*: 155°C (Luckenbach, 1980)

(c) *Spectroscopy data*: Ultra-violet (Bavin & Dewar, 1955; Paputa-Peck et al., 1983), nuclear magnetic resonance (Kaplan, 1981; Paputa-Peck et al., 1983) and mass (Schuetzle & Jensen, 1985) spectral data have been reported.

(d) *Solubility*: Very soluble in diethyl ether (Prager & Jacobson, 1922); soluble in ethanol and benzene at 15°C (Luckenbach, 1980); soluble in toluene and tetrahydrofluorenone (Chemsyn Science Laboratories, 1988)

(e) *Reactivity*: Reacts with ethanolic potassium hydroxide to form 1,1'-azoxypyrene; also reacts with zinc powder in ethanol in the presence of catalytic amounts of ammonium chloride or ammonia to form 1,1'-azoxypyrene or, without air, 1-aminopyrene and 1-hydroxylaminopyrene (Boit, 1965)

(f) *Stability*: Photodecomposition to 2-propanol is readily induced by ultra-violet/visible light (Stärk *et al.*, 1985).

**1.4 Technical products and impurities**

1-Nitropyrene is available for research purposes at 97% (Aldrich Chemical Co., 1988) or ≥99.5% purity with ≤0.1% total dinitropyrenes and pyrene (Chemsyn Science Laboratories, 1988). It is available at a purity of 99.68% as a reference material (Belliardo *et al.*, 1988).

# 2. Production, Use, Occurrence and Analysis

## 2.1 Production and use

(a) *Production*

1-Nitropyrene was first synthesized by Graebe in 1871 by heating pyrene with equal parts of nitric acid and water. It can also be obtained (in a mixture with dinitropyrenes) by the addition of potassium nitrite to a solution of pyrene in diethyl ether, followed by the slow addition of dilute sulfuric acid (Prager & Jacobson, 1922). This compound has also been synthesized by heating pyrene with nitric acid in acetic acid at 50°C (Boit, 1965). 1-Nitropyrene was the only mononitropyrene isomer produced when pyrene was reacted with nitrogen pentoxide in carbon tetrachloride, and only traces of other isomers were found (Pitts *et al.*, 1985).

1-Nitropyrene is formed as a result of the photochemical oxidation of 1-aminopyrene induced by ultra-violet A irradiation (Okinaka *et al.*, 1986).

Since 1972, one Japanese company has produced this compound by the reaction of pyrene with nitric acid. 1-Nitropyrene is reported in the 1985 *Toxic Substances Control Act Chemical Substance Inventory* (US Environmental Protection Agency, 1986).

(b) *Use*

1-Nitropyrene has been reported to be a chemical photosensitizer, increasing the spectral sensitivity of bis-azide compounds in the long-wavelength region (Tsunoda *et al.*, 1973). It has been reported that one Japanese company uses 1-nitropyrene as an intermediate in the production of 1-azidopyrene, which is used in photosensitive printing.

## 2.2 Occurrence

*(a) Engine exhaust*

1-Nitropyrene is one of the major nitroarenes in primary particulate emissions of diesel engines (Pitts, 1987). Substantially decreased amounts of 1-nitropyrene were reported in exhausts emitted from a single cylinder when nitrogen-free air was used in the diesel engine (Herr *et al.*, 1982). Illustrative data on 1-nitropyrene levels in the particles of exhaust emissions and in extracts of these particles are summarized in Table 1.

1-Nitropyrene has also been identified in used oil from a light-duty diesel engine at levels of 0.2 mg/kg after 8000 km and 0.5 mg/kg after 9000 km (Jensen *et al.*, 1986), and Manabe *et al.* (1984) found 0.4 mg/kg in used (4600 km) diesel engine oil and 0.2 mg/kg in used (3200 km) gasoline engine oil. Jensen *et al.* (1986) reported that oil was the source of a significant amount (16–80% depending on engine load) of extractable organic materials in diesel particulate emissions. Since 1-nitropyrene was not detected in new oil (on the basis of a detection limit of 0.1 mg/kg), they postulated that the nitropyrene found in used oil represents formation, scavenging during combustion or accumulation of the compound in oil during use. They concluded that the emission rate of 1-nitropyrene increases as oil ages with use. Emission rates of 1-nitropyrene in particles in vehicle engine exhausts are given in Table 2.

*(b) Other occurrence*

1-Nitropyrene is one of the most abundant mononitroarenes in the ambient atmosphere. Quantitative data on 1-nitropyrene levels in samples of airborne particulate matter are summarized in Table 3.

Nitroarenes occur in the emissions of numerous stationary combustion sources. 1-Nitropyrene was identified in Norway at more than 100 times the typical ambient air concentration in a potroom where Söderberg electrodes were used for aluminium reduction (Thrane & Stray, 1986). In addition, 1-nitropyrene was detected in stack gases from aluminium smelters and wood stoves in Denmark (Nielsen *et al.*, 1984) and in simulated stack gas. It was concluded that 1-nitropyrene is formed by reaction of pyrene in the presence of nitrogen and sulfur oxides during the sampling process (Brorström-Lundén & Lindskog, 1985).

1-Nitropyrene has been identified in coal fly-ash (Mumford & Lewtas, 1982), in fly-ash extracts of the combustion products of western low-sulfur coal collected in the stack of a commercial power plant (Harris *et al.*, 1984), and in both gas-phase and particulate condensates of flue gases from several coal-fired energy conversion plants (Olsen *et al.*, 1984). Since polycyclic aromatic hydrocarbons (PAH) were found mostly in the gaseous phase, it was concluded by the Working Group that the 1-nitropyrene originated in the oxidizer/combustion unit. 1-Nitropyrene was found in particles emitted from a wood

## Table 1. 1-Nitropyrene levels in exhaust particles and their extracts

| Sample | 1-Nitropyrene concentration | | Reference |
|---|---|---|---|
| | mg/kg extract | mg/kg particulate matter | |
| **Diesel** | | | |
| Car | – | 8.6 | Morita et al. (1982) |
|   1978 production model | – | 3.9 | Gibson (1983) |
|   1980 production model | – | 8.0 ± 2.4 | Gibson (1982) |
|   1982 production model | – | 7.6–24.5 | Gibson (1983) |
|   Mixed cars | – | 9.1 | Gibson (1983) |
| 4-Stroke, 6-cyclinder engines, typical of long-distance trucks | <2–39 | – | Rappaport et al. (1982) |
| 6-Cylinder engine | 870 | 93 | Pitts et al. (1982) |
| Passenger vehicle | 55 ± 11 150 ± 30 | – | Salmeen et al. (1982) |
| 1979 Passenger vehicle | 2030 ± 220 | – | Salmeen et al. (1982) |
| Light-duty engine | 2280 ± 230 | – | Schuetzle et al. (1982) |
| Passenger car | 75 ± 10 | – | Salmeen et al. (1984) |
| Bus | 70.5 | 30[a] | Nakagawa et al. (1983) |
| Passenger car | 107.2–589.3 | – | Nishioka et al. (1982) |
| Diesel-trap car | – | 14.2 | Gibson (1982) |
| Heavy-duty diesel (commercial mining engine) | | | Draper (1986) |
|   100% load, 1200 rpm | – | <0.12 | |
|   75% load, 1800 rpm | – | 5.0 | |
| Diesel vehicles (on road/mountain tunnel, Pennsylvania) | – | 2.1 | Gorse et al. (1983) |
| **Gasoline** | | | |
| Catalyst engine | – | 0.63 ± 0.52 | Gibson (1982) |
| No catalyst/unleaded | | 4.3 ± 3.2 | |
| No catalyst/leaded | – | 3.9 ± 1.3 | Gibson (1982) |
| Passenger car | 2.5 | – | Nishioka et al. (1982) |
| Spark ignition vehicles 75% catalyst equipped (on road/mountain tunnel, Pennsylvania) | – | 5 | Gorse et al. (1983) |

[a]Calculated by the Working Group for comparative purposes from data in the reference

## Table 2. Emission rates of 1-nitropyrene in exhaust particles of diesel and gasoline vehicles

| Sample[a] | 1-Nitropyrene particulate phase emission rate | | Reference |
|---|---|---|---|
| | μg/km[b] | μg/mile | |
| **Diesel** | | | |
| Production model car | (2.0 ± 0.8) | 3.2 ± 1.2 | Gibson (1982) |
| Diesel-trap car | (0.8) | 1.2 | Gibson (1982) |
| LDD/urban simulation (FTP) | 4.6 | – | Gorse et al. (1983) |
| LDD/highway simulation (HWFET) | 4.2 | – | Gorse et al. (1983) |
| HDD/direct-injection engines on road (Pennsylvania) | 0.49 ± 0.06 | – | Gorse et al. (1983) |
| LDD 22% fuel aromaticity | (2.6) | 4.1 | Schuetzle & Frazier |
| 55% fuel aromaticity | (2.3) | 3.7 | (1986) |
| **Gasoline** | | | |
| No catalyst car | (0.13 ± 0.08) | 0.20 ± 0.13[c] | Lang et al. (1981) |
| No catalyst/unleaded | (0.06 ± 0.06) | 0.10 ± 0.09 | Gibson (1982) |
| No catalyst/leaded | (0.11 ± 0.03) | 0.17 ± 0.05 | Gibson (1982) |
| Catalyst | (0.15 ± 0.26) | 0.24 ± 0.41[c] | Lang et al. (1981) |
| Catalyst | (0.03) | 0.05 | Gibson (1982) |
| Spark-ignition cars | 0.03 | – | Gorse et al. (1983) |

[a]LDD, light-duty diesel engine; FTP, Federal Test Procedure; HWFET, Highway Fuel Economy Test; HDD, heavy-duty diesel engine
[b]Figures in parentheses are conversions from reported figures to μg/km.
[c]Nitropyrene unspecified, presumed to be 1-nitropyrene

fireplace (0.11 mg/kg; Gibson, 1982) and from a coal-fired boiler (0.18 mg/kg; Gibson, 1983).

1-Nitropyrene was quantified in crude extracts of particles from gas burners (20.6 mg/kg) and from liquefied petroleum gas (LPG) burners (1.88 mg/kg), which are used widely for home heating and cooking in Japan (Tokiwa et al., 1985). 1-Nitropyrene was detected in Japanese grilled chicken (*yakitori*); the level varied with grilling time at 3.8, 19 and 43 μg/kg for 3, 5 and 7 min, respectively (Kinouchi et al., 1986a).

Toners for use in photocopy machines have been produced in quantity since the late 1950s and have seen widespread use. 'Long-flow' furnace black toner was first used in photocopy toners in 1967; its manufacture involved an oxidation process whereby nitration also occurred. Subsequent changes in the production technique reduced the total extractable nitropyrene content from an uncontrolled level of 5–100 mg/kg to below 0.3 mg/kg (Rosenkranz et al., 1980; Sanders, 1981; Butler et al., 1983), and toners produced from this carbon black since 1980 have not been found to contain detectable levels of mutagenicity or, hence, nitropyrenes (Rosenkranz et al., 1980; Butler et al., 1983).

## Table 3. 1-Nitropyrene levels in atmospheric airborne particles and air samples

| Sample | 1-Nitropyrene concentration | | Reference |
|---|---|---|---|
| | mg/kg particulate matter | ng/m$^3$ air sample | |
| Detroit, MI area, summer | 0.2–0.6 | 0.016–0.030 | Gibson (1982) |
| Japan, industrial | – | 0.021 | Morita et al. (1982) |
| Santiago, Chile, winter 1981 | 0.06–0.15 | 0.028–0.110 | Tokiwa et al. (1983) |
| Japan, industrial | | | Tokiwa et al. (1983) |
|   spring | – | 0.072 | |
|   summer | – | 0.022 | |
|   autumn | – | 0.051 | |
|   winter | – | 0.045 | |
| Denmark, rural winter, 1982 | – | <0.001–0.04 | Nielsen (1983) |
| Tunnel air (Allegheny mountain tunnel, PA) | – | 0.04–0.12 | Gorse et al. (1983) |
| Oslo, Norway, urban | – | 0.01–0.22 | Thrane & Stray (1986) |
| Tokyo, Japan, urban | 0.19–1.6 | 0.015–0.134 | Tanabe et al. (1986) |
| Michigan, urban, summer | 0.04–0.11 | 0.002–0.012 | Siak et al. (1985) |
| Riverside, CA, summer, 1984 | – | 0.008–0.03 | Pitts (1987) |
| Aurskog, Norway, winter 1984 | 0.15 | – | Ramdahl et al. (1986) |
| Claremont, CA, summer, 1985 | 0.36 | – | Ramdahl et al. (1986) |
| St Louis, MO | 0.16 | – | Ramdahl et al. (1986) |
| Washington DC | 0.20 | – | Ramdahl et al. (1986) |
| Bermuda, remote | | | Gibson (1986) |
|   summer, 1982 | 0.52 ± 0.29 | 0.010 | |
|   winter, 1983 | 0.72 ± 0.43 | 0.010 | |
| Delaware, rural, summer, 1982 | 0.54 ± 0.24 | 0.013 | Gibson (1986) |
| Warren, MI, suburban | | | Gibson (1986) |
|   winter, 1982 | 0.36 ± 0.15 | 0.015 | |
|   summer, 1984 | 0.35 ± 0.12 | 0.022 | |
| Detroit, MI, urban, summer, 1981 | 0.22 ± 0.20 | 0.030 | Gibson (1986) |
| River Rouge, MI, industrial, summer, 1982 | 0.59 ± 0.56 | 0.057 | Gibson (1986) |
| Dearborn, MI, industrial, summer, 1980 | 0.15 ± 0.13 | 0.029 | Gibson (1986) |
| Torrance, CA, winter | | | Arey et al. (1987) |
|   day-time | – | 0.04 | |
|   night-time | – | 0.03 | |

1-Nitropyrene was found at a level of 2.9 mg/kg in an extract of a pre-1979 sample of furnace black that had been aftertreated by an oxidation-nitration process (Sanders, 1981). One lot of this grade made in 1980 was found to contain 0.067 mg/kg mononitropyrene (Giammarise et al., 1982). In a more recent study, an undetermined level of 1-nitropyrene was detected in an extract of a formerly available commercial furnace black produced before 1980 (Ramdahl & Urdal, 1982).

1-Nitropyrene has been detected in the waste-water from gasoline service stations (Manabe et al., 1984) and in river sediment, at 25.2 μg/kg sediment (Sato et al., 1985).

## 2.3 Analysis

This section applies to nitroarenes in general.

### (a) Sampling and extraction

The sampling and extraction of nitroarenes from exhausts are described in the monograph on diesel and gasoline engine exhausts; the topic has also been reviewed by Chan and Gibson (1985).

### (b) Clean-up and separation of samples containing nitroarenes

In most enrichment procedures, nitroarenes appear in the so-called 'PAH fraction'. This fraction can be separated further by column chromatography on silica gel (Grimmer et al., 1987) or, more efficiently, by high-performance liquid chromatography (HPLC; Nielsen, 1983) using, e.g., normal-phase HPLC with silica gel columns (Nucleosil-Si-50-5) at room temperature with n-hexane:benzene (3:1) as eluent. Relative retention times (anthracene = 1.00) of 2.1–3.7 were found for mononitroarenes, which allows good separation from PAH, which have retention times of 0.78–1.26. Dinitroarenes have significantly longer retention times; other polar compounds such as cyano derivatives and aldehydes may interfere in the analysis.

A separation method for nitroarenes, consisting of silica gel filtration, chromatography on Sephadex LH 20 and subsequent semipreparative normal-phase HPLC, allows the fractionation of PAH, nitroarenes and dinitroarenes (D'Agostino et al., 1983; Fig. 1). Using sodium borohydride and cupric chloride, nitroarenes are converted into the corresponding amines, which are readily separable from PAH by chromatography on silica gel (Gibson et al., 1981). Another advantage of this method is that aminoarenes exhibit intense fluorescence spectra which facilitate their detection. This method has also been used to derivatize propionates from the corresponding aminoarenes with pentafluoropropionic anhydride (Fig. 2); propionates give high signal responses when an electron-capture detector is used with gas chromatography (Campbell & Lee, 1984).

### (c) Chemical analysis

Nitroarenes have been analysed by HPLC, gas chromatography and mass spectrometry; some thin-layer chromatography methods have also been described (e.g., Pitts et al., 1978).

**Fig. 1. Scheme for the isolation of polycyclic aromatic hydrocarbons (PAH) and nitroarenes in environmental samples**[a]

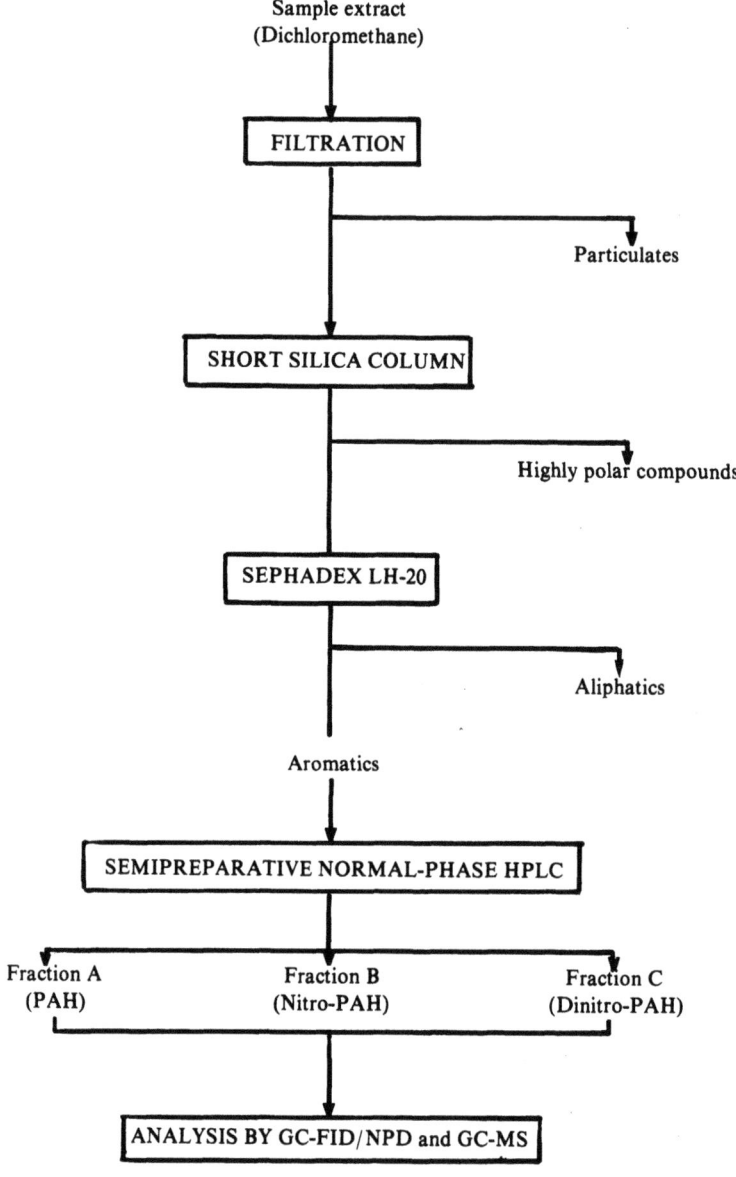

[a]From D'Agostino et al. (1983); HPLC, high-performance liquid chromatography; GC-FID/NPD, gas chromatography-flame ionization detection/nitrogen phosphorous detection; GC-MS, gas chromatography-mass spectrometry

**Fig. 2. Scheme for the separation of nitroarenes**[a]

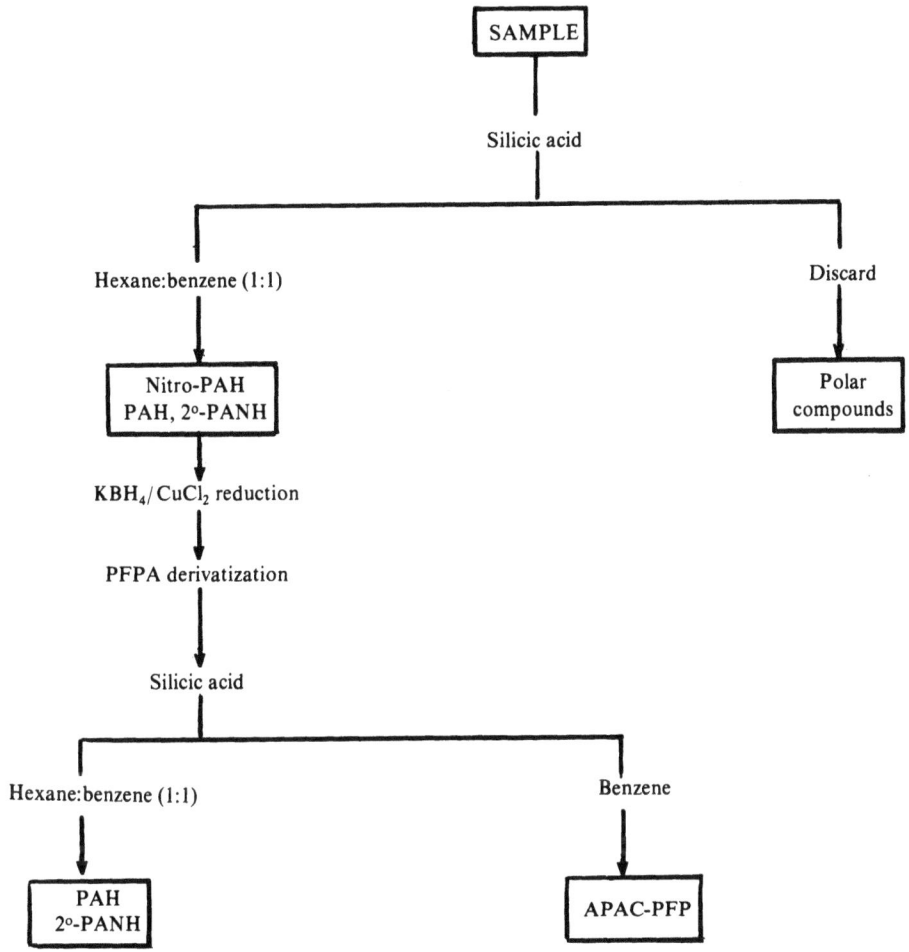

[a]From Campbell & Lee (1984); nitro-PAH, nitroarenes; PAH, polycyclic aromatic hydrocarbons; 2°-PANH, secondary azaarenes (e.g., carbazoles); PFPA, pentafluoropropionic anhydride; APAC-PFP, pentafluoropropylamide derivatives of aminoarenes

*(i) High-performance liquid chromatography*

Conditions for analytical, preparative and semipreparative liquid chromatography have been reviewed (Poole, 1985). Supports in microbore (packed microtubular), packed capillary and open tubular microcolumns using normal and reverse-phase HPLC have been used. Due to the poor sensitivity of ultra-violet detection, more sensitive and selective fluorescent detectors are favoured. Responses can be greatly increased by means of reductive electrochemical detection, which allows quantification over a linear range of $10^3$ with a sensitivity of 10–100 pg per compound (Rappaport *et al.*, 1982; Jin & Rappaport, 1983; MacCrehan & May, 1984). Conversion of nitroarenes by sodium borohydride/cupric chloride reduction to aminoarenes has also been used to increase detection sensitivity

(Gibson et al., 1981). Chiral stationary phases have been introduced into HPLC for the separation of geometric isomeric nitroarenes and their derivatives (Chou, 1986).

(ii) *Gas chromatography*

The various parameters involved in the gas chromatography of nitroarenes (support, stationary phase, working conditions) and in the relative retention times of many individual nitroarenes have been reviewed (White, 1985), together with the advantages of different detectors (Tomkins, 1985). Both the common carbon-dependent flame-ionization detector and nitrogen-phosphorous detectors have been used widely for the detection of nitroarenes, sometimes in combination (Ramdahl et al., 1982; Nielsen, 1983; Nielsen et al., 1983). Electron-capture detectors have been used preferentially when nitroarenes have been converted previously to aminoarenes and derivatized with either heptafluorobutyric anhydride (Morita et al., 1982) or pentafluoropropionic anhydride to the corresponding amides. Increased responses can be obtained when a thermionic ionization detector is used (Patterson et al., 1982). Further progress has been made by introducing the thermal energy analyser, which is highly selective for nitroarenes. Optimal responses were obtained at ≥800°C pyrolyser temperature, and detection limits of 30–80 pg were reported for mononitroarenes and of 25 pg for trinitro compounds (Yu, 1983).

(iii) *Mass spectrometry*

The use of mass spectrometry in the detection of nitroarenes has been reviewed, and the relative intensities of the key ions obtained with various mass spectrometric techniques have been tabulated (Schuetzle & Jensen, 1985). Electron impact ionization, recording full spectra or selected ions (selective ion monitoring), is used widely, and more than 50 nitroarenes have been identified tentatively in extracts of diesel exhaust by high-resolution mass spectrometry (Xu et al., 1982). More recently, chemical ionization was introduced into the analysis of nitroarenes, both as electron capture negative ion chemical ionization and as positive ion chemical ionization. A detection limit of 1 pg has been reported for 2-methyl-1-nitronaphthalene using negative ion chemical ionization (Ramdahl & Urdal, 1982).

Negative ion atmospheric pressure ionization mass spectrometry has also been applied to the analysis of nitroarenes and their metabolites, which, due to their high electron affinity, can be detected selectively by this technique; a good spectrum has been obtained with as little as 5 pg 1-nitropyrene (Korfmacher et al., 1984, 1987, 1988). With this method, the limit of detection for 1-nitropyrene was 0.5 pg (Korfmacher & Miller, 1984) and that for 1-nitronaphthalene, 0.3 pg (Korfmacher & Rushing, 1986).

Triple-quadrupole mass spectrometry has been used to analyse nitroarenes in diesel exhaust, and the presence of various dinitroarenes was demonstrated, in addition to the commonly found mononitroarenes (Henderson et al., 1983). Concentrations of dinitroarenes in diesel particulate extracts have been reported (Nishioka et al., 1982; Schuetzle et al., 1982).

In most studies, mass spectrometry has been used in combination with gas chromatography, but coupling with HPLC has also been reported (Levine et al., 1982).

(d) *Formation of nitroarenes during sample collection and loss during storage*

Nitroarenes may be formed to some extent during sample collection by reaction of PAH with nitrogen oxides, and various experiments have been undertaken to estimate the extent of this effect (see the monograph on diesel and gasoline engine exhausts, p. 80).

Conversion of pyrene into nitropyrene and of mononitropyrene into dinitropyrenes during long-term absorption on silica has been reported (Hughes *et al.*, 1980). Nitroarene concentrations in diesel extracts have been found to decrease significantly during storage, whereas concentrations in particles were more stable (Nishioka *et al.*, 1982).

## 3. Biological Data Relevant to the Evaluation of Carcinogenic Risk to Humans

### 3.1 Carcinogenicity studies in animals[1]

(a) *Oral administration*

*Rat*: A group of 36 female weanling CD rats received oral intubations of 10 μmol [2.5 mg]/kg bw 1-nitropyrene (purity, >99.9%) in dimethyl sulfoxide (DMSO; 1.7 μmol [0.5 mg]/ml DMSO) three times per week for four weeks (average total dose, 16 μmol [4.7 mg]/rat) and were sacrificed after 76–78 weeks or when moribund (King, 1988). A group of 36 females received DMSO only. The number of 1-nitropyrene-treated rats with mammary tumours (16/35; five with adenocarcinomas, nine with fibroadenomas) was not different from controls (12/35). [The Working Group noted the short duration of both treatment and observation.]

Groups of 40, 40 and 46 female specific-pathogen-free Fischer 344/Jcl rats, six weeks old, received intragastric instillations of 5, 10 and 20 mg/kg bw, respectively, of 1-nitropyrene (impurities: 0.11% 1,3-dinitropyrene, 0.27% 1,6-dinitropyrene and 0.23% 1,8-dinitropyrene) in olive oil twice a week for 55 weeks (Odagiri *et al.*, 1986). A group of 30 vehicle control rats received olive oil alone. Animals were killed when moribund or after 104 weeks, at which time the experiment was terminated; only rats surviving beyond experimental week 46, when the first tumour was observed, were evaluated. Mammary adenocarcinomas were induced in a dose-dependent manner in the three treated groups (in 2/36; 12/39 — $p < 0.001$; and 14/45 — $p < 0.001$, respectively); no adenocarcinoma was observed in vehicle controls. Clitoral gland tumours, most of which were diagnosed as squamous-cell carcinomas, developed in a dose-dependent manner in treated rats, and the numbers of rats with tumours in the high-dose (12/45; 11 with squamous-cell carcinomas) and intermediate-dose (11/39; nine with squamous-cell carcinomas) groups was significantly ($p < 0.001$) greater than that in controls (one adenoma). In addition, more animals in

---

[1]The Working Group was aware of studies in progress in rats by single subcutaneous injection and in mice by single subcutaneous and by intraperitoneal injection (IARC, 1988).

the treated groups had mononuclear-cell leukaemia (high-dose, 27/45; mid-dose, 22/39; and low-dose, 23/36; $p < 0.05$) than among vehicle controls (9/28). [The Working Group noted the presence of dinitropyrene impurities and could not ascertain their potential effect on the outcome of the experiment.]

*(b) Skin application*

*Mouse*: In a study of initiating activity, a group of 20 female CD-1 Charles River mice, aged 50—55 days, received ten applications of 0.1 mg 1-nitropyrene (purity, >99%) in 0.1 ml acetone onto shaved back skin every other day for 20 days (total dose, 1 mg; El-Bayoumy *et al.*, 1982). A group of 20 female mice receiving acetone alone served as controls. Starting ten days after initiation had been completed, all animals received applications of 2.5 μg 12-*O*-tetradecanoylphorbol 13-acetate in 0.1 ml acetone three times per week for 25 weeks. At the end of this time, 3/20 treated animals and 1/20 control animals had developed skin tumours (mainly papillomas). This difference was not statistically significant. [The Working Group noted the small number of animals used.]

In a study of initiating activity (Nesnow *et al.*, 1984), six groups of 39—40 male and 39—40 female SENCAR mice, seven weeks old, received a single dermal application of 0—3.0 mg 1-nitropyrene (purity, >99.5%) in 0.2 ml acetone; animals receiving 3.0 mg had two applications. A group of 40 males and 40 females received a single application of 0.05 mg benzo[*a*]pyrene and served as positive controls. One week after initiation, all mice received skin applications of 12-*O*-tetradecanoylphorbol 13-acetate in 0.2 ml acetone twice a week for 30 weeks. At the end of this period, no significant increase in the number of mice with skin papillomas was observed in the 1-nitropyrene-treated groups, although all mice in the benzo[*a*]pyrene-treated group that survived beyond week 31 developed skin papillomas.

*(c) Intratracheal instillation*

*Hamster*: A group of 34 male Syrian golden hamsters, eight weeks old, received intratracheal instillations of 2 mg 1-nitropyrene (purity, 98%; impurities: 0.008% 1,3-dinitropyrene, 0.6% 1,6-dinitropyrene plus 1,8-dinitropyrene, and 1.3% pyrene) suspended in 0.2 ml phosphate buffer solution once a week for 15 weeks (Yamamoto *et al.*, 1987). A further group received 2 mg benzo[*a*]pyrene and a vehicle control group of 19 animals received buffer solution alone. All hamsters in the 1-nitropyrene-treated and control groups had died within 663 and 684 days, respectively, following the initial instillation; after the 15 instillations, 24 and 16 animals in these groups, respectively, were still alive. Two lung adenomas were detected in 2/21 treated animals (the three others were cannibalized); in one animal, the adenoma co-existed with a squamous-cell papilloma in the trachea. No tumour was observed in the respiratory organs of control animals, but they occurred in 19/22 animals treated with benzo[*a*]pyrene.

*(d) Intrapulmonary administration*

*Rat*: A group of 32 male Fischer 344/DuCrj rats, 10-11 weeks old, received a single injection of 0.05 ml beeswax-tricaprylin containing 1.5 mg 1-nitropyrene (purity, >99.9%)

directly into the lower third of the left lung after left lateral thoracotomy (Maeda et al., 1986). A group of 19 rats received a single injection of 0.05 ml beeswax-tricaprylin containing 0.5 mg 3-methylcholanthrene [purity unspecified], and another group of 31 rats received beeswax-tricaprylin only. Animals were observed for 72 weeks after treatment, at which time the experiment was terminated. No squamous-cell carcinoma of the lung was induced in rats injected with 1-nitropyrene or in vehicle controls, but all 19 rats injected with 3-methylcholanthrene developed these tumours. No difference in the incidence of tumours in other organs was observed among the three groups. [The Working Group noted the short period of observation.]

(e) *Subcutaneous administration*

*Mouse*: A group of 20 male BALB/c mice, six weeks old, received subcutaneous injections of 0.1 mg 1-nitropyrene (purity, >99.9%) dissolved in 0.2 ml DMSO once a week for 20 weeks (total dose, 2 mg; Tokiwa et al., 1984). A group of 20 vehicle controls received injections of DMSO only. All animals were observed for 60 weeks or, for mice with tumours at the site of injection, until moribund. No subcutaneous tumour developed at the injection site in mice administered 1-nitropyrene or DMSO. In a group treated with the same dose of 1,6-dinitropyrene (see p. 219), 10/20 mice developed subcutaneous tumours. Lung tumours were found in 6/20 1-nitropyrene-treated and in 7/20 control mice. [The Working Group noted the small number of animals used and the short period of observation.]

*Rat*: A group of 20 male Fischer 344/DuCrj rats, eight weeks old, received subcutaneous injections of 2 mg 1-nitropyrene (purity, >99%) dissolved in 0.2 ml DMSO twice a week for ten weeks (Ohgaki et al., 1982). A control group of 20 male rats received injections of 0.2 ml DMSO only. The animals were observed for life; the last rats died on day 377. The first tumour in the treated group was seen after 162 days; 8/17 of the animals surviving beyond this time developed tumours, described as one extraskeletal osteosarcoma and seven malignant fibrous histiocytomas at the site of injection. Two of the malignant histiocytomas proved to be serially transplantable into the subcutis of the same strain over 14 generations. No tumour was observed in controls ($p < 0.003$). [The Working Group noted that the authors reported in a later publication (Ohgaki et al., 1985) that these findings were possibly due to contamination of the preparation of 1-nitropyrene with dinitropyrenes (about 0.8%) and not to 1-nitropyrene itself.]

A group of 20 male Fischer 344/DuCrj rats, six weeks old, received subcutaneous injections of 2 mg 1-nitropyrene (impurities: <0.05% each of 1,3-, 1,6 and 1,8-dinitropyrene, 1,3,6-trinitropyrene and 1,3,6,8-tetranitropyrene) dissolved in 0.2 ml DMSO twice a week for ten weeks (total dose, 40 mg); ten rats were treated with 0.2 mg 1-nitropyrene (total dose, 4 mg; Ohgaki et al., 1985). A further group of 20 rats received injections of 0.2 ml DMSO only. Observation was terminated on day 650. No tumour was found at the site of injection in treated or control animals. Two groups treated with total doses of 0.4 mg 1,8-dinitropyrene (see p. 235) or 4 mg 1,6-dinitropyrene (see p. 219) all developed sarcomas. [The Working Group noted the small number of animals used and the short period of observation.]

A group of 31 male and 32 female newborn Sprague-Dawley-derived CD rats received subcutaneous injections of 100 $\mu$mol[25 mg]/kg bw 1-nitropyrene (<0.02% dinitropyrenes) dissolved in DMSO once a week for eight weeks (Hirose *et al.*, 1984). Another group of 29 males and 31 females received injections of 50 $\mu$mol[12.5 mg]/kg bw 1-nitropyrene in DMSO. A further group of 28 male and 31 female rats receiving DMSO only served as controls. The experiment was terminated when animals were 62 weeks old. In the group injected with the higher dose of 1-nitropyrene, 10/31 males and 9/32 females developed sarcomas, primarily malignant fibrous histiocytomas, at the site of injection. Of the females, 15/32 also had mammary tumours (ten adenocarcinomas, seven fibroadenomas). In the group given the lower dose, 2/29 males and 3/31 females developed tumours at the site of injection, and mammary tumours were found in 7/31 (three adenocarcinomas, five fibroadenomas) females. No tumour was detected at the site of injection in control animals, but mammary tumours were found in 2/31 females. There was a dose-response relationship for the induction of tumours at the site of injection, and the incidence of tumours in males ($p < 0.001$) and females ($p < 0.01$) in the group given the higher dose of 1-nitropyrene was significantly different from that in controls. The average period of induction for tumours at the injection site was shorter in males given the high dose (262 days) than in males given the low dose (312 days); this response was not observed in females (288 and 285 days). There was a dose-related increase in the formation of mammary gland tumours in treated females, and the incidence of mammary tumours in the high-dose group was significantly different from that in controls ($p < 0.001$). The numbers of mammary tumours (29 and nine), especially adenocarcinomas (16 and four), were also dose-related. Although some tumours were observed in other organs, the incidences were not different between treated and control animals.

A group of 49 female newborn CD rats received subcutaneous injections of 1-nitropyrene (purity, >99.9%) dissolved in DMSO (1.7 $\mu$mol [0.4 mg]/ml DMSO) into the suprascapular region once a week for eight weeks (total dose, 6.3 $\mu$mol [1.6 mg]; King, 1988). Another group of 40 animals received DMSO alone. Rats were observed until moribund or up to 67 weeks, at which time no malignant fibrous histiocytoma was found in either group. The number of rats with mammary tumours did not differ significantly between treated (16/49) and control animals (8/40), but a higher prevalence of adenocarcinoma-bearing animals was observed in the treated group. [The Working Group noted the low dose used and the short observation period.]

A group of 29 female weanling CD rats received subcutaneous injections of 100 $\mu$mol [25 mg]/kg bw 1-nitropyrene (purity, >99.9%) dissolved in DMSO (70 $\mu$mol[17 mg]/ml DMSO) once a week for five weeks (total dose, 77 $\mu$mol[19 mg]/rat; King, 1988). Another group of 30 rats received DMSO alone. Rats were observed until moribund or up to 88 weeks, at which time more rats in the treated group had mammary adenocarcinomas and fibroadenomas (17/29) than controls (11/30; $p < 0.08$). [The Working Group noted the high and variable spontaneous incidence of mammary tumours in these studies.]

Groups of 48 female newborn CD rats and 55 female newborn Fischer 344 rats received subcutaneous injections of 100 $\mu$mol[25 mg]/kg bw 1-nitropyrene (purity, >99.9%) dissolved in DMSO (70 $\mu$mol[17 mg]/ml DMSO) once a week for eight weeks (total dose,

63 μmol[15.5 mg]; King, 1988). Groups of 47 CD and 55 Fischer 344 rats were injected with DMSO. Animals were sacrificed at 86 weeks. Mammary gland tumours developed in all groups, but the incidences did not differ between the treated and control groups. Four Fischer 344 rats injected with 1-nitropyrene had leukaemia, and this malignancy did not occur in controls ($p < 0.05$). [The Working Group noted the high and variable spontaneous incidence of mammary tumours in the CD rats and the unusually low incidence of leukaemia in control Fischer 344 rats.]

*(f) Intraperitoneal administration*

*Mouse*: Three groups of 15, 15 and 16 male and 14, 14 and 12 female A/J mice, six to eight weeks old, received 17 intraperitoneal injections of 1-nitropyrene (purity, >99%, with no dinitropyrenes (El-Bayoumy & Hecht, 1983); total doses, 175, 525 and 1575 mg/kg bw, respectively) in 0.1 ml trioctanoin over a period of six weeks (El-Bayoumy et al., 1984a). A group of 16 males and 16 females received injections of trioctanoin only. Mice were sacrificed 18 weeks after termination of the treatment at 24 weeks, and their lungs were examined. In the group given the highest dose of 1-nitropyrene, the number of male and female mice with lung tumours (22/28) was significantly higher ($p < 0.05$) than in controls (7/32); the mean number of lung tumours/mouse was also significantly increased (1.3 compared with 0.3 lung tumours/mouse; $p < 0.001$). The combined tumour incidences in the other two groups were not statistically different from that in controls, but the tumour incidence in males receiving the lowest dose was significantly greater (4/10). In each dose group, the numbers of mice with lung tumours and mean numbers of lung tumours/mouse were larger in males than in females. [The Working Group noted that studies conducted with strain A mice are usually considered to be of a screening nature and not definitive tests for carcinogenicity.]

Groups of 90 or 100 male and female newborn CD-1 mice received three intraperitoneal injections of 1-nitropyrene (purity, >99%; total doses, 700 or 2800 nmol [173 or 692 μg]) in 10, 20 and 40 μl DMSO on days 1, 8 and 15 after birth; a total dose of 560 nmol [140 μg] benzo[a]pyrene (purity, >99%); or three injections of DMSO only (Wislocki et al., 1986). Treatment of a second vehicle control group was begun ten weeks after that of the other groups. At 25–27 days, when the mice were weaned, 34 males and 50 females given 700 nmol 1-nitropyrene, 29 males and 26 females given 2800 nmol 1-nitropyrene, 37 males and 27 females in the positive control group, and 28 and 31 males and 45 and 34 females in the two vehicle control group were still alive. All remaining mice were killed after one year. Liver-cell tumours developed in 5/34 (two adenomas, three carcinomas) males treated with 700 nmol 1-nitropyrene and in 8/29 (three adenomas, five carcinomas) treated with 2800 nmol; the latter incidence was significantly greater than that in DMSO controls (2/28 and 5/45; $p < 0.05$). 1-Nitropyrene did not induce liver-cell tumours in females. The numbers of mice with lung tumours and with malignant lymphomas (1/29, 6/34) were not different from those in control mice. Benzo[a]pyrene induced liver-cell tumours in 18/37 males, but not in females. The numbers of benzo[a]pyrene-treated mice with lung tumours (males, 13/37; females, 13/27) were significantly greater than that in vehicle controls ($p < 0.005$). Of the vehicle controls, 2/28 and 5/45 males had liver tumours and 1/28 and 4/45 had lung tumours, and 0/31 and 0/34 females had liver tumours and 0/31 and 2/34 had lung tumours. [The Working Group noted the short observation period.]

*Rat*: A group of 36 female weanling CD rats received intraperitoneal injections of 10 μmol[2.5 mg]/kg bw 1-nitropyrene (purity, >99.9%) in DMSO (1.7 μmol[0.4 mg]/ml DMSO) three times per week for four weeks (total dose, 16 μmol (4 mg) per rat); 36 control animals received injections of DMSO only (King, 1988). Animals were sacrificed when moribund or after 76–78 weeks. Mammary tumours were found in 25/36 treated animals (14 adenocarcinomas, 19 fibroadenomas) and in 7/31 vehicle controls ($p < 0.0001$).

In a second study in the same laboratory (King, 1988), 29 female weanling CD rats received five weekly intraperitoneal injections of 100 μmol[25 mg]/kg bw 1-nitropyrene (purity, >99.9%) dissolved in DMSO (70 μmol[17 mg]/ml DMSO; total dose, 77 μmol[19 mg]/rat); 30 rats received DMSO alone. Animals were observed until moribund or up to 88 weeks. Mammary adenocarcinomas and fibroadenomas were observed in 17/29 treated rats and in 11/30 controls ($p < 0.08$). [The Working Group noted the inconsistent findings and the variations in the incidences of mammary tumours in controls.]

### 3.2 Other relevant data

(a) *Experimental systems*

(i) *Absorption, distribution, excretion and metabolism*

The kinetics and metabolism of 1-nitropyrene have been reviewed in recent articles on nitropyrenes (Beland *et al.*, 1985; Rosenkranz & Mermelstein, 1985; Rosenkranz & Howard, 1986; Tokiwa & Ohnishi, 1986). The major phase I metabolites identified are shown in Figure 3 (Beland *et al.*, 1985).

*Studies* in vivo

The principal metabolic pathways and metabolites in urine, faeces and bile have been identified in rats following oral, intravenous or intraperitoneal administration of radiolabelled 1-nitropyrene. Most administered 1-nitropyrene is accounted for by biliary excretion. For example, in one study on bile duct-cannulated rats, over 60% of the dose was excreted in bile over 24 h (Medinsky *et al.*, 1985). Most of this material is eventually excreted in the faeces, e.g., over 80% within 96 h (Ball, L.M. *et al.*, 1984a). Biliary metabolites have been characterized mainly as glucuronide and glutathione conjugates of oxidized nitropyrene metabolites (Howard *et al.*, 1985; Ohnishi *et al.*, 1986; Djurić *et al.*, 1989). Urinary metabolites are excreted in conjugated form, mainly with glucuronic acid (Ball, L.M. *et al.*, 1984a). In only one study in rats was excretion greater in urine than in faeces (Dutcher *et al.*, 1985).

*Effects of gut microflora*: The significance of gut microflora in the metabolism of 1-nitropyrene *in vivo* was demonstrated in several studies employing conventional (El-Bayoumy *et al.*, 1983; El-Bayoumy & Hecht, 1984; Kinouchi *et al.*, 1986b) and germ-free (El-Bayoumy *et al.*, 1984b; Kinouchi *et al.*, 1986b) or antibiotic-treated (Medinsky *et al.*, 1985) rats. Conventional but not germ-free or antibiotic-treated rats metabolized 1-nitropyrene to 1-aminopyrene.

## Fig. 3. Phase I metabolites of 1-nitropyrene[a]

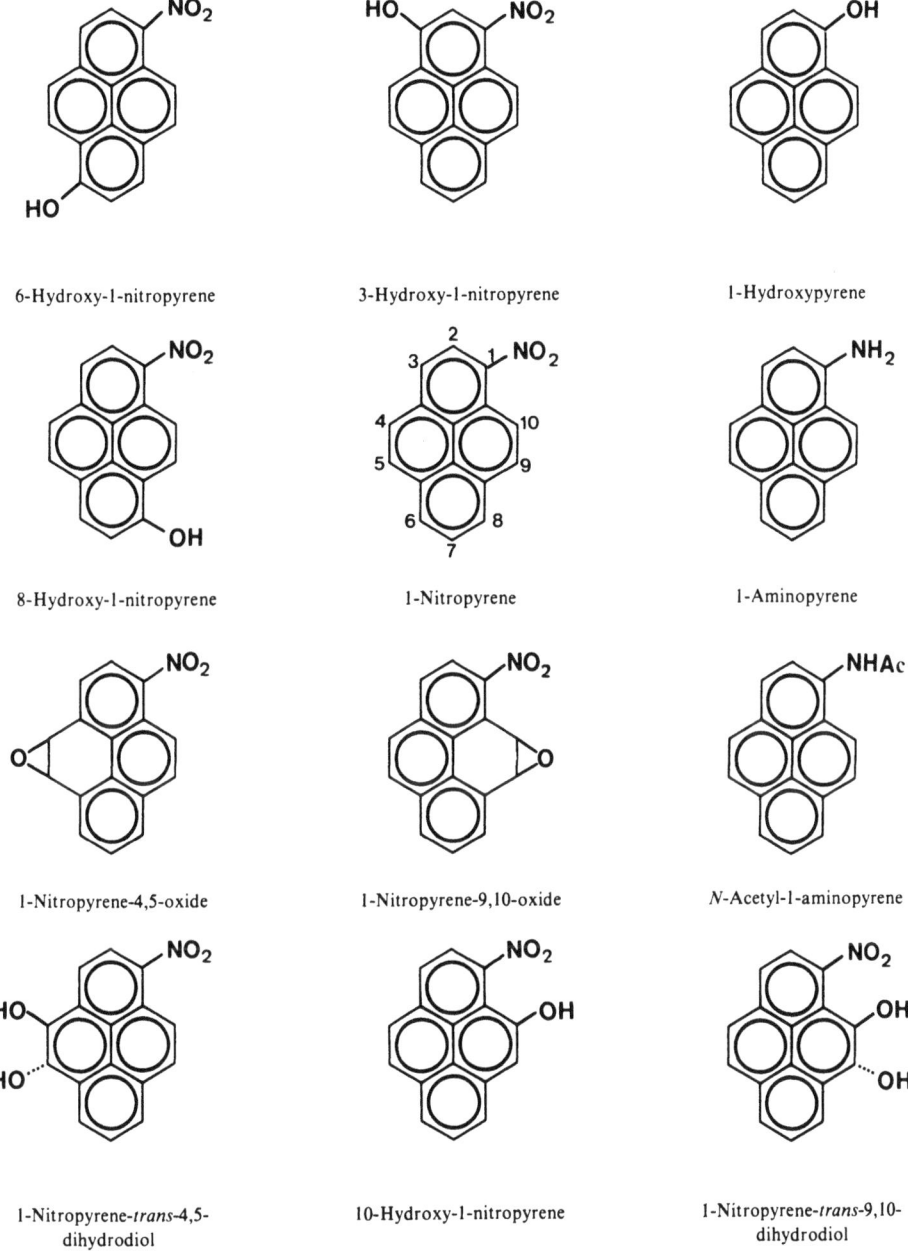

[a]From Beland et al. (1985)

*Effects of particle association*: Groups of Fischer 344 rats were exposed to [$^3$H]1-nitropyrene by nose-only inhalation, either as a coating (about 6% by mass) on relatively insoluble, ultrafine $^{67}$gallium oxide particles (6.2 mg/m$^3$) or as a homogeneous ultrafine aerosol (43 μg/m$^3$). Rats exposed to 1-nitropyrene on particles excreted the majority of the deposited radioactivity in the faeces (75 ± 18%), whereas animals exposed to 1-nitropyrene aerosol excreted a major portion of the radiolabel in the urine (76 ± 18%). There was no difference in the rates of lung clearance of 1-nitropyrene between the two groups. Most of the aerosol was cleared from the respiratory tract by direct absorption into the blood, while particle-associated nitropyrene was cleared by both blood absorption and mucociliary clearance followed by ingestion and faecal excretion (Sun *et al.*, 1983).

Male Fischer 344 rats were exposed by nose-only inhalation to various concentrations of [$^{14}$C]1-nitropyrene and [$^{14}$C]1-nitropyrene coated on diesel exhaust particles (50–1100 μg/m$^3$ 1-nitropyrene; particulate concentration, 70–7200 μ/m$^3$). Over the range of concentrations tested, the pathways for excretion of [$^{14}$C]1-nitropyrene in urine and faeces were independent of the concentration of nitropyrene, whether given alone or associated with diesel exhaust particles. In all cases, faecal excretion was the major route of elimination, about twice as much being excreted by this route as in the urine. The fractional deposition of [$^{14}$C]1-nitropyrene in the respiratory tract did not appear to be dependent on the concentration. Half-times for elimination of $^{14}$C in urine and faeces were about 15–20 h. Lungs of rats exposed to [$^{14}$C]1-nitropyrene coated on diesel exhaust particles contained nearly five times more $^{14}$C than lungs from rats exposed to [$^{14}$C]-1-nitropyrene alone within 1 h after exposure. This difference was increased to 80-fold at 94 h after exposure. The long-term half-time for clearance of $^{14}$C in the lungs of rats exposed to coated diesel particles was 36 days, in contrast to two days after exposure to 1-nitropyrene alone. The gastrointestinal absorption of the same 1-nitropyrene preparations was studied after an oral dose of 10 μg/kg bw. Within 1 h, >90% of $^{14}$C was found in nitropyrene metabolites (Bond *et al.*, 1986).

[The Working Group noted that, on the basis of lung retention, 1-nitropyrene coated on gallium oxide is a poor model for 1-nitropyrene coated on diesel particles.]

The overall excretion pattern of $^{14}$C was similar after intratracheal instillation of male Sprague-Dawley rats with [$^{14}$C]1-nitropyrene (8 nmol [2 μg]) either coated onto diesel particles (dose, 20 mg/kg bw), instilled along with unlabelled diesel particles, or administered alone (Ball *et al.*, 1986), and was also similar to that seen after intraperitoneal injection of [$^{14}$C]1-nitropyrene alone (Ball, L.M. *et al.*, 1984a). Lung retention was also similar to that following inhalation (described above). Protein-associated radioactivity has been observed in particle-treated lungs, with no detectable level of DNA adducts found up to 24 h after administration (Ball *et al.*, 1986).

*DNA binding*: DNA binding occurs in rat liver (Hsieh *et al.*, 1986) and in mouse lung (Mitchell, 1985a) after the administration of 1-nitropyrene. Less radioactivity was associated with lung macromolecules in antibiotic-treated rats than in controls (Ayres *et al.*, 1985). *N*-(Deoxyguanosin-8-yl)-1-aminopyrene has been identified in rat kidney, liver and mammary gland (Hashimoto & Shudo, 1985; Stanton *et al.*, 1985) and mouse lung (Mitchell, 1988); other unidentified adducts have been reported (Roy *et al.*, 1987; Mitchell,

1988). However, in another study, DNA was not bound in tissues of rats given 1-nitropyrene intraperitoneally (Djurić *et al.*, 1988).

*Factors affecting metabolism*: As reported in an abstract, newborn mice metabolized 1-nitropyrene more efficiently than older mice; the predominant metabolites were phenols and dihydrodiols (El-Bayoumy & Hecht, 1986).

Pretreatment with benzo[*a*]pyrene increased the radioactivity associated with DNA in the lungs of mice administered [$^{14}$C]1-nitropyrene (Mitchell, 1985a; Howard *et al.*, 1986); however, pretreatment with diesel extract had no effect (Howard *et al.*, 1986).

The capacity of liver microsomes to catalyse the oxidative metabolism of 1-nitropyrene was unchanged after rats were treated with 8 mg/kg bw 1-nitropyrene. Liver cytosolic and microsomal nitroreductase activities toward 1-nitropyrene were increased two-fold. DNA binding of 1-nitropyrene *in vitro* was two-fold higher in the presence of cytosol from 1-nitropyrene-pretreated rats (Djurić *et al.*, 1988).

*Studies* in vitro

*Perfused organs*: In isolated perfused and ventilated rat lungs, the major metabolites of [$^{14}$C]1-nitropyrene were 3-, 6-, and 8-hydroxy-1-nitropyrene; smaller quantities of 10-hydroxy-1-nitropyrene, 1-aminopyrene and *N*-acetyl-1-aminopyrene were also detected. Pretreatment with 3-methylcholanthrene increased the rate of metabolism ten-fold and the extent of radioactivity associated with tissue macromolecules 20-fold (Bond & Mauderly, 1984). Pretreatment of rats with diesel exhaust (particles, 7.4 mg/m$^3$) for four weeks increased the rate of metabolism in perfused lung and in nasal tissue two-fold and the extent of radioactivity associated with tissue macromolecules in the perfused lung four-fold (Bond *et al.*, 1985).

In isolated perfused rat livers, N-acetyl-1-aminopyrene was the major metabolite of [$^{14}$C]1-nitropyrene; smaller quantities of 1-aminopyrene and hydroxy-1-nitropyrenes were detected (Bond *et al.*, 1984).

*Cultured cells*: Chinese hamster ovary cells, Chinese hamster lung fibroblasts, calf thymus cells, rabbit alveolar macrophages, rabbit epithelial cells and human diploid fibroblasts catalysed the reduction of 1-nitropyrene to an intermediate which bound to DNA, giving an adduct identified as *N*-(deoxyguanosin-8-yl)-1-aminopyrene (Heflich *et al.*, 1985b; Jackson *et al.*, 1985; Beland *et al.*, 1986; Edwards *et al.*, 1986a; Heflich *et al.*, 1986a; Patton *et al.*, 1986; Gallagher *et al.*, 1988; Maher *et al.*, 1988). Incubation of rabbit lung and tracheal tissues with [$^{14}$C]1-nitropyrene resulted in association of the radioactivity with cellular DNA (King *et al.*, 1983).

Primary rat hepatocytes, Chinese hamster V79 cells and human hepatoma HepG2 cells catalysed the conversion of 1-nitropyrene into 1-aminopyrene (Salmeen *et al.*, 1983; Eddy *et al.*, 1987). Oxidized metabolites were also detected with the latter cell line (Eddy *et al.*, 1987).

*Subcellular fractions*: Cytosolic preparations from the livers of rats (Nachtman & Wei, 1982; Djurić *et al.*, 1985, 1986a, 1988), rabbits (Tatsumi *et al.*, 1986) and dogs (Djurić *et al.*, 1985) catalysed the reduction of 1-nitropyrene to 1-aminopyrene. Postmitochondrial supernatants of rat liver, lung and nasal tissue and of rabbit and hamster lung and liver catalysed both the oxidation and reduction of 1-nitropyrene (Nachtman & Wei, 1982; Bond, 1983; El-Bayoumy & Hecht, 1983; Ball, L.M. et al., 1984b; King et al., 1984; Saito et al., 1984a; Belisario et al., 1986; Dybing et al., 1986; Tatsumi et al., 1986). Guinea-pig liver microsomes also catalysed the oxidation of 1-nitropyrene (Fifer et al., 1986). In some instances, this metabolism was accompanied by binding to exogenous DNA (Ball & Lewtas, 1985; Djurić et al., 1985, 1986b; Dybing et al., 1986; Djurić et al., 1988). Following incubation of [$^3$H]1-nitropyrene with calf thymus DNA, bovine xanthine oxidase and hypoxanthine at 37°C, covalent binding to DNA was shown to be proportional to the amount of reducing enzyme present (Howard & Beland, 1982).

*Bacteria*: Several strains of bacterial and gut microflora from animals and humans have been shown to reduce 1-nitropyrene (Kinouchi et al., 1982; El-Bayoumy et al., 1983; Howard et al., 1983a; Cerniglia, 1985; Heflich et al., 1985b; Manning et al., 1986). In some instances, this metabolism was accompanied by the formation of a DNA adduct identified as *N*-(deoxyguanosin-8-yl)-1-aminopyrene.

(ii) *Toxic effects*

Groups of male and female specific-pathogen-free Fischer 344 rats that received single oral doses of up to 5 g/kg bw 1-nitropyrene as a fine powder suspension in 2% gelatin showed no mortality or histological damage in a wide range of organs examined when the animals were killed 4 or 14 days after administration (Marshall et al., 1982).

Topical application and intraperitoneal administration of 1-nitropyrene to rats induced cutaneous and hepatic drug and carcinogen metabolism (Asokan et al., 1985, 1986; Belisario et al., 1988; Mukhtar et al., 1988) and nitroreductase activity (Chou et al., 1986; Djurić et al., 1988).

Intraperitoneal injection of 1-nitropyrene (105 μmol[26 mg]/kg bw) into female Sprague-Dawley rats induced an oncofetal protein (Hanausek-Walaszek et al., 1985). Superoxide radical was generated on incubation of rat lung microsomes with 1-nitropyrene (Nachtman, 1986).

(iii) *Genetic and related effects*

The genetic and related effects of nitroarenes and of their metabolites have been reviewed (Rosenkranz & Mermelstein, 1983; Beland et al., 1985; Rosenkranz & Mermelstein, 1985; Tokiwa & Ohnishi, 1986).

[It is to be noted that, on occasion, 1-nitropyrene contains small quantities of dinitropyrenes (e.g., Odagiri et al., 1986; Yamamoto et al., 1987). Due to the potent mutagenicity of dinitropyrenes (Mermelstein et al., 1981), their presence may affect the results. The Working Group has indicated in the text studies in which the purity of the compound tested was less than 99%.]

1-Nitropyrene induced DNA damage in *Escherichia coli* (at 0.5–2 μg/ml; Ohta et al., 1984) and *Salmonella typhimurium* (lowest effective dose, 0.02 μg/ml; Nakamura et al., 1987). It preferentially inhibited the growth of DNA repair-deficient *Bacillus subtilis* (at 0.2–1.0 μg/disc; Horikawa et al., 1986).

1-Nitropyrene was mutagenic to *E. coli* WP2 *uvrA* pKM101 (Tokiwa et al., 1984 (0.125–1 μg/plate); McCoy et al., 1985a (0.3–33 μg/plate)) and to *S. typhimurium* TA96,

TA97, TA98, TA100, TA102, TA104, TA1537 and TA1538 (Rosenkranz et al., 1980; Wang et al., 1980; Löfroth, 1981; Mermelstein et al., 1981; Pederson & Siak, 1981; Tokiwa et al., 1981a, b; Pitts et al., 1982; McCoy et al., 1983a; Tokiwa et al., 1984; Ball, L.M. et al., 1984b; Heflich et al., 1985a,b; McCoy et al., 1985b; Rosenkranz et al., 1985; Tokiwa et al., 1985).

The urine of male rats receiving 10 mg/kg bw 1-nitropyrene intraperitoneally was mutagenic to S. typhimurium in the presence of $\beta$-glucuronidase and an exogenous metabolic system from rat liver (Ball, L.M. et al., 1984a); the bile of treated rats was mutagenic in the presence and in the absence of an exogenous metabolic system (Morotomi et al., 1985).

1-Nitropyrene (at up to 0.5 mg/ml) did not induce gene conversion or recombination in the yeast Saccharomyces cerevisiae D4 (McCoy et al., 1983b, 1984).

1-Nitropyrene induced single-strand DNA breaks, as determined by alkaline elution, in primary mouse hepatocytes (at 10–200 $\mu$M; Møller & Thorgeirsson, 1985), in Chinese hamster DON lung fibroblasts (at 0.25–48 $\mu$g/ml; Edwards et al., 1986b) and V79 cells (tested at 15 and 30 $\mu$M; Saito et al., 1984b) and in cultured rat hepatoma cells (at 10–50 $\mu$M; Møller & Thorgeirsson, 1985).

1-Nitropyrene induced unscheduled DNA synthesis in cultured hepatocytes from mice ($3.5 \times 10^{-3}$–$3.5 \times 10^{-2}$ mg/ml; Mori et al., 1987), rats (Mori et al., 1987 ($3.5 \times 10^{-3}$–$3.5 \times 10^{-2}$ mg/ml); Kornbrust & Barfknecht, 1984 ($5 \times 10^{-7}$–$10^{-4}$ M, 97% pure)) and hamsters (Kornbrust & Barfknecht, 1984 ($5 \times 10^{-7}$–$10^{-4}$ M, 97% pure)). It was reported in an abstract to induce unscheduled DNA synthesis in human hepatocytes (Yoshimi et al., 1987). It also induced unscheduled DNA synthesis in human ($10^{-4}$ M; Sugimura & Takayama, 1983) and rat (10–100 $\mu$M; Doolittle & Butterworth, 1984) tracheal epithelial cells, in human hepatoma-derived HepG2 cells (Eddy et al., 1986, 1987) and in rabbit lung Clara, but not alveolar type II, cells (Haugen et al., 1986).

1-Nitropyrene preferentially killed DNA repair-deficient human xeroderma pigmentosum fibroblasts (Patton et al., 1986 (20% survival at 25 $\mu$M); Maher et al., 1988). This compound induced the synthesis of viral DNA in polyoma virus-transformed rat fibroblasts (at 10–30 $\mu$g/ml; Lambert & Weinstein, 1987).

1-Nitropyrene (at 33–60 $\mu$M) induced mutations at the 6-thioguanine locus of human diploid fibroblasts (Patton et al., 1986; Maher et al., 1988) and human hepatoma-derived HepG2 cells (at 2–20 $\mu$M; Eddy et al., 1986, 1987) and had a marginal mutagenic effect on cultured Chinese hamster CHO cells (Marshall et al., 1982 (at 2–20 $\mu$g/ml)) and V79 cells (Ball, J.C. et al., 1984 (2–40.5 $\mu$M); Berry et al., 1985 (only dose tested, 50 $\mu$M)), although no effect was observed in other studies with Chinese hamster CHO cells (Heflich et al., 1985b, 1986a,b). The marginal effects were increased by the presence of an exogenous metabolic system from rat liver (Li & Dutcher, 1983 (20 $\mu$g/ml tested); Berry et al., 1985 (50 $\mu$M tested)).

1-Nitropyrene (purity, 95%) was reported to be mutagenic to mouse lymphoma L5178Y cells at the $TK^{+/-}$ locus in the presence of an exogenous metabolic system (Lewtas, 1982). It did not induce mutation to diphtheria toxin resistance (at up to 20 $\mu$g/ml; Nakayasu et al., 1982) or to ouabain resistance (at 1–10 $\mu$g/ml; Takayama et al., 1983) in cultured Chinese hamster lung fibroblasts.

1-Nitropyrene (1–30 μM) induced sister chromatid exchange in cultured Chinese hamster CHO cells in the presence and absence of an exogenous metabolic system (Nachtman & Wolff, 1982) and was reported in an abstract to induce sister chromatid exchange in V79 cells (Heidemann & Miltenburger, 1983) and in CHO cells in the absence of an exogenous metabolic system (Lewtas, 1982; purity, 95%). It induced chromosomal aberrations, including chromosome and chromatid deletions and asymmetrical exchanges, in Chinese hamster DON lung fibroblasts (at 3.8–60 μg/ml; Lafi & Parry, 1987) and, as reported in an abstract, in Chinese hamster lung fibroblasts (Matsuoka et al., 1987).

1-Nitropyrene (at 4–41 μM) induced morphological transformation in Syrian hamster embryo cells (DiPaolo et al., 1983) and transformation (induction of growth in soft agar and invasiveness in chicken embryo skin cultures) in normal human fibroblasts (at 3–33 μM) under anaerobic conditions (Howard et al., 1983b; Kumari et al., 1984).

In mice, intratracheal instillation of 1-nitropyrene (at 10–100 mg/kg bw) induced damage in lung DNA as determined by alkaline elution (Mitchell, 1984, 1985a,b[abstract]; Mitchell, 1986 [abstract]).

Oral administration of 1-nitropyrene (at 0.5–5 g/kg bw) to rats induced a slight increase in the incidence of sister chromatid exchange in bone-marrow cells (Marshall et al., 1982). It was reported in an abstract that increases in sister chromatid exchange and micronuclei frequency occurred in Chinese hamsters receiving 125 and 1000 mg/kg bw 1-nitropyrene, respectively (Heidemann & Miltenburger, 1983).

*(b) Humans*

No data were available to the Working Group.

### 3.3 Epidemiological studies and case reports of carcinogenicity to humans

No data were available to the Working Group.

## 4. Summary of Data Reported and Evaluation

### 4.1 Exposure data

1-Nitropyrene has been detected in some carbon blacks, in stack gases from coal-fired power plants and aluminium smelters and in particulate emissions from other stationary sources and from diesel and gasoline engines. 1-Nitropyrene also occurs at low concentrations in ambient air.

## 4.2 Experimental data[1]

1-Nitropyrene was tested for carcinogenicity by oral administration in rats, by skin application in mice, by intratracheal instillation in hamsters, by intrapulmonary administration in rats, by subcutaneous injection in mice and in newborn and young rats and by intraperitoneal injection in newborn and young mice and in rats. Two experiments by oral administration to rats were considered to be inadequate for evaluation. One experiment on mouse skin gave negative results; the other was considered to be inadequate. Following either intratracheal instillation in hamsters or intrapulmonary administration in rats, negative results were obtained.

One study by subcutaneous injection in young mice gave negative results, however the group was quite small. In one study in newborn rats, 1-nitropyrene produced sarcomas at the site of injection and an increased incidence of mammary tumours, including adenocarcinomas. In two other studies using newborn rats (including one using two different strains), no tumour was observed at the site of injection and there was no increase in the total number of mammary tumours. Two studies with young rats given subcutaneous injections of 1-nitropyrene yielded negative results, but the groups were small and the observation periods relatively short.

In a screening test by intraperitoneal injection using strain A mice, lung tumour incidence and the number of adenomas per mouse were significantly increased. One study using intraperitoneal injection in newborn mice showed an increase in the incidence of liver-cell tumours in males. One study on weanling rats showed an increased incidence of mammary tumours; a second study from the same laboratory showed a nonsignificant increase in the incidence of mammary tumours.

## 4.3 Human data

No data were available to the Working Group.

## 4.4 Other relevant data

The association of 1-nitropyrene with diesel particles led to a substantial reduction in clearance of the compound from the lungs of rats.

Metabolism of 1-nitropyrene led to DNA adduct formation in cultured human and mammalian cells and in animals. 1-Nitropyrene induced DNA damage and sister chromatid exchange in rodents; DNA damage, mutations and transformation in cultured human cells; and DNA damage, sister chromatid exchange, chromosomal aberrations, mutation and transformation in cultured animal cells. It was not recombinogenic to yeast but induced DNA damage and mutation in bacteria.

---

[1]Subsequent to the meeting, the Secretariat became aware of a newly published study (El-Bayoumy *et al.*, 1988) describing the induction of mammary adenocarcinomas in female Sprague-Dawley rats given 1-nitropyrene (purity, >99.9%) by gavage from birth to 16 weeks of age.

## Summary table of genetic and related effects of 1-nitropyrene

| Nonmammalian systems | | | | | | | | | | | | Mammalian systems | | | | | | | | | | | | | | | | | | | | |
|---|---|---|---|---|---|---|---|---|---|---|---|---|---|---|---|---|---|---|---|---|---|---|---|---|---|---|---|---|---|---|---|---|
| Prokaryotes | | | | Lower eukaryotes | | | | Plants | | | | Insects | | | In vitro | | | | | | | | | | | | | | In vivo | | | |
| | | | | | | | | | | | | | | | Animal cells | | | | | | Human cells | | | | | | | | Animals | | | Humans |
| D | G | D | R | G | A | D | G | C | R | G | C | A | | | D | G | S | M | C | A | T | I | D | G | S | M | C | A | T | I | D | G | S | M | C | DL | A | D | S | M | C | A |
| + | + | | – | | | | | | | | | | | | + | + | + | ±  | ±  | | | ±  | + | + | + | | | | ±  | | + | + | ±  | | | | | | | | |

A, aneuploidy; C, chromosomal aberrations; D, DNA damage; DL, dominant lethal mutation; G, gene mutation; I, inhibition of intercellular communication; M, micronuclei; R, mitotic recombination and gene conversion; S, sister chromatid exchange; T, cell transformation

*In completing the tables, the following symbols indicate the consensus of the Working Group with regard to the results for each endpoint:*
+ considered to be positive for the specific endpoint and level of biological complexity
±  considered to be positive, but only one valid study was available to the Working Group
– considered to be negative

## 4.5 Evaluation[1]

There is *sufficient evidence* for the carcinogenicity in experimental animals of 1-nitropyrene.

No data were available from studies in humans on the carcinogenicity of 1-nitropyrene.

**Overall evaluation**

1-Nitropyrene *is possibly carcinogenic to humans (Group 2B)*.

# 5. References

Aldrich Chemical Co. (1988) *Aldrich Catalog/Handbook of Fine Chemicals 1988*–1989, Milwaukee, WI, p. 1127

Arey, J., Zielinska, B., Atkinson, R. & Winer, A.M. (1987) Polycyclic aromatic hydrocarbon and nitroarene concentrations in ambient air during a wintertime high-$NO_x$ episode in the Los Angeles basin. *Atmos. Environ.*, 21, 1437–1444

Asokan, P., Das, M., Rosenkranz, H.S., Bickers, D.R. & Mukhtar, H. (1985) Topically applied nitropyrenes are potent inducers of cutaneous and hepatic monooxygenases. *Biochem. biophys. Res. Commun.*, 129, 134–140

Asokan, P., Das, M., Bik, D.P., Howard, P.C., McCoy, G.D., Rosenkranz, H.S., Bickers, D.R. & Mukhtar, H. (1986) Comparative effects of topically applied nitrated arenes and their nonnitrated parent arenes on cutaneous and hepatic drug and carcinogen metabolism in neonatal rats. *Toxicol. appl. Pharmacol.*, 86, 33–43

Ayres, P.H., Sun, J.D. & Bond, J.A. (1985) Contribution of intestinal microfloral metabolism to the total macromolecular covalent binding of 1-nitropyrene in the lung and liver of the rat. *Toxicology*, 36, 263–273

Ball, J.C., Zacmanidis, P. & Salmeen, I.T. (1984) The reduction of 1-nitropyrene to 1-aminopyrene does not correlate with the mutagenicity of 1-nitropyrene in V79 Chinese hamster cells. In: Cooke, M.W. & Dennis, A.J., eds, *Polynuclear Aromatic Hydrocarbons, 8th International Symposium, Mechanisms, Methods and Metabolism*, Columbus, OH, Battelle, pp. 113–120

Ball, L.M. & Lewtas, J. (1985) Rat liver subcellular fractions catalyze aerobic binding of 1-nitro[$^{14}$C]pyrene to DNA. *Environ. Health Perspect.*, 62, 193–196

Ball, L.M., Kohan, M.J., Inmon, J., Claxton, L.D. & Lewtas, J. (1984a) Metabolism of 1-nitro[$^{14}$C]pyrene *in vivo* in the rat and mutagenicity of urinary metabolites. *Carcinogenesis*, 5, 1557–1564

Ball, L.M., Kohan, M.J., Claxton, L.D. & Lewtas, J. (1984b) Mutagenicity of derivatives and metabolites of 1-nitropyrene: activation by rat liver S9 and bacterial enzymes. *Mutat. Res.*, 138, 113–125

---

[1]For definitions of the italicized terms, see Preamble, pp. 25–28.

Ball, L.M., King, L.C., Jackson, M.A. & Lewtas, J. (1986) In vivo metabolism, disposition and macromolecular binding of 1-nitro[$^{14}$C]pyrene vapor-coated onto diesel particles. In: Cooke, M.W. & Dennis, A.J., eds, *Polynuclear Aromatic Hydrocarbons, 9th International Symposium, Chemistry, Characterization and Carcinogenesis*, Columbus, OH, Battelle, pp. 53–64

Bavin, P.M.G. & Dewar, M.J.S. (1955) Absorption spectra of nitro- and fluoro-derivatives of phenanthrene, triphenylene and pyrene. *J. chem. Soc.*, 4486–4487

Beland, F.A., Heflich, R.H., Howard, P.C. & Fu, P.P. (1985) The in vitro metabolic activation of nitro polycyclic aromatic hydrocarbons. In: Harvey, R.G., ed., *Polycyclic Hydrocarbons and Carcinogenesis (ACS Symposium Series No. 283)*, Washington DC, American Chemical Society, pp. 371–396

Beland, F.A., Ribovich, M., Howard, P.C., Heflich, R.H., Kurian, P. & Milo, G.E. (1986) Cytotoxicity, cellular transformation and DNA adducts in normal human diploid fibroblasts exposed to 1-nitrosopyrene, a reduced derivative of the environmental contaminant, 1-nitropyrene. *Carcinogenesis*, 7, 1279–1283

Belisario, M.A., Carrano, L., de Giulio, A. & Buonocore, V. (1986) Role of rat liver inducibile enzymes in in vitro metabolic transformation of 1-nitropyrene. *Toxicol. Lett.*, 32, 89–96

Belisario, M.A., Borgia, R., Pecce, R. & de Lorenzo, F. (1988) Induction of hepatic drug-metabolizing enzymes in rats treated with 1-nitropyrene. *Environ. Res.*, 45, 91–100

Belliardo, J.J., Jacob, J. & Lindsey, A.S. (1988) *The Certification of the Purity of Seven Nitro-polycyclic Aromatic Compounds. CRM Nos 305, 306, 307, 308, 310, 311, 312, BCR Information, Reference Materials (EUR 11254EN)*, Brussels, Commission of the European Communities, p. III

Berry, D.L., Schoofs, G.M. & Vance, W.A. (1985) Mutagenicity of nitrofluoranthenes, 3-aminofluoranthene and 1-nitropyrene in Chinese hamster V79 cells. *Carcinogenesis*, 6, 1403–1407

Boit, H.G., ed. (1965) *Beilsteins Handbuch der Organischen Chemie*, Vol. 5, 4th ed., 3rd Suppl. (*Syst. No. 487*), Berlin (West), Springer Verlag, p. 2286

Bond, J.A. (1983) Bioactivation and biotransformation of 1-nitropyrene in liver, lung and nasal tissue of rats. *Mutat. Res.*, 124, 315–324

Bond, J.A. & Mauderly, J.L. (1984) Metabolism and macromolecular covalent binding of [$^{14}$C]-1-nitropyrene in isolated perfused and ventilated rat lungs. *Cancer Res.*, 44, 3924–3929

Bond, J.A., Medinsky, M.A. & Dutcher, J.S. (1984) Metabolism of 1-[$^{14}$C]nitropyrene in isolated perfused rat livers. *Toxicol. appl. Pharmacol.*, 75, 531–538

Bond, J.A., Mauderly, J.L., Henderson, R.F. & McClellan, R.O. (1985) Metabolism of 1-[$^{14}$C]nitropyrene in respiratory tract tissue of rats exposed to diesel exhaust. *Toxicol. appl. Pharmacol.*, 79, 461–470

Bond, J.A., Sun, J.D., Medinsky, M.A., Jones, R.K. & Yeh, H.C. (1986) Deposition, metabolism, and excretion of 1-[$^{14}$C]nitropyrene and 1-[$^{14}$C]nitropyrene coated on diesel exhaust particles as influenced by exposure concentration. *Toxicol. appl. Pharmacol.*, 85, 102–117

Brorström-Lundén, E. & Lindskog, A. (1985) Degradation of polycyclic aromatic hydrocarbons during simulated stack gas sampling. *Environ. Sci. Technol.*, 19, 313–316

Butler, M.A., Evans, D.L., Giammarise, A.T., Kiriazides, D.K., Marsh, D., McCoy, E.C., Mermelstein, R., Murphy, C.B. & Rosenkranz, H.S. (1983) Application of *Salmonella* assay to carbon blacks and toners. In: Cooke, M. & Dennis, A.J., eds, *Polynuclear Aromatic Hydrocarbons, 7th International Symposium, Formation, Metabolism and Measurement*, Columbus, OH, Battelle, pp. 225—241

Campbell, R.M. & Lee, M.L. (1984) Capillary column gas chromatographic determination of nitro polycyclic aromatic compounds in particulate extracts. *Anal. Chem.*, 56, 1026—1030

Cerniglia, C.E. (1985) Metabolism of 1-nitropyrene and 6-nitrobenzo(a)pyrene by intestinal microflora. In: *Germfree Research: Microflora Control and Its Application to the Biomedical Sciences*, New York, Alan R. Liss, pp. 133—137

Chan, T.L. & Gibson, T.L. (1985) Sampling and atmospheric chemistry of particles containing nitrated polycyclic aromatic hydrocarbons. In: White, C.M., ed., *Nitrated Polycyclic Aromatic Hydrocarbons*, Heidelberg, A. Hüthig Verlag, pp. 237—266

Chemsyn Science Laboratories (1988) *1-Nitropyrene (Product Code U1005)*, Lenexa, KS, pp. 90—93

Chou, M.W. (1986) High performance liquid chromatographic separation of nitro-polycyclic aromatic hydrocarbons and their oxidized derivatives. In: Cooke, M. & Dennis, A.J., eds, *Polynuclear Aromatic Hydrocarbons, 9th International Symposium, Chemistry, Characterization and Carcinogenesis*, Columbus, OH, Battelle Press, pp. 145—153

Chou, M.W., Wang, B., Von Tungeln, L.S., Beland, F.A. & Fu, P.P. (1986) Induction of rat hepatic microsomal enzyme activities by environmental nitropolycyclic aromatic hydrocarbons (Abstract No. 451). *Proc. Am. Assoc. Cancer Res.*, 27, 114

D'Agostino, P.A., Narine, D.R., McCarry, B.E. & Quilliam, M.A. (1983) Clean-up and analysis of nitrated polycyclic aromatic hydrocarbons in environmental samples. In: Cooke, M. & Dennis, A.J., eds, *Polynuclear Aromatic Hydrocarbons, 7th International Symposium, Formation, Metabolism and Measurement*, Columbus, OH, Battelle, pp. 365—377

DiPaolo, J.A., DeMarinis, A.J., Chow, F.L., Garner, R.C., Martin, C.N. & Doniger, J. (1983) Nitration of carcinogenic and non-carcinogenic polycyclic aromatic hydrocarbons results in products able to induce transformation of Syrian hamster cells. *Carcinogenesis*, 4, 357—359

Djurić, Z., Fifer, E.K. & Beland, S.A. (1985) Acetyl coenzyme A-dependent binding of carcinogenic and mutagenic dinitropyrenes to DNA. *Carcinogenesis*, 6, 941—944

Djurić, Z., Yamazoe, Y. & Beland, F.A. (1986a) Effects of nitroreductase induction on DNA-binding of 1-nitropyrene and 1,6-dinitropyrene *in vivo* and *in vitro* (Abstract No. 448). *Proc. Am. Assoc. Cancer Res.*, 27, 114

Djurić, Z., Fifer, E.K., Howard, P.C. & Beland, F.A. (1986b) Oxidative microsomal metabolism of 1-nitropyrene and DNA-binding of oxidized metabolites following nitroreduction. *Carcinogenesis*, 7, 1073—1070

Djurić, Z., Fifer, E.K., Yamazoe, Y. & Beland, F.A. (1988) DNA binding by 1-nitropyrene and 1,6-dinitropyrene *in vitro* and *in vivo*: effects of nitroreductase induction. *Carcinogenesis*, 9, 357—364

Djurić, Z., Coles, B., Fifer, E.K., Ketterer, B. & Beland, F.A. (1989) In vivo and in vitro formation of glutathione conjugates from the K-region epoxides of 1-nitropyrene. *Carcinogenesis* (in press)

Doolittle, D.J. & Butterworth, B.E. (1984) Assessment of chemically-induced DNA repair in rat tracheal epithelial cells. *Carcinogenesis*, 5, 773—779

Draper, W.M. (1986) Quantitation of nitro- and dinitropolycyclic aromatic hydrocarbons in diesel exhaust particulate matter. *Chemosphere*, 15, 437—447

Dutcher, J.S., Sun, J.D., Bechtold, W.E. & Unkefer, C.J. (1985) Excretion and metabolism of 1-nitropyrene in rats after oral or intraperitoneal administration. *Fundam. appl. Toxicol., 5*, 287–296

Dybing, E., Dahl, J.E., Beland, F.A. & Thorgeirsson, S.S. (1986) Formation of reactive 1-nitropyrene metabolites by lung microsomes and isolated lung cells. *Cell Biol. Toxicol., 2*, 341–355

Eddy, E.P., McCoy, E.C., Rosenkranz, H.S. & Mermelstein, R. (1986) Dichotomy in the mutagenicity and genotoxicity of nitropyrenes: apparent effect of the number of electrons involved in nitroreduction. *Mutat. Res., 161*, 109–111

Eddy, E.P., Howard, P.C., McCoy, E.C. & Rosenkrantz, H.S. (1987) Mutagenicity, unscheduled DNA synthesis, and metabolism of 1-nitropyrene in the human hepatoma cell line HepG2. *Cancer Res., 47*, 3163–3168

Edwards, M.J., Batmanghelich, S., Smith, K. & Parry, J.M. (1986a) Nitropyrene induced DNA damage, toxicity and DNA-adduct formation in mammalian cells (Abstract G3). *Br. J. Cancer, 54*, 369

Edwards, M.J., Parry, J.M., Batmanghelich, S. & Smith, K. (1986b) Toxicity and DNA damage induced by 1-nitropyrene and its derivatives in Chinese hamster lung fibroblasts. *Mutat. Res., 163*, 81–89

El-Bayoumy, K. & Hecht, S.S. (1983) Identification and mutagenicity of metabolites of 1-nitropyrene formed by rat liver. *Cancer Res., 43*, 3132–3137

El-Bayoumy, K. & Hecht, S.S. (1984) Metabolism of 1-nitro($U$-4,5,9,10-$^{14}$C)pyrene in the F344 rat. *Cancer Res., 44*, 4317–4322

El-Bayoumy, K. & Hecht, S.S. (1986) The metabolism of 1-nitropyrene in newborn mice (Abstract No. 454). *Proc. Am. Assoc. Cancer Res., 27*, 115

El-Bayoumy, K., Hecht, S.S. & Hoffmann, D. (1982) Comparative tumor initiating activity on mouse skin of 6-nitrobenzo[a]pyrene, 6-nitrochrysene, 3-nitroperylene, 1-nitropyrene and their parent hydrocarbons. *Cancer Lett., 16*, 333–337

El-Bayoumy, K., Sharma, C., Louis, Y.M., Reddy, B. & Hecht, S.S. (1983) The role of intestinal microflora in the metabolic reduction of 1-nitropyrene to 1-aminopyrene in conventional and germfree rats and in humans. *Cancer Lett., 19*, 311–316

El-Bayoumy, K., Hecht, S.S., Sackl, T. & Stoner, G.D. (1984a) Tumorigenicity and metabolism of 1-nitropyrene in A/J mice. *Carcinogenesis, 5*, 1449–1452

El-Bayoumy, K., Reddy, B. & Hecht, S.S. (1984b) Identification of ring oxidized metabolites of 1-nitropyrene in the feces and urine of germfree F344 rats. *Carcinogenesis, 5*, 1371–1373

El-Bayoumy, K., Rivenson, A., Johnson, B., DiBello, J., Little, P. & Hecht, S.S. (1988) Comparative tumorigenicity of 1-nitropyrene, 1-nitrosopyrene, and 1-aminopyrene administered by gavage to Sprague-Dawley rats. *Cancer Res., 48*, 4256–4260

Fifer, E.K., Howard, P.C., Heflich, R.M. & Beland, F.A. (1986) Synthesis and mutagenicity of 1-nitropyrene 4,5-oxide and 1-nitropyrene 9,10-oxide, microsomal metabolites of 1-nitropyrene. *Mutagenesis, 1*, 433–438

Gallagher, J.E., Robertson, I.G.C., Jackson, M.A., Dietrich, A.M., Ball, L.M. & Lewtas, J. (1988) $^{32}$P-Postlabelling analysis of DNA adducts of two nitrated polycyclic aromatic hydrocarbons in rabbit tracheal epithelial cells. In: King, C.M., Romano, L.J. & Schuetzle, D., eds, *Carcinogenic and Mutagenic Responses to Aromatic Amines and Nitroarenes*, Amsterdam, Elsevier, pp. 277–281

Giammarise, A.T., Evans, D.L., Butler, M.A., Murphy, C.B., Kiriazides, D.K., Marsh, D. & Mermelstein, R. (1982) Improved methodology for carbon black extraction. In: Cooke, M., Dennis, A.J. & Fischer, G.L., eds, *Polynuclear Aromatic Hydrocarbons, 6th International Symposium, Physical and Biological Chemistry*, Columbus, OH, Battelle, pp. 325–334

Gibson, T.L. (1982) Nitro derivatives of polynuclear aromatic hydrocarbons in airborne and source particulate matter. *Atmos. Environ.*, 16, 2037–2040

Gibson, T.L. (1983) Sources of direct-acting nitroarene mutagens in airborne particulate matter. *Mutat. Res.*, 122, 115–121

Gibson, T.L. (1986) Sources of nitroaromatic mutagens in atmosphere polycyclic organic matter. *J. Air Pollut. Control Assoc.*, 36, 1022–1025

Gibson, T.L., Ricci, A.I. & Williams, R.L. (1981) Measurement of polynuclear aromatic hydrocarbons, their derivatives, and their reactivity in diesel automobile exhaust. In: Cooke, M. & Dennis, A.J., eds, *Polynuclear Aromatic Hydrocarbons, 5th International Symposium, Chemical Analysis and Biological Fate*, Columbus, OH, Battelle, pp. 707–717

Gorse, R.A., Jr, Riley, T.L., Ferris, F.C., Pero, A.M. & Skewes, L.M. (1983) 1-Nitropyrene concentration and bacterial mutagenicity in on-road vehicle particulate emissions. *Environ. Sci. Technol.*, 17, 198–202

Grimmer, G., Brune, H., Deutsch-Wenzel, R., Dettbarn, G., Jacob, J., Naujack, K.-W., Mohr, U. & Ernst, H. (1987) Contribution of polycyclic aromatic hydrocarbons and nitro-derivatives to the carcinogenic impact of diesel engine exhaust condensate evaluated by implantation into the lungs of rats. *Cancer Lett.*, 37, 173–180

Hanausek-Walaszek, M., Walaszek, Z. & Webb, T.E. (1985) Chemical carcinogens as specific inducers of a 60-kilodalton oncofetal protein in rats. *Carcinogenesis*, 6, 1725–1730

Harris, W.R., Chess, E.K., Okamoto, D., Remsen, J.F. & Later, D.W. (1984) Contribution of nitropyrene to the mutagenic activity of coal fly ash. *Environ. Mutagenesis*, 6, 131–144

Hashimoto, Y. & Shudo, K. (1985) Modification of nucleic acids with 1-nitropyrene in the rat: identification of the modified nucleic acid base. *Jpn. J. Cancer Res. (Gann)*, 76, 253–256

Haugen, A., Aune, T. & Deilhaug, T. (1986) Nitropyrene-induced DNA repair in Clara cells and alveolar type-II cells isolated from rabbit lung. *Mutat. Res.*, 175, 259–262

Heflich, R.H., Howard, P.C. & Beland, F.A. (1985a) 1-Nitrosopyrene: an intermediate in the metabolic activation of 1-nitropyrene to a mutagen in *Salmonella typhimurium* TA1538. *Mutat. Res.*, 149, 25–32

Heflich, R.M., Fifer, E.K., Djurić, Z. & Beland, F.A. (1985b) DNA adduct formation and mutation induction by nitropyrenes in *Salmonella* and Chinese hamster ovary cells: relationships with nitroreduction and acetylation. *Environ. Health Perspect.*, 62, 135–143

Heflich, R.H., Fullerton, N.F. & Beland, F.A. (1986a) An examination of the weak mutagenic response of 1-nitropyrene in Chinese hamster ovary cells. *Mutat. Res.*, 161, 99–108

Heflich, R.H., Fifer, E.K., Djurić, Z. & Beland, F.A. (1986b) Mutation induction and DNA adduct formation by 1,8-dinitropyrene in Chinese hamster ovary cells. *Progr. clin. Biol. Res.*, 209A, 265–273

Heidemann, A. & Miltenburger, H.G. (1983) Investigations on the mutagenic activity of fractions from diesel exhaust particulate matter in mammalian cells *in vivo* and *in vitro* (Abstract No. 15). *Mutat. Res.*, 113, 339

Henderson, T.R., Sun, J.D., Royer, R.E., Clark, C.R., Li, A.P., Harvey, T.M., Hunt, D.H., Fulford, J.E., Lovette, A.M. & Davidson, W.R. (1983) Triple-quadrupole mass spectrometry studies of nitroaromatic emissions from different diesel engines. *Environ. Sci. Technol.*, 17, 443–449

Herr, J.D., Dukovich, M., Lestz, S.S., Yergey, J.A., Risby, T.H. & Tejada, S.B. (1982) *The Role of Nitrogen in the Observed Direct Microbial Mutagenic Activity for Diesel Engine Combustion in a Single-cylinder CI Engine (Paper No. 820467)*, Warrendale, PA, Society of Automotive Engineers

Hirose, M., Lee, M.-S., Wang, C.Y. & King, C.M. (1984) Induction of rat mammary gland tumors by 1-nitropyrene, a recently recognized environmental mutagen. *Cancer Res.*, 44, 1158–1162

Horikawa, K., Sera, N., Tokiwa, H. & Kada, T. (1986) Results of the *rec*-assay of nitropyrenes in the *Bacillus subtilis* test system. *Mutat. Res.*, 174, 89–92

Howard, P.C. & Beland, F.A. (1982) Xanthine oxidase catalyzed binding of 1-nitropyrene to DNA. *Biochem. biophys. Res. Commun.*, 104, 727–732

Howard, P.C., Beland, F.A. & Cerniglia, C.E. (1983a) Formation of DNA adducts *in vitro* and in *Salmonella typhimurium* upon metabolic reduction of the environmental mutagen 1-nitropyrene. *Cancer Res.*, 43, 2052–2058

Howard, P.C., Gerrard, J.A., Milo, G.E., Fu, P.P., Beland, F.A. & Kadlubar, F.F. (1983b) Transformation of normal human skin fibroblasts by 1-nitropyrene and 6-nitrobenzo[*a*]pyrene. *Carcinogenesis*, 4, 353–355

Howard, P.C., Flammang, T.J. & Beland, F.A. (1985) Comparison of the in vitro and in vivo hepatic metabolism of the carcinogen 1-nitropyrene. *Carcinogenesis*, 6, 243–249

Howard, A.J., Mitchell, C.E., Dutcher, J.S., Henderson, T.R. & McClellan, R.O. (1986) Binding of nitropyrenes and benzo[*a*]pyrene to mouse lung deoxyribonucleic acid after pretreatment with inducing agents. *Biochem. Pharmacol.*, 35, 2129–2134

Hsieh, L.L., Wong, D., Heisig, V., Santella, R.M., Mauderly, J.L., Mitchell, C.E., Wolff, R.K. & Jeffrey, A.M. (1986) Analysis of genotoxic components in diesel engine emissions. In: Ishinishi, N., Koizumi, A., McClellan, R.O. & Stöber, W., eds, *Carcinogenic and Mutagenic Effects of Diesel Engine Exhaust*, Amsterdam, Elsevier, pp. 223–232

Hughes, M.M., Natusch, D.F.S., Taylor, D.R. & Zeller, M.V. (1980) Chemical transformations of particulate polycyclic organic matter. In: Bjørseth, A. & Dennis, A.J., eds, *Polynuclear Aromatic Hydrocarbons, 4th International Symposium, Chemistry and Biological Effects*, Columbus, OH, Battelle, pp. 1–8

IARC (1984) *IARC Monographs on the Evaluation of the Carcinogenic Risk of Chemicals to Humans*, Vol. 33, *Polynuclear Aromatic Compounds, Part 2, Carbon Blacks, Mineral Oils and Some Nitroarenes*, Lyon, pp. 209–222

IARC (1988) *Information Bulletin on the Survey of Chemicals Being Tested for Carcinogenicity*, No. 13, Lyon, pp. 21, 171

Jackson, M.A., King, L.C., Ball, L.M., Ghayourmanesh, S., Jeffrey, A.M. & Lewtas, J. (1985) Nitropyrene: DNA binding and adduct formation in respiratory tissues. *Environ. Health Perspect.*, 62, 203–207

Jensen, T.E., Richert, J.F.O., Cleary, A.C., LaCourse, D.L. & Gorse, R.A., Jr (1986) 1-Nitropyrene in used diesel engine oil. *J. Air Pollut. Control Assoc.*, 36, 1255–1256

Jin, Z. & Rappaport, S.M. (1983) Microbore liquid chromatography with electrochemical detection for determination of nitro-substituted polynuclear aromatic hydrocarbons in diesel soot. *Anal. Chem.*, 55, 1778–1781

Kaplan, S. (1981) Carbon-13 chemical shift assignments of the nitration products of pyrene. *Org. magn. Resonance, 15*, 197–199

King, C.M. (1988) *Metabolism and Biological Effects of Nitropyrene and Related Compounds (Research Report No. 16)*, Cambridge, MA, Health Effects Institute

King, L.C., Jackson, M., Ball, L.M. & Lewtas, J. (1983) Binding of 1-nitro[$^{14}$C]pyrene to DNA and protein in cultured lung macrophages and respiratory tissues. *Cancer Lett., 19*, 241–246

King, L.C., Kohan, M.J., Ball, L.M. & Lewtas, J. (1984) Mutagenicity of 1-nitropyrene metabolites from lung S9. *Cancer Lett., 22*, 255–262

Kinouchi, I., Manabe, Y., Wakisaka, K. & Ohnishi, Y. (1982) Biotransformation of 1-nitropyrene in intestinal anaerobic bacteria. *Microbiol. Immunol., 26*, 993–1005

Kinouchi, T., Tsutsui, H. & Ohnishi, Y. (1986a) Detection of 1-nitropyrene in yakitori (grilled chicken). *Mutat. Res., 171*, 105–113

Kinouchi, T., Morotomi, M., Mutai, M., Fifer, E.K., Beland, F.A. & Ohnishi, Y. (1986b) Metabolism of 1-nitropyrene in germ-free and conventional rats. *Jpn. J. Cancer Res. (Gann), 77*, 356–369

Korfmacher, W.A. & Miller, D.W. (1984) Analysis of 1- and 4-nitropyrene and 1-nitropyrene-d$_9$ via fused silica GC combined with negative ion atmospheric pressure ionization mass spectrometry. *J. high Resol. Chromatogr. Chromatogr. Commun., 7*, 581–583

Korfmacher, W.A. & Rushing, L.G. (1986) Analysis of seven nitronaphthalene compounds via fused silica gas chromatography combined with negative ion atmospheric pressure ionization mass spectrometry. *J. high Resol. Chromatogr. Chromatogr. Commun., 9*, 293–296

Korfmacher, W.A., Fu, P.P. & Mitchum, R.K. (1984) Characterization of nitro-polycyclic aromatic hydrocarbons by negative ion atmospheric pressure ionization mass spectrometry. In: Cooke, M. & Dennis, A.J., eds, *Polynuclear Aromatic Hydrocarbons, 8th International Symposium, Mechanisms, Methods and Metabolism*, Columbus, OH, Battelle, pp. 749–762

Korfmacher, W.A., Rushing, L.G., Engelbach, R.J., Freeman, J.P., Djurić, Z., Fifer, E.K. & Beland, F.A. (1987) Analysis of three aminonitropyrene isomers via fused silica gas chromatography combined with negative ion atmospheric pressure ionization mass spectrometry. *J. high Resol. Chromatogr. Chromatogr. Commun., 10*, 43–45

Korfmacher, W.A., Djurić, Z., Fifer, E.K. & Beland, F.A. (1988) Characterization of nitro-polycyclic aromatic hydrocarbon metabolites via methane enhanced negative ion mass spectrometry. *Spectrosc. int. J., 6*, 1–16

Kornbrust, D.J. & Barfknecht, J.R. (1984) Comparison of rat and hamster hepatocyte primary culture/DNA repair assays. *Environ. Mutagenesis, 6*, 1–11

Kumari, H.L., Kurian, P., Beland, F., Howard, P., Kamat, P., Witiak, D.T. & Milo, G.E. (1984) Early events of the carcinogenesis process in human foreskin fibroblasts. In: Cooke, M. & Dennis, A.J., eds, *Polynuclear Aromatic Hydrocarbons, 8th International Symposium, Mechanisms, Methods and Metabolism*, Columbus, OH, Battelle, pp. 771–783

Lafi, A. & Parry, J.M. (1987) Chromosome aberrations induced by nitro-, nitroso- and aminopyrenes in cultured Chinese hamster cells. *Mutagenesis, 2*, 23–26

Lambert, M.E. & Weinstein, I.B. (1987) Nitropyrenes are inducers of polyoma viral DNA synthesis. *Mutat. Res., 183*, 203–211

Lang, J.M., Snow, L., Carlson, R., Black, F., Zweidinger, R. & Tejada, S. (1981) *Characterization of Particulate Emissions from In-use Gasoline-fueled Motor Vehicles (Paper No. 811186)*, Warrendale, PA, Society of Automotive Engineers

Levine, S.P., Skewes, L.M., Abrams, L.D. & Palmer, A.G., III (1982) High performance semi-preparative liquid chromatography and liquid chromatography-mass spectrometry of diesel engine emission particulate extracts. In: Cooke, M., Dennis, A.J. & Fisher, G.L., eds, *Polynuclear Aromatic Hydrocarbons, 6th International Symposium, Physical and Biological Chemistry*, Columbus, OH, Battelle, pp. 439-448

Lewtas, J. (1982) Mutagenic activity of diesel emissions. In: Lewtas, J., ed., *Toxicological Effects of Emissions from Diesel Engines*, Amsterdam, Elsevier, pp. 243-264

Li, A.P. & Dutcher, J.S. (1983) Mutagenicity of mono-, di- and tri-nitropyrenes in Chinese hamster ovary cells. *Mutat. Res.*, 119, 387-392

Löfroth, G. (1981) Comparison of the mutagenic activity in carbon particulate matter and in diesel and gasoline engine exhaust. In: Waters, M.D., Sandhu, S.S., Lewtas Huisingh, J., Claxton, L. & Nesnow, S., eds, *Application of Short-term Bioassays in the Analysis of Complex Environmental Mixtures, II*, New York, Plenum, pp. 319-336

Luckenbach, R., ed. (1980) *Beilsteins Handbuch der Organischen Chemie*, Vol. 5, 4th ed., 4th Suppl. (*Syst. No. 487*), Berlin (West), Springer Verlag, p. 2471

MacCrehan, W.A. & May, W.E. (1984) Determination of nitro-polynuclear aromatic hydrocarbons in diesel soot by liquid chromatography with fluorescence and electrochemical detection. In: Cooke, M. & Dennis, A.J., eds, *Polynuclear Aromatic Hydrocarbons, 8th International Symposium, Mechanisms, Methods and Metabolism*, Columbus, OH, Battelle, pp. 857-869

Maeda, T., Izumi, K., Otsuka, H., Manabe, Y., Kinouchi, T. & Ohnishi, Y. (1986) Induction of squamous cell carcinoma in the rat lung by 1,6-dinitropyrene. *J. natl Cancer Inst.*, 76, 693-701

Maher, V.M., Patton, J.D. & McCormick, J.J. (1988) Mutagenicity of 1-nitropyrene and related polycyclic aromatic carcinogens in human cells and the role of DNA repair. In: King, C.M., Romano, L.J. & Schuetzle, D., eds, *Carcinogenic and Mutagenic Responses to Aromatic Amines and Nitroarenes*, Amsterdam, Elsevier, pp. 351-359

Manabe, Y., Kinouchi, T., Wakisaka, K., Tahara, I. & Ohnishi, Y. (1984) Mutagenic 1-nitropyrene in wastewater from oil-water separating tanks of gasoline stations and in used crankcase oil. *Environ. Mutagenesis*, 6, 669-681

Manning, B.W., Cerniglia, C.E. & Federle, T.W. (1986) Biotransformation of 1-nitropyrene to 1-aminopyrene and N-formyl-1-aminopyrene in the human intestinal microbiota. *J. Toxicol. environ. Health*, 18, 339-346

Marshall, T.C., Royer, R.E., Li, A.P., Kusewitt, D.F. & Brooks, A.L. (1982) Acute and genetic toxicity of 1-nitropyrene and its fate after single oral doses to rats. *J. Toxicol. environ. Health*, 10, 373-384

Matsuoka, A., Sofuni, T., Sato, S., Miyata, N. & Ishidate, M., Jr (1987) In vitro clastogenicity of nitropyrenes and nitrofluorenes (Abstract No. 25). *Mutat. Res.*, 182, 366-367

McCoy, E.C., Anders, M. & Rosenkranz, H.S. (1983a) The basis of the insensitivity of *Salmonella typhimurium* strain TA98/1,8-$DNP_6$ to the mutagenic action of nitroarenes. *Mutat. Res.*, 121, 17-23

McCoy, E.C., Anders, M., Rosenkranz, H.S. & Mermelstein, R. (1983b) Apparent absence of recombinogenic activity of nitropyrenes for yeast. *Mutat. Res.*, 116, 119-127

McCoy, E.C., Anders, M., McCartney, M., Howard, P.C., Beland, F.A. & Rosenkranz, H.S. (1984) The recombinogenic inactivity of 1-nitropyrene for yeast is due to a deficiency in a functional nitroreductase. *Mutat. Res.*, 139, 115-118

McCoy, E.C., Anders, M., Rosenkranz, H.S. & Mermelstein, R. (1985a) Mutagenicity of nitropyrenes for *Escherichia coli*: requirement for increased cell permeability. *Mutat. Res.*, *142*, 163—167

McCoy, E.C., Holloway, M., Frierson, M., Klopman, G., Mermelstein, R. & Rosenkranz, H.S. (1985b) Genetic and quantum chemical basis of the mutagenicity of nitroarenes for adenine-thymine base pairs. *Mutat. Res.*, *149*, 311—319

Medinsky, M.A., Shelton, H., Bond, J.A. & McClellan, R.O. (1985) Biliary excretion and enterohepatic circulation of 1-nitropyrene metabolites in Fischer-344 rats. *Biochem. Pharmacol.*, *34*, 2325—2330

Mermelstein, R., Kiriazides, D.K., Butler, M., McCoy, E.C. & Rosenkranz, H.S. (1981) The extraordinary mutagenicity of nitropyrenes in bacteria. *Mutat. Res.*, *89*, 187—196

Mitchell, C.E. (1984) Damage and repair of mouse lung deoxyribonucleic acid induced by 1-nitropyrene. In: Guilmette, R.A. & Medinsky, M.A., eds, *Inhalation Toxicology Research Institute Annual Report 1983*—1984, Albuquerque, NM, Lovelace Biomedical and Environmental Research Institute, pp. 320—322

Mitchell, C.E. (1985a) Effect of aryl hydrocarbon hydroxylase induction on the in vivo covalent binding of 1-nitropyrene, benzo[*a*]pyrene, 2-aminoanthracene, and phenanthridone to mouse lung deoxyribonucleic acid. *Biochem. Pharmacol.*, *34*, 545—551

Mitchell, C.E. (1985b) Genotoxicity of 1-nitropyrene in mouse lung after intratracheal instillation (Abstract No. 2999). *Fed. Proc.*, *44*, 924

Mitchell, C.E. (1986) The relationship of 1-nitropyrene-induced DNA damage in mouse lung and covalent binding to DNA (Abstract No. 403). *Proc. Am. Assoc. Cancer Res.*, *27*, 102

Mitchell, C.E. (1988) Formation of DNA adducts in mouse tissues after intratracheal instillation of 1-nitropyrene. *Carcinogenesis*, *9*, 857—860

Møller, M.E. & Thorgeirsson, S.S. (1985) DNA damage induced by nitropyrenes in primary mouse hepatocytes and in rat H4-II-E hepatoma cells. *Mutat. Res.*, *151*, 137—146

Mori, H., Sugie, S., Yoshimi, N., Kinouchi, T. & Ohnishi, Y. (1987) Genotoxicity of a variety of nitroarenes and other nitro compounds in DNA-repair tests with rat and mouse hepatocytes. *Mutat. Res.*, *190*, 159—167

Morita, K., Fukamachi, K. & Tokiwa, H. (1982) Studies on aromatic nitro compounds in air. II. Determination of aromatic nitro compounds in airborne particulates by gas chromatography (Jpn.). *Bunseki Kagaku*, *31*, 255—260 [*Chem. Abstr.*, *97*, 11089q]

Morotomi, M., Nanno, M., Watanabe, T., Sakurai, T. & Mutai, M. (1985) Mutagenic activation of biliary metabolites of 1-nitropyrene by intestinal microflora. *Mutat. Res.*, *149*, 171—178

Mukhtar, H., Asokan, P., Das, M., Bik, D.P., Howard, P.C., McCoy, G.D., Rosenkranz, H.S. & Bickers, D.R. (1988) Nitroarenes are inducers of cutaneous and hepatic monooxygenases in neonatal rats: comparison with the parent arenes. In: Cook, M. & Dennis, A.J., eds, *Polynuclear Aromatic Hydrocarbons, 10th International Symposium, A Decade of Progress*, Columbus, OH, Battelle, pp. 581—594

Mumford, J.L. & Lewtas, J. (1982) Mutagenicity and cytotoxicity of coal fly ash from fluidized-bed and conventional combustion. *J. Toxicol. environ. Health*, *10*, 565—586

Nachtman, J.P. (1986) Superoxide generation by 1-nitropyrene in rat lung microsomes. *Res. Commun. chem. Pathol. Pharmacol.*, *51*, 73—80

Nachtman, J.P. & Wei, E.T. (1982) Evidence for enzymatic reduction of 1-nitropyrene by rat liver fractions. *Experientia*, *38*, 837–838

Nachtman, J.P. & Wolff, S. (1982) Activity of nitro-polynuclear aromatic hydrocarbons in the sister chromatid exchange assay with and without metabolic activation. *Environ. Mutagenesis*, *4*, 1–5

Nakagawa, R., Kitamori, S., Horikawa, K., Nakashima, K. & Tokiwa, H. (1983) Identification of dinitropyrenes in diesel-exhaust particles. Their probable presence as the major mutagens. *Mutat. Res.*, *124*, 201–211

Nakamura, S.-I., Oda, Y., Shimada, T., Oki, I. & Sugimoto, K. (1987) SOS-inducing activity of chemical carcinogens and mutagens in *Salmonella typhimurium* TA1535/pSK1002: examination with 151 chemicals. *Mutat. Res.*, *192*, 239–246

Nakayasu, M., Sakamoto, H., Wakabayashi, K., Terada, M., Sugimura, T. & Rosenkranz, H.S. (1982) Potent mutagenic activity of nitropyrenes on Chinese hamster lung cells with diphtheria toxin resistance as a selective marker. *Carcinogenesis*, *3*, 917–922

Nesnow, S., Triplett, L.L. & Slaga, T.J. (1984) Tumor initiating activities of 1-nitropyrene and its nitrated products in SENCAR mice. *Cancer Lett.*, *23*, 1–8

Nielsen, T. (1983) Isolation of polycyclic aromatic hydrocarbons and nitro derivatives in complex mixtures by liquid chromatography. *Anal. Chem.*, *55*, 286–290

Nielsen, T., Seitz, B., Hansen, A.M., Keiding, K. & Westerberg, B. (1983) The presence of nitro-PAH in samples of airborne particulate matter. In: Cooke, M. & Dennis, A.J., eds, *Polynuclear Aromatic Hydrocarbons, 7th International Symposium, Formation, Metabolism and Measurement*, Columbus, OH, Battelle, pp. 961–970

Nielsen, T., Seitz, B. & Ramdahl, T. (1984) Occurrence of nitro-PAH in the atmosphere in a rural area. *Atmos. Environ.*, *18*, 2159–2165

Nishioka, M.G., Petersen, B.A. & Lewtas, J. (1982) Comparison of nitro-aromatic content and direct-acting mutagenicity of diesel emissions. In: Cooke, M., Dennis, A.J. & Fisher, G.L., eds, *Polynuclear Aromatic Hydrocarbons, 6th International Symposium, Physical and Biological Chemistry*, Columbus, OH, Battelle, pp. 603–613

Odagiri, Y., Adachi, S., Katayama, H., Matsushita, H. & Takemoto, K. (1986) Carcinogenic effects of a mixture of nitropyrenes in F344 rats following its repeated oral administrations. In: Ishinishi, N., Koizumi, A., McClellan, R.O. & Stöber, W., eds, *Carcinogenic and Mutagenic Effects of Diesel Engine Exhaust*, Amsterdam, Elsevier, pp. 291–307

Ohgaki, H., Matsukura, N., Morino, K., Kawachi, T., Sugimura, T., Morita, K., Tokiwa, H. & Hirota, T. (1982) Carcinogenicity in rats of the mutagenic compounds 1-nitropyrene and 3-nitrofluoranthene. *Cancer Lett.*, *15*, 1–7

Ohgaki, H., Hasegawa, H., Kato, T., Negishi, C., Sato, S. & Sugimura, T. (1985) Absence of carcinogenicity of 1-nitropyrene, correction of previous results, and new demonstration of carcinogenicity of 1,6-dinitropyrene in rats. *Cancer Lett.*, *25*, 239–245

Ohnishi, Y., Kinouchi, T., Nishifuji, K., Fifer, E.K. & Beland, F.A. (1986) Metabolism of mutagenic 1-nitropyrene in rats. In: Ishinishi, N., Koizumi, A., McClellan, R.O. & Stöber, W., eds, *Carcinogenic and Mutagenic Effects of Diesel Engine Exhaust*, Amsterdam, Elsevier, pp. 171–183

Ohta, T., Nakamura, N., Moriya, M., Shirasu, Y. & Kada, T. (1984) The SOS-function-inducing activity of chemical mutagens in *Escherichia coli*. *Mutat. Res.*, *131*, 101–109

Okinaka, R.T., Nickols, J.W., Strniste, G.F. & Whaley, T.W. (1986) Photochemical transformation of primary aromatic amines into 'direct-acting' mutagens. In: Cooke, M. & Dennis, A.J., eds, *Polynuclear Aromatic Hydrocarbons, 9th International Symposium, Chemistry, Characterization and Carcinogenesis*, Columbus, OH, Battelle, pp. 717–728

Olsen, K.B., Kalkwarf, D.R. & Veverka, C., Jr (1984) Analysis and collection of PAHs in the flue gas of energy conversion facilities. In: Cooke, M. & Dennis, A.J., eds, *Polynuclear Aromatic Hydrocarbons, 8th International Symposium, Mechanisms, Methods and Metabolism*, Columbus, OH, Battelle, pp. 973–986

Paputa-Peck, M.C., Marano, R.S., Schuetzle, D., Riley, T.L., Hampton, C.V., Prater, T.J., Skewes, L.M., Jensen, T.E., Ruehle, P.H., Bosch, L.C. & Duncan, W.P. (1983) Determination of nitrated polynuclear aromatic hydrocarbons in particulate extracts by capillary column gas chromatography with nitrogen selective detection. *Anal. Chem.*, 55, 1946–1954

Patterson, P.L., Gatten, R.A. & Ontiveros, C. (1982) An improved thermionic ionization detector for gas chromatography. *J. chromatogr. Sci.*, 20, 97–102

Patton, J.D., Maher, V.M. & McCormick, J.J. (1986) Cytotoxic and mutagenic effects of 1-nitropyrene and 1-nitrosopyrene in diploid human fibroblasts. *Carcinogenesis*, 7, 89–93

Pederson, T.C. & Siak, J.C. (1981) The role of nitroaromatic compounds in the direct-acting mutagenicity of diesel particle extracts. *J. appl. Toxicol.*, 1, 54–60

Pitts, J.N., Jr (1987) Nitration of gaseous polycyclic aromatic hydrocarbons in simulated and ambient urban atmospheres: a source of mutagenic nitroarenes. *Atmos. Environ.*, 21, 2531–2547

Pitts, J.N., Jr, Lokensgard, D.M., Harper, W., Fisher, T.S., Mejia, V., Schuler, J.J., Scorziell, G.M. & Katzenstein, Y.A. (1982) Mutagens in diesel exhaust particulate. Identification and direct activities of 6-nitrobenzo[a]pyrene, 9-nitroanthracene, 1-nitropyrene and 5H-phenanthro[4,5-bcd]pyran-5-one. *Mutat. Res.*, 103, 241–249

Pitts, J.N., Jr, Sweetman, J.A., Zielinska, B., Atkinson, R., Winer, A.M. & Harger, W.P. (1985) Formation of nitroarenes from the reaction of polycyclic aromatic hydrocarbons with dinitrogen pentaoxide. *Environ. Sci. Technol.*, 19, 1115–1121

Poole, C.F. (1985) Liquid chromatography of nitrated polycyclic aromatic hydrocarbons. In: White, C.M., ed., *Nitrated Polycyclic Aromatic Hydrocarbons*, Heidelberg, A. Hüthig Verlag, pp. 299–329

Prager, B. & Jacobson, P., eds (1922) *Beilsteins Handbuch der Organischen Chemie*, 4th ed., Vol. 5 (*Syst. No. 487*), Berlin (West), Springer Verlag, p. 694

Ramdahl, T. & Urdal, K. (1982) Determination of nitrated polycyclic aromatic hydrocarbons by fused silica capillary gas chromatography/negative ion chemical ionization mass spectrometry. *Anal. Chem.*, 54, 2256–2260

Ramdahl, T., Kveseth, K. & Becher, G. (1982) Analysis of nitrated polycyclic aromatic hydrocarbons by glass capillary gas chromatography using different detectors. *J. high Resol. Chromatogr. Chromatogr. Commun.*, 5, 19–26

Ramdahl, T., Zielinska, B., Arey, J., Atkinson, R., Winer, A.M. & Pitts, J.N., Jr (1986) Ubiquitous occurrence of 2-nitrofluoranthene and 2-nitropyrene in air. *Nature*, 321, 425–427

Rappaport, S.M., Jin, Z.L. & Xu, X.B. (1982) High-performance liquid chromatography with reductive electrochemical detection of mutagenic nitrosubstituted polynuclear aromatic hydrocarbons in diesel exhausts. *J. Chromatogr.*, 240, 145–154

Rosenkranz, H.S. & Howard, P.C. (1986) Structural basis of the activity of nitrated polycyclic aromatic hydrocarbons. In: Ishinishi, N., Koizumi, A., McClellan, R.O. & Stöber, W., eds, *Carcinogenic and Mutagenic Effects of Diesel Engine Exhaust*, Amsterdam, Elsevier, pp. 141-168

Rosenkranz, H.S. & Mermelstein, R. (1983) Mutagenicity and genotoxicity of nitroarenes. All nitro-containing chemicals were not created equal. *Mutat. Res.*, 114, 217-267

Rosenkranz, H.S. & Mermelstein, R. (1985) The genotoxicity, metabolism and carcinogenicity of nitrated polycyclic aromatic hydrocarbons. *J. environ. Sci. Health*, C3, 221-272

Rosenkranz, H.S., McCoy, E.C., Sanders, D.R., Butler, M., Kiriazides, D.K. & Mermelstein, R. (1980) Nitropyrenes: isolation, identification, and reduction of mutagenic impurities in carbon black and toners. *Science*, 209, 1039-1043

Rosenkranz, H.S., McCoy, E.C., Frierson, M. & Klopman, G. (1985) The role of DNA sequence and structure of the electrophile on the mutagenicity of nitroarenes and arylamine derivatives. *Environ. Mutagenesis*, 7, 645-653

Roy, A.K., El-Bayoumy, K. & Hecht, S.S. (1987) DNA binding study of 1-nitropyrene by $^{32}$P-postlabelling technique (Abstract No. 391). *Proc. Am. Assoc. Cancer Res.*, 28, 99

Saito, K., Kamataki, T. & Kato, R. (1984a) Participation of cytochrome P-450 in reductive metabolism of 1-nitropyrene by rat liver microsomes. *Cancer Res.*, 44, 3169-3173

Saito, K., Mita, S., Kamataki, T. & Kato, R. (1984b) DNA single-strand breaks by nitropyrenes and related compounds in Chinese hamster V79 cells. *Cancer Lett.*, 24, 121-127

Salmeen, I., Durisin, A.M., Prater, T.J., Riley, T. & Schuetzle, D. (1982) Contribution of 1-nitropyrene to direct-acting Ames assay mutagenicities of diesel particulate extracts. *Mutat. Res.*, 104, 17-23

Salmeen, I., Zacmanidis, P. & Ball, J. (1983) 1-Nitropyrene reduction by *Salmonella typhimurium*, V79 Chinese hamster and primary rat liver cells. *Mutat. Res.*, 122, 23-28

Salmeen, I.T., Pero, A.M., Zator, R., Schuetzle, D. & Riley, T.L. (1984) Ames assay chromatograms and the identification of mutagens in diesel particle extracts. *Environ. Sci. Technol.*, 18, 375-382

Sanders, D.R. (1981) Nitropyrenes: the isolation of trace mutagenic impurities from the toluene extract of an aftertreated carbon black. In: Cooke, M. & Dennis, A.J., eds, *Polynuclear Aromatic Hydrocarbons, 5th International Symposium, Chemical Analysis and Biological Fate*, Columbus, OH, Battelle, pp. 145-158

Sato, T., Kato, K., Ose, Y., Nagase, H. & Ishikawa, T. (1985) Nitroarenes in Suimon River sediment. *Mutat. Res.*, 157, 135-143

Schuetzle, D. & Frazier, J.A. (1986) Factors influencing the emission of vapor and particulate phase components from diesel engines. In: Ishinishi, N., Koizumi, A., McClellan, R.O. & Stöber, eds, *Carcinogenic and Mutagenic Effects of Diesel Engine Exhaust*, Amsterdam, Elsevier, pp. 41-63

Schuetzle, D. & Jensen, T.E. (1985) Analysis of nitrated polycyclic aromatic hydrocarbons (nitro-PAH) by mass spectrometry. In: White, C.M., ed., *Nitrated Polycyclic Aromatic Hydrocarbons*, Heidelberg, A. Hüthig Verlag, pp. 121-167

Schuetzle, D., Riley, T.L., Prater, T.J., Harvey, T.M. & Hunt, D.F. (1982) Analysis of nitrated polycyclic aromatic hydrocarbons in diesel particulates. *Anal. Chem.*, 54, 265-271

Siak, J., Chan, T.L., Gibson, T.L. & Wolff, G.T. (1985) Contribution to bacterial mutagenicity from nitro-PAH compounds in ambient aerosols. *Atmos. Environ.*, 19, 369-376

Stanton, C.A., Chow, F.L., Phillips, D.H., Grover, P.L., Garner, R.C. & Martin, C.N. (1985) Evidence for *N*-(deoxyguanosin-8-yl)-1-aminopyrene as a major DNA adduct in female rats treated with 1-nitropyrene. *Carcinogenesis*, *6*, 535–538

Stärk, G., Stauff, J., Miltenburger, H.G. & Stumm-Fischer, I. (1985) Photodecomposition of 1-nitropyrene and other direct acting mutagens extracted from diesel-exhaust particulates. *Mutat. Res.*, *155*, 27–33

Sugimura, T. & Takayama, S. (1983) Biological actions of nitroarenes in short-term tests on *Salmonella*, cultured mammalian cells and cultured human tracheal tissues: possible basis for regulatory control. *Environ. Health Perspect.*, *47*, 171–176

Sun, J.D., Wolff, R.K., Aberman, H.M. & McClellan, R.O. (1983) Inhalation of 1-nitropyrene associated with ultrafine insoluble particles or as a pure aerosol: a comparison of deposition and biological fate. *Toxicol. appl. Pharmacol.*, *69*, 185–198

Takayama, S., Tanaka, M., Katoh, Y., Terada, M. & Sugimura, T. (1983) Mutagenicity of nitropyrenes in Chinese hamster V79 cells. *Gann*, *74*, 338–341

Tanabe, K., Matsushita, H., Kuo, C.-T. & Imamiya, S. (1986) Determination of carcinogenic nitroarenes in airborne particulates by high performance liquid chromatography. *Taiku Osen Gakkaishi (J. Jpn. Soc. Air Pollut.)*, *21*, 535–544

Tatsumi, K., Kitamura, S. & Narai, N. (1986) Reductive metabolism of aromatic nitro compounds including carcinogens by rabbit liver preparations. *Cancer Res.*, *46*, 1089–1093

Thrane, K.E. & Stray, H. (1986) Organic air pollutants in an aluminum reduction plant. *Sci. total Environ.*, *53*, 111–131

Tokiwa, H. & Ohnishi, Y. (1986) Mutagenicity and carcinogenicity of nitroarenes and their sources in the environment. *CRC crit. Rev. Toxicol.*, *17*, 23–60

Tokiwa, H., Nakagawa, R., Morita, K. & Ohnishi, Y. (1981a) Mutagenicity of nitro derivatives induced by exposure of aromatic compounds to nitrogen dioxide. *Mutat. Res.*, *85*, 195–205

Tokiwa, H., Nakagawa, R. & Ohnishi, Y. (1981b) Mutagenic assay of aromatic nitro compounds with *Salmonella typhimurium*. *Mutat. Res.*, *91*, 321–325

Tokiwa, H., Kitamori, S., Nakagawa, R., Horikawa, K. & Matamala, L. (1983) Demonstration of a powerful mutagenic dinitropyrene in airborne particulate matter. *Mutat. Res.*, *121*, 107–116

Tokiwa, H., Otofuji, T., Horikawa, K., Kitamori, S., Otsuka, H., Manabe, Y., Kinouchi, T. & Ohnishi, Y. (1984) 1,6-Dinitropyrene: mutagenicity in *Salmonella* and carcinogenicity in BALB/c mice. *J. natl Cancer Inst.*, *73*, 1359–1363

Tokiwa, H., Nakagawa, R. & Horikawa, K. (1985) Mutagenic/carcinogenic agents in indoor pollutants, the dinitropyrenes generated by kerosene heaters and fuel gas and liquefied petroleum gas burners. *Mutat. Res.*, *157*, 39–47

Tomkins, B.A. (1985) Chromatographic detectors used for the determination of nitrated polycyclic aromatic hydrocarbons. In: White, C.M., ed., *Nitrated Polycyclic Aromatic Hydrocarbons*, Heidelberg, A. Hüthig Verlag, pp. 87–120

Tsunoda, T., Yamaoka, T. & Nagamatsu, G. (1973) Spectral sensitization of bisazide compounds. *Photogr. Sci. Eng.*, *17*, 390–393

US Environmental Protection Agency (1986) *Toxic Substances Control Act Chemical Substance Inventory*, 1985 ed., Vol. III, *Substance Name Index* (*EPA-560/7-85-002c*), Washington, DC, Office of Toxic Substances

Wang, C.Y., Lee, M.-S., King, C.M. & Warner, P.O. (1980) Evidence for nitroaromatics as direct-acting mutagens of airborne particulates. *Chemosphere*, *9*, 83–87

White, C.M. (1985) Analysis of nitrated polycyclic aromatic hydrocarbons by gas chromatography. In: White, C.M., ed., *Nitrated Polycyclic Aromatic Hydrocarbons*, Heidelberg, A. Hüthig Verlag, pp. 1–86

Wislocki, P.G., Bagan, E.S., Lu, A.Y.H., Dooley, K.L., Fu, P.P., Han-Hsu, H., Beland, F.A. & Kadlubar, F.F. (1986) Tumorigenicity of nitrated derivatives of pyrene, benz[a]anthracene, chrysene and benzo[a]pyrene in the newborn mouse assay. *Carcinogenesis*, *7*, 1317–1322

Xu, X.B., Nachtman, J.P., Jin, Z.L., Wei, E.T., Rappaport, S.M. & Burlingame, A.L. (1982) Isolation and identification of mutagenic nitro-PAH in diesel-exhaust particulates. *Anal. chim. Acta*, *136*, 163–174

Yamamoto, A., Inamasu, T., Hisanaga, A., Kitamori, S. & Ishinishi, N. (1987) Comparative study on the carcinogenicity of 1-nitropyrene and benzo[a]pyrene to the lung of Syrian golden hamsters induced by intermittent intratracheal instillations. *J. Jpn. Soc. Air Pollut.*, *22*, 29–35

Yoshimi, N., Sugie, S., Mori, H., Kinouchi, T. & Ohnishi, Y. (1987) Genotoxicity of various nitroarenes in DNA repair tests with human hepatocytes (Abstract No. 73). *Mutat. Res.*, *182*, 384

Yu, W.C. (1983) Trace level determination of nitro-PAHs by capillary gas chromatography with a chemiluminescent detector. In: Cooke, M. & Dennis, A.J., eds, *Polynuclear Aromatic Hydrocarbons, 7th International Symposium, Formation, Metabolism and Measurement*, Columbus, OH, Battelle, pp. 1267–1277

# 2-NITROPYRENE

## 1. Chemical and Physical Data

### 1.1 Synonyms

*Chem. Abstr. Services Reg. No.*: 789-07-1
*Chem. Abstr. Name*: Pyrene, 2-nitro-
*IUPAC Systematic Name*: 2-Nitropyrene

### 1.2 Structural and molecular formulae and molecular weight

$C_{16}H_9NO_2$                Mol. wt: 247.3

### 1.3 Chemical and physical properties of the pure substance

(a) *Description*: Yellow crystalline solid (Chemsyn Science Laboratories, 1988)

(b) *Melting-point*: 197–199°C (Paputa-Peck *et al.*, 1983); 201–202.5°C (Bolton, 1964)

(c) *Spectroscopy data*: Nuclear magnetic resonance and ultra-violet spectral data have been reported (Paputa-Peck *et al.*, 1983).

(d) *Solubility*: Soluble in toluene and benzene (Chemsyn Science Laboratories, 1988)

### 1.4 Technical products and impurities

2-Nitropyrene is available for research purposes at ≥95% purity (Chemsyn Science Laboratories, 1988)

## 2. Production, Use, Occurrence and Analysis

### 2.1 Production and use

*(a) Production*

2-Nitropyrene can be synthesized by the photoinduced reaction of pyrene with nitrogen dioxide in which monodisperse pyrene on silica particles in nitrogen reacts with nitrogen dioxide in the presence of light (Ramdahl *et al.*, 1986).

No evidence was found that 2-nitropyrene has been produced for other than laboratory use.

*(b) Use*

No evidence was found that 2-nitropyrene has been used for commercial applications.

### 2.2 Occurrence

2-Nitropyrene has been reported to be one of the most abundant nitroarenes in ambient particulate matter (Arey *et al.*, 1987). It was the third most abundant mononitroarene in ambient particles collected in both urban and rural areas of Los Angeles, CA, USA, in winter and in summer (Pitts, 1987). 2-Nitropyrene may result from atmospheric tranformation of pyrene, including the gas-phase reaction of pyrene with nitrogen pentoxide at night and the hydroxyl radical-initiated reaction of pyrene with nitrogen oxides in the day (Arey *et al.*, 1987; Pitts, 1987). 2-Nitropyrene is the only mononitropyrene formed by the hydroxyl radical-initiated reaction (Arey *et al.*, 1986). Atmospheric transformation of pyrene to mononitropyrene, induced in the presence of nitrogen dioxide, is reported to be enhanced in the presence of sulfur dioxide (Tokiwa & Ohnishi, 1986). 2-Nitropyrene was identified in airborne particles in rural Denmark (Nielsen *et al.*, 1984).

A level of 0.17 mg/kg particulate matter was found in an air sample taken in Aurskog, Norway, in winter 1984, and 0.08 mg/kg particulate matter in a sample taken in Claremont, CA, USA, in summer 1985 (Ramdahl *et al.*, 1986). Pitts (1987) reported 0–0.02 mg/kg particulate matter in an air sample taken in Riverside, CA, in summer 1984. A level of 0.04 ng/m$^3$ was found in a day-time sample of ambient air taken in the winter in Torrance, CA, calculated as the sum of the concentrations on the filter and on three polyurethane foam plugs. A night-time sample contained 0.03 ng/m$^3$ (Arey *et al.*, 1987).

Toners for use in photocopy machines have been produced in quantity since the late 1950s and have seen widespread use. 'Long-flow' furnace black was first used in photocopy toners in 1967; its manufacture involved an oxidation whereby some nitration also occurred. Subsequent changes in the production technique reduced the total extractable nitropyrene content from an uncontrolled level of 5–100 mg/kg to below 0.3 mg/kg (Rosenkranz *et al.*, 1980; Sanders, 1981; Butler *et al.*, 1983), and toners produced from this carbon black since 1980 have not been found to contain detectable levels of mutagenicity or, hence, nitropyrenes (Rosenkranz et al., 1980; Butler et al., 1983).

## 2.3 Analysis

See the monograph on 1-nitropyrene.

# 3. Biological Data Relevant to the Evaluation of Carcinogenic Risk to Humans

## 3.1 Carcinogenicity studies in animals

*Intraperitoneal injection*

*Rat*: In a study reported as an abstract, female CD rats [initial number unspecified], 30 days of age, received intraperitoneal injections of 67 $\mu$mol[16.5 mg]/kg bw 2-nitropyrene [purity unspecified] three times per week for four weeks (Imaida et al., 1985). Surviving rats were killed at 62 weeks. The incidence of mammary tumours [unspecified] was reported to be not significantly different from that in controls (4/29). [The Working Group noted the short periods of treatment and observation and the inadequate reporting of the data.]

## 3.2 Other relevant data

(a) *Experimental systems*

(i) *Absorption, distribution, excretion and metabolism*
No data were available to the Working Group.

(ii) *Toxic effects*
No data were available to the Working Group.

(iii) *Genetic and related effects*
The genetic and related effects of nitroarenes and of their metabolites have been reviewed (Rosenkranz & Mermelstein, 1983; Beland et al., 1985; Rosenkranz & Mermelstein, 1985; Tokiwa & Ohnishi, 1986).

2-Nitropyrene was mutagenic to *Salmonella typhimurium* TA98 and TA100 in the absence of an exogenous metabolic system (Greibrokk et al., 1984).

(b) *Humans*

No data were available to the Working Group.

### 3.3 Epidemiological studies and case reports of carcinogenicity in humans

No data were available to the Working Group.

## 4. Summary of Data Reported and Evaluation

### 4.1 Exposure data

2-Nitropyrene has been measured at low concentrations in ambient air.

### 4.2 Experimental data

No adequate data were available to the Working Group to evaluate the carcinogenicity of 2-nitropyrene in experimental animals.

### 4.3 Human data

No data were available to the Working Group.

### 4.4 Other relevant data

2-Nitropyrene was mutagenic to bacteria.

### 4.5 Evaluation[1]

There is *inadequate evidence* for the carcinogenicity in experimental animals of 2-nitropyrene.

No data were available from studies in humans on the carcinogenicity of 2-nitropyrene.

**Overall evaluation**

2-Nitropyrene *is not classifiable as to its carcinogenicity to humans (Group 3)*.

---

[1]For definitions of the italicized terms, see Preamble, pp. 25–28.

## Summary table of genetic and related effects of 2-nitropyrene

| Nonmammalian systems | | | | | | | | | | | | | | | Mammalian systems | | | | | | | | | | | | | | | | | | |
|---|---|---|---|---|---|---|---|---|---|---|---|---|---|---|---|---|---|---|---|---|---|---|---|---|---|---|---|---|---|---|---|---|---|
| Prokaryotes | | | | Lower eukaryotes | | | | Plants | | | | Insects | | | In vitro | | | | | | | | | | | | | In vivo | | | | | |
| | | | | | | | | | | | | | | | Animal cells | | | | | | | | Human cells | | | | | | Animals | | | | Humans | | |
| D | G | D | R | G | A | D | G | C | R | G | C | A | D | G | S | M | C | A | T | I | D | G | S | M | C | A | T | I | D | G | S | M | C | DL | A | D | S | M | C | A |
| +¹ | | | | | | | | | | | | | | | | | | | | | | | | | | | | | | | | | | | | | | | | |

A, aneuploidy; C, chromosomal aberrations; D, DNA damage; DL, dominant lethal mutation; G, gene mutation; I, inhibition of intercellular communication; M, micronuclei; R, mitotic recombination and gene conversion; S, sister chromatid exchange; T, cell transformation

+¹, considered to be positive, but only one valid study was available to the Working Group

## 5. References

Arey, J., Zielinska, B., Atkinson, R., Winer, A.M., Ramdahl, T. & Pitts, J.N., Jr (1986) The formation of nitro-PAH from the gas-phase reactions of fluoranthene and pyrene with the OH radical in the presence of $NO_x$. *Atmos. Environ.*, 20, 2339–2345

Arey, J., Zielinska, B., Atkinson, R. & Winer, A.M. (1987) Polycyclic aromatic hydrocarbon and nitroarene concentrations in ambient air during a wintertime high-$NO_x$ episode in the Los Angeles basin. *Atmos. Environ.*, 21, 1437–1444

Beland, F.A., Heflich, R.H., Howard, P.C. & Fu, P.P. (1985) The in vitro metabolic activation of nitro polycyclic aromatic hydrocarbons. In: Harvey, R.G., ed., *Polycyclic Hydrocarbons and Carcinogenesis (ACS Symposium Series No. 283)*, Washington DC, American Chemical Society, pp. 371–396

Bolton, R. (1964) Tetrahydropyrene as a source of 2-pyrenyl derivatives. *J. chem. Soc.*, 4637–4638

Butler, M.A., Evans, D.L., Giammarise, A.T., Kiriazides, D.K., Marsh, D., McCoy, E.C., Mermelstein, R., Murphy, C.B. & Rosenkranz, H.S. (1983) Application of *Salmonella* assay to carbon blacks and toners. In: Cooke, M. & Dennis, A.J., eds, *Polynuclear Aromatic Hydrocarbons, 7th International Symposium, Formation, Metabolism and Measurement*, Columbus, OH, Battelle, pp. 225–241

Chemsyn Science Laboratories (1988) *2-Nitropyrene (Product Code U1012)*, Lenexa, KS, p. 94

Greibrokk, T., Löfroth, G., Nilsson, L., Toftgård, R., Carlstedt-Duke, J. & Gustafsson, J.-Å. (1984) Nitroarenes: mutagenicity in the Ames *Salmonella*/microsome assay and affinity to the TCDD-receptor protein. In: Rickert, D.E., ed., *Toxicity of Nitroaromatic Compounds*, Washington DC, Hemisphere, pp. 167–183

Imaida, K., Hirose, M., Lee, M.-S., Wang, C.Y. & King, C.M. (1985) Comparative carcinogenicities of 1-, 2-, and 4-nitropyrenes (NP) and structurally related compounds for female CD rats following intraperitoneal injection (Abstract No. 366). *Proc. Am. Assoc. Cancer Res.*, 26, 93

Nielsen, T., Seitz, B. & Ramdahl, T. (1984) Occurrence of nitro-PAH in the atmosphere in a rural area. *Atmos. Environ.*, 18, 2159–2165

Paputa-Peck, M.C., Marano, R.S., Schuetzle, D., Riley, T.L., Hampton, C.V., Prater, T.J., Skewes, L.M., Jensen, T.E., Ruehle, P.H., Bosch, L.C. & Duncan, W.P. (1983) Determination of nitrated polynuclear aromatic hydrocarbons in particulate extracts by capillary column gas chromatography with nitrogen selective detection. *Anal. Chem.*, 55, 1946–1954

Pitts, J.N., Jr (1987) Nitration of gaseous polycyclic aromatic hydrocarbons in simulated and ambient urban atmospheres: a source of mutagenic nitroarenes. *Atmos. Environ.*, 21, 2531–2547

Ramdahl, T., Zielinska, B., Arey, J., Atkinson, R., Winer, A.M. & Pitts, J.N., Jr (1986) Ubiquitous occurrence of 2-nitrofluoranthene and 2-nitropyrene in air. *Nature*, 321, 425–427

Rosenkranz, H.S. & Mermelstein, R. (1983) Mutagenicity and genotoxicity of nitroarenes: all nitro-containing chemicals were not created equal. *Mutat. Res.*, 114, 217–267

Rosenkranz, H.S. & Mermelstein, R. (1985) The genotoxicity, metabolism and carcinogenicity of nitrated polycyclic aromatic hydrocarbons. *J. environ. Sci. Health*, C3, 221–272

Rosenkranz, H.S., McCoy, E.C., Sanders, D.R., Butler, M., Kiriazides, D.K. & Mermelstein, R. (1980) Nitropyrenes: isolation, identification, and reduction of mutagenic impurities in carbon black and toners. *Science*, 209, 1039–1043

Sanders, D.R. (1981) Nitropyrenes: the isolation of trace mutagenic impurities from the toluene extract of an aftertreated carbon black. In: Cooke, M. & Dennis, A.J., eds, *Polynuclear Aromatic Hydrocarbons, 5th International Symposium, Chemical Analysis and Biological Fate*, Columbus, OH, Battelle, pp. 145–158

Tokiwa, H. & Ohnishi, Y. (1986) Mutagenicity and carcinogenicity of nitroarenes and their sources in the environment. *CRC crit. Rev. Toxicol., 17*, 23–60

# 4-NITROPYRENE

## 1. Chemical and Physical Data

### 1.1 Synonyms

*Chem. Abstr. Services Reg. No.*: 57835-92-4
*Chem. Abstr. Name*: Pyrene, 4-nitro-
*IUPAC Systematic Name*: 4-Nitropyrene

### 1.2 Structural and molecular formulae and molecular weight

$C_{16}H_9NO_2$    Mol. wt: 247.3

### 1.3 Chemical and physical properties of the pure substance

(a) *Description*: Slender orange needles (Bavin, 1959)

(b) *Melting-point*: 190–192°C (Paputa-Peck *et al.*, 1983); 196–197.5°C (Bavin, 1959)

(c) *Spectroscopy data*: Nuclear magnetic resonance and ultra-violet spectral data have been reported (Paputa-Peck *et al.*, 1983).

### 1.4 Technical products and impurities

No data were available to the Working Group.

## 2. Production, Use, Occurrence and Analysis

### 2.1 Production and use

*(a) Production*

4-Nitropyrene can be produced by the electrophilic nitration of pyrene. No evidence was found that 4-nitropyrene has been produced for other than laboratory use.

*(b) Use*

No evidence was found that 4-nitropyrene has been used for commercial applications.

### 2.2 Occurrence

4-Nitropyrene was found in a sample of ambient airborne particulates collected in Torrance, CA, USA (Korfmacher *et al.*, 1987).

Toners for use in photocopy machines have been produced in quantity since the late 1950s and have seen widespread use. 'Long-flow' furnace black was first used in photocopy toners in 1967; its manufacture involved an oxidation whereby some nitration also occurred. Subsequent changes in the production technique reduced the total extractable nitropyrene content from an uncontrolled level of 5–100 mg/kg to below 0.3 mg/kg (Rosenkranz *et al.*, 1980; Sanders, 1981; Butler *et al.*, 1983), and toners produced from this carbon black since 1980 have not been found to contain detectable levels of mutagenicity or, hence, nitropyrenes (Rosenkranz *et al.*, 1980; Butler *et al.*, 1983).

### 2.3 Analysis

See the monograph on 1-nitropyrene

## 3. Biological Data Relevant to the Evaluation of Carcinogenic Risk to Humans

### 3.1 Carcinogenicity studies in animals

*(a) Subcutaneous administration*

*Rat*: A group of female newborn CD rats [initial numbers unspecified] received subcutaneous injections of 0.1 mmol[25 mg]/kg bw 4-nitropyrene [purity unspecified] dissolved in dimethyl sulfoxide (DMSO) once a week for eight weeks (total dose, 63 $\mu$mol [15.6 mg]; King, 1988). A group of rats received DMSO alone. Animals were sacrificed when moribund or at 86 weeks. A statistically significant increase ($p < 0.005$) in the number of rats with mammary tumours was observed in the treated group (20/27; 18 adenocarcinomas, 14 fibroadenomas; induction period, 263 days) compared with controls (17/47; 16 fibroadenomas; induction period, 502 days). Ten rats developed other malignant tumours (malignant fibrous histiocytomas, leukaemias and ear-duct tumours [numbers unspecified]) that were not observed in controls.

*(b) Intraperitoneal administration*

*Mouse*: Groups of 90 or 100 male and female newborn CD-1 mice received three intraperitoneal injections of 4-nitropyrene (total dose, 2800 nmol [692 $\mu$g]; purity, >99%) in 10, 20 and 40 $\mu$l DMSO on days 1, 8 and 15 of age; a total dose of 560 nmol [140 $\mu$g] benzo[*a*]pyrene (purity, >99%); or three injections of DMSO only (Wislocki *et al.*, 1986). Treatment of a second vehicle control group was begun ten weeks after that of the other groups. At 25–27 days, when the mice were weaned, 29 male and 29 female treated mice, 37 male and 27 female positive controls, and 28 and 31 males and 45 and 34 females in the two vehicle control groups were still alive. All remaining mice were killed after one year. Liver-cell tumours developed in 24/29 treated males (four adenomas, 20 carcinomas; $p < 0.005$) and 2/29 treated females (one adenoma and one carcinoma). Male mice also had a higher multiplicity of liver tumours than controls, with an average of 6.0 nodules per tumour-bearing animal. Lung tumours occurred in 11/29 treated males (ten adenomas, one carcinoma; $p < 0.005$) and 9/29 treated females (eight adenomas, one carcinoma; $p < 0.005$). Benzo[*a*]pyrene induced liver-cell tumours in 18/37 males but not in females, and lung adenomas in 13/37 males and 13/27 females ($p < 0.005$). Of the vehicle controls, 2/28 and 5/45 males had liver adenomas and 1/28 and 4/45 had lung tumours, and 0/31 and 0/34 females had liver tumours and 0/31 and 2/34 had lung tumours.

*Rat*: In a study reported as an abstract, female CD rats [initial number unspecified], 30 days of age, received intraperitoneal injections of 67 $\mu$mol [16.5 mg]/kg bw 4-nitropyrene [purity unspecified] three times per week for four weeks (Imaida *et al.*, 1985). Surviving rats were killed at 62 weeks. The incidence of mammary tumours (17/29) was significantly different from that in controls (4/29; $p < 0.001$).

## 3.2 Other relevant data

*(a) Experimental systems*

(i) *Absorption, distribution, excretion and metabolism*

It was reported in an abstract that rat liver microsomes catalysed the conversion of 4-nitropyrene to 4-nitropyrene 9,10-dione, 8-hydroxy-4-nitropyrene and 4-nitropyrene-1,6-hydroquinone (Fu *et al.*, 1986).

(ii) *Toxic effects*

No data were available to the Working Group.

(iii) *Genetic and related effects*

The genetic and related effects of nitroarenes and of their metabolites have been reviewed (Rosenkranz & Mermelstein, 1983; Beland *et al.*, 1985; Rosenkranz & Mermelstein, 1985; Tokiwa & Ohnishi, 1986).

4-Nitropyrene (0.1–2.0 µg/disc) preferentially inhibited the growth of DNA repair-deficient *Bacillus subtilis* (Horikawa *et al.*, 1986; Tokiwa *et al.*, 1987) and was mutagenic to *Salmonella typhimurium* TA98 and TA100 (Fu *et al.*, 1985).

(b) *Humans*

No data were available to the Working Group.

### 3.3 Epidemiological studies and case reports of carcinogenicity in humans

No data were available to the Working Group.

## 4. Summary of Data Reported and Evaluation

### 4.1 Exposure data

4-Nitropyrene was detected at a low concentration in ambient air in one study.

### 4.2 Experimental data

4-Nitropyrene was tested for carcinogenicity in newborn rats by subcutaneous injection, producing an increase in the incidence of mammary tumours. It was also tested by intraperitoneal injection in newborn mice, producing an increase in the incidence of liver-cell tumours in males and of lung tumours in animals of each sex. A study by intraperitoneal injection was inadequately reported.

### 4.3 Human data

No data were available to the Working Group.

### 4.4 Other relevant data

4-Nitropyrene induced DNA damage and mutation in bacteria.

## Summary table of genetic and related effects of 4-nitropyrene

| Nonmammalian systems | | | | | | | | | | | | | | | Mammalian systems | | | | | | | | | | | | | | | | | | | | | |
|---|---|---|---|---|---|---|---|---|---|---|---|---|---|---|---|---|---|---|---|---|---|---|---|---|---|---|---|---|---|---|---|---|---|---|---|
| Proka-ryotes | | | | Lower eukaryotes | | | | | Plants | | | Insects | | | In vitro | | | | | | | | | | | | | | In vivo | | | | | | |
| | | | | | | | | | | | | | | | Animal cells | | | | | | | Human cells | | | | | | | Animals | | | | Humans | | |
| D | G | R | D | G | A | D | G | C | R | A | D | G | C | A | D | G | S | M | C | A | T | I | D | G | S | M | C | A | T | I | D | G | S | M | C | A | D | S | M | C | A |
| + | ±  | | | | | | | | | | | | | | | | | | | | | | | | | | | | | | | | | | | | | | | | |

A, aneuploidy; C, chromosomal aberrations; D, DNA damage; DL, dominant lethal mutation; G, gene mutation; I, inhibition of intercellular communication; M, micronuclei; R, mitotic recombination and gene conversion; S, sister chromatid exchange; T, cell transformation

*In completing the table, the following symbols indicate the consensus of the Working Group with regard to the results for each endpoint:*
+   considered to be positive for the specific endpoint and level of biological complexity
±   considered to be positive, but only one valid study was available to the Working Group

## 4.5 Evaluation[1]

There is *sufficient evidence* for the carcinogenicity in experimental animals of 4-nitropyrene.

No data were available from studies in humans on the carcinogenicity of 4-nitropyrene.

4-Nitropyrene *is possibly carcinogenic to humans (Group 2B)*.

# 5. References

Bavin, P.M.G. (1959) 4-Nitropyrene. *Can. J. Chem.*, 37, 1614–1615

Beland, F.A., Heflich, R.H., Howard, P.C. & Fu, P.P. (1985) The in vitro metabolic activation of nitro polycyclic aromatic hydrocarbons. In: Harvey, R.G., ed., *Polycyclic Hydrocarbons and Carcinogenesis (ACS Symposium Series No. 283)*, Washington DC, American Chemical Society, pp. 371–396

Butler, M.A., Evans, D.L., Giammarise, A.T., Kiriazides, D.K., Marsh, D., McCoy, E.C., Mermelstein, R., Murphy, C.B. & Rosenkranz, H.S. (1983) Application of *Salmonella* assay to carbon blacks and toners. In: Cooke, M. & Dennis, A.J., eds, *Polynuclear Aromatic Hydrocarbons, 7th International Symposium, Formation, Metabolism and Measurement*, Columbus, OH, Battelle, pp. 225–241

Fu, P.P., Chou, M.W., Miller, D.W., White, G.L., Heflich, R.H. & Beland, F.A. (1985) The orientation of the nitro substituent predicts the direct-acting bacterial mutagenicity of nitrated polycyclic aromatic hydrocarbons. *Mutat. Res.*, 143, 173–181

Fu, P.P., Von Tungeln, L.S., Unruh, L.E. & Heflich, R.H. (1986) In vitro metabolism of 4-nitropyrene to a new type of mutagenic metabolite (Abstract No. 157). *Pharmacologist*, 28, 120

Horikawa, K., Sera, N., Tokiwa, H. & Kada, T. (1986) Results of the *rec*-assay of nitropyrenes in the *Bacillus subtilis* test system. *Mutat. Res.*, 174, 89–92

Imaida, K., Hirose, M., Lee, M.-S., Wang, C.Y. & King, C.M. (1985) Comparative carcinogenicities of 1-, 2-, and 4-nitropyrenes (NP) and structurally related compounds for female CD rats following intraperitoneal injection (Abstract No. 366). *Proc. Am. Assoc. Cancer Res.*, 26, 93

King, C.M. (1988) *Metabolism and Biological Effects of Nitropyrene and Related Compounds (Research Report No. 16)*, Cambridge, MA, Health Effects Institute

Korfmacher, W.A., Rushing, L.G., Arey, J., Zielinska, B. & Pitts, J.N., Jr (1987) Identification of mononitropyrenes and mononitrofluoranthenes in air particulate matter *via* fused silica gas chromatography combined with negative ion atmospheric pressure ionization mass spectrometry. *J. high Resol. Chromatogr. Chromatogr. Commun.*, 10, 641–646

Paputa-Peck, M.C., Marano, R.S., Schuetzle, D., Riley, T.L., Hampton, C.V., Prater, T.J., Skewes, L.M., Jensen, T.E., Ruehle, P.H., Bosch, L.C. & Duncan, W.P. (1983) Determination of nitrated polynuclear aromatic hydrocarbons in particulate extracts by capillary column gas chromatography with nitrogen selective detection. *Anal. Chem.*, 55, 1946–1954

---

[1]For definitions of the italicized terms, see Preamble, pp. 25–28.

Rosenkranz, H.S. & Mermelstein, R. (1983) Mutagenicity and genotoxicity of nitroarenes: all nitro-containing chemicals were not created equal. *Mutat. Res.*, *114*, 217–267

Rosenkranz, H.S. & Mermelstein, R. (1985) The genotoxicity, metabolism and carcinogenicity of nitrated polycyclic aromatic hydrocarbons. *J. environ. Sci. Health*, *C3*, 221–272

Rosenkranz, H.S., McCoy, E.C., Sanders, D.R., Butler, M., Kiriazides, D.K. & Mermelstein, R. (1980) Nitropyrenes: isolation, identification, and reduction of mutagenic impurities in carbon black and toners. *Science*, *209*, 1039–1043

Sanders, D.R. (1981) Nitropyrenes: the isolation of trace mutagenic impurities from the toluene extract of an aftertreated carbon black. In: Cooke, M. & Dennis, A.J., eds, *Polynuclear Aromatic Hydrocarbons, 5th International Symposium, Chemical Analysis and Biological Fate*, Columbus, OH, Battelle, pp. 145–158

Tokiwa, H. & Ohnishi, Y. (1986) Mutagenicity and carcinogenicity of nitroarenes and their sources in the environment. *CRC crit. Rev. Toxicol.*, *17*, 23–60

Tokiwa, H., Nakagawa, R., Horikawa, K. & Ohkubo, A. (1987) The nature of the mutagenicity and carcinogenicity of nitrated, aromatic compounds in the environment. *Environ. Health Perspect.*, *73*, 191–199

Wislocki, P.G., Bagan, E.S., Lu, A.Y.H., Dooley, K.L., Fu, P.P., Han-Hsu, H., Beland, F.A. & Kadlubar, F.F. (1986) Tumorigenicity of nitrated derivatives of pyrene, benz[a]anthracene, chrysene and benzo[a]pyrene in the newborn mouse assay. *Carcinogenesis*, *7*, 1317–1322

# SUMMARY OF FINAL EVALUATIONS

| Agent | Degree of evidence for carcinogenicity[a] | | Overall evaluation[b] |
|---|---|---|---|
| | Humans | Animals | |
| Diesel engine exhaust | Limited | | 2A |
|   Whole diesel engine exhaust | | Sufficient | |
|   Gas-phase diesel engine exhaust (with particles removed) | | Inadequate | |
|   Extracts of diesel engine exhaust particles | | Sufficient | |
| Gasoline engine exhaust | Inadequate | | 2B |
|   Whole gasoline engine exhaust | | Inadequate | |
|   Condensates/extracts of gasoline engine exhaust | | Sufficient | |
| Engine exhaust (unspecified as from diesel or gasoline engines) | Limited | | |
| 3,7-Dinitrofluoranthene | No data | Limited | 3 |
| 3,9-Dinitrofluoranthene | No data | Limited | 3 |
| 1,3-Dinitropyrene | No data | Limited | 3 |
| 1,6-Dinitropyrene | No data | Sufficient | 2B |
| 1,8-Dinitropyrene | No data | Sufficient | 2B |
| 7-Nitrobenz[a]anthracene | No data | Limited | 3 |
| 6-Nitrobenzo[a]pyrene | No data | Limited | 3 |
| 6-Nitrochrysene | No data | Sufficient | 2B |
| 2-Nitrofluorene | No data | Sufficient | 2B |
| 1-Nitronaphthalene | No data | Inadequate | 3 |
| 2-Nitronaphthalene | No data | Inadequate | 3 |
| 3-Nitroperylene | No data | Inadequate | 3 |
| 1-Nitropyrene | No data | Sufficient | 2B |
| 2-Nitropyrene | No data | Inadequate | 3 |
| 4-Nitropyrene | No data | Sufficient | 2B |

[a]For definitions of the degrees of evidence, see pp. 25–27 of the Preamble of this volume.

[b]For definitions of the groups, see pp. 27–28 of the Preamble to this volume.

# APPENDIX 1

# ACTIVITY PROFILES FOR GENETIC AND RELATED TESTS

# APPENDIX 1
# ACTIVITY PROFILES FOR GENETIC AND RELATED TESTS

*Methods*

The x-axis of the activity profile represents the bioassays in phylogenetic sequence by endpoint, and the values on the y-axis represent the logarithmically transformed lowest effective doses (LED) and highest ineffective doses (HID) tested. The term 'dose', as used in this report, does not take into consideration length of treatment or exposure and may therefore be considered synonymous with concentration. In practice, the concentrations used in all the in-vitro tests were converted to $\mu$g/ml, and those for in-vivo tests were expressed as mg/kg bw. Because dose units are plotted on a log scale, differences in molecular weights of compounds do not, in most cases, greatly influence comparisons of their activity profiles. Conventions for dose conversions are given below.

Profile-line height (the magnitude of each bar) is a function of the LED or HID, which is associated with the characteristics of each individual test system — such as population size, cell-cycle kinetics and metabolic competence. Thus, the detection limit of each test system is different, and, across a given activity profile, responses will vary substantially. No attempt is made to adjust or relate responses in one test system to those of another.

Line heights are derived as follows: for negative test results, the highest dose tested without appreciable toxicity is defined as the HID. If there was evidence of extreme toxicity, the next highest dose is used. A single dose tested with a negative result is considered to be equivalent to the HID. Similarly, for positive results, the LED is recorded. If the original data were analysed statistically by the author, the dose recorded is that at which the response was significant ($p < 0.05$). If the available data were not analysed statistically, the dose required to produce an effect is estimated as follows: when a dose-related positive response is observed with two or more doses, the lower of the doses is taken as the LED; a single dose resulting in a positive response is considered to be equivalent to the LED.

In order to accommodate both the wide range of doses encountered and positive and negative responses on a continuous scale, doses are transformed logarithmically, so that effective (LED) and ineffective (HID) doses are represented by positive and negative numbers, respectively. The response, or logarithmic dose unit ($LDU_{ij}$), for a given test system $i$ and chemical $j$ is represented by the expressions

$$LDU_{ij} = -\log_{10}(\text{dose}), \text{ for HID values}; LDU \leq 0$$

and  (1)

$$LDU_{ij} = -\log_{10}(\text{dose} \times 10^{-5}), \text{ for LED values}; LDU \geq 0.$$

These simple relationships define a dose range of 0 to −5 logarithmic units for ineffective doses (1−100 000 μg/ml or mg/kg bw) and 0 to +8 logarithmic units for effective doses (100 000−0.001 μg/ml or mg/kg bw). A scale illustrating the LDU values is shown in Figure 1. Negative responses at doses less than 1 μg/ml (mg/kg bw) are set equal to 1. Effectively, an LED value ⩾100 000 or an HID value ⩽1 produces an LDU = 0; no quantitative information is gained from such extreme values. The dotted lines at the levels of log dose units 1 and −1 define a 'zone of uncertainty' in which positive results are reported at such high doses (between 10 000 and 100 000 μg/ml or mg/kg bw) or negative results are reported at such low dose levels (1 to 10 μg/ml or mg/kg bw) as to call into question the adequacy of the test.

**Fig. 1. Scale of log dose units used on the y-axis of activity profiles**

| Positive (μg/ml or mg/kg bw) | | Log dose units | |
|---|---|---|---|
| 0.001 | ................................. | 8 | ---- |
| 0.01 | ................................. | 7 | -- |
| 0.1 | ................................. | 6 | -- |
| 1.0 | ................................. | 5 | -- |
| 10 | ................................. | 4 | -- |
| 100 | ................................. | 3 | -- |
| 1000 | ................................. | 2 | -- |
| 10 000 | ................................. | 1 | -- |
| 100 000 | ............. 1 ............... | 0 | ---- |
| | 10 ............... | −1 | -- |
| | 100 ............... | −2 | -- |
| | 1000 ............... | −3 | -- |
| | 10 000 ............... | −4 | -- |
| | 100 000 ............... | −5 | ---- |

Negative (μg/ml or mg/kg bw)

LED and HID are expressed as μg/ml or mg/kg bw.

In practice, an activity profile is computer generated. A data entry programme is used to store abstracted data from published reports. A sequential file (in ASCII) is created for each compound, and a record within that file consists of the name and Chemical Abstracts Service number of the compound, a three-letter code for the test system (see below), the qualitative test result (with and without an exogenous metabolic system), dose (LED or HID), citation number and additional source information. An abbreviated citation for each publication is stored in a segment of a record accessing both the test data file and the citation file. During processing of the data file, an average of the logarithmic values of the data subset is calculated, and the length of the profile line represents this average value. All dose values are plotted for each profile line, regardless of whether results are positive or negative. Results obtained in the absence of an exogenous metabolic system are indicated by a bar (−), and results obtained in the presence of an exogenous metabolic system are indicated by an upward-directed arrow ( ↑ ). When all results for a given assay are either positive or negative, the mean of the LDU values is plotted as a solid line; when conflicting data are reported for the same assay (i.e., both positive and negative results), the majority data are shown by a solid line and the minority data by a dashed line (drawn to the extreme conflicting response). In the few cases in which the numbers of positive and negative results are equal, the solid line is drawn in the positive direction and the maximal negative response is indicated with a dashed line.

Profile lines are identified by three-letter code words representing the commonly used tests. Code words for most of the test systems in current use in genetic toxicology were defined for the US Environmental Protection Agency's GENE-TOX Program (Waters, 1979; Waters & Auletta, 1981). For this publication, codes were redefined in a manner that should facilitate inclusion of additional tests in the future. If a test system is not defined precisely, a general code is used that best defines the category of the test. Naming conventions are described below.

*Dose conversions for activity profiles*

Doses are converted to $\mu g/ml$ for in-vitro tests and to mg/kg bw per day for in-vivo experiments.

1. In-vitro test systems

    (a) Weight/volume converts directly to $\mu g/ml$.

    (b) Molar (M) concentration $\times$ molecular weight = mg/ml = $10^3$ $\mu g/ml$; mM concentration $\times$ molecular weight = $\mu g/ml$.

    (c) Soluble solids expressed as % concentration are assumed to be in units of mass per volume (i.e., 1% = 0.01 g/ml = 10 000 $\mu g/ml$; also, 1 ppm = 1 $\mu g/ml$).

    (d) Liquids and gases expressed as % concentration are assumed to be given in units of volume per volume. Liquids are converted to weight per volume using the density (D) of the solution (D = g/ml). If the bulk of the solution is water, then D = 1.0 g/ml. Gases are converted from volume to mass using the ideal gas law, PV = nRT. For exposure at 20–37°C at standard atmospheric pressure, 1% (v/v) = 0.4 $\mu g/ml \times$ molecular weight of the gas. Also, 1 ppm (v/v) = $4 \times 10^{-5}$ $\mu g/ml \times$ molecular weight.

    (e) For microbial plate tests, concentrations reported as weight/plate are divided by top agar volume (if volume is not given, a 2-ml top agar is assumed). For spot tests, in which concentrations are reported as weight or weight/disc, a 1-ml volume is used as a rough approximation.

(f) Conversion of asbestos concentrations given in µg/cm² are based on the area (A) of the dish and the volume of medium per dish; i.e., for a 100-mm dish: A = $\pi R^2$ = $\pi \times$ (5 cm)² = 78.5 cm². If the volume of medium is 10 ml, then 78.5 cm² = 10 ml and 1 cm² = 0.13 ml.

2. In-vitro systems using in-vivo activation

For the body fluid-urine (BF–) test, the concentration used is the dose (in mg/kg bw) of the compound administered to test animals or patients.

3. In-vivo test systems

(a) Doses are converted to mg/kg bw per day of exposure, assuming 100% absorption. Standard values are used for each sex and species of rodent, including body weight and average intake per day, as reported by Gold *et al.* (1984). For example, in a test using male mice fed 50 ppm of the agent in the diet, the standard food intake per day is 12% of body weight, and the conversion is dose = 50 ppm × 12% = 6 mg/kg bw per day.

Standard values used for humans are: weight — males, 70 kg; females, 55 kg; surface area, 1.7 m²; inhalation rate, 20 l/min for light work, 30 l/min for mild exercise.

(b) When reported, the dose at the target site is used. For example, doses given in studies of lymphocytes of humans exposed *in vivo* are the measured blood concentrations in µg/ml.

*Codes for test systems*

For specific nonmammalian test systems, the first two letters of the three-symbol code word define the test organism (e.g., SA– for *Salmonella typhimurium*, EC– for *Escherichia coli*). In most cases, the first two letters accurately represent the scientific name of the organism. If the species is not known, the convention used is –S–. The third symbol may be used to define the tester strain (e.g., SA8 for *S. typhimurium* TA1538, ECW for *E. coli* WP2*uvrA*). When strain designation is not indicated, the third letter is used to define the specific genetic endpoint under investigation (e.g., ––D for differential toxicity, ––F for forward mutation, ––G for gene conversion or genetic crossing-over, ––N for aneuploidy, ––R for reverse mutation, ––U for unscheduled DNA synthesis). The third letter may also be used to define the general endpoint under investigation when a more complete definition is not possible or relevant (e.g., ––M for mutation, ––C for chromosomal aberration).

For mammalian test systems, the first letter of the three-letter code word defines the genetic endpoint under investigation: A–– for aneuploidy, B–– for binding, C–– for chromosomal aberration, D–– for DNA strand breaks, G–– for gene mutation, I–– for inhibition of intercellular communication, M–– for micronucleus formation, R–– for DNA repair, S–– for sister chromatid exchange, T–– for cell transformation and U–– for unscheduled DNA synthesis.

For animal (i.e., nonhuman) test systems *in vitro*, when the cell type is not specified, the code letters –IA are used. For such assays *in vivo*, when the animal species is not specified, the code letters –VA are used. Commonly used animal species are identified by the third letter (e.g., ——C for Chinese hamster, ——M for mouse, ——R for rat, ——S for Syrian hamster).

For test systems using human cells *in vitro*, when the cell type is not specified, the code letters –IH are used. For assays on humans *in vivo*, when the cell type is not specified, the code letters –VH are used. Otherwise, the second letter specifies the cell type under investigation (e.g., –BH for bone marrow, –LH for lymphocytes).

Some other specific coding conventions used for mammalian systems are as follows: BF– for body fluids, HM– for host-mediated, ——L for leucocytes or lymphocytes *in vitro* (–AL, animals; –HL, humans), –L– for leucocytes *in vivo* (–LA, animals; –LH, humans), ——T for transformed cells.

Note that these are examples of major conventions used to define the assay code words. The alphabetized listing of codes must be examined to confirm a specific code word. As might be expected from the limitation to three symbols, some codes do not fit the naming conventions precisely. In a few cases, test systems are defined by first-letter code words, for example: MST, mouse spot test; SLP, mouse specific locus test, postspermatogonia; SLO, mouse specific locus test, other stages; DLM, dominant lethal test in mice; DLR, dominant lethal test in rats; MHT, mouse heritable translocation test.

The genetic activity profiles and listings that follow were prepared in collaboration with Environmental Health Research and Testing Inc. (EHRT) under contract to the US Environmental Protection Agency; EHRT also determined the doses used. The references cited in each genetic activity profile listing can be found in the list of references in the appropriate monograph.

*References*

Garrett, N.E., Stack, H.F., Gross, M.R. & Waters, M.D. (1984) An analysis of the spectra of genetic activity produced by known or suspected human carcinogens. *Mutat. Res.*, *134*, 89–111

Gold, L.S., Sawyer, C.B., Magaw, R., Backman, G.M., de Veciana, M., Levinson, R., Hooper, N.K., Havender, W.R., Bernstein, L., Peto, R., Pike, M.C. & Ames, B.N. (1984) A carcinogenic potency database of the standardized results of animal bioassays. *Environ. Health Perspect.*, *58*, 9–319

Waters, M.D. (1979) *The GENE-TOX program*. In: Hsie, A.W., O'Neill, J.P. & McElheny, V.K., eds, *Mammalian Cell Mutagenesis: The Maturation of Test Systems* (*Banbury Report 2*), Cold Spring Harbor, NY, CHS Press, pp. 449–467

Waters, M.D. & Auletta, A. (1981) The GENE-TOX program: genetic activity evaluation. *J. chem. Inf. comput. Sci.*, *21*, 35–38

# TABLE 1. ALPHABETICAL LIST OF TEST SYSTEM CODE WORDS

| Endpoint | Code | Definition |
|---|---|---|
| C | ACC | *Allium cepa*, chromosomal aberrations |
| A | AIA | Aneuploidy, animal cells *in vitro* |
| A | AIH | Aneuploidy, human cells *in vitro* |
| G | ANF | *Aspergillus nidulans*, forward mutation |
| R | ANG | *Aspergillus nidulans*, genetic crossing-over |
| A | ANN | *Aspergillus nidulans*, aneuploidy |
| G | ANR | *Aspergillus nidulans*, reverse mutation |
| G | ASM | *Arabidopsis* species, mutation |
| A | AVA | Aneuploidy, animal cells *in vivo* |
| A | AVH | Aneuploidy, human cells *in vivo* |
| F | BFA | Body fluids from animals, microbial mutagenicity |
| F | BFH | Body fluids from humans, microbial mutagenicity |
| D | BHD | Binding (covalent) to DNA, human cells *in vivo* |
| D | BHP | Binding (covalent) to RNA or protein, human cells *in vivo* |
| D | BID | Binding (covalent) to DNA *in vitro* |
| D | BIP | Binding (covalent) to RNA or protein *in vitro* |
| G | BPF | Bacteriophage, forward mutation |
| G | BPR | Bacteriophage, reverse mutation |
| D | BRD | Other DNA repair-deficient bacteria, differential toxicity |
| D | BSD | *Bacillus subtilis rec* strains, differential toxicity |
| G | BSM | *Bacillus subtilis*, multigene test |
| D | BVD | Binding (covalent) to DNA, animal cells *in vivo* |
| D | BVP | Binding (covalent) to RNA or protein, animal cells *in vivo* |
| C | CBA | Chromosomal aberrations, animal bone-marrow cells *in vivo* |
| C | CBH | Chromosomal aberrations, human bone-marrow cells *in vivo* |
| C | CCC | Chromosomal aberrations, spermatocytes treated *in vivo*, spermatocytes observed |
| C | CGC | Chromosomal aberrations, spermatogonia treated *in vivo*, spermatocytes observed |
| C | CGG | Chromosomal aberrations, spermatogonia treated *in vivo*, spermatogonia observed |
| C | CHF | Chromosomal aberrations, human fibroblasts *in vitro* |
| C | CHL | Chromosomal aberrations, human lymphocytes *in vitro* |
| C | CHT | Chromosomal aberrations, transformed human cells *in vitro* |
| C | CIA | Chromosomal aberrations, other animal cells *in vitro* |
| C | CIC | Chromosomal aberrations, Chinese hamster cells *in vitro* |
| C | CIH | Chromosomal aberrations, other human cells *in vitro* |
| C | CIM | Chromosomal aberrations, mouse cells *in vitro* |
| C | CIR | Chromosomal aberrations, rat cells *in vitro* |
| C | CIS | Chromosomal aberrations, Syrian hamster cells *in vitro* |
| C | CIT | Chromosomal aberrations, transformed animal cells *in vitro* |
| C | CLA | Chromosomal aberrations, animal leucocytes *in vivo* |
| C | CLH | Chromosomal aberrations, human lymphocytes *in vivo* |
| C | COE | Chromosomal aberrations, oocytes or embryos treated *in vivo* |
| C | CVA | Chromosomal aberrations, other animal cells *in vivo* |
| C | CVH | Chromosomal aberrations, other human cells *in vivo* |
| D | DIA | DNA strand breaks, cross-links or related damage, animal cells *in vitro* |
| D | DIH | DNA strand breaks, cross-links or related damage, human cells *in vitro* |
| C | DLM | Dominant lethal test, mice |
| C | DLR | Dominant lethal test, rats |
| C | DMC | *Drosophila melanogaster*, chromosomal aberrations |
| R | DMG | *Drosophila melanogaster*, genetic crossing-over or recombination |
| C | DMH | *Drosophila melanogaster*, heritable translocation test |
| C | DML | *Drosophila melanogaster*, dominant lethal test |
| G | DMM | *Drosophila melanogaster*, somatic mutation (and recombination) |
| A | DMN | *Drosophila melanogaster*, aneuploidy |
| G | DMX | *Drosophila melanogaster*, sex-linked recessive lethal mutations |
| D | DVA | DNA strand breaks, cross-links or related damage, animal cells *in vivo* |
| D | DVH | DNA strand breaks, cross-links or related damage, human cells *in vivo* |
| G | EC2 | *Escherichia coli* WP2, reverse mutation |
| D | ECB | *Escherichia coli* (or *E. coli* DNA), strand breaks, cross-links or related damage; DNA repair |
| D | ECD | *Escherichia coli pol* A/W3110-P3478 differential toxicity (spot test) |
| G | ECF | *Escherichia coli pol* A/W3110-P3478, forward mutation |
| G | ECK | *Escherichia coli* K12, forward or reverse mutation |
| D | ECL | *Escherichia coli pol* A/W3110-P3478, differential toxicity (liquid suspension test) |
| G | ECR | *Escherichia coli* (other miscellaneous strains), reverse mutation |
| G | ECW | *Escherichia coli* WP2 *uvrA*, reverse mutation |
| D | ERD | *Escherichia coli rec* strains, differential toxicity |
| G | G51 | Gene mutation, mouse lymphoma L5178Y cells *in vitro*, all other loci |

**Table 1 (contd)**

| Endpoint | Code | Definition | Endpoint | Code | Definition |
|---|---|---|---|---|---|
| G | G9O | Gene mutation, Chinese hamster lung V79 cells, ouabain resistance | D | RVA | DNA repair exclusive of unscheduled DNA synthesis, animal cells in vivo |
| G | GCL | Gene mutation, Chinese hamster lung cells exclusive of V79 in vitro | G | SA0 | Salmonella typhimurium TA100, reverse mutation |
| G | GCO | Gene mutation, Chinese hamster ovary cells in vitro | G | SA2 | Salmonella typhimurium TA102, reverse mutation |
| G | G9H | Gene mutation, Chinese hamster lung V79 cells, hprt locus | G | SA3 | Salmonella typhimurium TA1530, reverse mutation |
| G | GHT | Gene mutation, transformed human cells | G | SA4 | Salmonella typhimurium TA104, reverse mutation |
| G | GIA | Gene mutation, other animal cells in vitro | G | SA5 | Salmonella typhimurium TA1535, reverse mutation |
| G | GIH | Gene mutation, human cells in vitro | G | SA7 | Salmonella typhimurium TA1537, reverse mutation |
| G | GML | Gene mutation, mouse lymphoma cells exclusive of L5178Y in vitro | G | SA8 | Salmonella typhimurium TA1538, reverse mutation |
| G | G5T | Gene mutation, mouse lymphoma L5178Y cells in vitro, TK locus | G | SA9 | Salmonella typhimurium TA98, reverse mutation |
| G | GVA | Gene mutation, animal cells in vivo | D | SAD | Salmonella typhimurium, DNA repair-deficient strains, differential toxicity |
| H | HMA | Host-mediated assay, animal cells in animal hosts | G | SAF | Salmonella typhimurium, forward mutation |
| H | HMH | Host-mediated assay, human cells in animal hosts | G | SAS | Salmonella typhimurium (other miscellaneous strains), reverse mutation |
| H | HMM | Host-mediated assay, microbial cells in animal hosts | G | SCF | Saccharomyces cerevisiae, forward mutation |
| C | HSC | Hordeum species, chromosomal aberrations | R | SCG | Saccharomyces cerevisiae, gene conversion |
| G | HSM | Hordeum species, mutation | R | SCH | Saccharomyces cerevisiae, homozygosis by mitotic recombination or gene conversion |
| I | ICH | Inhibition of intercellular communication, human cells in vitro | A | SCN | Saccharomyces cerevisiae, aneuploidy |
| I | ICR | Inhibition of intercellular communication, animal cells in vitro | G | SCR | Saccharomyces cerevisiae, reverse mutation |
| G | KPF | Klebsiella pneumonia, forward mutation | G | SGR | Streptomyces griseoflavus, reverse mutation |
| G | MAF | Micrococcus aureus, forward mutation | S | SHF | Sister chromatid exchange, human fibroblasts in vitro |
| C | MHT | Mouse heritable translocation test | S | SHL | Sister chromatid exchange, human lymphocytes in vitro |
| M | MIA | Micronucleus test, animal cells in vitro | S | SHT | Sister chromatid exchange, transformed human cells in vitro |
| M | MIH | Micronucleus test, human cells in vitro | S | SIA | Sister chromatid exchange, other animal cells in vitro |
| G | MST | Mouse spot test | S | SIC | Sister chromatid exchange, Chinese hamster cells in vitro |
| M | MVA | Micronucleus test, other animals in vivo | S | SIH | Sister chromatid exchange, other human cells in vitro |
| M | MVC | Micronucleus test, hamsters in vivo | S | SIM | Sister chromatid exchange, mouse cells in vivo |
| M | MVH | Micronucleus test, human cells in vivo | S | SIR | Sister chromatid exchange, rat cells in vivo |
| M | MVM | Micronucleus test, mice in vivo | S | SIS | Sister chromatid exchange, Syrian hamster cells in vitro |
| M | MVR | Micronucleus test, rats in vivo | S | SIT | Sister chromatid exchange, transformed animal cells in vitro |
| G | NCF | Neurospora crassa, forward mutation | S | SLH | Sister chromatid exchange, human lymphocytes in vivo |
| A | NCN | Neurospora crassa, aneuploidy | G | SLO | Mouse specific locus test, other stages |
| G | NCR | Neurospora crassa, reverse mutation | G | SLP | Mouse specific locus test, postspermatogonia |
| C | PLC | Plants (other), chromosomal aberrations | P | SPF | Sperm morphology, F1 mice |
| M | PLI | Plants (other), micronuclei | P | SPH | Sperm morphology, humans in vivo |
| G | PLM | Plants (other), mutation | P | SPM | Sperm morphology, mice |
| S | PLS | Plants (other), sister chromatid exchanges | P | SPR | Sperm morphology, rats |
| D | PLU | Plants, unscheduled DNA synthesis | D | SSB | Saccharomyces species, DNA strand breaks, cross-links or related damage |
| D | PRB | Prophage induction, SOS repair test or DNA strand breaks, cross-links or related damage | D | SSD | Saccharomyces species, DNA repair-deficient strains, differential toxicity |
| C | PSC | Paramecium species, chromosomal aberrations | G | STF | Streptomyces coelicolor, forward mutation |
| G | PSM | Paramecium species, mutation | G | STR | Streptomyces coelicolor, reverse mutation |
| D | RIA | DNA repair exclusive of unscheduled DNA synthesis, animal cells in vitro | | | |
| D | RIH | DNA repair exclusive of unscheduled DNA synthesis, human cells in vitro | | | |

## Table 1 (contd)

| Endpoint | Code | Definition |
|---|---|---|
| S | SVA | Sister chromatid exchange, animal cells *in vivo* |
| S | SVH | Sister chromatid exchange, other human cells *in vivo* |
| D | SZD | *Schizosaccharomyces pombe*, DNA repair-deficient strains, differential toxicity |
| G | SZF | *Schizosaccharomyces pombe*, forward mutation |
| R | SZG | *Schizosaccharomyces pombe*, gene conversion |
| G | SZR | *Schizosaccharomyces pombe*, reverse mutation |
| T | TBM | Cell transformation, BALB/c 3T3 mouse cells |
| T | TCL | Cell transformation, other established cell lines |
| T | TCM | Cell transformation, C3H 10T1/2 mouse cells |
| T | TCS | Cell transformation, Syrian hamster embryo cells, clonal assay |
| T | TEV | Cell transformation, other viral enhancement systems |
| T | TFS | Cell transformation, Syrian hamster embryo cells, focus assay |
| T | TIH | Cell transformation, human cells *in vitro* |
| T | TPM | Cell transformation, mouse prostate cells |
| T | T7R | Cell transformation, SA7/rat cells |
| T | TRR | Cell transformation, RLV/Fischer rat embryo cells |
| T | T7S | Cell transformation, SA7/Syrian hamster embryo cells |
| C | TSC | *Tradescantia* species, chromosomal aberrations |
| M | TSI | *Tradescantia* species, micronuclei |
| G | TSM | *Tradescantia* species, mutation |
| T | TVI | Cell transformation, treated *in vivo*, scored *in vitro* |
| D | UBH | Unscheduled DNA synthesis, human bone-marrow cells *in vivo* |
| D | UHF | Unscheduled DNA synthesis, human fibroblasts *in vitro* |
| D | UHL | Unscheduled DNA synthesis, human lymphocytes *in vitro* |
| D | UHT | Unscheduled DNA synthesis, transformed human cells *in vitro* |
| D | UIA | Unscheduled DNA synthesis, other animal cells *in vitro* |
| D | UIH | Unscheduled DNA synthesis, other human cells *in vitro* |
| D | UPR | Unscheduled DNA synthesis, rat hepatocytes *in vivo* |
| D | URP | Unscheduled DNA synthesis, rat primary hepatocytes |
| D | UVA | Unscheduled DNA synthesis, other animal cells *in vivo* |
| D | UVC | Unscheduled DNA synthesis, hamster cells *in vivo* |
| D | UVH | Unscheduled DNA synthesis, other human cells *in vivo* |
| D | UVM | Unscheduled DNA synthesis, mouse cells *in vivo* |
| D | UVR | Unscheduled DNA synthesis, other rat cells *in vivo* |
| C | VFC | *Vicia faba*, chromosomal aberrations |
| S | VFS | *Vicia faba*, sister chromatid exchange |

# APPENDIX 1

DINITROFLUORANTHENE, 3,7-
105735-71-5

| TEST CODE | END POINT | RESULTS NO ACT | ACT | DOSE (LED OR HID) | SHORT CITATION |
|---|---|---|---|---|---|
| 1 BSD | D | + | 0 | 0.0200 | TOKIWA ET AL., 1986 |
| 2 BSD | D | + | 0 | 0.0100 | NAKAGAWA ET AL., 1987 |
| 3 SA0 | G | + | 0 | 0.0010 | NAKAGAWA ET AL., 1987 |
| 4 SA7 | G | + | 0 | 0.0010 | NAKAGAWA ET AL., 1987 |
| 5 SA8 | G | + | 0 | 0.0005 | NAKAGAWA ET AL., 1987 |
| 6 SA9 | G | + | 0 | 0.0001 | NAKAGAWA ET AL., 1987 |
| 7 SAS | G | + | 0 | 0.0003 | NAKAGAWA ET AL., 1987 |

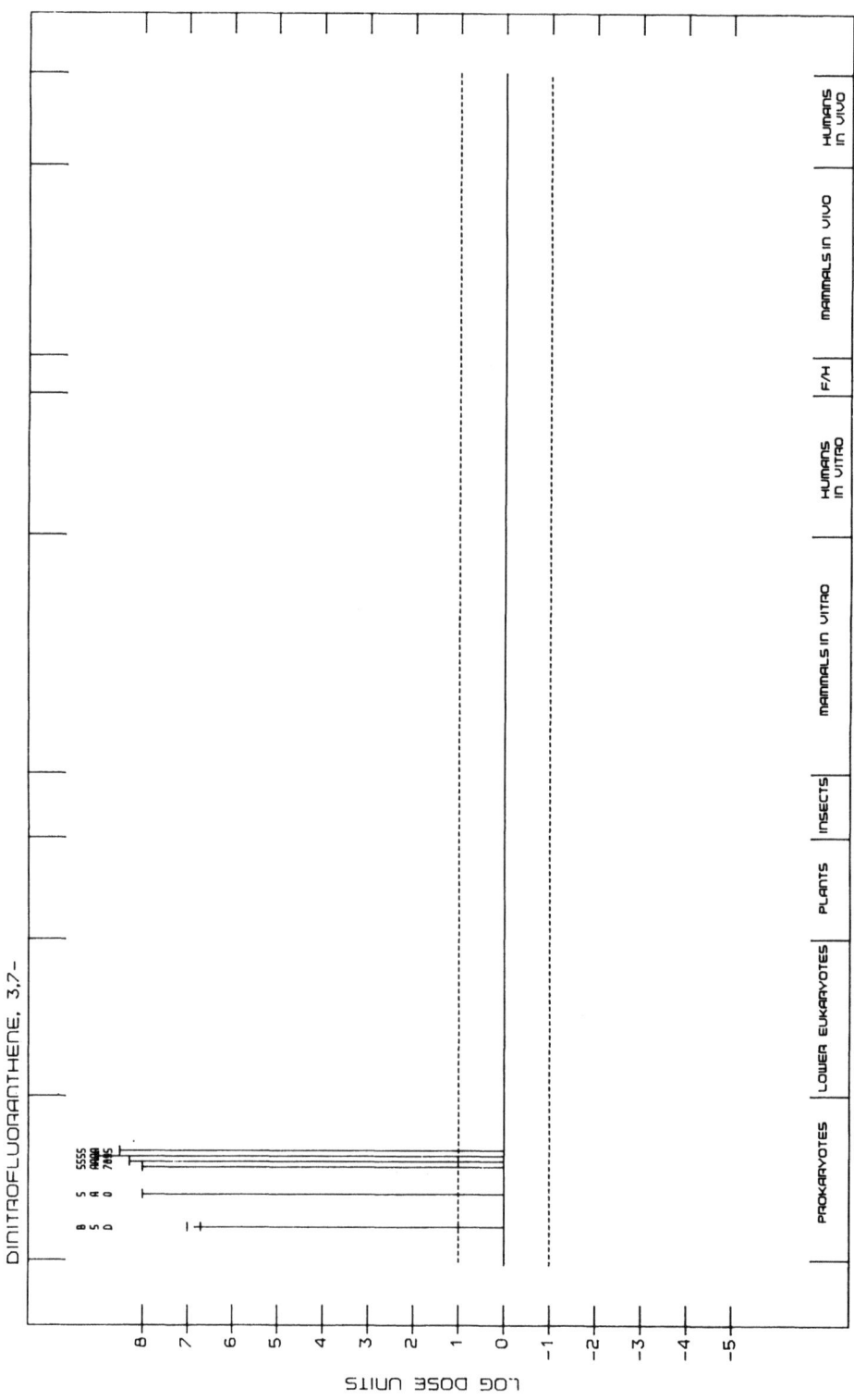

# APPENDIX 1

DINITROFLUORANTHENE, 3,9-
22506-53-2

| | TEST CODE | END POINT | RESULTS NO ACT | RESULTS ACT | DOSE (LED OR HID) | SHORT CITATION |
|---|---|---|---|---|---|---|
| 1 | BSD | D | + | 0 | 0.0200 | TOKIWA ET AL., 1986 |
| 2 | BSD | D | + | 0 | 0.0100 | NAKAGAWA ET AL., 1987 |
| 3 | SA0 | G | + | 0 | 0.0010 | NAKAGAWA ET AL., 1987 |
| 4 | SA7 | G | + | 0 | 0.0010 | NAKAGAWA ET AL., 1987 |
| 5 | SA8 | G | + | 0 | 0.0001 | NAKAGAWA ET AL., 1987 |
| 6 | SA9 | G | + | 0 | 0.0001 | NAKAGAWA ET AL., 1987 |
| 7 | SAS | G | + | 0 | 0.0003 | NAKAGAWA ET AL., 1987 |

# 390 IARC MONOGRAPHS VOLUME 46

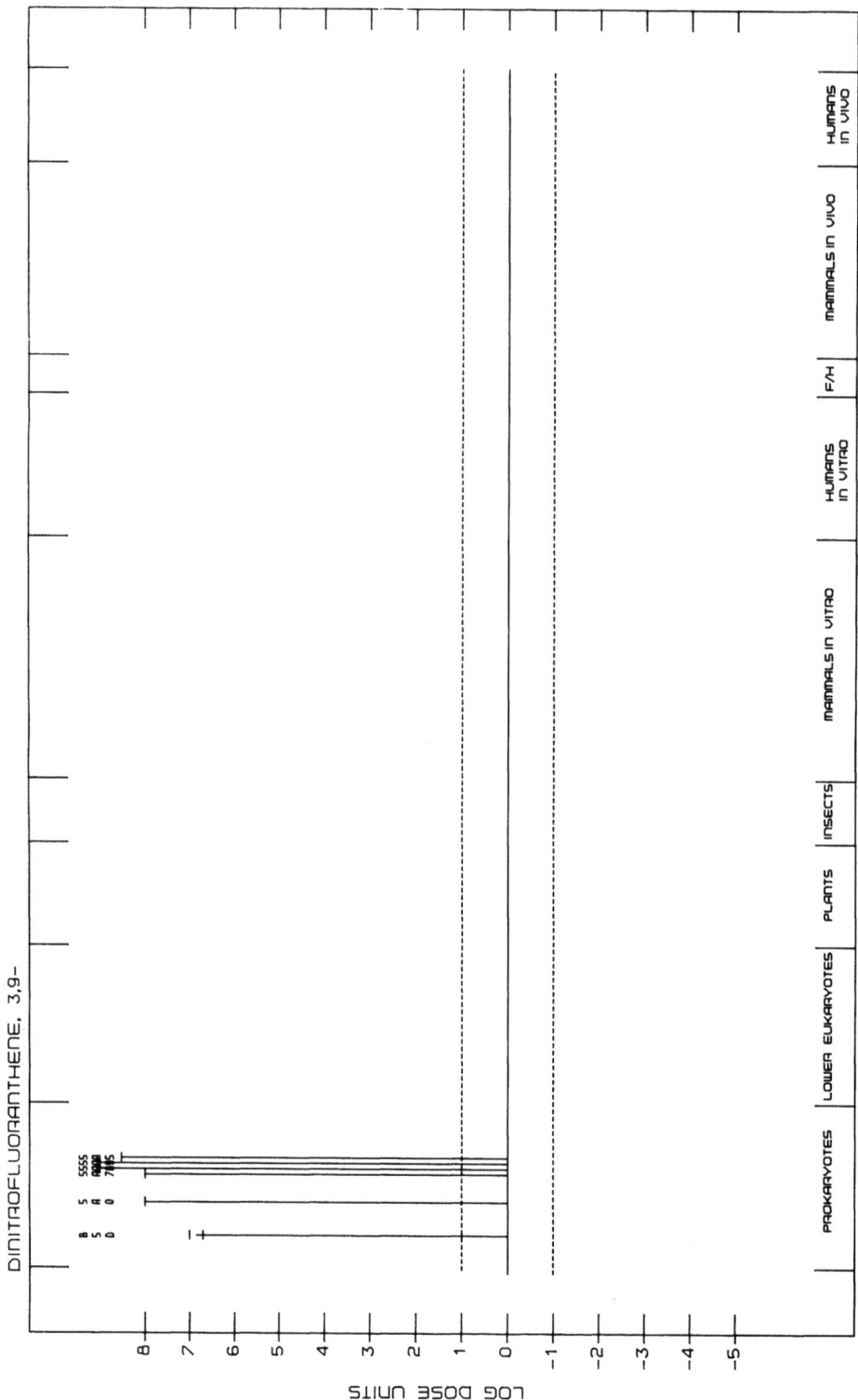

# APPENDIX 1

DINITROPYRENE, 1,3-
75321-20-9

| TEST CODE | END POINT | RESULTS NO ACT | ACT | DOSE (LED OR HID) | SHORT CITATION |
|---|---|---|---|---|---|
| 1 SAD | D | + | 0 | 0.0015 | NAKAMURA ET AL., 1987 |
| 2 BSD | D | + | 0 | 0.0300 | HORIKAWA ET AL., 1986 |
| 3 BSD | D | + | 0 | 0.1000 | TOKIWA ET AL., 1986 |
| 4 SA0 | G | + | 0 | 0.0012 | MERMELSTEIN ET AL., 1981 |
| 5 SA0 | G | + | 0 | 0.0000 | ROSENKRANZ ET AL., 1985 |
| 6 SA0 | G | + | 0 | 0.0000 | MCCOY ET AL., 1985b |
| 7 SA2 | G | + | 0 | 0.0000 | MCCOY ET AL., 1985b |
| 8 SA4 | G | + | 0 | 0.0000 | MCCOY ET AL., 1985b |
| 9 SA5 | G | − | 0 | 0.0125 | MERMELSTEIN ET AL., 1981 |
| 10 SA7 | G | + | 0 | 0.0001 | MERMELSTEIN ET AL., 1981 |
| 11 SA8 | G | + | 0 | 0.0004 | MERMELSTEIN ET AL., 1981 |
| 12 SA9 | G | + | 0 | 0.0001 | MERMELSTEIN ET AL., 1981 |
| 13 SA9 | G | + | 0 | 0.0000 | PEDERSON & SIAK, 1981 |
| 14 SA9 | G | + | 0 | 0.0000 | ROSENKRANZ ET AL., 1985 |
| 15 SA9 | G | + | 0 | 0.0000 | TOKIWA ET AL., 1985 |
| 16 SA9 | G | + | 0 | 0.0000 | LOFROTH, 1981 |
| 17 SA9 | G | + | 0 | 0.0010 | MOROTOMI & WATANABE, 1984 |
| 18 SA9 | G | + | 0 | 0.0000 | MCCOY ET AL., 1985b |
| 19 SAS | G | + | 0 | 0.0000 | ROSENKRANZ ET AL., 1985 |
| 20 SAS | G | + | 0 | 0.0000 | MCCOY ET AL., 1985b |
| 21 ECW | G | − | 0 | 0.0125 | MERMELSTEIN ET AL., 1981 |
| 22 ECW | G | + | 0 | 0.0100 | MCCOY ET AL., 1985a |
| 23 SCG | R | − | 0 | 500.0000 | MCCOY ET AL., 1983 |
| 24 DIA | D | (+) | 0 | 5.8000 | MOLLER & THORGEIRSSON, 1985 |
| 25 URP | D | + | 0 | 0.1000 | MORI ET AL., 1987 |
| 26 UIA | D | + | 0 | 1.0000 | MORI ET AL., 1987 |
| 27 GCL | G | + | 0 | 0.6700 | NAKAYASU ET AL., 1982 |
| 28 GCO | G | (+) | + | 2.0000 | LI & DUTCHER, 1983 |
| 29 G9O | G | + | 0 | 10.0000 | TAKAYAMA ET AL., 1983 |
| 30 G9O | G | + | 0 | 10.0000 | KATOH ET AL., 1984 |
| 31 UHT | D | + | 0 | 0.0000 | EDDY ET AL., 1986 |
| 32 GIH | G | + | 0 | 0.0000 | EDDY ET AL., 1986 |
| 33 BID | * | (+) | 0 | 1.0000 | HSIEH ET AL., 1986 |

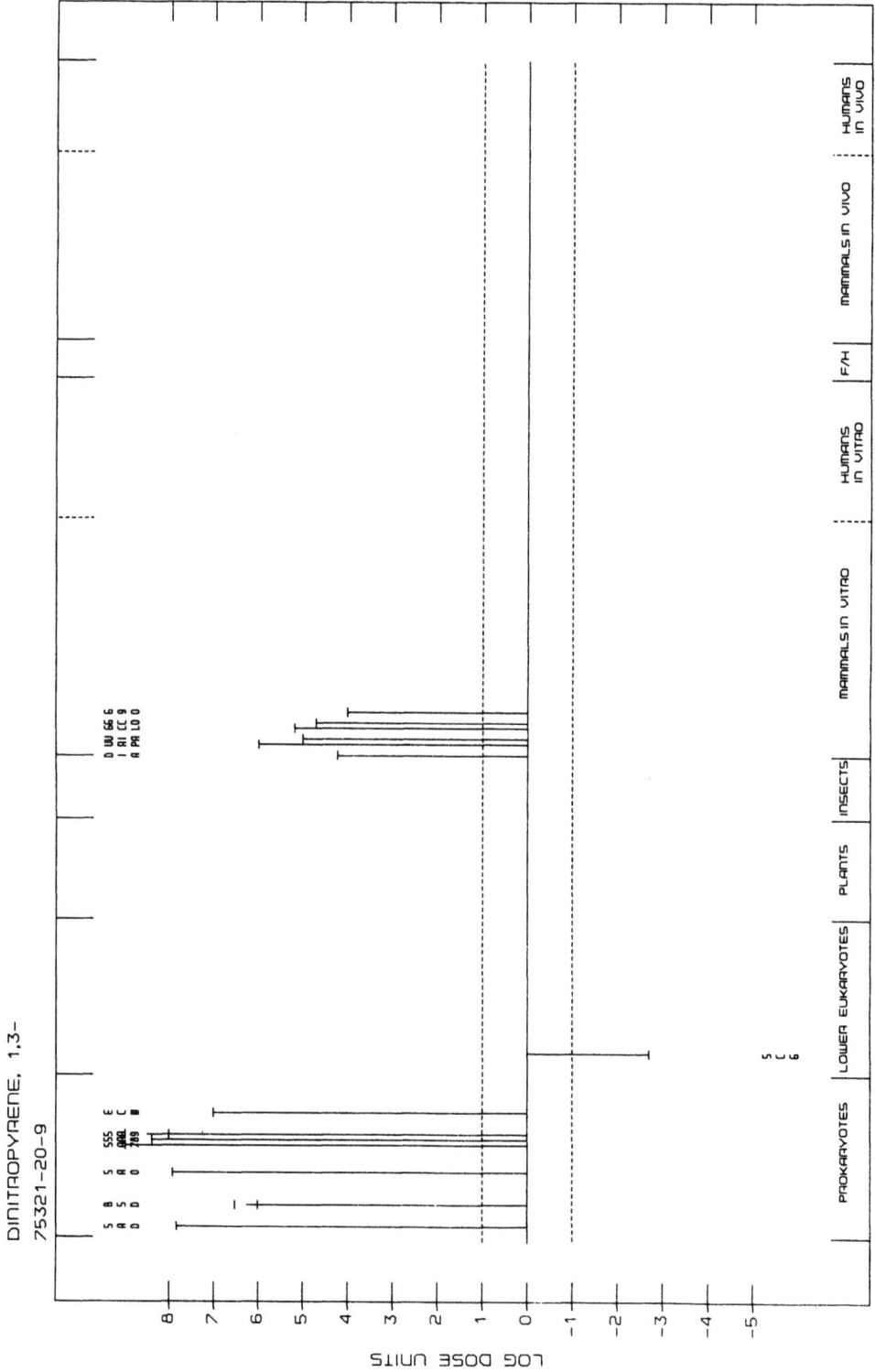

# APPENDIX 1

DINITROPYRENE, 1,6-
42397-64-8

| TEST CODE | END POINT | RESULTS NO ACT | ACT | DOSE (LED OR HID) | SHORT CITATION |
|---|---|---|---|---|---|
| 1 SAD | D | + | 0 | 0.0050 | NAKAMURA ET AL., 1987 |
| 2 BSD | D | + | 0 | 0.0200 | HORIKAWA ET AL., 1986 |
| 3 BSD | D | + | 0 | 0.0400 | TOKIWA ET AL., 1986 |
| 4 SA0 | G | + | 0 | 0.0006 | TOKIWA ET AL., 1984 |
| 5 SA0 | G | + | + | 0.0025 | EL-BAYOUMY & HECHT, 1986 |
| 6 SA0 | G | + | + | 0.0050 | TOKIWA ET AL., 1981 |
| 7 SA0 | G | + | 0 | 0.0000 | ROSENKRANZ ET AL., 1985 |
| 8 SA2 | G | + | 0 | 0.1500 | MCCOY ET AL., 1985b |
| 9 SA4 | G | + | 0 | 0.0000 | MCCOY ET AL., 1985b |
| 10 SA5 | G | − | 0 | 0.0125 | MERMELSTEIN ET AL., 1981 |
| 11 SA7 | G | + | 0 | 0.0003 | TOKIWA ET AL., 1984 |
| 12 SA7 | G | + | 0 | 0.0001 | MERMELSTEIN ET AL., 1981 |
| 13 SA8 | G | + | 0 | 0.0006 | TOKIWA ET AL., 1984 |
| 14 SA8 | G | + | 0 | 0.0001 | MERMELSTEIN ET AL., 1981 |
| 15 SA9 | G | + | 0 | 0.0003 | TOKIWA ET AL., 1984 |
| 16 SA9 | G | + | 0 | 0.0001 | MERMELSTEIN ET AL., 1981 |
| 17 SA9 | G | + | + | 0.0050 | TOKIWA ET AL., 1981 |
| 18 SA9 | G | + | 0 | 0.0050 | ASHBY ET AL., 1983 |
| 19 SA9 | G | + | + | 0.0025 | EL-BAYOUMY & HECHT, 1986 |
| 20 SA9 | G | + | 0 | 0.0008 | FIFER ET AL., 1986 |
| 21 SA9 | G | + | 0 | 0.0000 | LOFROTH, 1981 |
| 22 SA9 | G | + | 0 | 0.0000 | ROSENKRANZ ET AL., 1985 |
| 23 SA9 | G | + | 0 | 0.0000 | TOKIWA ET AL., 1985 |
| 24 SA9 | G | + | 0 | 0.0000 | FU ET AL., 1986 |
| 25 SA9 | G | + | 0 | 0.0010 | MOROTOMI & WATANABE, 1984 |
| 26 SA9 | G | + | 0 | 0.0000 | NAKAYASU ET AL., 1982 |
| 27 SAS | G | + | 0 | 0.0000 | ROSENKRANZ ET AL., 1985 |
| 28 SAS | G | + | 0 | 0.0000 | MCCOY ET AL., 1985b |
| 29 ECW | G | + | 0 | 0.0012 | TOKIWA ET AL., 1984 |
| 30 ECW | G | + | 0 | 0.0400 | MCCOY ET AL., 1985a |
| 31 SCG | R | − | 0 | 500.0000 | MCCOY ET AL., 1983 |
| 32 SCG | R | + | 0 | 1.6000 | WILCOX & PARRY, 1981 |
| 33 SCG | R | + | + | 0.0000 | WILCOX ET AL., 1982 |
| 34 DIA | D | + | 0 | 4.4000 | SAITO ET AL., 1984b |
| 35 DIA | D | (+) | 0 | 5.8000 | MOLLER & THORGEIRSSON, 1985 |
| 36 URP | D | + | 0 | 0.0100 | MORI ET AL., 1987 |
| 37 URP | D | + | 0 | 0.0150 | BUTTERWORTH ET AL., 1983 |
| 38 UIA | D | + | 0 | 0.0150 | DOOLITTLE & BUTTERWORTH, 1984 |
| 39 UIA | D | + | 0 | 0.6300 | HAUGEN ET AL., 1986 |
| 40 UIA | D | − | 0 | 1.5000 | WORKING & BUTTERWORTH, 1984 |
| 41 UIA | D | + | 0 | 1.1000 | MORI ET AL., 1987 |
| 42 GCL | G | + | 0 | 0.5700 | NAKAYASU ET AL., 1982 |
| 43 GCO | G | (+) | + | 0.5000 | LI & DUTCHER, 1983 |
| 44 GCO | G | + | 0 | 0.0500 | EDGAR & BROOKER, 1985 |
| 45 GCO | G | (+) | 0 | 1.5000 | FIFER ET AL., 1986 |
| 46 G9O | G | + | 0 | 0.1000 | KATOH ET AL., 1984 |
| 47 SIC | S | + | 0 | 0.0500 | EDGAR & BROOKER, 1985 |
| 48 CIC | C | + | 0 | 0.0500 | EDGAR & BROOKER, 1985 |
| 49 CIR | C | + | 0 | 0.0100 | DANFORD ET AL., 1982 |
| 50 CIR | C | + | 0 | 0.0100 | WILCOX ET AL., 1982 |

DINITROPYRENE, 1,6-
42397-64-8

| TEST CODE | END POINT | RESULTS NO ACT | ACT | DOSE (LED OR HID) | SHORT CITATION |
|---|---|---|---|---|---|
| 51 UHT | D | – | 0 | 0.0000 | EDDY ET AL., 1986 |
| 52 UIH | D | + | 0 | 29.0000 | SUGIMURA & TAKAYAMA, 1983 |
| 53 UIH | D | + | 0 | 1.5000 | DOOLITTLE ET AL., 1985 |
| 54 UIH | D | + | 0 | 0.0150 | BUTTERWORTH ET AL., 1983 |
| 55 GIH | G | – | 0 | 0.0000 | EDDY ET AL., 1986 |
| 56 CHF | C | + | 0 | 0.0200 | WILCOX ET AL., 1982 |
| 57 UPR | D | – | 0 | 50.0000 | BUTTERWORTH ET AL., 1983 |
| 58 UVR | D | – | 0 | 50.0000 | WORKING & BUTTERWORTH, 1984 |
| 59 BVD | * | + | 0 | 0.2000 | DJURIC ET AL., 1988 |
| 60 BID | * | 0 | + | 5.9000 | DJURIC ET AL., 1988 |
| 61 BID | * | + | 0 | 1.0000 | HSIEH ET AL.,1986 |
| 62 BVD | * | + | 0 | 3.4000 | DELCLOS ET AL., 1987 |

# APPENDIX 1

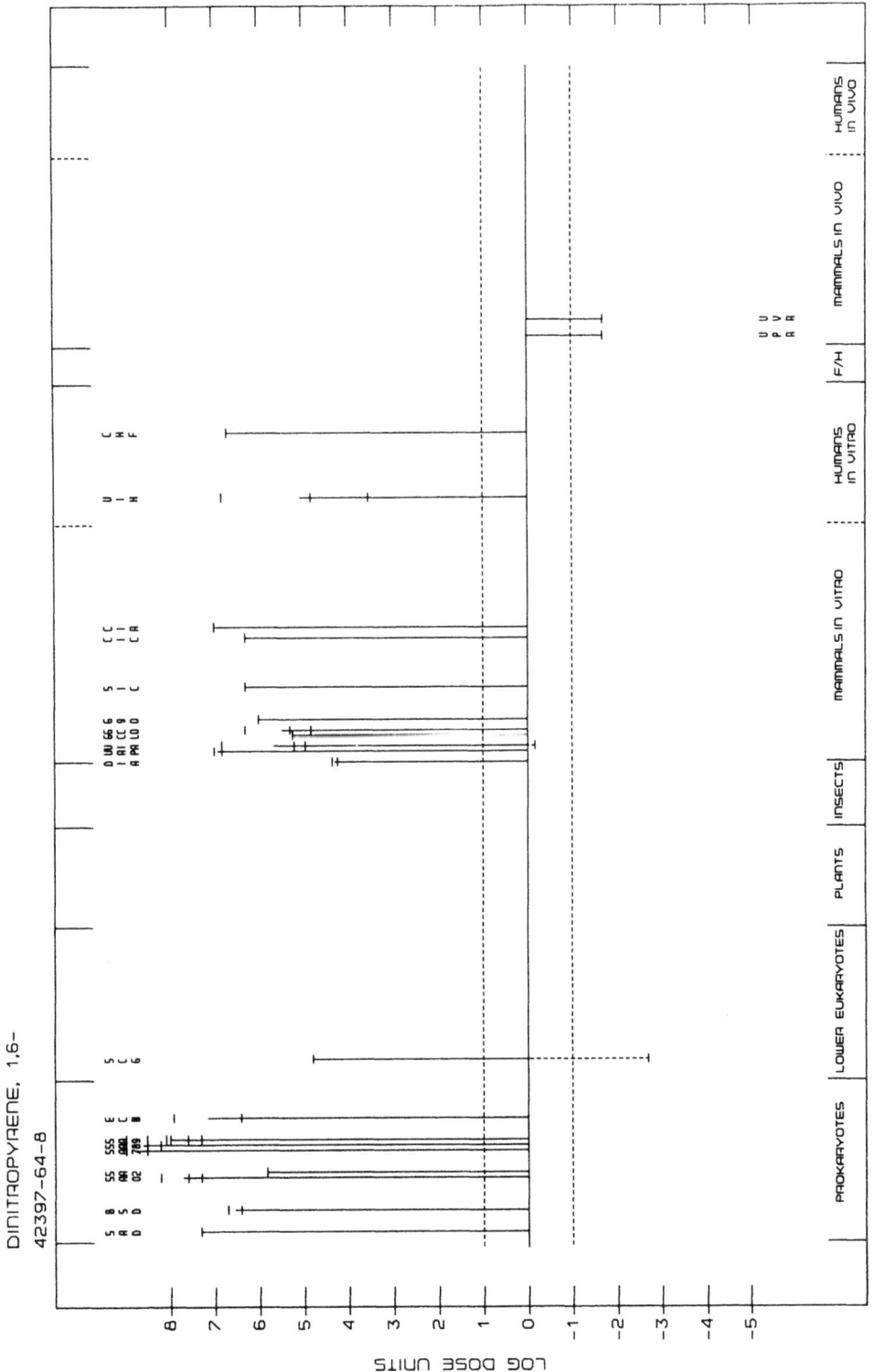

DINITROPYRENE, 1,8-
42397-65-9

| TEST CODE | END POINT | RESULTS NO ACT | ACT | DOSE (LED OR HID) | SHORT CITATION |
|---|---|---|---|---|---|
| 1 SAD | D | + | 0 | 0.0030 | NAKAMURA ET AL., 1987 |
| 2 BSD | D | + | 0 | 0.0100 | HORIKAWA ET AL., 1986 |
| 3 BSD | D | + | 0 | 0.0200 | TOKIWA ET AL., 1986 |
| 4 SA0 | G | + | 0 | 0.0000 | ROSENKRANZ ET AL., 1985 |
| 5 SA0 | G | + | + | 0.0050 | TOKIWA ET AL., 1981 |
| 6 SA2 | G | + | 0 | 0.0400 | MCCOY ET AL., 1985b |
| 7 SA4 | G | + | 0 | 0.0000 | MCCOY ET AL., 1985b |
| 8 SA5 | G | − | 0 | 0.0125 | MERMELSTEIN ET AL., 1981 |
| 9 SA7 | G | + | 0 | 0.0001 | MERMELSTEIN ET AL., 1981 |
| 10 SA8 | G | + | 0 | 0.0001 | MERMELSTEIN ET AL., 1981 |
| 11 SA9 | G | + | + | 0.0050 | TOKIWA ET AL., 1981 |
| 12 SA9 | G | + | 0 | 0.0008 | FIFER ET AL., 1986 |
| 13 SA9 | G | + | 0 | 0.0001 | MERMELSTEIN ET AL., 1981 |
| 14 SA9 | G | + | 0 | 0.0000 | PEDERSON & SIAK, 1981 |
| 15 SA9 | G | + | 0 | 0.0000 | ROSENKRANZ ET AL., 1985 |
| 16 SA9 | G | + | 0 | 0.0000 | TOKIWA ET AL., 1985 |
| 17 SA9 | G | + | 0 | 0.0000 | HOLLOWAY ET AL., 1987 |
| 18 SA9 | G | + | 0 | 0.0000 | LOFROTH, 1981 |
| 19 SA9 | G | + | 0 | 0.0000 | PITTS ET AL., 1984 |
| 20 SA9 | G | + | 0 | 0.0000 | ZIELINSKA ET AL., 1987 |
| 21 SA9 | G | + | 0 | 0.0010 | MOROTOMI & WATANABE, 1984 |
| 22 SA9 | G | + | 0 | 0.0000 | NAKAYASU ET AL., 1982 |
| 23 SA9 | G | + | 0 | 0.0000 | HEFLICH ET AL., 1985 |
| 24 SAS | G | + | 0 | 0.0000 | ROSENKRANZ ET AL., 1985 |
| 25 SAS | G | + | 0 | 0.0000 | HEFLICH ET AL., 1985 |
| 26 SAS | G | + | 0 | 0.0000 | MCCOY ET AL., 1985b |
| 27 ECW | G | − | 0 | 0.0300 | MERMELSTEIN ET AL., 1981 |
| 28 ECW | G | + | 0 | 0.0125 | MCCOY ET AL., 1985a |
| 29 SCG | R | + | 0 | 1.6000 | WILCOX & PARRY, 1981 |
| 30 SCG | R | − | 0 | 500.0000 | MCCOY ET AL., 1983 |
| 31 SCG | R | + | + | 0.0000 | WILCOX ET AL., 1982 |
| 32 DIA | D | (+) | 0 | 4.4000 | SAITO ET AL., 1984b |
| 33 DIA | D | + | 0 | 1.5000 | MOLLER & THORGEIRSSON, 1985 |
| 34 UIA | D | + | 0 | 0.1000 | MORI ET AL., 1987 |
| 35 UIA | D | + | 0 | 0.6300 | HAUGEN ET AL., 1986 |
| 36 GCL | G | + | 0 | 0.7500 | NAKAYASU ET AL., 1982 |
| 37 GCO | G | + | 0 | 0.0500 | EDGAR & BROOKER, 1985 |
| 38 GCO | G | + | 0 | 1.5000 | HEFLICH ET AL., 1986b |
| 39 GCO | G | (+) | + | 0.2000 | LI & DUTCHER, 1983 |
| 40 G9O | G | + | 0 | 0.0500 | TAKAYAMA ET AL., 1983 |
| 41 G9O | G | + | 0 | 0.1000 | KATOH ET AL., 1984 |
| 42 G5T | G | + | 0 | 0.1000 | EDGAR, 1985 |
| 43 G51 | G | + | 0 | 0.0250 | COLE ET AL., 1982 |
| 44 G51 | G | + | 0 | 0.1000 | ARLETT, 1984 |
| 45 SIC | S | + | 0 | 0.0500 | EDGAR & BROOKER, 1985 |
| 46 SIC | S | + | + | 0.3000 | NACHTMAN & WOLFF, 1982 |
| 47 CIC | C | + | 0 | 0.0500 | EDGAR & BROOKER, 1985 |
| 48 CIR | C | + | 0 | 0.0100 | WILCOX ET AL., 1982 |
| 49 CIR | C | + | 0 | 0.0400 | DANFORD ET AL., 1982 |
| 50 TCS | T | + | 0 | 1.0000 | DIPAOLO ET AL., 1983 |

# APPENDIX 1

DINITROPYRENE, 1,8-
42397-65-9

| TEST CODE | END POINT | RESULTS NO ACT | ACT | DOSE (LED OR HID) | SHORT CITATION |
|---|---|---|---|---|---|
| 51 UHT | D | − | 0 | 0.0000 | EDDY ET AL., 1986 |
| 52 GIH | G | − | 0 | 0.0000 | EDDY ET AL., 1986 |
| 53 GIH | G | − | 0 | 2.5000 | ARLETT, 1984 |
| 54 MIH | M | − | 0 | 2.5000 | ARLETT, 1984 |
| 55 CHF | C | + | 0 | 0.3100 | WILCOX ET AL., 1982 |
| 56 BVD | * | + | 0 | 1.0000 | HEFLICH ET AL., 1986a |
| 57 BID | * | + | 0 | 1.0000 | HSIEH ET AL., 1986 |
| 58 BID | * | + | 0 | 2.9000 | HEFLICH ET AL., 1986b |
| 59 BID | * | + | 0 | 0.9000 | HEFLICH ET AL., 1985 |
| 60 BID | * | + | 0 | 0.0100 | ANDREWS ET AL., 1986 |

# 398 IARC MONOGRAPHS VOLUME 46

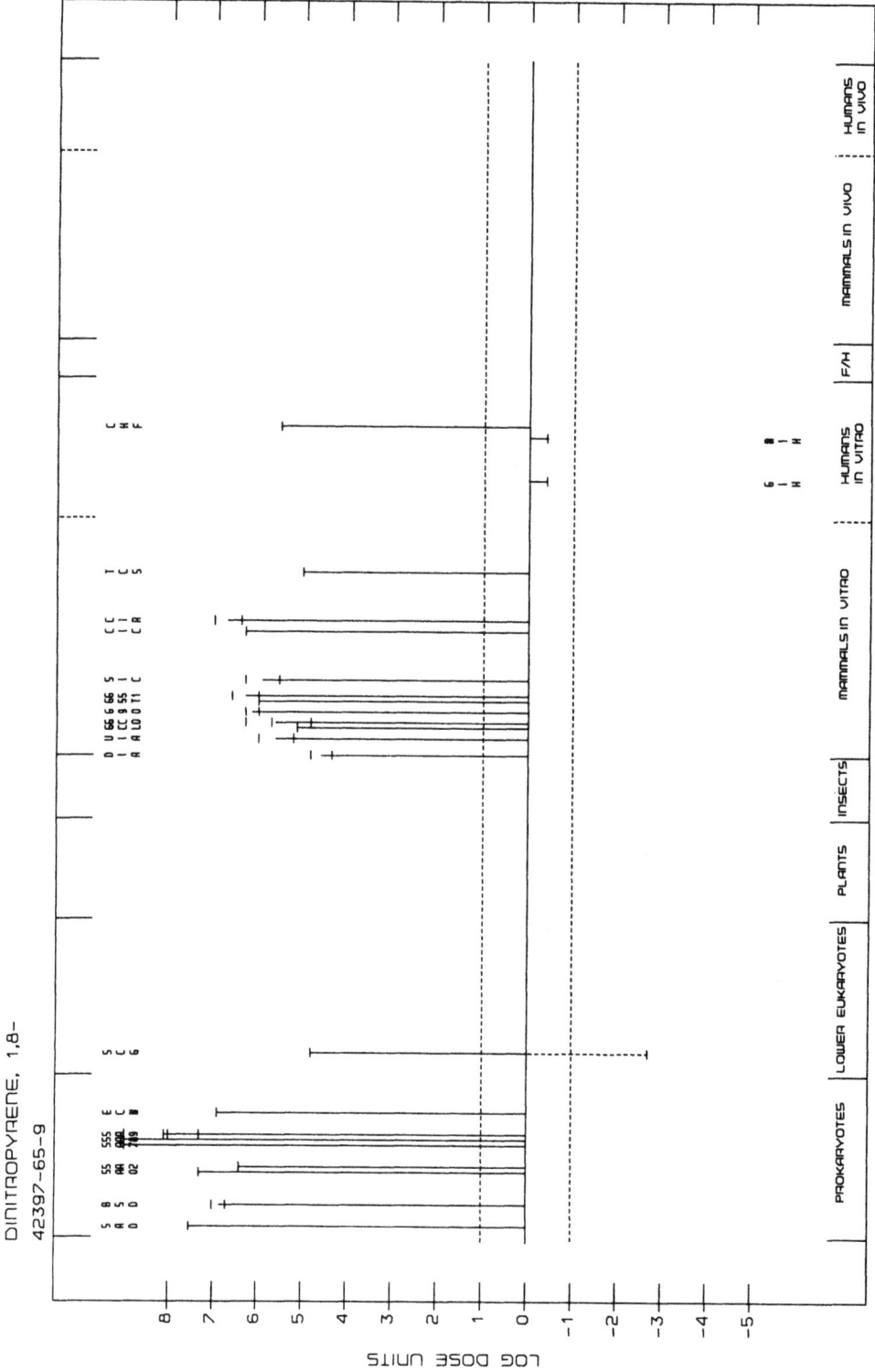

# APPENDIX 1

NITROBENZO[A]ANTHRACENE, 7-
20268-51-3

| TEST CODE | END POINT | RESULTS NO ACT | ACT | DOSE (LED OR HID) | SHORT CITATION |
|---|---|---|---|---|---|
| 1 SA0 | G | - | - | 0.0000 | GREIBROKK ET AL., 1984 |
| 2 SA9 | G | - | - | 0.0000 | GREIBROKK ET AL., 1984 |
| 3 SA9 | G | - | 0 | 4.0000 | WHITE ET AL., 1985 |
| 4 SAS | G | - | 0 | 4.0000 | WHITE ET AL., 1985 |

# 400　IARC MONOGRAPHS VOLUME 46

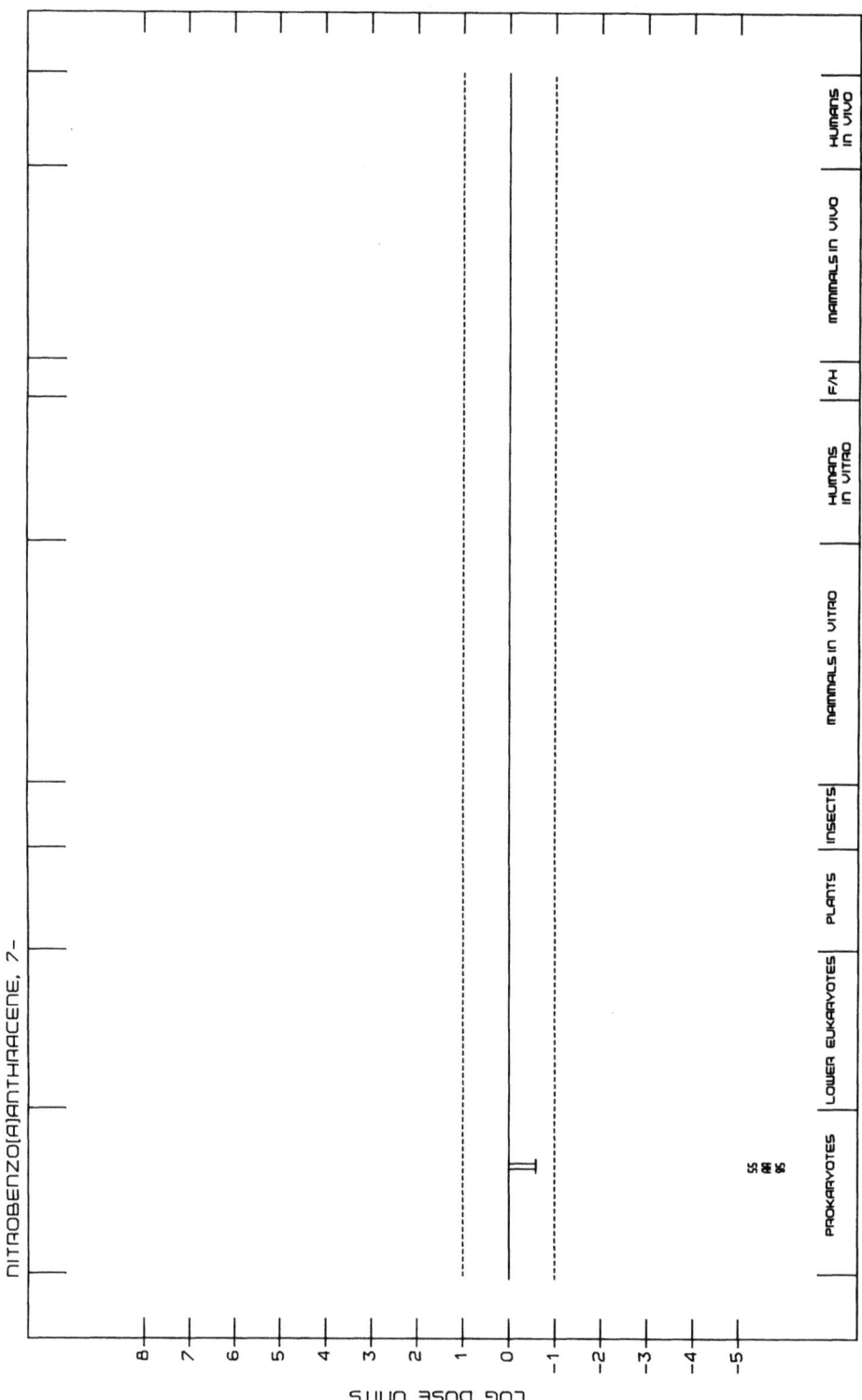

# APPENDIX 1

NITROBENZO[A]PYRENE, 6-
63041-90-7

| TEST CODE | END POINT | RESULTS NO ACT | RESULTS ACT | DOSE (LED OR HID) | SHORT CITATION |
|---|---|---|---|---|---|
| 1 SA0 | G | - | + | 0.7000 | FU ET AL., 1982a |
| 2 SA0 | G | - | + | 0.7500 | CHOU ET AL., 1984 |
| 3 SA0 | G | + | + | 10.0000 | TOKIWA ET AL., 1981 |
| 4 SA0 | G | - | + | 0.1000 | LOFROTH ET AL., 1984 |
| 5 SA9 | G | - | + | 0.7000 | FU ET AL., 1982a |
| 6 SA9 | G | - | + | 0.7500 | CHOU ET AL., 1984 |
| 7 SA9 | G | + | + | 10.0000 | TOKIWA ET AL., 1981 |
| 8 SA9 | G | - | + | 0.2000 | LOFROTH ET AL., 1984 |
| 9 SA9 | G | - | + | 0.1500 | ANDERSON ET AL., 1987 |
| 10 SA9 | G | - | - | 2.5000 | HASS ET AL., 1986a |
| 11 SA9 | G | + | + | 0.7500 | WANG ET AL., 1978 |
| 12 SA9 | G | - | + | 0.0000 | PITTS ET AL., 1982 |
| 13 SA9 | G | - | 0 | 5.0000 | WHITE ET AL., 1985 |
| 14 SAS | G | - | + | 0.0000 | PITTS ET AL., 1982 |
| 15 GCO | G | + | 0 | 1.0000 | CHOU ET AL., 1984 |
| 16 GCO | G | - | + | 5.0000 | HASS ET AL., 1986b |
| 17 TBM | T | + | 0 | 1.2000 | SALA ET AL., 1987 |
| 18 TCM | T | - | 0 | 2.4000 | SALA ET AL., 1987 |
| 19 TCS | T | + | 0 | 1.0000 | DIPAOLO ET AL., 1983 |
| 20 TCS | T | + | 0 | 0.6000 | SALA ET AL., 1987 |
| 21 TIH | T | + | 0 | 1.2000 | HOWARD ET AL., 1983b |
| 22 BVD | * | + | 0 | 2.0000 | GARNER ET AL., 1985 |
| 23 BID | * | + | 0 | 0.5000 | GARNER ET AL., 1985 |

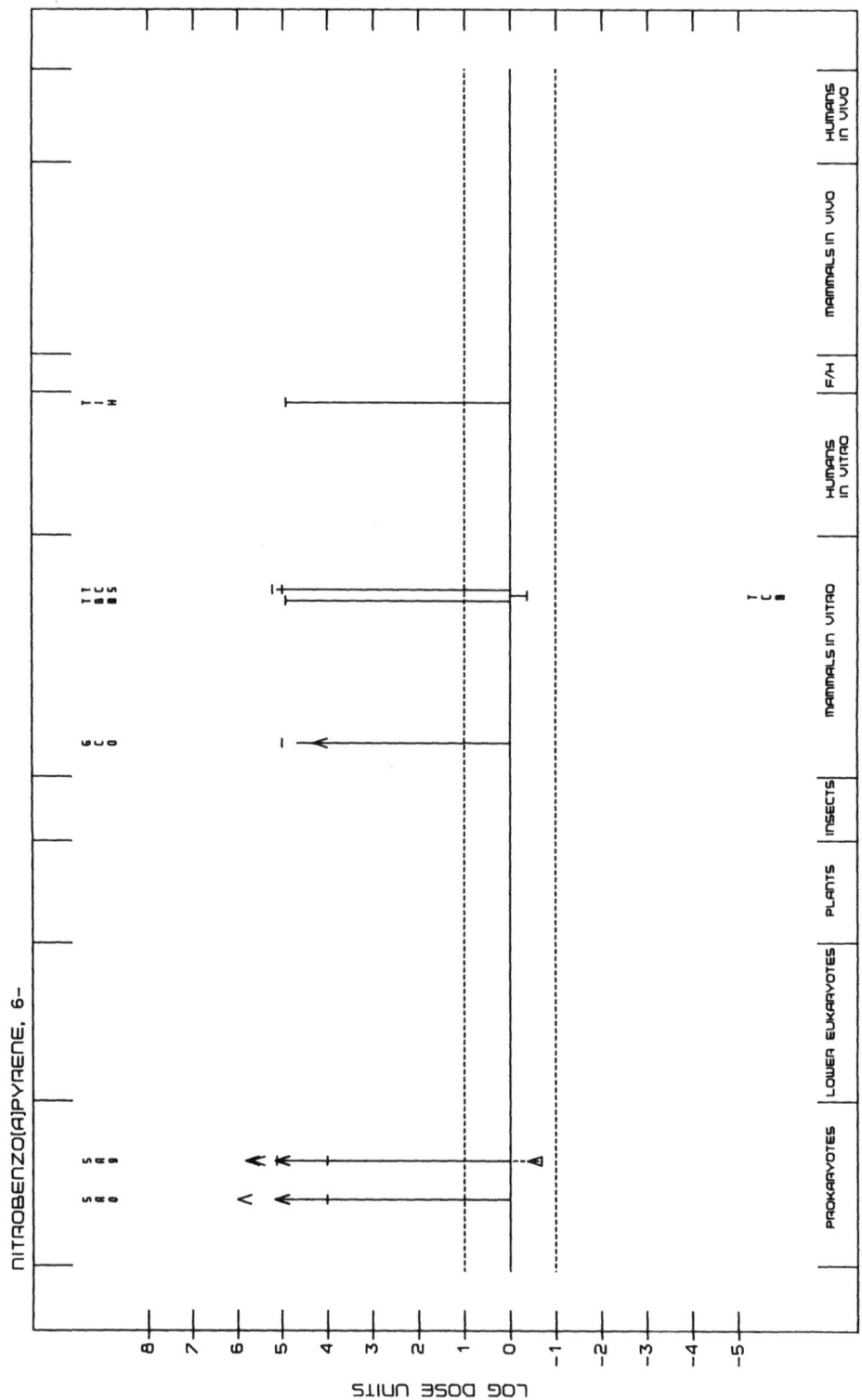

# APPENDIX 1

NITROCHRYSENE, 6-
7496-02-8

| TEST CODE | END POINT | RESULTS NO ACT | ACT | DOSE (LED OR HID) | SHORT CITATION |
|---|---|---|---|---|---|
| 1 BSD | D | + | 0 | 0.5000 | TOKIWA ET AL., 1987 |
| 2 SA0 | G | + | + | 0.0000 | GREIBROKK ET AL., 1984 |
| 3 SA0 | G | + | + | 0.0000 | SUGIMURA & TAKAYAMA, 1983 |
| 4 SA0 | G | + | + | 0.2500 | TOKIWA ET AL., 1981b |
| 5 SA0 | G | + | + | 0.2500 | EL-BAYOUMY & HECHT, 1984 |
| 6 SA9 | G | + | 0 | 0.0000 | PEDERSON & SIAK, 1981 |
| 7 SA9 | G | + | + | 12.5000 | TOKIWA ET AL., 1981a |
| 8 SA9 | G | + | + | 0.5000 | GREIBROKK ET AL., 1984 |
| 9 SA9 | G | + | + | 0.0000 | SUGIMURA & TAKAYAMA, 1983 |
| 10 SA9 | G | + | + | 0.2500 | TOKIWA ET AL., 1981b |
| 11 SA9 | G | + | + | 0.2500 | EL-BAYOUMY & HECHT, 1984 |
| 12 TBM | T | - | 0 | 10.8000 | SALA ET AL., 1987 |
| 13 TCS | T | + | 0 | 1.0000 | DIPAOLO ET AL., 1983 |
| 14 TCS | T | + | 0 | 3.6000 | SALA ET AL., 1987 |
| 15 BVD | * | + | 0 | 11.0000 | DELCLOS ET AL., 1988 |
| 16 BID | * | + | 0 | 2.7000 | DELCLOS ET AL., 1987a |

404                    IARC MONOGRAPHS VOLUME 46

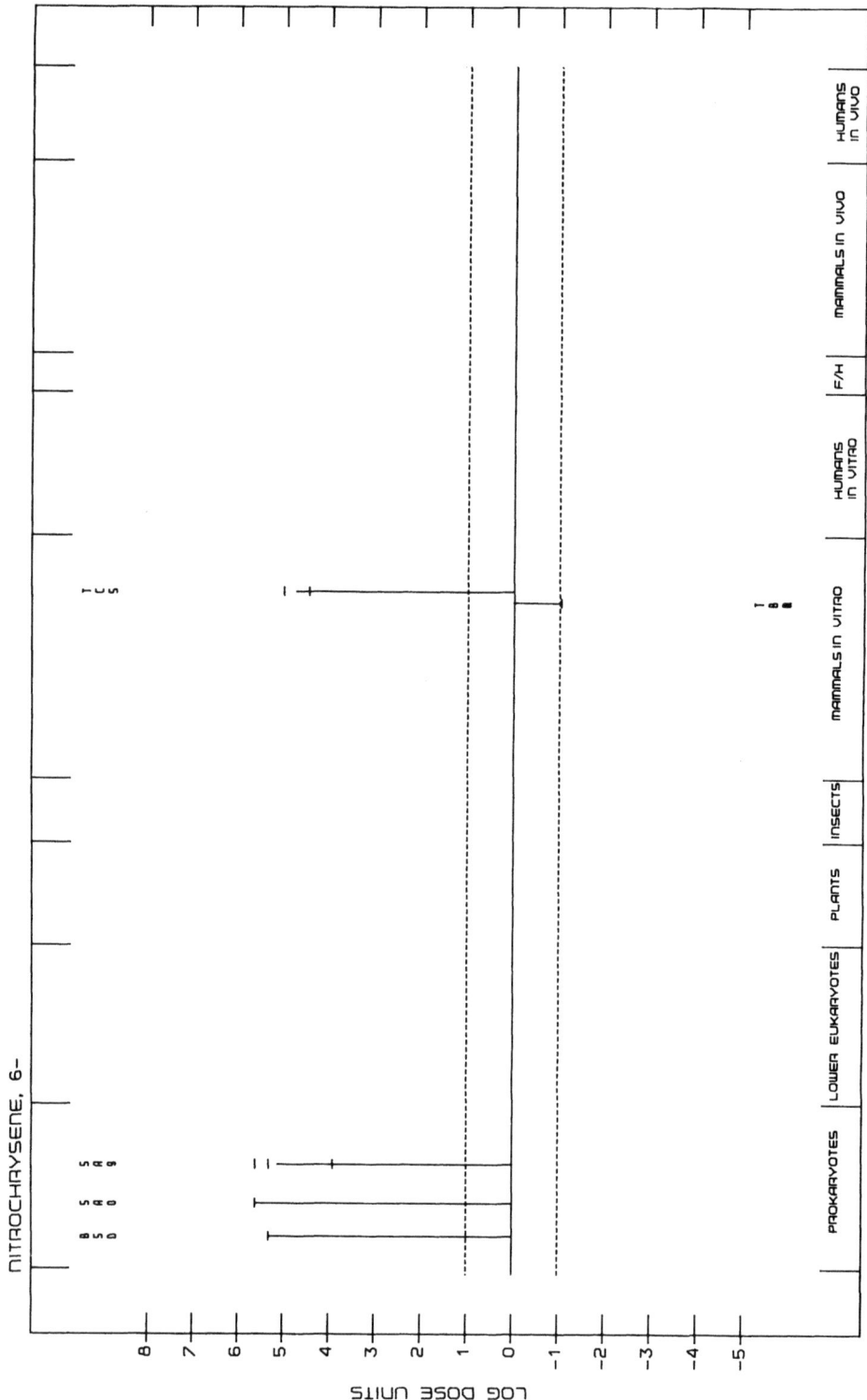

# APPENDIX 1

NITROFLUORENE, 2-
607-57-8

| | TEST CODE | END POINT | RESULTS NO ACT | ACT | DOSE (LED OR HID) | SHORT CITATION |
|---|---|---|---|---|---|---|
| 1 | PRB | D | + | 0 | 31.0000 | NAKAMURA ET AL., 1987 |
| 2 | PRB | D | + | 0 | 30.0000 | MAMBER ET AL., 1986 |
| 3 | PRB | D | + | 0 | 50.0000 | OHTA ET AL., 1984 |
| 4 | PRB | D | + | 0 | 21.0000 | QUILLARDET ET AL., 1985 |
| 5 | PRB | D | + | 0 | 105.0000 | MARZIN ET AL., 1986 |
| 6 | PRB | D | + | + | 125.0000 | HO & HO, 1981 |
| 7 | PRB | D | - | - | 1000.0000 | MAMBER ET AL., 1984 |
| 8 | ECL | D | + | 0 | 10.0000 | ROSENKRANZ & POIRIER, 1979 |
| 9 | ERD | D | 0 | + | 31.0000 | MCCARROLL ET AL., 1981a |
| 10 | ERD | D | + | 0 | 120.0000 | MAMBER ET AL., 1983 |
| 11 | ERD | D | + | 0 | 0.0000 | DOUDNEY ET AL., 1981 |
| 12 | BSD | D | 0 | + | 20.0000 | MCCARROLL ET AL., 1981b |
| 13 | BSD | D | + | 0 | 0.0000 | SUTER & JAEGER, 1982 |
| 14 | SAF | G | - | - | 2.5000 | XU ET AL., 1984 |
| 15 | SAF | G | + | 0 | 0.5000 | HERA & PUEYO, 1986 |
| 16 | SA0 | G | - | 0 | 1250.0000 | PURCHASE ET AL., 1978 |
| 17 | SA0 | G | + | 0 | 5.0000 | MCCOY ET AL., 1981 |
| 18 | SA0 | G | + | + | 1.7000 | DUNKEL ET AL., 1984 |
| 19 | SA0 | G | + | 0 | 5.0000 | SAKAMOTO ET AL., 1980 |
| 20 | SA5 | G | - | 0 | 1250.0000 | PURCHASE ET AL., 1978 |
| 21 | SA5 | G | - | ? | 167.0000 | DUNKEL ET AL., 1984 |
| 22 | SA5 | G | - | 0 | 5.0000 | SAKAMOTO ET AL., 1980 |
| 23 | SA5 | G | - | - | 12.5000 | ROSENKRANZ & POIRIER, 1979 |
| 24 | SA5 | G | - | 0 | 167.0000 | MCCOY ET AL., 1981 |
| 25 | SA7 | G | + | 0 | 17.0000 | MCCOY ET AL., 1981 |
| 26 | SA7 | G | + | + | 0.5000 | DUNKEL ET AL., 1984 |
| 27 | SA8 | G | + | 0 | 50.0000 | PURCHASE ET AL., 1978 |
| 28 | SA8 | G | + | 0 | 1.7000 | MCCOY ET AL., 1981 |
| 29 | SA8 | G | + | + | 0.1500 | DUNKEL ET AL., 1984 |
| 30 | SA8 | G | + | 0 | 5.0000 | SAKAMOTO ET AL., 1980 |
| 31 | SA8 | G | + | + | 12.5000 | ROSENKRANZ & POIRIER, 1979 |
| 32 | SA8 | G | + | 0 | 0.0000 | VANCE ET AL., 1987 |
| 33 | SA9 | G | + | 0 | 50.0000 | PURCHASE ET AL., 1978 |
| 34 | SA9 | G | + | 0 | 0.5000 | MCCOY ET AL., 1981 |
| 35 | SA9 | G | + | + | 0.1500 | DUNKEL ET AL., 1984 |
| 36 | SA9 | G | + | 0 | 5.0000 | SAKAMOTO ET AL., 1980 |
| 37 | SA9 | G | + | 0 | 0.3000 | XU ET AL., 1984 |
| 38 | SA9 | G | + | + | 0.0000 | PITTS ET AL., 1982 |
| 39 | SA9 | G | + | + | 0.0000 | VANCE ET AL., 1987 |
| 40 | SA9 | G | + | 0 | 1.0000 | ROSENKRANZ & MERMELSTEIN, 1983 |
| 41 | SA9 | G | + | 0 | 0.0000 | PEDERSON & SIAK, 1981 |
| 42 | SA9 | G | + | 0 | 1.0000 | WANG ET AL., 1980 |
| 43 | SAS | G | + | 0 | 50.0000 | MCCOY ET AL., 1981 |
| 44 | SAS | G | + | 0 | 0.6500 | RUIZ-RUBIO ET AL., 1984 |
| 45 | SAS | G | + | 0 | 5.0000 | SAKAMOTO ET AL., 1980 |
| 46 | SAS | G | + | + | 0.0000 | PITTS ET AL., 1982 |
| 47 | ECW | G | - | 0 | 25.0000 | MITCHELL & GILBERT, 1985 |
| 48 | ECW | G | - | - | 167.0000 | DUNKEL ET AL., 1984 |
| 49 | ECW | G | - | 0 | 5.0000 | SAKAMOTO ET AL., 1980 |
| 50 | EC2 | G | - | 0 | 5.0000 | SAKAMOTO ET AL., 1980 |

NITROFLUORENE, 2-
607-57-8

| TEST CODE | END POINT | RESULTS NO ACT | ACT | DOSE (LED OR HID) | SHORT CITATION |
|---|---|---|---|---|---|
| 51 ECR | G | (+) | 0 | 25.0000 | MITCHELL & GILBERT, 1984 |
| 52 ECR | G | + | 0 | 25.0000 | MITCHELL & GILBERT, 1985 |
| 53 ECR | G | − | 0 | 5.0000 | SAKAMOTO ET AL., 1980 |
| 54 SCH | R | + | + | 50000.0000 | SIMMON, 1979 |
| 55 SCH | R | − | 0 | 100.0000 | MITCHELL, 1980 |
| 56 ANR | G | − | 0 | 2000.0000 | BIGNAMI ET AL., 1982 |
| 57 TSM | G | + | 0 | 0.0000 | SCHAIRER & SAUTKULIS, 1982 |
| 58 URP | D | − | 0 | 211.0000 | PROBST ET AL., 1981 |
| 59 URP | D | + | 0 | 10.0000 | MORI ET AL., 1987 |
| 60 UIA | D | + | 0 | 10.0000 | MORI ET AL., 1987 |
| 61 G5T | G | + | 0 | 4.2000 | AMACHER ET AL., 1979 |
| 62 G5T | G | + | 0 | 250.0000 | OBERLY ET AL., 1984 |
| 63 SIC | S | + | + | 2.1000 | NACHTMAN & WOLFF, 1982 |
| 64 TCS | T | 0 | + | 20.0000 | POILEY ET AL., 1979 |
| 65 BFA | F | + | 0 | 0.0000 | BEIJE & MOLLER, 1988 |
| 66 HMM | H | + | 0 | 125.0000 | SIMMON ET AL., 1979 |
| 67 SVA | S | − | + | 125.0000 | NEAL & PROBST, 1983 |

# APPENDIX 1

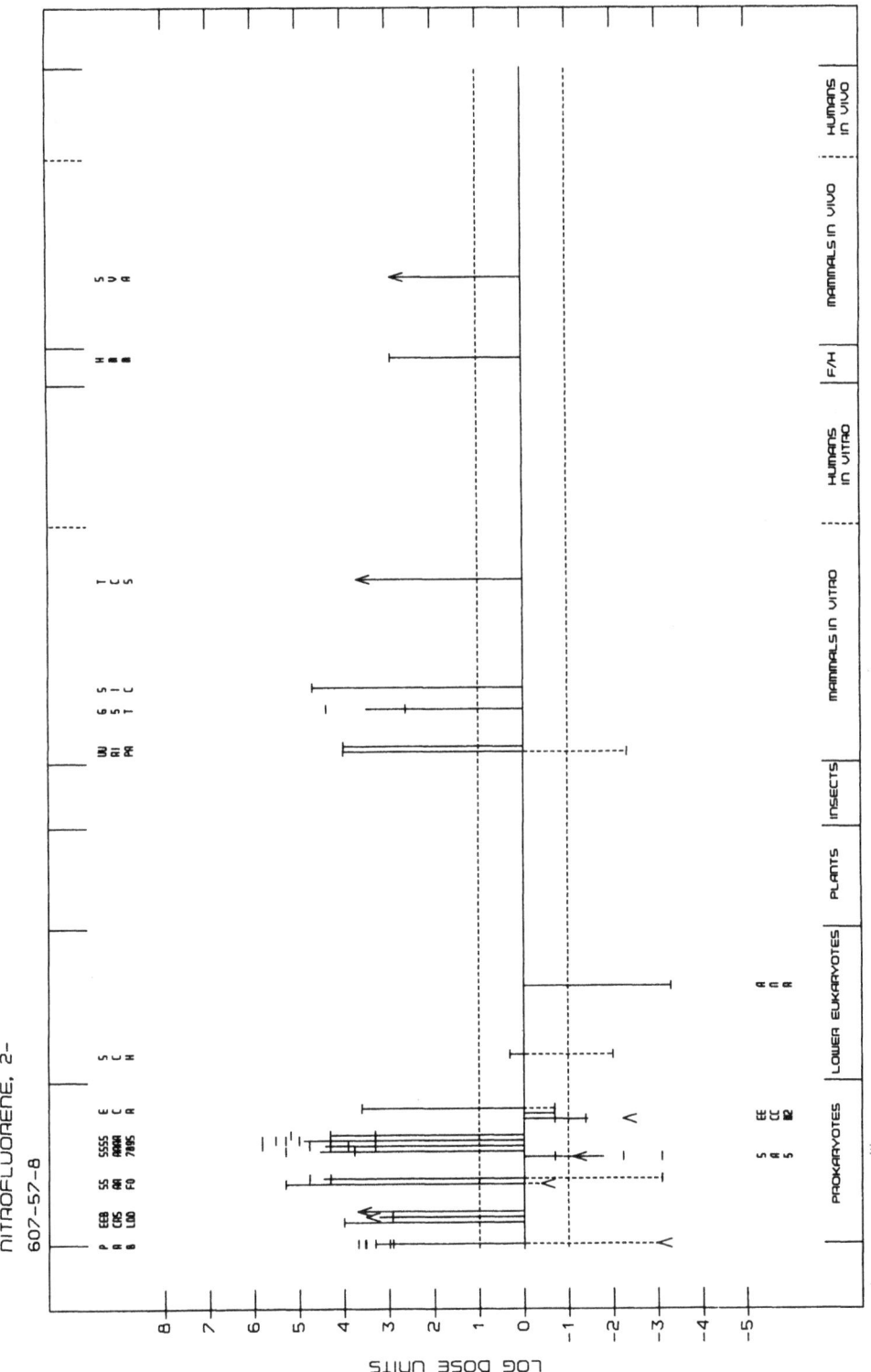

NITRONAPHTHALENE, 1-
86-57-7

| | TEST CODE | END POINT | RESULTS NO ACT | ACT | DOSE (LED OR HID) | SHORT CITATION |
|---|---|---|---|---|---|---|
| 1 | PRB | D | (+) | 0 | 19.0000 | NAKAMURA ET AL., 1987 |
| 2 | BSD | D | + | 0 | 100.0000 | TOKIWA ET AL., 1987 |
| 3 | SA0 | G | + | + | 5.0000 | DUNKEL ET AL., 1985 |
| 4 | SA0 | G | + | + | 5.0000 | TOKIWA ET AL., 1981 |
| 5 | SA0 | G | + | 0 | 17.0000 | MCCOY ET AL., 1981 |
| 6 | SA0 | G | + | + | 12.5000 | EL-BAYOUMI ET AL., 1981 |
| 7 | SA0 | G | + | 0 | 10.0000 | LOFROTH ET AL., 1984 |
| 8 | SA0 | G | + | + | 5.0000 | MORTELMANS ET AL., 1986 |
| 9 | SA0 | G | + | + | 0.0000 | MATSUDA, 1981 |
| 10 | SA5 | G | (+) | + | 16.7000 | DUNKEL ET AL., 1985 |
| 11 | SA5 | G | - | 0 | 50.0000 | MCCOY ET AL., 1981 |
| 12 | SA5 | G | - | (+) | 50.0000 | MORTELMANS ET AL., 1986 |
| 13 | SA7 | G | - | - | 167.0000 | DUNKEL ET AL., 1985 |
| 14 | SA7 | G | - | 0 | 167.0000 | MCCOY ET AL., 1981 |
| 15 | SA7 | G | - | - | 50.0000 | MORTELMANS ET AL., 1986 |
| 16 | SA8 | G | (+) | + | 16.7000 | DUNKEL ET AL., 1985 |
| 17 | SA9 | G | + | + | 16.7000 | DUNKEL ET AL., 1985 |
| 18 | SA9 | G | + | (+) | 100.0000 | TOKIWA ET AL., 1981 |
| 19 | SA9 | G | (+) | 0 | 50.0000 | MCCOY ET AL., 1981 |
| 20 | SA9 | G | + | 0 | 13.0000 | VANCE & LEVIN, 1984 |
| 21 | SA9 | G | + | + | 25.0000 | EL-BAYOUMI ET AL., 1981 |
| 22 | SA9 | G | (+) | + | 50.0000 | MORTELMANS ET AL., 1986 |
| 23 | SA9 | G | (+) | + | 0.0000 | MATSUDA, 1981 |
| 24 | SA9 | G | + | 0 | 0.0000 | SCRIBNER ET AL., 1979 |
| 25 | SAS | G | - | 0 | 0.0000 | ROSENKRANZ ET AL., 1985 |
| 26 | ECW | G | - | - | 167.0000 | DUNKEL ET AL., 1985 |
| 27 | DMX | G | - | 0 | 400.0000 | VALENCIA ET AL., 1985 |
| 28 | SIC | S | - | 0 | 0.0000 | SHELBY & STASIEWICZ, 1984 |
| 29 | CIC | C | + | 0 | 0.0000 | SHELBY & STASIEWICZ, 1984 |

# APPENDIX 1

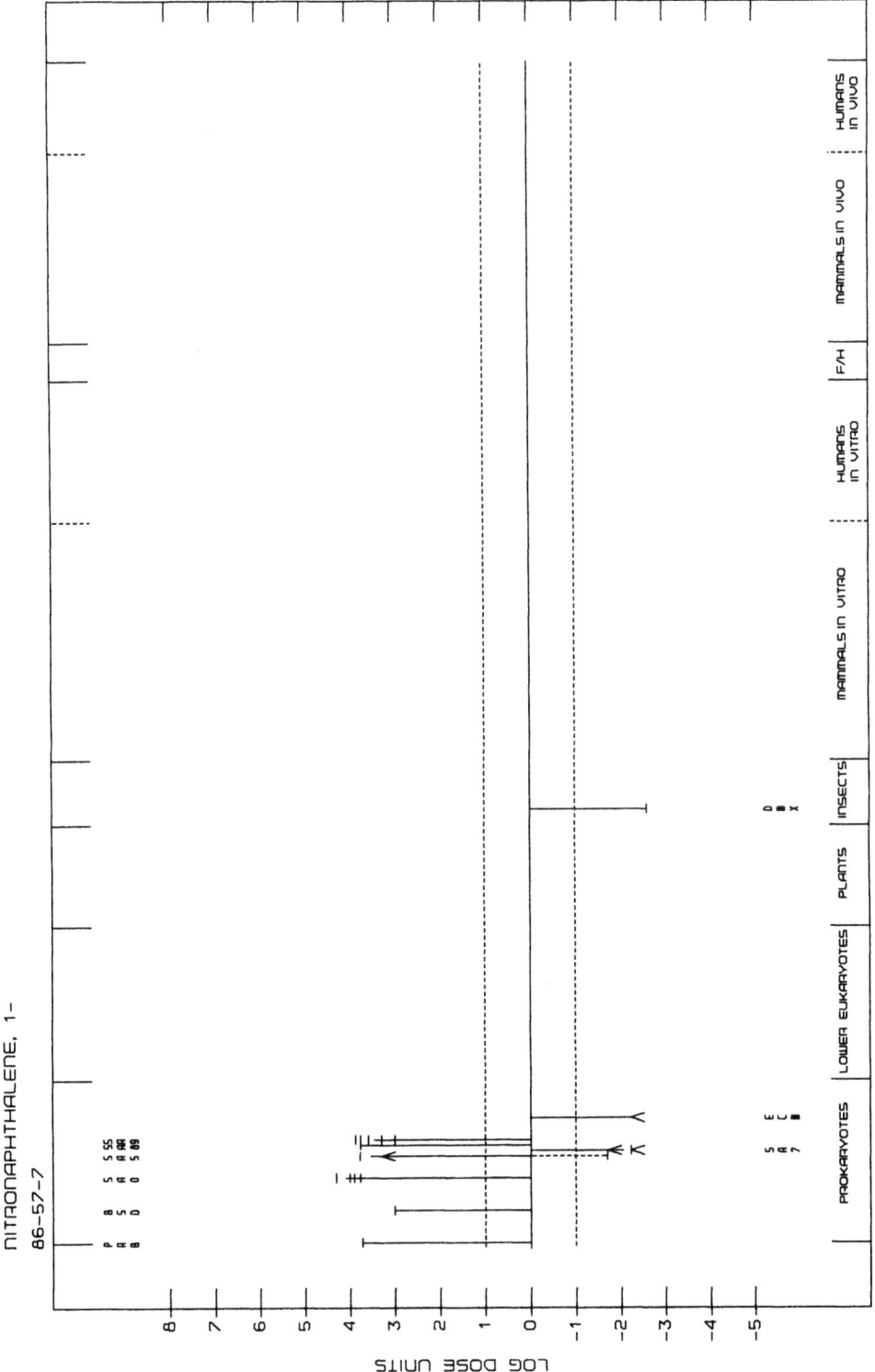

NITRONAPHTHALENE, 2-
581-89-5

| TEST CODE | END POINT | RESULTS NO ACT | RESULTS ACT | DOSE (LED OR HID) | SHORT CITATION |
|---|---|---|---|---|---|
| 1 PRB | D | + | 0 | 6.0000 | NAKAMURA ET AL., 1987 |
| 2 ECL | D | + | 0 | 5.0000 | ROSENKRANZ & POIRIER, 1979 |
| 3 ECL | D | + | + | 0.0000 | DE FLORA ET AL., 1984 |
| 4 BSD | D | + | 0 | 100.0000 | TOKIWA ET AL., 1987 |
| 5 SA0 | G | + | + | 3.1200 | DE FLORA, 1979 |
| 6 SA0 | G | + | 0 | 2.5000 | SCRIBNER ET AL., 1979 |
| 7 SA0 | G | + | 0 | 150.0000 | SIMMON, 1979a |
| 8 SA0 | G | + | + | 12.5000 | EL-BAYOUMI ET AL., 1981 |
| 9 SA0 | G | + | 0 | 5.0000 | MCCOY ET AL., 1981 |
| 10 SA0 | G | + | 0 | 50.0000 | MCCANN ET AL., 1975 |
| 11 SA0 | G | + | + | 0.0000 | DE FLORA ET AL., 1984 |
| 12 SA0 | G | + | 0 | 10.0000 | MOROTOMI & WATANABE, 1984 |
| 13 SA0 | G | + | + | 0.0000 | DE FLORA, 1981 |
| 14 SA5 | G | + | + | 25.0000 | ROSENKRANZ & POIRIER, 1979 |
| 15 SA5 | G | + | 0 | 2.5000 | SCRIBNER ET AL., 1979 |
| 16 SA5 | G | + | 0 | 150.0000 | SIMMON, 1979a |
| 17 SA5 | G | + | 0 | 5.0000 | MCCOY ET AL., 1981 |
| 18 SA5 | G | + | 0 | 50.0000 | MCCANN ET AL., 1975 |
| 19 SA5 | G | + | - | 0.0000 | DE FLORA ET AL., 1984 |
| 20 SA5 | G | + | + | 0.0000 | DE FLORA, 1981 |
| 21 SA7 | G | + | 0 | 150.0000 | SIMMON, 1979a |
| 22 SA7 | G | + | 0 | 50.0000 | MCCOY ET AL., 1981 |
| 23 SA7 | G | + | + | 0.0000 | DE FLORA ET AL., 1984 |
| 24 SA8 | G | + | 0 | 12.5000 | SCRIBNER ET AL., 1979 |
| 25 SA8 | G | + | 0 | 150.0000 | SIMMON, 1979a |
| 26 SA8 | G | + | + | 0.0000 | DE FLORA ET AL., 1984 |
| 27 SA9 | G | + | 0 | 25.0000 | WANG ET AL., 1978 |
| 28 SA9 | G | + | 0 | 12.5000 | SCRIBNER ET AL., 1979 |
| 29 SA9 | G | + | 0 | 150.0000 | SIMMON, 1979a |
| 30 SA9 | G | 0 | + | 25.0000 | HO ET AL., 1981 |
| 31 SA9 | G | + | 0 | 50.0000 | LOFROTH, 1981 |
| 32 SA9 | G | + | 0 | 16.7000 | MCCOY ET AL., 1981 |
| 33 SA9 | G | + | + | 0.0000 | DE FLORA ET AL., 1984 |
| 34 SA9 | G | + | 0 | 87.0000 | WANG ET AL., 1980 |
| 35 SAS | G | - | 0 | 0.0000 | ROSENKRANZ ET AL., 1985 |
| 36 SCH | R | + | + | 10000.0000 | SIMMON, 1979b |
| 37 URP | D | - | 0 | 15.0000 | MORI ET AL., 1987 |
| 38 UIA | D | - | 0 | 15.0000 | MORI ET AL., 1987 |
| 39 TCS | T | + | 0 | 1.0000 | PIENTA, 1980 |
| 40 HMM | H | + | 0 | 125.0000 | SIMMON ET AL., 1979 |

# APPENDIX 1

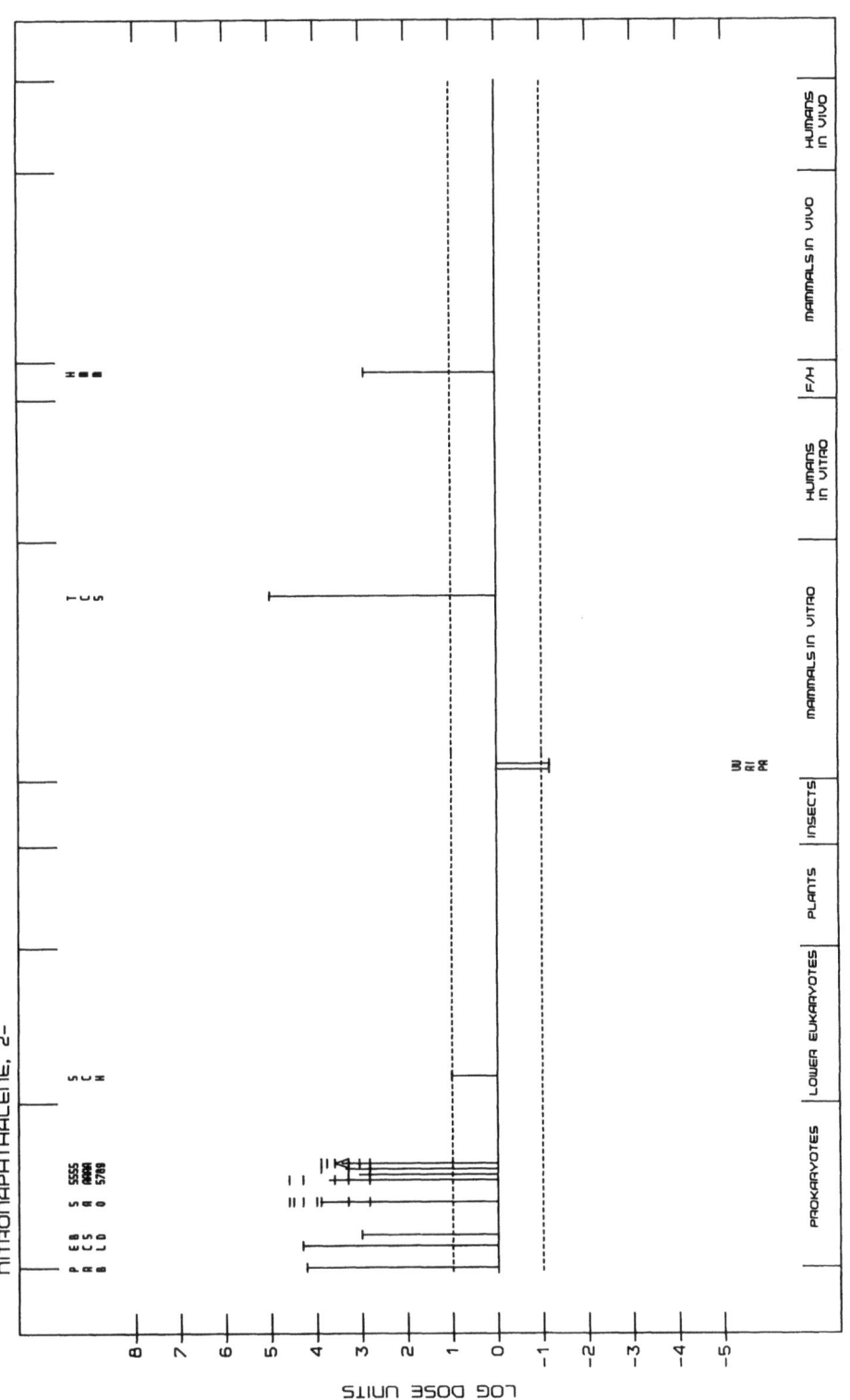

NITROPERYLENE, 3-
20589-63-3

| TEST CODE | END POINT | RESULTS NO ACT | ACT | DOSE (LED OR HID) | SHORT CITATION |
|---|---|---|---|---|---|
| 1 SA0 | G | − | + | 0.0000 | GREIBROKK ET AL., 1984 |
| 2 SA0 | G | − | + | 0.1000 | LOFROTH ET AL., 1984 |
| 3 SA9 | G | 0 | + | 0.1000 | HO ET AL., 1981 |
| 4 SA9 | G | − | + | 0.0000 | GREIBROKK ET AL., 1984 |
| 5 SA9 | G | − | + | 0.0750 | ANDERSON ET AL., 1987 |
| 6 SA9 | G | − | + | 0.0000 | PITTS, 1983 |
| 7 SA9 | G | (+) | + | 0.0500 | LOFROTH ET AL., 1984 |

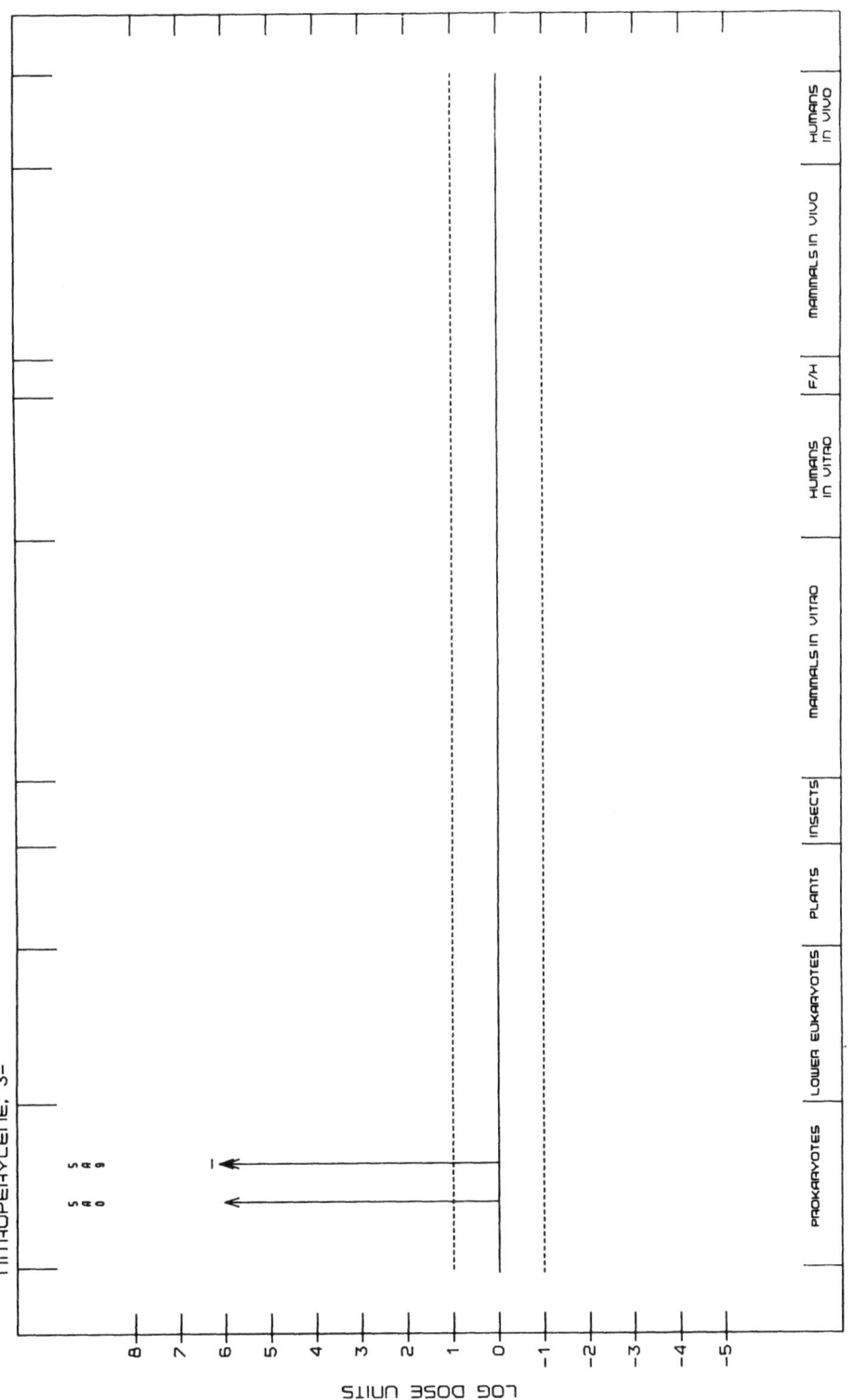

NITROPYRENE, 1-
5522-43-0

| | TEST CODE | END POINT | RESULTS NO ACT | ACT | DOSE (LED OR HID) | SHORT CITATION |
|---|---|---|---|---|---|---|
| 1 | PRB | D | + | 0 | 0.5000 | OHTA ET AL., 1984 |
| 2 | PRB | D | + | 0 | 0.0200 | NAKAMURA ET AL., 1987 |
| 3 | BSD | D | + | 0 | 0.2000 | HORIKAWA ET AL., 1986 |
| 4 | SA0 | G | + | 0 | 0.1300 | TOKIWA ET AL., 1984 |
| 5 | SA0 | G | + | 0 | 0.0000 | ROSENKRANZ ET AL., 1980 |
| 6 | SA0 | G | + | 0 | 0.1700 | MERMELSTEIN ET AL., 1981 |
| 7 | SA0 | G | + | 0 | 0.0000 | MCCOY ET AL., 1985b |
| 8 | SA0 | G | + | 0 | 0.0000 | MCCOY ET AL., 1983a |
| 9 | SA0 | G | + | 0 | 0.0000 | ROSENKRANZ ET AL., 1985 |
| 10 | SA0 | G | + | + | 0.0300 | TOKIWA ET AL., 1981 |
| 11 | SA2 | G | + | 0 | 0.0000 | MCCOY ET AL., 1985b |
| 12 | SA4 | G | + | 0 | 0.0000 | MCCOY ET AL., 1985b |
| 13 | SA7 | G | + | 0 | 0.5000 | TOKIWA ET AL., 1984 |
| 14 | SA7 | G | + | 0 | 0.0000 | ROSENKRANZ ET AL., 1980 |
| 15 | SA7 | G | + | 0 | 0.0150 | MERMELSTEIN ET AL., 1981 |
| 16 | SA8 | G | + | 0 | 0.0620 | TOKIWA ET AL., 1984 |
| 17 | SA8 | G | + | 0 | 0.0000 | ROSENKRANZ ET AL., 1980 |
| 18 | SA8 | G | + | 0 | 0.0150 | MERMELSTEIN ET AL., 1981 |
| 19 | SA8 | G | + | - | 0.0600 | TOKIWA ET AL., 1981a |
| 20 | SA8 | G | + | 0 | 6.0000 | HEFLICH ET AL., 1985a |
| 21 | SA9 | G | + | 0 | 0.0620 | TOKIWA ET AL., 1984 |
| 22 | SA9 | G | + | 0 | 0.0000 | ROSENKRANZ ET AL., 1980 |
| 23 | SA9 | G | + | 0 | 0.0050 | MERMELSTEIN ET AL., 1981 |
| 24 | SA9 | G | + | 0 | 0.0000 | MCCOY ET AL., 1985b |
| 25 | SA9 | G | + | + | 0.0500 | TOKIWA ET AL., 1981a |
| 26 | SA9 | G | + | 0 | 0.0000 | LOFROTH, 1981 |
| 27 | SA9 | G | + | 0 | 0.0000 | HEFLICH ET AL., 1985 |
| 28 | SA9 | G | + | 0 | 0.0000 | TOKIWA ET AL., 1985 |
| 29 | SA9 | G | + | 0 | 0.0000 | MCCOY ET AL., 1983a |
| 30 | SA9 | G | + | + | 0.0300 | BALL, LM ET AL., 1984b |
| 31 | SA9 | G | + | 0 | 0.0000 | ROSENKRANZ ET AL., 1985 |
| 32 | SA9 | G | + | 0 | 0.0500 | PEDERSON & SIAK, 1981 |
| 33 | SA9 | G | + | + | 0.0000 | PITTS ET AL., 1982 |
| 34 | SA9 | G | + | 0 | 0.0600 | WANG ET AL., 1980 |
| 35 | SA9 | G | + | + | 0.0700 | TOKIWA ET AL., 1981 |
| 36 | SAS | G | + | 0 | 0.0000 | HEFLICH ET AL., 1985 |
| 37 | SAS | G | + | + | 0.1500 | BALL, LM ET AL., 1984b |
| 38 | SAS | G | + | 0 | 0.0000 | ROSENKRANZ ET AL., 1985 |
| 39 | ECW | G | (+) | 0 | 0.3000 | MCCOY ET AL., 1985a |
| 40 | ECW | G | (+) | 0 | 0.5000 | TOKIWA ET AL., 1984 |
| 41 | SCG | R | - | 0 | 500.0000 | MCCOY ET AL., 1983 |
| 42 | SCH | R | - | 0 | 500.0000 | MCCOY ET AL., 1984 |
| 43 | DIA | D | + | 0 | 2.5000 | MOLLER & THORGEIRSSON, 1985 |
| 44 | DIA | D | + | - | 10.0000 | EDWARDS ET AL., 1986b |
| 45 | DIA | D | + | 0 | 3.7000 | SAITO ET AL., 1984b |
| 46 | URP | D | + | 0 | 0.2500 | KORNBRUST & BARFKNECHT, 1984 |
| 47 | URP | D | + | 0 | 35.0000 | MORI ET AL., 1987 |
| 48 | UIA | D | + | 0 | 3.5000 | MORI ET AL., 1987 |
| 49 | UIA | D | + | 0 | 2.5000 | KORNBRUST & BARFKNECHT, 1984 |
| 50 | UIA | D | + | 0 | 2.5000 | DOOLITTLE & BUTTERWORTH, 1984 |

# APPENDIX 1

NITROPYRENE, 1-
5522-43-0

| TEST CODE | END POINT | RESULTS NO ACT | ACT | DOSE (LED OR HID) | SHORT CITATION |
|---|---|---|---|---|---|
| 51 UIA | D | + | 0 | 1.2500 | HAUGEN ET AL., 1986 |
| 52 GCL | G | - | - | 20.0000 | NAKAYASU ET AL., 1982 |
| 53 GCO | G | (+) | (+) | 0.0000 | MARSHALL ET AL., 1982 |
| 54 GCO | G | - | 0 | 15.0000 | HEFLICH ET AL., 1986a |
| 55 GCO | G | - | 0 | 5.0000 | HEFLICH ET AL., 1986b |
| 56 GCO | G | (+) | + | 20.0000 | LI & DUTCHER, 1983 |
| 57 GCO | G | - | 0 | 15.0000 | HEFLICH ET AL., 1985 |
| 58 G9H | G | - | + | 0.5000 | BALL, JC ET AL., 1984 |
| 59 G9H | G | - | + | 12.4000 | BERRY ET AL., 1985 |
| 60 G9O | G | - | 0 | 10.0000 | TAKAYAMA ET AL., 1983 |
| 61 G5T | G | - | + | 0.0000 | LEWTAS, 1982 |
| 62 SIC | S | (+) | + | 0.7000 | NACHTMAN & WOLFF, 1982 |
| 63 SIC | S | (+) | - | 0.0000 | LEWTAS, 1982 |
| 64 CIT | C | + | 0 | 15.0000 | LAFI & PARRY, 1987 |
| 65 TCS | T | + | 0 | 1.0000 | DIPAOLO ET AL., 1983 |
| 66 UHT | D | + | 0 | 0.0000 | EDDY ET AL., 1986 |
| 67 UHT | D | + | 0 | 0.5000 | EDDY ET AL., 1987 |
| 68 UIH | D | + | 0 | 24.7000 | SUGIMURA & TAKAYAMA, 1983 |
| 69 GIH | G | + | 0 | 12.4000 | PATTON ET AL., 1986 |
| 70 TIH | T | + | 0 | 0.7000 | HOWARD ET AL., 1983b |
| 71 TIH | T | + | 0 | 0.0000 | KUMARI ET AL., 1984 |
| 72 BFA | F | - | + | 10.0000 | BALL, LM ET AL., 1984a |
| 73 BFA | F | + | + | 4.0000 | MOROTOMI ET AL., 1985 |
| 74 DVA | D | + | 0 | 50.0000 | MITCHELL, 1984 |
| 75 RVA | D | + | 0 | 50.0000 | MITCHELL, 1984 |
| 76 SVA | S | + | 0 | 500.0000 | MARSHALL ET AL., 1982 |
| 77 GHT | G | + | 0 | 0.0000 | EDDY ET AL., 1986 |
| 78 GHT | G | + | 0 | 1.0000 | EDDY ET AL., 1987 |
| 79 BID | * | + | 0 | 4.9000 | HOWARD & BELAND, 1982 |
| 80 BVD | * | + | 0 | 10.0000 | HOWARD ET AL., 1986 |
| 81 BID | * | + | 0 | 15.0000 | HEFLICH ET AL., 1985 |
| 82 BVD | * | + | 0 | 25.0000 | HASHIMOTO & SHUDO, 1985 |
| 83 BVD | * | + | 0 | 25.0000 | STANTON ET AL., 1985 |
| 84 BVD | * | + | 0 | 1.0000 | MITCHELL, 1988 |
| 85 BVD | * | - | 0 | 30.0000 | DJURIC ET AL., 1988 |
| 86 BID | * | 0 | (+) | 5.0000 | DJURIC ET AL., 1988 |
| 87 BID | * | + | 0 | 2.0000 | JACKSON ET AL., 1985 |
| 88 BID | * | + | 0 | 12.0000 | PATTON ET AL., 1986 |
| 89 BID | * | + | 0 | 2.0000 | BELAND ET AL., 1986 |
| 90 BID | * | + | 0 | 2.5000 | GALLAGHER ET AL., 1988 |
| 91 BID | * | (+) | 0 | 14.8000 | HEFLICH ET AL., 1986a |
| 92 BID | * | + | 0 | 0.5000 | HOWARD ET AL., 1983a |

# 416 IARC MONOGRAPHS VOLUME 46

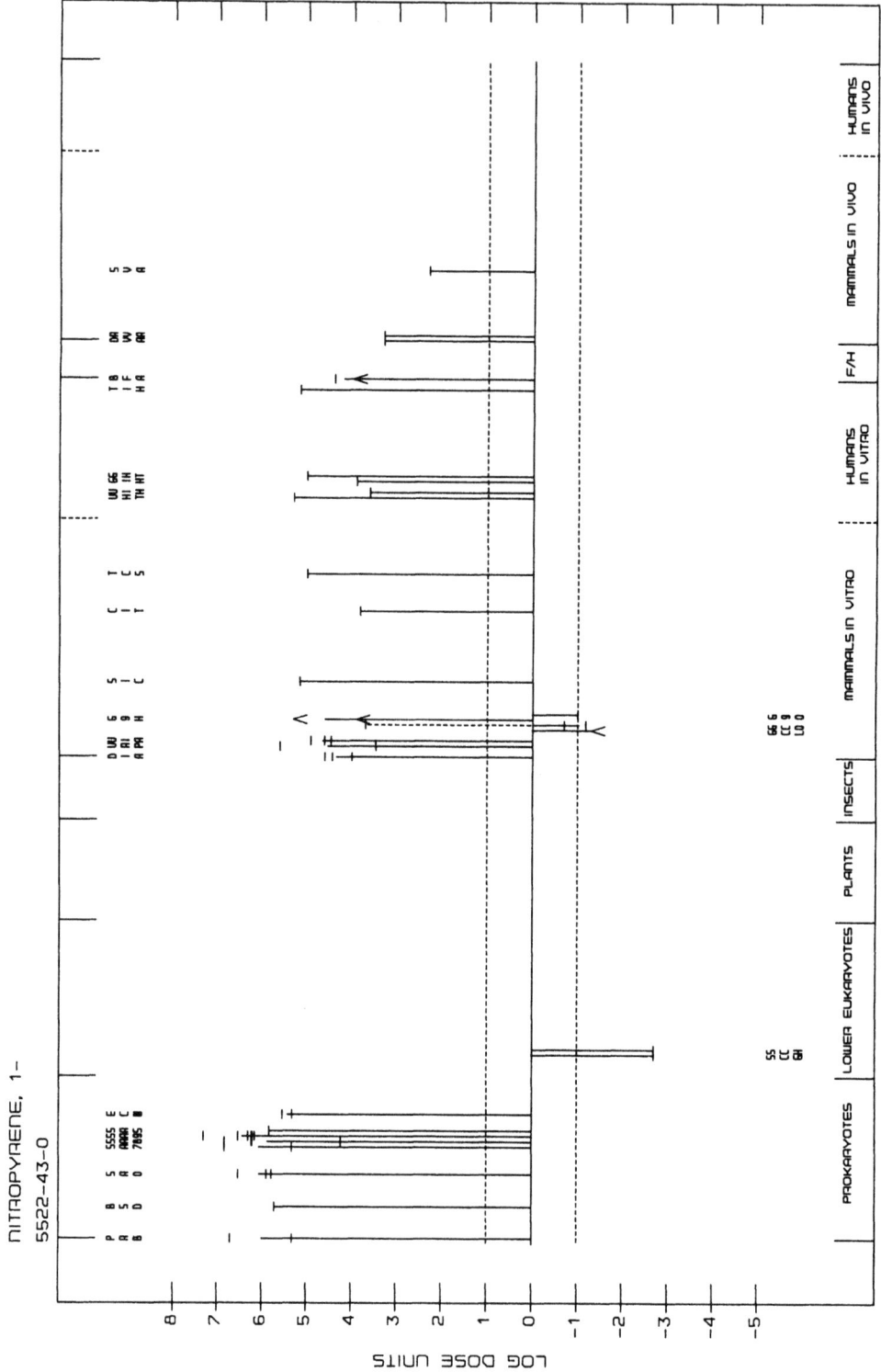

NITROPYRENE, 2-
789-07-1

| TEST CODE | END POINT | RESULTS NO ACT | ACT | DOSE (LED OR HID) | SHORT CITATION |
|---|---|---|---|---|---|
| 1 SA0 | G | + | 0 | 0.0000 | GREIBROKK ET AL., 1984 |
| 2 SA9 | G | + | 0 | 0.0000 | GREIBROKK ET AL., 1984 |

NITROPYRENE, 4-
57835-92-4

| TEST CODE | END POINT | RESULTS NO ACT | ACT | DOSE (LED OR HID) | SHORT CITATION |
|---|---|---|---|---|---|
| 1 BSD | D | + | 0 | 0.2000 | TOKIWA ET AL., 1987 |
| 2 BSD | D | + | 0 | 0.0100 | HORIKAWA ET AL., 1986 |
| 3 SA0 | G | + | 0 | 0.0000 | FU ET AL., 1985 |
| 4 SA9 | G | + | 0 | 0.0000 | FU ET AL., 1985 |

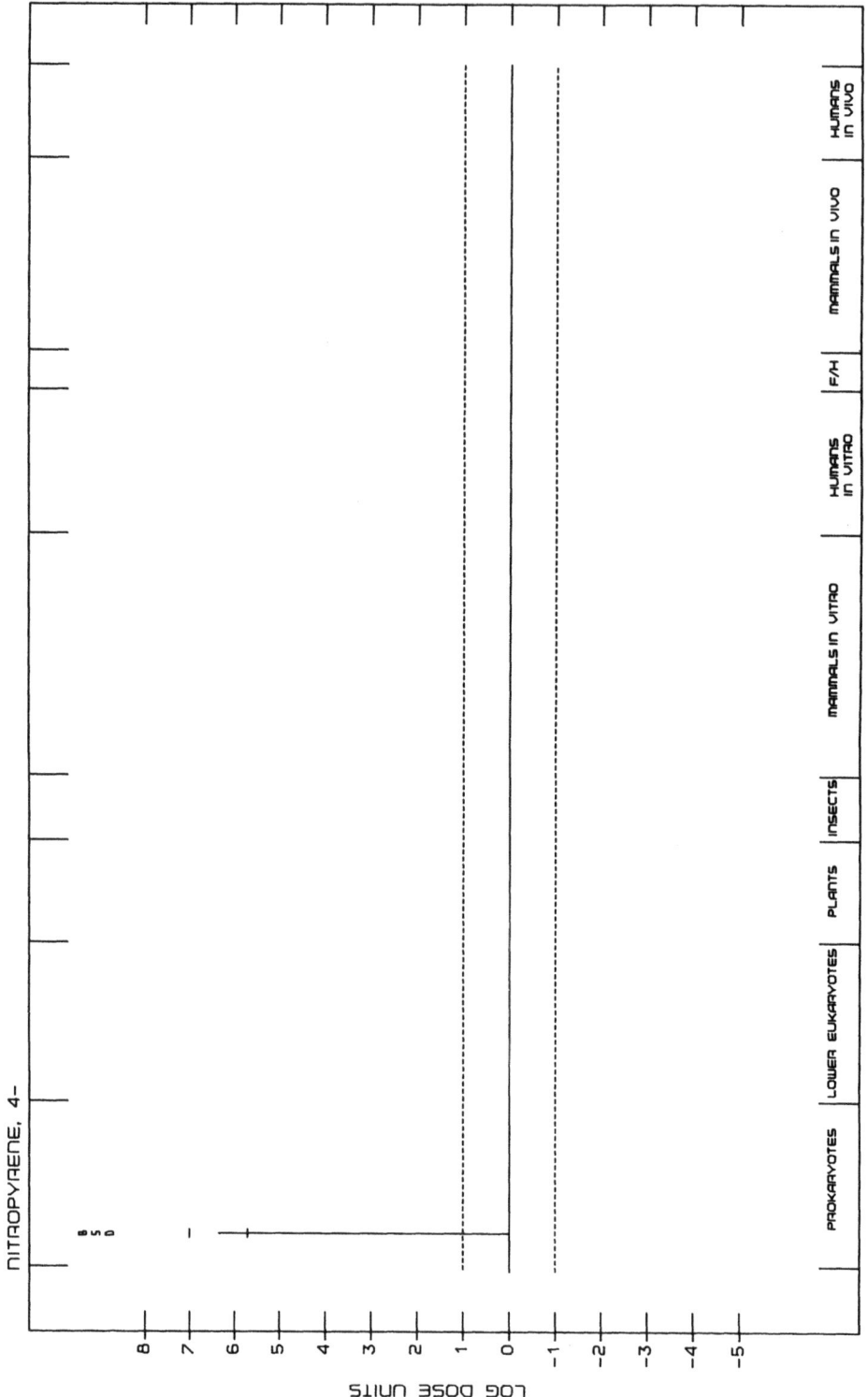

## SUPPLEMENTARY CORRIGENDA TO VOLUMES 1–45

Corrigenda to Volumes 1–43 are listed in Volume 42 pp. 251–264, in Volume 43 p. 261 and in Volume 45 p. 283.

**Volume 44**

p. 95        para 4 line 3        *replace* (0.5–425 g/l) *by* (0.5–4 µg/l)

# CUMULATIVE CROSS INDEX TO *IARC MONOGRAPHS ON THE EVALUATION OF CARCINOGENIC RISKS TO HUMANS*

The volume, page and year are given. References to corrigenda are given in parentheses.

A

| | |
|---|---|
| A-α-C | *40*, 245 (1986) |
| | *Suppl. 7*, 56 (1987) |
| Acetaldehyde | *36*, 101 (1985) (*corr. 42*, 263) |
| | *Suppl. 7*, 77 (1987) |
| Acetaldehyde formylmethylhydrazone (*see* Gyromitrin) | |
| Acetamide | *7*, 197 (1974) |
| | *Suppl. 7*, 389 (1987) |
| Acridine orange | *16*, 145 (1978) |
| | *Suppl. 7*, 56 (1987) |
| Acriflavinium chloride | *13*, 31 (1977) |
| | *Suppl. 7*, 56 (1987) |
| Acrolein | *19*, 479 (1979) |
| | *36*, 133 (1985) |
| | *Suppl. 7*, 78 (1987) |
| Acrylamide | *39*, 41 (1986) |
| | *Suppl. 7*, 56 (1987) |
| Acrylic acid | *19*, 47 (1979) |
| | *Suppl. 7*, 56 (1987) |
| Acrylic fibres | *19*, 86 (1979) |
| | *Suppl. 7*, 56 (1987) |
| Acrylonitrile | *19*, 73 (1979) |
| | *Suppl. 7*, 79 (1987) |
| Acrylonitrile-butadiene-styrene copolymers | *19*, 91 (1979) |
| | *Suppl. 7*, 56 (1987) |
| Actinolite (*see* Asbestos) | |
| Actinomycins | *10*, 29 (1976) (*corr. 42*, 255) |
| | *Suppl. 7*, 80 (1987) |
| Adriamycin | *10*, 43 (1976) |
| | *Suppl. 7*, 82 (1987) |

| | |
|---|---|
| AF-2 | *31*, 47 (1983) |
| | *Suppl. 7*, 56 (1987) |
| Aflatoxins | *1*, 145 (1972) (*corr. 42*, 251) |
| | *10*, 51 (1976) |
| | *Suppl. 7*, 83 (1987) |
| Aflatoxin $B_1$ (*see* Aflatoxins) | |
| Aflatoxin $B_2$ (*see* Aflatoxins) | |
| Aflatoxin $G_1$ (*see* Aflatoxins) | |
| Aflatoxin $G_2$ (*see* Aflatoxins) | |
| Aflatoxin $M_1$ (*see* Aflatoxins) | |
| Agaritine | *31*, 63 (1983) |
| | *Suppl. 7*, 56 (1987) |
| Alcohol drinking | *44* |
| Aldrin | *5*, 25 (1974) |
| | *Suppl. 7*, 88 (1987) |
| Allyl chloride | *36*, 39 (1985) |
| | *Suppl. 7*, 56 (1987) |
| Allyl isothiocyanate | *36*, 55 (1985) |
| | *Suppl. 7*, 56 (1987) |
| Allyl isovalerate | *36*, 69 (1985) |
| | *Suppl. 7*, 56 (1987) |
| Aluminium production | *34*, 37 (1984) |
| | *Suppl. 7*, 89 (1987) |
| Amaranth | *8*, 41 (1975) |
| | *Suppl. 7*, 56 (1987) |
| 5-Aminoacenaphthene | *16*, 243 (1978) |
| | *Suppl. 7*, 56 (1987) |
| 2-Aminoanthraquinone | *27*, 191 (1982) |
| | *Suppl. 7*, 56 (1987) |
| *para*-Aminoazobenzene | *8*, 53 (1975) |
| | *Suppl. 7*, 390 (1987) |
| *ortho*-Aminoazotoluene | *8*, 61 (1975) (*corr. 42*, 254) |
| | *Suppl. 7*, 56 (1987) |
| *para*-Aminobenzoic acid | *16*, 249 (1978) |
| | *Suppl. 7*, 56 (1987) |
| 4-Aminobiphenyl | *1*, 74 (1972) (*corr. 42*, 251) |
| | *Suppl. 7*, 91 (1987) |
| 2-Amino-3,4-dimethylimidazo[4,5-*f*]quinoline (*see* MeIQ) | |
| 2-Amino-3,8-dimethylimidazo[4,5-*f*]quinoxaline (*see* MeIQx) | |
| 3-Amino-1,4-dimethyl-5*H*-pyrido[4,3-*b*]indole (*see* Trp-P-1) | |
| 2-Aminodipyrido[1,2-*a*:3′,2′-*d*]imidazole (*see* Glu-P-2) | |
| 1-Amino-2-methylanthraquinone | *27*, 199 (1982) |
| | *Suppl. 7*, 57 (1987) |
| 2-Amino-3-methylimidazo[4,5-*f*]quinoline (*see* IQ) | |
| 2-Amino-6-methyldipyrido[1,2-*a*:3′,2′-*d*]-imidazole (*see* Glu-P-1) | |
| 2-Amino-3-methyl-9*H*-pyrido[2,3-*b*]indole (*see* MeA-α-C) | |
| 3-Amino-1-methyl-5*H*-pyrido[4,3-*b*]indole (*see* Trp-P-2) | |

| | |
|---|---|
| 2-Amino-5-(5-nitro-2-furyl)-1,3,4-thiadiazole | 7, 143 (1974) |
| | *Suppl. 7*, 57 (1987) |
| 4-Amino-2-nitrophenol | *16*, 43 (1978) |
| | *Suppl. 7*, 57 (1987) |
| 2-Amino-5-nitrothiazole | *31*, 71 (1983) |
| | *Suppl. 7*, 57 (1987) |
| 2-Amino-9H-pyrido[2,3-b]indole (see A-α-C) | |
| 11-Aminoundecanoic acid | *39*, 239 (1986) |
| | *Suppl. 7*, 57 (1987) |
| Amitrole | 7, 31 (1974) |
| | *41*, 293 (1986) |
| | *Suppl. 7*, 92 (1987) |
| Ammonium potassium selenide (see Selenium and selenium compounds) | |
| Amorphous silica (see also Silica) | *Suppl. 7*, 341 (1987) |
| Amosite (see Asbestos) | |
| Anabolic steroids (see Androgenic (anabolic) steroids) | |
| Anaesthetics, volatile | *11*, 285 (1976) |
| | *Suppl. 7*, 93 (1987) |
| Analgesic mixtures containing phenacetin (see also Phenacetin) | *Suppl. 7*, 310 (1987) |
| Androgenic (anabolic) steroids | *Suppl. 7*, 96 (1987) |
| Angelicin and some synthetic derivatives (see also Angelicins) | *40*, 291 (1986) |
| Angelicin plus ultraviolet radiation (see also Angelicin and some synthetic derivatives) | *Suppl. 7*, 57 (1987) |
| Angelicins | *Suppl. 7*, 57 (1987) |
| Aniline | *4*, 27 (1974) (*corr. 42*, 252) |
| | *27*, 39 (1982) |
| | *Suppl. 7*, 99 (1987) |
| *ortho*-Anisidine | *27*, 63 (1982) |
| | *Suppl. 7*, 57 (1987) |
| *para*-Anisidine | *27*, 65 (1982) |
| | *Suppl. 7*, 57 (1987) |
| Anthanthrene | *32*, 95 (1983) |
| | *Suppl. 7*, 57 (1987) |
| Anthophyllite (see Asbestos) | |
| Anthracene | *32*, 105 (1983) |
| | *Suppl. 7*, 57 (1987) |
| Anthranilic acid | *16*, 265 (1978) |
| | *Suppl. 7*, 57 (1987) |
| ANTU (see 1-Naphthylthiourea) | |
| Apholate | *9*, 31 (1975) |
| | *Suppl. 7*, 57 (1987) |
| Aramite® | *5*, 39 (1974) |
| | *Suppl. 7*, 57 (1987) |
| Areca nut (see Betel quid) | |
| Arsanilic acid (see Arsenic and arsenic compounds) | |

Arsenic and arsenic compounds                                   *1*, 41 (1972)
                                                                *2*, 48 (1973)
                                                                *23*, 39 (1980)
                                                                *Suppl. 7*, 100 (1987)
Arsenic pentoxide (*see* Arsenic and arsenic compounds)
Arsenic sulphide (*see* Arsenic and arsenic compounds)
Arsenic trioxide (*see* Arsenic and arsenic compounds)
Arsine (*see* Arsenic and arsenic compounds)
Asbestos                                                        *2*, 17 (1973) (*corr. 42*, 252)
                                                                *14* (1977) (*corr. 42*, 256)
                                                                *Suppl. 7*, 106 (1987) (*corr. 45*, 283)
Attapulgite                                                     *42*, 159 (1987)
                                                                *Suppl. 7*, 117 (1987)
Auramine (technical-grade)                                      *1*, 69 (1972) (*corr. 42*, 251)
                                                                *Suppl. 7*, 118 (1987)
Auramine, manufacture of (*see also* Auramine, technical-grade) *Suppl. 7*, 118 (1987)
Aurothioglucose                                                 *13*, 39 (1977)
                                                                *Suppl. 7*, 57 (1987)
5-Azacytidine                                                   *26*, 37 (1981)
                                                                *Suppl. 7*, 57 (1987)
Azaserine                                                       *10*, 73 (1976) (*corr. 42*, 255)
                                                                *Suppl. 7*, 57 (1987)
Azathioprine                                                    *26*, 47 (1981)
                                                                *Suppl. 7*, 119 (1987)
Aziridine                                                       *9*, 37 (1975)
                                                                *Suppl. 7*, 58 (1987)
2-(1-Aziridinyl)ethanol                                         *9*, 47 (1975)
                                                                *Suppl. 7*, 58 (1987)
Aziridyl benzoquinone                                           *9*, 51 (1975)
                                                                *Suppl. 7*, 58 (1987)
Azobenzene                                                      *8*, 75 (1975)
                                                                *Suppl. 7*, 58 (1987)

# B

Barium chromate (*see* Chromium and chromium compounds)
Basic chromic sulphate (*see* Chromium and chromium compounds)
BCNU (*see* Bischloroethyl nitrosourea)
Benz[*a*]acridine                                               *32*, 123 (1983)
                                                                *Suppl. 7*, 58 (1987)
Benz[*c*]acridine                                               *3*, 241 (1973)
                                                                *32*, 129 (1983)
                                                                *Suppl. 7*, 58 (1987)
Benzal chloride (*see also* α-Chlorinated toluenes)             *29*, 65 (1982)
                                                                *Suppl. 7*, 148 (1987)
Benz[*a*]anthracene                                             *3*, 45 (1973)
                                                                *32*, 135 (1983)
                                                                *Suppl. 7*, 58 (1987)

| | |
|---|---|
| Benzene | 7, 203 (1974) (*corr.* 42, 254) |
| | 29, 93, 391 (1982) |
| | *Suppl. 7*, 120 (1987) |
| Benzidine | *1*, 80 (1972) |
| | 29, 149, 391 (1982) |
| | *Suppl. 7*, 123 (1987) |
| Benzidine-based dyes | *Suppl. 7*, 125 (1987) |
| Benzo[*b*]fluoranthene | *3*, 69 (1973) |
| | *32*, 147 (1983) |
| | *Suppl. 7*, 58 (1987) |
| Benzo[*j*]fluoranthene | *3*, 82 (1973) |
| | *32*, 155 (1983) |
| | *Suppl. 7*, 58 (1987) |
| Benzo[*k*]fluoranthene | *32*, 163 (1983) |
| | *Suppl. 7*, 58 (1987) |
| Benzo[*ghi*]fluoranthene | *32*, 171 (1983) |
| | *Suppl. 7*, 58 (1987) |
| Benzo[*a*]fluorene | *32*, 177 (1983) |
| | *Suppl. 7*, 58 (1987) |
| Benzo[*b*]fluorene | *32*, 183 (1983) |
| | *Suppl. 7*, 58 (1987) |
| Benzo[*c*]fluorene | *32*, 189 (1983) |
| | *Suppl. 7*, 58 (1987) |
| Benzo[*ghi*]perylene | *32*, 195 (1983) |
| | *Suppl. 7*, 58 (1987) |
| Benzo[*c*]phenanthrene | *32*, 205 (1983) |
| | *Suppl. 7*, 58 (1987) |
| Benzo[*a*]pyrene | *3*, 91 (1973) |
| | *32*, 211 (1983) |
| | *Suppl. 7*, 58 (1987) |
| Benzo[*e*]pyrene | *3*, 137 (1973) |
| | *32*, 225 (1983) |
| | *Suppl. 7*, 58 (1987) |
| *para*-Benzoquinone dioxime | 29, 185 (1982) |
| | *Suppl. 7*, 58 (1987) |
| Benzotrichloride (*see also* α-Chlorinated toluenes) | 29, 73 (1982) |
| | *Suppl. 7*, 148 (1987) |
| Benzoyl chloride | 29, 83 (1982) (*corr.* 42, 261) |
| | *Suppl. 7*, 126 (1987) |
| Benzoyl peroxide | *36*, 267 (1985) |
| | *Suppl. 7*, 58 (1987) |
| Benzyl acetate | *40*, 109 (1986) |
| | *Suppl. 7*, 58 (1987) |
| Benzyl chloride (*see also* α-Chlorinated toluenes) | *11*, 217 (1976) (*corr.* 42, 256) |
| | 29, 49 (1982) |
| | *Suppl. 7*, 148 (1987) |
| Benzyl violet 4B | *16*, 153 (1978) |
| | *Suppl. 7*, 58 (1987) |
| Bertrandite (*see* Beryllium and beryllium compounds) | |

Beryllium and beryllium compounds                                  *1*, 17 (1972)
                                                                   *23*, 143 (1980) (*corr. 42*, 260)
                                                                   *Suppl. 7*, 127 (1987)

Beryllium acetate (*see* Beryllium and beryllium compounds)
Beryllium acetate, basic (*see* Beryllium and beryllium compounds)
Beryllium-aluminium alloy (*see* Beryllium and beryllium
  compounds)
Beryllium carbonate (*see* Beryllium and beryllium compounds)
Beryllium chloride (*see* Beryllium and beryllium compounds)
Beryllium-copper alloy (*see* Beryllium and beryllium compounds)
Beryllium-copper-cobalt alloy (*see* Beryllium and beryllium
  compounds)
Beryllium fluoride (*see* Beryllium and beryllium compounds)
Beryllium hydroxide (*see* Beryllium and beryllium compounds)
Beryllium-nickel alloy (*see* Beryllium and beryllium compounds)
Beryllium oxide (*see* Beryllium and beryllium compounds)
Beryllium phosphate (*see* Beryllium and beryllium compounds)
Beryllium silicate (*see* Beryllium and beryllium compounds)
Beryllium sulphate (*see* Beryllium and beryllium compounds)
Beryl ore (*see* Beryllium and beryllium compounds)
Betel quid                                                          *37*, 141 (1985)
                                                                    *Suppl. 7*, 128 (1987)

Betel-quid chewing (*see* Betel quid)
BHA (*see* Butylated hydroxyanisole)
BHT (*see* Butylated hydroxytoluene)
Bis(1-aziridinyl)morpholinophosphine sulphide                       *9*, 55 (1975)
                                                                    *Suppl. 7*, 58 (1987)
Bis(2-chloroethyl)ether                                             *9*, 117 (1975)
                                                                    *Suppl. 7*, 58 (1987)
*N,N*-Bis(2-chloroethyl)-2-naphthylamine                            *4*, 119 (1974) (*corr. 42*, 253)
                                                                    *Suppl. 7*, 130 (1987)
Bischloroethyl nitrosourea (*see also* Chloroethyl nitrosoureas)    *26*, 79 (1981)
                                                                    *Suppl. 7*, 150 (1987)
1,2-Bis(chloromethoxy)ethane                                        *15*, 31 (1977)
                                                                    *Suppl. 7*, 58 (1987)
1,4-Bis(chloromethoxymethyl)benzene                                 *15*, 37 (1977)
                                                                    *Suppl. 7*, 58 (1987)
Bis(chloromethyl)ether                                              *4*, 231 (1974) (*corr. 42*, 253)
                                                                    *Suppl. 7*, 131 (1987)
Bis(2-chloro-1-methylethyl)ether                                    *41*, 149 (1986)
                                                                    *Suppl. 7*, 59 (1987)
Bitumens                                                            *35*, 39 (1985)
                                                                    *Suppl. 7*, 133 (1987)
Bleomycins                                                          *26*, 97 (1981)
                                                                    *Suppl. 7*, 134 (1987)
Blue VRS                                                            *16*, 163 (1978)
                                                                    *Suppl. 7*, 59 (1987)

| | |
|---|---|
| Boot and shoe manufacture and repair | 25, 249 (1981) |
| | *Suppl. 7*, 232 (1987) |
| Bracken fern | 40, 47 (1986) |
| | *Suppl. 7*, 135 (1987) |
| Brilliant Blue FCF | 16, 171 (1978) (*corr. 42*, 257) |
| | *Suppl. 7*, 59 (1987) |
| 1,3-Butadiene | 39, 155 (1986) (*corr. 42*, 264) |
| | *Suppl. 7*, 136 (1987) |
| 1,4-Butanediol dimethanesulphonate | 4, 247 (1974) |
| | *Suppl. 7*, 137 (1987) |
| *n*-Butyl acrylate | 39, 67 (1986) |
| | *Suppl. 7*, 59 (1987) |
| Butylated hydroxyanisole | 40, 123 (1986) |
| | *Suppl. 7*, 59 (1987) |
| Butylated hydroxytoluene | 40, 161 (1986) |
| | *Suppl. 7*, 59 (1987) |
| Butyl benzyl phthalate | 29, 193 (1982) (*corr. 42*, 261) |
| | *Suppl. 7*, 59 (1987) |
| β-Butyrolactone | 11, 225 (1976) |
| | *Suppl. 7*, 59 (1987) |
| γ-Butyrolactone | 11, 231 (1976) |
| | *Suppl. 7*, 59 (1987) |

C

| | |
|---|---|
| Cabinet-making (*see* Furniture and cabinet-making) | |
| Cadmium acetate (*see* Cadmium and cadmium compounds) | |
| Cadmium and cadmium compounds | 2, 74 (1973) |
| | 11, 39 (1976) (*corr. 42*, 255) |
| | *Suppl. 7*, 139 (1987) |
| Cadmium chloride (*see* Cadmium and cadmium compounds) | |
| Cadmium oxide (*see* Cadmium and cadmium compounds) | |
| Cadmium sulphate (*see* Cadmium and cadmium compounds) | |
| Cadmium sulphide (*see* Cadmium and cadmium compounds) | |
| Calcium arsenate (*see* Arsenic and arsenic compounds) | |
| Calcium chromate (*see* Chromium and chromium compounds) | |
| Calcium cyclamate (*see* Cyclamates) | |
| Calcium saccharin (*see* Saccharin) | |
| Cantharidin | 10, 79 (1976) |
| | *Suppl. 7*, 59 (1987) |
| Caprolactam | 19, 115 (1979) (*corr. 42*, 258) |
| | 39, 247 (1986) (*corr. 42*, 264) |
| | *Suppl. 7*, 390 (1987) |
| Captan | 30, 295 (1983) |
| | *Suppl. 7*, 59 (1987) |
| Carbaryl | 12, 37 (1976) |
| | *Suppl. 7*, 59 (1987) |

| | |
|---|---|
| Carbazole | 32, 239 (1983) |
| | Suppl. 7, 59 (1987) |
| 3-Carbethoxypsoralen | 40, 317 (1986) |
| | Suppl. 7, 59 (1987) |
| Carbon blacks | 3, 22 (1973) |
| | 33, 35 (1984) |
| | Suppl. 7, 142 (1987) |
| Carbon tetrachloride | 1, 53 (1972) |
| | 20, 371 (1979) |
| | Suppl. 7, 143 (1987) |
| Carmoisine | 8, 83 (1975) |
| | Suppl. 7, 59 (1987) |
| Carpentry and joinery | 25, 139 (1981) |
| | Suppl. 7, 378 (1987) |
| Carrageenan | 10, 181 (1976) (corr. 42, 255) |
| | 31, 79 (1983) |
| | Suppl. 7, 59 (1987) |
| Catechol | 15, 155 (1977) |
| | Suppl. 7, 59 (1987) |
| CCNU (see 1-(2-Chloroethyl)-3-cyclohexyl-1-nitrosourea) | |
| Ceramic fibres (see Man-made mineral fibres) | |
| Chemotherapy, combined, including alkylating agents (see MOPP and other combined chemotherapy including alkylating agents) | |
| Chlorambucil | 9, 125 (1975) |
| | 26, 115 (1981) |
| | Suppl. 7, 144 (1987) |
| Chloramphenicol | 10, 85 (1976) |
| | Suppl. 7, 145 (1987) |
| Chlordane (see also Chlordane/Heptachlor) | 20, 45 (1979) (corr. 42, 258) |
| Chlordane/Heptachlor | Suppl. 7, 146 (1987) |
| Chlordecone | 20, 67 (1979) |
| | Suppl. 7, 59 (1987) |
| Chlordimeform | 30, 61 (1983) |
| | Suppl. 7, 59 (1987) |
| Chlorinated dibenzodioxins (other than TCDD) | 15, 41 (1977) |
| | Suppl. 7, 59 (1987) |
| α-Chlorinated toluenes | Suppl. 7, 148 (1987) |
| Chlormadinone acetate (see also Progestins; Combined oral contraceptives) | 6, 149 (1974) |
| | 21, 365 (1979) |
| Chlornaphazine (see N,N-Bis(2-chloroethyl)-2-naphthylamine) | |
| Chlorobenzilate | 5, 75 (1974) |
| | 30, 73 (1983) |
| | Suppl. 7, 60 (1987) |
| Chlorodifluoromethane | 41, 237 (1986) |
| | Suppl. 7, 149 (1987) |
| 1-(2-Chloroethyl)-3-cyclohexyl-1-nitrosourea (see also Chloroethyl nitrosoureas) | 26, 137 (1981) (corr. 42, 260) |
| | Suppl. 7, 150 (1987) |

| | |
|---|---|
| 1-(2-Chloroethyl)-3-(4-methylcyclohexyl)-1-nitrosourea (*see also* Chloroethyl nitrosoureas) | *Suppl. 7*, 150 (1987) |
| Chloroethyl nitrosoureas | *Suppl. 7*, 150 (1987) |
| Chlorofluoromethane | *41*, 229 (1986) |
| | *Suppl. 7*, 60 (1987) |
| Chloroform | *1*, 61 (1972) |
| | *20*, 401 (1979) |
| | *Suppl. 7*, 152 (1987) |
| Chloromethyl methyl ether (technical-grade) (*see also* Bis(chloromethyl) ether) | *4*, 239 (1974) |
| (4-Chloro-2-methylphenoxy)-acetic acid (*see* MCPA) | |
| Chlorophenols | *Suppl. 7*, 154 (1987) |
| Chlorophenols (occupational exposures to) | *41*, 319 (1986) |
| Chlorophenoxy herbicides | *Suppl. 7*, 156 (1987) |
| Chlorophenoxy herbicides (occupational exposures to) | *41*, 357 (1986) |
| 4-Chloro-*ortho*-phenylenediamine | *27*, 81 (1982) |
| | *Suppl. 7*, 60 (1987) |
| 4-Chloro-*meta*-phenylenediamine | *27*, 82 (1982) |
| | *Suppl. 7*, 60 (1987) |
| Chloroprene | *19*, 131 (1979) |
| | *Suppl. 7*, 160 (1987) |
| Chloropropham | *12*, 55 (1976) |
| | *Suppl. 7*, 60 (1987) |
| Chloroquine | *13*, 47 (1977) |
| | *Suppl. 7*, 60 (1987) |
| Chlorothalonil | *30*, 319 (1983) |
| | *Suppl. 7*, 60 (1987) |
| *para*-Chloro-*ortho*-toluidine (*see also* Chlordimeform) | *16*, 277 (1978) |
| | *30*, 65 (1983) |
| | *Suppl. 7*, 60 (1987) |
| Chlorotrianisene (*see also* Nonsteroidal oestrogens) | *21*, 139 (1979) |
| 2-Chloro-1,1,1-trifluoroethane | *41*, 253 (1986) |
| | *Suppl. 7*, 60 (1987) |
| Cholesterol | *10*, 99 (1976) |
| | *31*, 95 (1983) |
| | *Suppl. 7*, 161 (1987) |
| Chromic acetate (*see* Chromium and chromium compounds) | |
| Chromic chloride (*see* Chromium and chromium compounds) | |
| Chromic oxide (*see* Chromium and chromium compounds | |
| Chromic phosphate (*see* Chromium and chromium compounds) | |
| Chromite ore (*see* Chromium and chromium compounds) | |
| Chromium and chromium compounds | *2*, 100 (1973) |
| | *23*, 205 (1980) |
| | *Suppl. 7*, 165 (1987) |
| Chromium carbonyl (*see* Chromium and chromium compounds) | |
| Chromium potassium sulphate (*see* Chromium and chromium compounds) | |
| Chromium sulphate (*see* Chromium and chromium compounds) | |

Chromium trioxide (see Chromium and chromium compounds)
Chrysene                                                         3, 159 (1973)
                                                                 32, 247 (1983)
                                                                 Suppl. 7, 60 (1987)
Chrysoidine                                                      8, 91 (1975)
                                                                 Suppl. 7, 169 (1987)
Chrysotile (see Asbestos)
CI Disperse Yellow 3                                             8, 97 (1975)
                                                                 Suppl. 7, 60 (1987)
Cinnamyl anthranilate                                            16, 287 (1978)
                                                                 31, 133 (1983)
                                                                 Suppl. 7, 60 (1987)
Cisplatin                                                        26, 151 (1981)
                                                                 Suppl. 7, 170 (1987)
Citrinin                                                         40, 67 (1986)
                                                                 Suppl. 7, 60 (1987)
Citrus Red No. 2                                                 8, 101 (1975) (corr. 42, 254)
                                                                 Suppl. 7, 60 (1987)
Clofibrate                                                       24, 39 (1980)
                                                                 Suppl. 7, 171 (1987)
Clomiphene citrate                                               21, 551 (1979)
                                                                 Suppl. 7, 172 (1987)
Coal gasification                                                34, 65 (1984)
                                                                 Suppl. 7, 173 (1987)
Coal-tar pitches (see also Coal-tars)                            Suppl. 7, 174 (1987)
Coal-tars                                                        35, 83 (1985)
                                                                 Suppl. 7, 175 (1987)
Cobalt-chromium alloy (see Chromium and chromium
    compounds)
Coke production                                                  34, 101 (1984)
                                                                 Suppl. 7, 176 (1987)
Combined oral contraceptives (see also Oestrogens, progestins    Suppl. 7, 297 (1987)
    and combinations)
Conjugated oestrogens (see also Steroidal oestrogens)            21, 147 (1979)
Contraceptives, oral (see Combined oral contraceptives;
    Sequential oral contraceptives)
Copper 8-hydroxyquinoline                                        15, 103 (1977)
                                                                 Suppl. 7, 61 (1987)
Coronene                                                         32, 263 (1983)
                                                                 Suppl. 7, 61 (1987)
Coumarin                                                         10, 113 (1976)
                                                                 Suppl. 7, 61 (1987)
Creosotes (see also Coal-tars)                                   Suppl. 7, 177 (1987)
meta-Cresidine                                                   27, 91 (1982)
                                                                 Suppl. 7, 61 (1987)
para-Cresidine                                                   27, 92 (1982)
                                                                 Suppl. 7, 61 (1987)

| | |
|---|---|
| Crocidolite (*see* Asbestos) | |
| Crude oil | *45*, 119 (1989) |
| Crystalline silica (*see also* Silica) | *Suppl. 7*, 341 (1987) |
| Cycasin | *1*, 157 (1972) (*corr. 42*, 251) |
| | *10*, 121 (1976) |
| | *Suppl. 7*, 61 (1987) |
| Cyclamates | *22*, 55 (1980) |
| | *Suppl. 7*, 178 (1987) |
| Cyclamic acid (*see* Cyclamates) | |
| Cyclochlorotine | *10*, 139 (1976) |
| | *Suppl. 7*, 61 (1987) |
| Cyclohexylamine (*see* Cyclamates) | |
| Cyclopenta[*cd*]pyrene | *32*, 269 (1983) |
| | *Suppl. 7*, 61 (1987) |
| Cyclopropane (*see* Anaesthetics, volatile) | |
| Cyclophosphamide | *9*, 135 (1975) |
| | *26*, 165 (1981) |
| | *Suppl. 7*, 182 (1987) |

# D

| | |
|---|---|
| 2,4-D (*see also* Chlorophenoxy herbicides; Chlorophenoxy herbicides, occupational exposures to) | *15*, 111 (1977) |
| Dacarbazine | *26*, 203 (1981) |
| | *Suppl. 7*, 184 (1987) |
| D & C Red No. 9 | *8*, 107 (1975) |
| | *Suppl. 7*, 61 (1987) |
| Dapsone | *24*, 59 (1980) |
| | *Suppl. 7*, 185 (1987) |
| Daunomycin | *10*, 145 (1976) |
| | *Suppl. 7*, 61 (1987) |
| DDD (*see* DDT) | |
| DDE (*see* DDT) | |
| DDT | *5*, 83 (1974) (*corr. 42*, 253) |
| | *Suppl. 7*, 186 (1987) |
| Diacetylaminoazotoluene | *8*, 113 (1975) |
| | *Suppl. 7*, 61 (1987) |
| *N,N'*-Diacetylbenzidine | *16*, 293 (1978) |
| | *Suppl. 7*, 61 (1987) |
| Diallate | *12*, 69 (1976) |
| | *30*, 235 (1983) |
| | *Suppl. 7*, 61 (1987) |
| 2,4-Diaminoanisole | *16*, 51 (1978) |
| | *27*, 103 (1982) |
| | *Suppl. 7*, 61 (1987) |

| | |
|---|---|
| 4,4'-Diaminodiphenyl ether | *16*, 301 (1978);<br>*29*, 203 (1982) |
| *Suppl. 7*, 61 (1987) | |
| 1,2-Diamino-4-nitrobenzene | *16*, 63 (1978) |
| | *Suppl. 7*, 61 (1987) |
| 1,4-Diamino-2-nitrobenzene | *16*, 73 (1978) |
| | *Suppl. 7*, 61 (1987) |
| 2,6-Diamino-3-(phenylazo)pyridine (*see* Phenazopyridine hydrochloride) | |
| 2,4-Diaminotoluene (*see also* Toluene diisocyanates) | *16*, 83 (1978) |
| | *Suppl. 7*, 61 (1987) |
| 2,5-Diaminotoluene (*see also* Toluene diisocyanates) | *16*, 97 (1978) |
| | *Suppl. 7*, 61 (1987) |
| *ortho*-Dianisidine (*see* 3,3'-Dimethoxybenzidine) | |
| Diazepam | *13*, 57 (1977) |
| | *Suppl. 7*, 189 (1987) |
| Diazomethane | *7*, 223 (1974) |
| | *Suppl. 7*, 61 (1987) |
| Dibenz[*a,h*]acridine | *3*, 247 (1973) |
| | *32*, 277 (1983) |
| | *Suppl. 7*, 61 (1987) |
| Dibenz[*a,j*]acridine | *3*, 254 (1973) |
| | *32*, 283 (1983) |
| | *Suppl. 7*, 61 (1987) |
| Dibenz[*a,c*]anthracene | *32*, 289 (1983) (*corr. 42*, 262) |
| | *Suppl. 7*, 61 (1987) |
| Dibenz[*a,h*]anthracene | *3*, 178 (1973) (*corr. 43*, 261) |
| | *32*, 299 (1983) |
| | *Suppl. 7*, 61 (1987) |
| Dibenz[*a,j*]anthracene | *32*, 309 (1983) |
| | *Suppl. 7*, 61 (1987) |
| 7*H*-Dibenzo[*c,g*]carbazole | *3*, 260 (1973) |
| | *32*, 315 (1983) |
| | *Suppl. 7*, 61 (1987) |
| Dibenzodioxins, chlorinated (other than TCDD) [*see* Chlorinated dibenzodioxins (other than TCDD)] | |
| Dibenzo[*a,e*]fluoranthene | *32*, 321 (1983) |
| | *Suppl. 7*, 61 (1987) |
| Dibenzo[*h,rst*]pentaphene | *3*, 197 (1973) |
| | *Suppl. 7*, 62 (1987) |
| Dibenzo[*a,e*]pyrene | *3*, 201 (1973) |
| | *32*, 327 (1983) |
| | *Suppl. 7*, 62 (1987) |
| Dibenzo[*a,h*]pyrene | *3*, 207 (1973) |
| | *32*, 331 (1983) |
| | *Suppl. 7*, 62 (1987) |

| | |
|---|---|
| Dibenzo[*a,i*]pyrene | *3*, 215 (1973) |
| | *32*, 337 (1983) |
| | *Suppl. 7*, 62 (1987) |
| Dibenzo[*a,l*]pyrene | *3*, 224 (1973) |
| | *32*, 343 (1983) |
| | *Suppl. 7*, 62 (1987) |
| 1,2-Dibromo-3-chloropropane | *15*, 139 (1977) |
| | *20*, 83 (1979) |
| | *Suppl. 7*, 191 (1987) |
| Dichloroacetylene | *39*, 369 (1986) |
| | *Suppl. 7*, 62 (1987) |
| *ortho*-Dichlorobenzene | *7*, 231 (1974) |
| | *29*, 213 (1982) |
| | *Suppl. 7*, 192 (1987) |
| *para*-Dichlorobenzene | *7*, 231 (1974) |
| | *29*, 215 (1982) |
| | *Suppl. 7*, 192 (1987) |
| 3,3'-Dichlorobenzidine | *4*, 49 (1974) |
| | *29*, 239 (1982) |
| | *Suppl. 7*, 193 (1987) |
| *trans*-1,4-Dichlorobutene | *15*, 149 (1977) |
| | *Suppl. 7*, 62 (1987) |
| 3,3'-Dichloro-4,4'-diaminodiphenyl ether | *16*, 309 (1978) |
| | *Suppl. 7*, 62 (1987) |
| 1,2-Dichloroethane | *20*, 429 (1979) |
| | *Suppl. 7*, 62 (1987) |
| Dichloromethane | *20*, 449 (1979) |
| | *41*, 43 (1986) |
| | *Suppl. 7*, 194 (1987) |
| 2,4-Dichlorophenol (*see* Chlorophenols; Chlorophenols, occupational exposures to) | |
| (2,4-Dichlorophenoxy)acetic acid (*see* 2,4-D) | |
| 2,6-Dichloro-*para*-phenylenediamine | *39*, 325 (1986) |
| | *Suppl. 7*, 62 (1987) |
| 1,2-Dichloropropane | *41*, 131 (1986) |
| | *Suppl. 7*, 62 (1987) |
| 1,3-Dichloropropene (technical-grade) | *41*, 113 (1986) |
| | *Suppl. 7*, 195 (1987) |
| Dichlorvos | *20*, 97 (1979) |
| | *Suppl. 7*, 62 (1987) |
| Dicofol | *30*, 87 (1983) |
| | *Suppl. 7*, 62 (1987) |
| Dicyclohexylamine (*see* Cyclamates) | |
| Dieldrin | *5*, 125 (1974) |
| | *Suppl. 7*, 196 (1987) |
| Dienoestrol (*see also* Nonsteroidal oestrogens) | *21*, 161 (1979) |

| | |
|---|---|
| Diepoxybutane | *11*, 115 (1976) (*corr. 42*, 255) |
| | *Suppl. 7*, 62 (1987) |
| Diesel and gasoline engine exhausts | *46*, 41 (1989) |
| Diesel fuels | *45*, 219 (1989) |
| Diethyl ether (*see* Anaesthetics, volatile) | |
| Di(2-ethylhexyl)adipate | *29*, 257 (1982) |
| | *Suppl. 7*, 62 (1987) |
| Di(2-ethylhexyl)phthalate | *29*, 269 (1982) (*corr. 42*, 261) |
| | *Suppl. 7*, 62 (1987) |
| 1,2-Diethylhydrazine | *4*, 153 (1974) |
| | *Suppl. 7*, 62 (1987) |
| Diethylstilboestrol | *6*, 55 (1974) |
| | *21*, 173 (1979) (*corr. 42*, 259) |
| | *Suppl. 7*, 273 (1987) |
| Diethylstilboestrol dipropionate (*see* Diethylstilboestrol) | |
| Diethyl sulphate | *4*, 277 (1974) |
| | *Suppl. 7*, 198 (1987) |
| Diglycidyl resorcinol ether | *11*, 125 (1976) |
| | *36*, 181 (1985) |
| | *Suppl. 7*, 62 (1987) |
| Dihydrosafrole | *1*, 170 (1972) |
| | *10*, 233 (1976) |
| | *Suppl. 7*, 62 (1987) |
| Dihydroxybenzenes (*see* Catechol; Hydroquinone; Resorcinol) | |
| Dihydroxymethylfuratrizine | *24*, 77 (1980) |
| | *Suppl. 7*, 62 (1987) |
| Dimethisterone (*see also* Progestins; Sequential oral contraceptives) | *6*, 167 (1974) |
| | *21*, 377 (1979) |
| Dimethoxane | *15*, 177 (1977) |
| | *Suppl. 7*, 62 (1987) |
| 3,3'-Dimethoxybenzidine | *4*, 41 (1974) |
| | *Suppl. 7*, 198 (1987) |
| 3,3'-Dimethoxybenzidine-4,4'-diisocyanate | *39*, 279 (1986) |
| | *Suppl. 7*, 62 (1987) |
| *para*-Dimethylaminoazobenzene | *8*, 125 (1975) |
| | *Suppl. 7*, 62 (1987) |
| *para*-Dimethylaminoazobenzenediazo sodium sulphonate | *8*, 147 (1975) |
| | *Suppl. 7*, 62 (1987) |
| *trans*-2-[(Dimethylamino)methylimino]-5-[2-(5-nitro-2-furyl)-vinyl]-1,3,4-oxadiazole | *7*, 147 (1974) (*corr. 42*, 253) |
| | *Suppl. 7*, 62 (1987) |
| 4,4'-Dimethylangelicin plus ultraviolet radiation (*see also* Angelicin and some synthetic derivatives) | *Suppl. 7*, 57 (1987) |
| 4,5'-Dimethylangelicin plus ultraviolet radiation (*see also* Angelicin and some synthetic derivatives) | *Suppl. 7*, 57 (1987) |
| Dimethylarsinic acid (*see* Arsenic and arsenic compounds) | |
| 3,3'-Dimethylbenzidine | *1*, 87 (1972) |
| | *Suppl. 7*, 62 (1987) |

| | |
|---|---|
| Dimethylcarbamoyl chloride | *12*, 77 (1976) |
| | *Suppl. 7*, 199 (1987) |
| 1,1-Dimethylhydrazine | *4*, 137 (1974) |
| | *Suppl. 7*, 62 (1987) |
| 1,2-Dimethylhydrazine | *4*, 145 (1974) (*corr. 42*, 253) |
| | *Suppl. 7*, 62 (1987) |
| 1,4-Dimethylphenanthrene | *32*, 349 (1983) |
| | *Suppl. 7*, 62 (1987) |
| Dimethyl sulphate | *4*, 271 (1974) |
| | *Suppl. 7*, 200 (1987) |
| 3,7-Dinitrofluoranthene | *46*, 189 |
| 3,9-Dinitrofluoranthene | *46*, 195 |
| 1,3-Dinitropyrene | *46*, 201 |
| 1,6-Dinitropyrene | *46*, 215 |
| 1,8-Dinitropyrene | *33*, 171 (1984) |
| | *Suppl. 7*, 63 (1987) |
| | *46*, 231 |
| Dinitrosopentamethylenetetramine | *11*, 241 (1976) |
| | *Suppl. 7*, 63 (1987) |
| 1,4-Dioxane | *11*, 247 (1976) |
| | *Suppl. 7*, 201 (1987) |
| 2,4′-Diphenyldiamine | *16*, 313 (1978) |
| | *Suppl. 7*, 63 (1987) |
| Direct Black 38 (*see also* Benzidine-based dyes) | *29*, 295 (1982) (*corr. 42*, 261) |
| Direct Blue 6 (*see also* Benzidine-based dyes) | *29*, 311 (1982) |
| Direct Brown 95 (*see also* Benzidine-based dyes) | *29*, 321 (1982) |
| Disulfiram | *12*, 85 (1976) |
| | *Suppl. 7*, 63 (1987) |
| Dithranol | *13*, 75 (1977) |
| | *Suppl. 7*, 63 (1987) |
| Divinyl ether (*see* Anaesthetics, volatile) | |
| Dulcin | *12*, 97 (1976) |
| | *Suppl. 7*, 63 (1987) |

E

| | |
|---|---|
| Endrin | *5*, 157 (1974) |
| | *Suppl. 7*, 63 (1987) |
| Enflurane (*see* Anaesthetics, volatile) | |
| Eosin | *15*, 183 (1977) |
| | *Suppl. 7*, 63 (1987) |
| Epichlorohydrin | *11*, 131 (1976) (*corr. 42*, 256) |
| | *Suppl. 7*, 202 (1987) |
| 1-Epoxyethyl-3,4-epoxycyclohexane | *11*, 141 (1976) |
| | *Suppl. 7*, 63 (1987) |
| 3,4-Epoxy-6-methylcyclohexylmethyl-3,4-epoxy-6-methyl-cyclohexane carboxylate | *11*, 147 (1976) |
| | *Suppl. 7*, 63 (1987) |

| | |
|---|---|
| cis-9,10-Epoxystearic acid | *11*, 153 (1976) |
| | *Suppl. 7*, 63 (1987) |
| Erionite | *42*, 225 (1987) |
| | *Suppl. 7*, 203 (1987) |
| Ethinyloestradiol (*see also* Steroidal oestrogens) | *6*, 77 (1974) |
| | *21*, 233 (1979) |
| Ethionamide | *13*, 83 (1977) |
| | *Suppl. 7*, 63 (1987) |
| Ethyl acrylate | *19*, 57 (1979) |
| | *39*, 81 (1986) |
| | *Suppl. 7*, 63 (1987) |
| Ethylene | *19*, 157 (1979) |
| | *Suppl. 7*, 63 (1987) |
| Ethylene dibromide | *15*, 195 (1977) |
| | *Suppl. 7*, 204 (1987) |
| Ethylene oxide | *11*, 157 (1976) |
| | *36*, 189 (1985) (*corr. 42*, 263) |
| | *Suppl. 7*, 205 (1987) |
| Ethylene sulphide | *11*, 257 (1976) |
| | *Suppl. 7*, 63 (1987) |
| Ethylene thiourea | *7*, 45 (1974) |
| | *Suppl. 7*, 207 (1987) |
| Ethyl methanesulphonate | *7*, 245 (1974) |
| | *Suppl. 7*, 63 (1987) |
| N-Ethyl-N-nitrosourea | *1*, 135 (1972) |
| | *17*, 191 (1978) |
| | *Suppl. 7*, 63 (1987) |
| Ethyl selenac (*see also* Selenium and selenium compounds) | *12*, 107 (1976) |
| | *Suppl. 7*, 63 (1987) |
| Ethyl tellurac | *12*, 115 (1976) |
| | *Suppl. 7*, 63 (1987) |
| Ethynodiol diacetate (*see also* Progestins; Combined oral contraceptives) | *6* 173 (1974) |
| | *21*, 387 (1979) |
| Eugenol | *36*, 75 (1985) |
| | *Suppl. 7*, 63 (1987) |
| Evans blue | *8*, 151 (1975) |
| | *Suppl. 7*, 63 (1987) |

F

| | |
|---|---|
| Fast Green FCF | *16*, 187 (1978) |
| | *Suppl. 7*, 63 (1987) |
| Ferbam | *12*, 121 (1976) (*corr. 42*, 256) |
| | *Suppl. 7*, 63 (1987) |
| Ferric oxide | *1*, 29 (1972) |
| | *Suppl. 7*, 216 (1987) |
| Ferrochromium (*see* Chromium and chromium compounds) | |

| | |
|---|---|
| Fluometuron | *30*, 245 (1983) |
| | *Suppl. 7*, 63 (1987) |
| Fluoranthene | *32*, 355 (1983) |
| | *Suppl. 7*, 63 (1987) |
| Fluorene | *32*, 365 (1983) |
| | *Suppl. 7*, 63 (1987) |
| Fluorides (inorganic, used in drinking-water) | *27*, 237 (1982) |
| | *Suppl. 7*, 208 (1987) |
| 5-Fluorouracil | *26*, 217 (1981) |
| | *Suppl. 7*, 210 (1987) |
| Fluorspar (*see* Fluorides) | |
| Fluosilicic acid (*see* Fluorides) | |
| Fluroxene (*see* Anaesthetics, volatile) | |
| Formaldehyde | *29*, 345 (1982) |
| | *Suppl. 7*, 211 (1987) |
| 2-(2-Formylhydrazino)-4-(5-nitro-2-furyl)thiazole | *7*, 151 (1974) (*corr. 42*, 253) |
| | *Suppl. 7*, 63 (1987) |
| Fuel oils (heating oils) | *45*, 239 (1989) |
| Furazolidone | *31*, 141 (1983) |
| | *Suppl. 7*, 63 (1987) |
| Furniture and cabinet-making | *25*, 99 (1981) |
| | *Suppl. 7*, 380 (1987) |
| 2-(2-Furyl)-3-(5-nitro-2-furyl)acrylamide (*see* AF-2) | |
| Fusarenon-X | *11*, 169 (1976) |
| | *31*, 153 (1983) |
| | *Suppl. 7*, 64 (1987) |

G

| | |
|---|---|
| Gasoline | *45*, 159 (1989) |
| Gasoline engine exhaust (*see* Diesel and gasoline engine exhausts) | |
| Glass fibres (*see* Man-made mineral fibres) | |
| Glasswool (*see* Man-made mineral fibres) | |
| Glass filaments (*see* Man-made mineral fibres) | |
| Glu-P-1 | *40*, 223 (1986) |
| | *Suppl. 7*, 64 (1987) |
| Glu-P-2 | *40*, 235 (1986) |
| | *Suppl. 7*, 64 (1987) |
| L-Glutamic acid, 5-[2-(4-hydroxymethyl)phenylhydrazide] (*see* Agaratine) | |
| Glycidaldehyde | *11*, 175 (1976) |
| | *Suppl. 7*, 64 (1987) |
| Glycidyl oleate | *11*, 183 (1976) |
| | *Suppl. 7*, 64 (1987) |
| Glycidyl stearate | *11*, 187 (1976) |
| | *Suppl. 7*, 64 (1987) |
| Griseofulvin | *10*, 153 (1976) |
| | *Suppl. 7*, 391 (1987) |
| Guinea Green B | *16*, 199 (1978) |
| | *Suppl. 7*, 64 (1987) |

| | |
|---|---|
| Gyromitrin | *31*, 163 (1983) |
| | *Suppl. 7*, 391 (1987) |
| **H** | |
| Haematite | *1*, 29 (1972) |
| | *Suppl. 7*, 216 (1987) |
| Haematite and ferric oxide | *Suppl. 7*, 216 (1987) |
| Haematite mining, underground, with exposure to radon | *1*, 29 (1972) |
| | *Suppl. 7*, 216 (1987) |
| Hair dyes, epidemiology of | *16*, 29 (1978) |
| | *27*, 307 (1982) |
| Halothane (*see* Anaesthetics, volatile) | |
| α-HCH (*see* Hexachlorocyclohexanes) | |
| β-HCH (*see* Hexachlorocyclohexanes) | |
| γ-HCH (*see* Hexachlorocyclohexanes) | |
| Heating oils (*see* Fuel oils) | |
| Heptachlor (*see also* Chlordane/Heptachlor) | *5*, 173 (1974) |
| | *20*, 129 (1979) |
| Hexachlorobenzene | *20*, 155 (1979) |
| | *Suppl. 7*, 219 (1987) |
| Hexachlorobutadiene | *20*, 179 (1979) |
| | *Suppl. 7*, 64 (1987) |
| Hexachlorocyclohexanes | *5*, 47 (1974) |
| | *20*, 195 (1979) (*corr. 42*, 258) |
| | *Suppl. 7*, 220 (1987) |
| Hexachlorocyclohexane, technical-grade (*see* Hexachlorocyclohexanes) | |
| Hexachloroethane | *20*, 467 (1979) |
| | *Suppl. 7*, 64 (1987) |
| Hexachlorophene | *20*, 241 (1979) |
| | *Suppl. 7*, 64 (1987) |
| Hexamethylphosphoramide | *15*, 211 (1977) |
| | *Suppl. 7*, 64 (1987) |
| Hexoestrol (*see* Nonsteroidal oestrogens) | |
| Hycanthone mesylate | *13*, 91 (1977) |
| | *Suppl. 7*, 64 (1987) |
| Hydralazine | *24*, 85 (1980) |
| | *Suppl. 7*, 222 (1987) |
| Hydrazine | *4*, 127 (1974) |
| | *Suppl. 7*, 223 (1987) |
| Hydrogen peroxide | *36*, 285 (1985) |
| | *Suppl. 7*, 64 (1987) |
| Hydroquinone | *15*, 155 (1977) |
| | *Suppl. 7*, 64 (1987) |
| 4-Hydroxyazobenzene | *8*, 157 (1975) |
| | *Suppl. 7*, 64 (1987) |
| 17α-Hydroxyprogesterone caproate (*see also* Progestins) | *21*, 399 (1979) (*corr. 42*, 259) |
| 8-Hydroxyquinoline | *13*, 101 (1977) |
| | *Suppl. 7*, 64 (1987) |

8-Hydroxysenkirkine                                        *10*, 265 (1976)
                                                            *Suppl. 7*, 64 (1987)

I

Indeno[1,2,3-*cd*]pyrene                                   *3*, 229 (1973)
                                                            *32*, 373 (1983)
                                                            *Suppl. 7*, 64 (1987)
IQ                                                          *40*, 261 (1986)
                                                            *Suppl. 7*, 64 (1987)
Iron and steel founding                                    *34*, 133 (1984)
                                                            *Suppl. 7*, 224 (1987)
Iron-dextran complex                                       *2*, 161 (1973)
                                                            *Suppl. 7*, 226 (1987)
Iron-dextrin complex                                       *2*, 161 (1973) (*corr. 42*, 252)
                                                            *Suppl. 7*, 64 (1987)
Iron oxide (*see* Ferric oxide)
Iron oxide, saccharated (*see* Saccharated iron oxide)
Iron sorbitol-citric acid complex                          *2*, 161 (1973)
                                                            *Suppl. 7*, 64 (1987)
Isatidine                                                   *10*, 269 (1976)
                                                            *Suppl. 7*, 65 (1987)

Isoflurane (*see* Anaesthetics, volatile)
Isoniazid (*see* Isonicotinic acid hydrazide)
Isonicotinic acid hydrazide                                *4*, 159 (1974)
                                                            *Suppl. 7*, 227 (1987)
Isophosphamide                                              *26*, 237 (1981)
                                                            *Suppl. 7*, 65 (1987)
Isopropyl alcohol                                           *15*, 223 (1977)
                                                            *Suppl. 7*, 229 (1987)
Isopropyl alcohol manufacture (strong-acid process)         *Suppl. 7*, 229 (1987)
  (*see also* Isopropyl alcohol)
Isopropyl oils                                              *15*, 223 (1977)
                                                            *Suppl. 7*, 229 (1987)
Isosafrole                                                  *1*, 169 (1972)
                                                            *10*, 232 (1976)
                                                            *Suppl. 7*, 65 (1987)

J

Jacobine                                                    *10*, 275 (1976)
                                                            *Suppl. 7*, 65 (1987)
Jet fuel                                                    *45*, 203 (1989)
Joinery (*see* Carpentry and joinery)

K

Kaempferol                                                  *31*, 171 (1983)
                                                            *Suppl. 7*, 65 (1987)

Kepone (*see* Chlordecone)

## L

Lasiocarpine                                            *10*, 281 (1976)
                                                        *Suppl. 7*, 65 (1987)
Lauroyl peroxide                                        *36*, 315 (1985)
                                                        *Suppl. 7*, 65 (1987)
Lead acetate (*see* Lead and lead compounds)
Lead and lead compounds                                 *1*, 40 (1972) (*corr. 42*, 251)
                                                        *2*, 52, 150 (1973)
                                                        *12*, 131 (1976)
                                                        *23*, 40, 208, 209, 325 (1980)
                                                        *Suppl. 7*, 230 (1987)
Lead arsenate (*see* Arsenic and arsenic compounds)
Lead carbonate (*see* Lead and lead compounds)
Lead chloride (*see* Lead and lead compounds)
Lead chromate (*see* Chromium and chromium compounds)
Lead chromate oxide (*see* Chromium and chromium compounds)
Lead naphthenate (*see* Lead and lead compounds)
Lead nitrate (*see* Lead and lead compounds)
Lead oxide (*see* Lead and lead compounds)
Lead phosphate (*see* Lead and lead compounds)
Lead subacetate (*see* Lead and lead compounds)
Lead tetroxide (*see* Lead and lead compounds)
Leather goods manufacture                               *25*, 279 (1981)
                                                        *Suppl. 7*, 235 (1987)
Leather industries                                      *25*, 199 (1981)
                                                        *Suppl. 7*, 232 (1987)
Leather tanning and processing                          *25*, 201 (1981)
                                                        *Suppl. 7*, 236 (1987)
Ledate (*see also* Lead and lead compounds)             *12*, 131 (1976)
Light Green SF                                          *16*, 209 (1978)
                                                        *Suppl. 7*, 65 (1987)
Lindane (*see* Hexachlorocyclohexanes)
The lumber and sawmill industries (including logging)   *25*, 49 (1981)
                                                        *Suppl. 7*, 383 (1987)
Luteoskyrin                                             *10*, 163 (1976)
                                                        *Suppl. 7*, 65 (1987)
Lynoestrenol (*see also* Progestins; Combined oral contraceptives)   *21*, 407 (1979)

## M

Magenta                                                 *4*, 57 (1974) (*corr. 42*, 252)
                                                        *Suppl. 7*, 238 (1987)
Magenta, manufacture of (*see also* Magenta)            *Suppl. 7*, 238 (1987)
Malathion                                               *30*, 103 (1983)
                                                        *Suppl. 7*, 65 (1987)
Maleic hydrazide                                        *4*, 173 (1974) (*corr. 42*, 253)
                                                        *Suppl. 7*, 65 (1987)

| | |
|---|---|
| Malonaldehyde | 36, 163 (1985) |
| | Suppl. 7, 65 (1987) |
| Maneb | 12, 137 (1976) |
| | Suppl. 7, 65 (1987) |
| Man-made mineral fibres | 43, 39 (1988) |
| Mannomustine | 9, 157 (1975) |
| | Suppl. 7, 65 (1987) |
| MCPA (see also Chlorophenoxy herbicides; Chlorophenoxy herbicides, occupational exposures) | 30, 255 (1983) |
| MeA-α-C | 40, 253 (1986) |
| | Suppl. 7, 65 (1987) |
| Medphalan | 9, 168 (1975) |
| | Suppl. 7, 65 (1987) |
| Medroxyprogesterone acetate | 6, 157 (1974) |
| | 21, 417 (1979) (corr. 42, 259) |
| | Suppl. 7, 289 (1987) |
| Megestrol acetate (see also Progestins; Combined oral contraceptives) | 21, 431 (1979) |
| MeIQ | 40, 275 (1986) |
| | Suppl. 7, 65 (1987) |
| MeIQx | 40, 283 (1986) |
| | Suppl. 7, 65 (1987) |
| Melamine | 39, 333 (1986) |
| | Suppl. 7, 65 (1987) |
| Melphalan | 9, 167 (1975) |
| | Suppl. 7, 239 (1987) |
| 6-Mercaptopurine | 26, 249 (1981) |
| | Suppl. 7, 240 (1987) |
| Merphalan | 9, 169 (1975) |
| | Suppl. 7, 65 (1987) |
| Mestranol (see also Steroidal oestrogens) | 6, 87 (1974) |
| | 21, 257 (1979) (corr. 42, 259) |
| Methanearsonic acid, disodium salt (see Arsenic and arsenic compounds) | |
| Methanearsonic acid, monosodium salt (see Arsenic and arsenic compounds) | |
| Methotrexate | 26, 267 (1981) |
| | Suppl. 7, 241 (1987) |
| Methoxsalen (see 8-Methoxypsoralen) | |
| Methoxychlor | 5, 193 (1974) |
| | 20, 259 (1979) |
| | Suppl. 7, 66 (1987) |
| Methoxyflurane (see Anaesthetics, volatile) | |
| 5-Methoxypsoralen | 40, 327 (1986) |
| | Suppl. 7, 242 (1987) |
| 8-Methoxypsoralen (see also 8-Methoxypsoralen plus ultraviolet radiation) | 24, 101 (1980) |
| 8-Methoxypsoralen plus ultraviolet radiation | Suppl. 7, 243 (1987) |

| | |
|---|---|
| Methyl acrylate | *19*, 52 (1979) |
| | *39*, 99 (1986) |
| | *Suppl. 7*, 66 (1987) |
| 5-Methylangelicin plus ultraviolet radiation (*see also* Angelicin and some synthetic derivatives) | *Suppl. 7*, 57 (1987) |
| 2-Methylaziridine | *9*, 61 (1975) |
| | *Suppl. 7*, 66 (1987) |
| Methylazoxymethanol acetate | *1*, 164 (1972) |
| | *10*, 131 (1976) |
| | *Suppl. 7*, 66 (1987) |
| Methyl bromide | *41*, 187 (1986) (*corr. 45*, 283) |
| | *Suppl. 7*, 245 (1987) |
| Methyl carbamate | *12*, 151 (1976) |
| | *Suppl. 7*, 66 (1987) |
| Methyl-CCNU [*see* 1-(2-Chloroethyl)-3-(4-methyl-cyclohexyl)-1-nitrosourea] | |
| Methyl chloride | *41*, 161 (1986) |
| | *Suppl. 7*, 246 (1987) |
| 1-, 2-, 3-, 4-, 5- and 6-Methylchrysenes | *32*, 379 (1983) |
| | *Suppl. 7*, 66 (1987) |
| $N$-Methyl-$N$,4-dinitrosoaniline | *1*, 141 (1972) |
| | *Suppl. 7*, 66 (1987) |
| 4,4'-Methylene bis(2-chloroaniline) | *4*, 65 (1974) (*corr. 42*, 252) |
| | *Suppl. 7*, 246 (1987) |
| 4,4'-Methylene bis($N,N$-dimethyl)benzenamine | *27*, 119 (1982) |
| | *Suppl. 7*, 66 (1987) |
| 4,4'-Methylene bis(2-methylaniline) | *4*, 73 (1974) |
| | *Suppl. 7*, 248 (1987) |
| 4,4'-Methylenedianiline | *4*, 79 (1974) (*corr. 42*, 252) |
| | *39*, 347 (1986) |
| | *Suppl. 7*, 66 (1987) |
| 4,4'-Methylenediphenyl diisocyanate | *19*, 314 (1979) |
| | *Suppl. 7*, 66 (1987) |
| 2-Methylfluoranthene | *32*, 399 (1983) |
| | *Suppl. 7*, 66 (1987) |
| 3-Methylfluoranthene | *32*, 399 (1983) |
| | *Suppl. 7*, 66 (1987) |
| Methyl iodide | *15*, 245 (1977) |
| | *41*, 213 (1986) |
| | *Suppl. 7*, 66 (1987) |
| Methyl methacrylate | *19*, 187 (1979) |
| | *Suppl. 7*, 66 (1987) |
| Methyl methanesulphonate | *7*, 253 (1974) |
| | *Suppl. 7*, 66 (1987) |
| 2-Methyl-1-nitroanthraquinone | *27*, 205 (1982) |
| | *Suppl. 7*, 66 (1987) |

| | |
|---|---|
| *N*-Methyl-*N'*-nitro-*N*-nitrosoguanidine | *4*, 183 (1974) |
| | *Suppl. 7*, 248 (1987) |
| 3-Methylnitrosaminopropionaldehyde (*see* 3-(*N*-Nitrosomethylamino)propionaldehyde) | |
| 3-Methylnitrosaminopropionitrile (*see* 3-(*N*-Nitrosomethylamino)propionitrile) | |
| 4-(Methylnitrosamino)-4-(3-pyridyl)-1-butanal (*see* 4-(*N*-Nitrosomethylamino)-4-(3-pyridyl)-1-butanal) | |
| 4-(Methylnitrosamino)-1-(3-pyridyl)-1-butanone (*see* 4-(*N*-Nitrosomethylamino)-1-(3-pyridyl)-1-butanone) | |
| *N*-Methyl-*N*-nitrosourea | *1*, 125 (1972) |
| | *17*, 227 (1978) |
| | *Suppl. 7*, 66 (1987) |
| *N*-Methyl-*N*-nitrosourethane | *4*, 211 (1974) |
| | *Suppl. 7*, 66 (1987) |
| Methyl parathion | *30*, 131 (1983) |
| | *Suppl. 7*, 392 (1987) |
| 1-Methylphenanthrene | *32*, 405 (1983) |
| | *Suppl. 7*, 66 (1987) |
| 7-Methylpyrido[3,4-*c*]psoralen | *40*, 349 (1986) |
| | *Suppl. 7*, 71 (1987) |
| Methyl red | *8*, 161 (1975) |
| | *Suppl. 7*, 66 (1987) |
| Methyl selenac (*see also* Selenium and selenium compounds) | *12*, 161 (1976) |
| | *Suppl. 7*, 66 (1987) |
| Methylthiouracil | *7*, 53 (1974) |
| | *Suppl. 7*, 66 (1987) |
| Metronidazole | *13*, 113 (1977) |
| | *Suppl. 7*, 250 (1987) |
| Mineral oils | *3*, 30 (1973) |
| | *33*, 87 (1984) (*corr. 42*, 262) |
| | *Suppl. 7*, 252 (1987) |
| Mirex | *5*, 203 (1974) |
| | *20*, 283 (1979) (*corr. 42*, 258) |
| | *Suppl. 7*, 66 (1987) |
| Mitomycin C | *10*, 171 (1976) |
| | *Suppl. 7*, 67 (1987) |
| MNNG (*see N*-Methyl-*N'*-nitro-*N*-nitrosoguanidine) | |
| MOCA (*see* 4,4'-Methylene bis(2-chloroaniline)) | |
| Modacrylic fibres | *19*, 86 (1979) |
| | *Suppl. 7*, 67 (1987) |
| Monocrotaline | *10*, 291 (1976) |
| | *Suppl. 7*, 67 (1987) |
| Monuron | *12*, 167 (1976) |
| | *Suppl. 7*, 67 (1987) |
| MOPP and other combined chemotherapy including alkylating agents | *Suppl. 7*, 254 (1987) |

5-(Morpholinomethyl)-3-[(5-nitrofurfurylidene)amino]-2-     7, 161 (1974)
oxazolidinone                                                Suppl. 7, 67 (1987)
Mustard gas                                                  9. 181 (1975) (corr. 42, 254)
                                                             Suppl. 7, 259 (1987)

Myleran (see 1,4-Butanediol dimethanesulphonate)

N

Nafenopin                                                    24, 125 (1980)
                                                             Suppl. 7, 67 (1987)
1,5-Naphthalenediamine                                       27, 127 (1982)
                                                             Suppl. 7, 67 (1987)
1,5-Naphthalene diisocyanate                                 19, 311 (1979)
                                                             Suppl. 7, 67 (1987)
1-Naphthylamine                                              4, 87 (1974) (corr. 42, 253)
                                                             Suppl. 7, 260 (1987)
2-Naphthylamine                                              4, 97 (1974)
                                                             Suppl. 7, 261 (1987)
1-Naphthylthiourea                                           30, 347 (1983)
                                                             Suppl. 7, 263 (1987)

Nickel acetate (see Nickel and nickel compounds)
Nickel ammonium sulphate (see Nickel and nickel compounds)
Nickel and nickel compounds                                  2, 126 (1973) (corr. 42, 252)
                                                             11, 75 (1976)
                                                             Suppl. 7, 264 (1987)
                                                             (corr. 45, 283)

Nickel carbonate (see Nickel and nickel compounds)
Nickel carbonyl (see Nickel and nickel compounds)
Nickel chloride (see Nickel and nickel compounds)
Nickel-gallium alloy (see Nickel and nickel compounds)
Nickel hydroxide (see Nickel and nickel compounds)
Nickelocene (see Nickel and nickel compounds)
Nickel oxide (see Nickel and nickel compounds)
Nickel subsulphide (see Nickel and nickel compounds)
Nickel sulphate (see Nickel and nickel compounds)
Niridazole                                                   13, 123 (1977)
                                                             Suppl. 7, 67 (1987)
Nithiazide                                                   31, 179 (1983)
                                                             Suppl. 7, 67 (1987)
5-Nitroacenaphthene                                          16, 319 (1978)
                                                             Suppl. 7, 67 (1987)
5-Nitro-ortho-anisidine                                      27, 133 (1982)
                                                             Suppl. 7, 67 (1987)
9-Nitroanthracene                                            33, 179 (1984)
                                                             Suppl. 7, 67 (1987)
7-Nitrobenz[a]anthracene                                     46, 247
6-Nitrobenzo[a]pyrene                                        33, 187 (1984)
                                                             Suppl. 7, 67 (1987)
                                                             46, 255

| | |
|---|---|
| 4-Nitrobiphenyl | *4*, 113 (1974) |
| | *Suppl. 7*, 67 (1987) |
| 6-Nitrochrysene | *33*, 195 (1984) |
| | *Suppl. 7*, 67 (1987) |
| | *46*, 267 |
| Nitrofen (technical-grade) | *30*, 271 (1983) |
| | *Suppl. 7*, 67 (1987) |
| 3-Nitrofluoranthene | *33*, 201 (1984) |
| | *Suppl. 7*, 67 (1987) |
| 2-Nitrofluorene | *46*, 277 |
| 5-Nitro-2-furaldehyde semicarbazone | *7*, 171 (1974) |
| | *Suppl. 7*, 67 (1987) |
| 1-[(5-Nitrofurfurylidene)amino]-2-imidazolidinone | *7*, 181 (1974) |
| | *Suppl. 7*, 67 (1987) |
| *N*-[4-(5-Nitro-2-furyl)-2-thiazolyl]acetamide | *1*, 181 (1972) |
| | *7*, 185 (1974) |
| | *Suppl. 7*, 67 (1987) |
| Nitrogen mustard | *9*, 193 (1975) |
| | *Suppl. 7*, 269 (1987) |
| Nitrogen mustard *N*-oxide | *9*, 209 (1975) |
| | *Suppl. 7*, 67 (1987) |
| 1-Nitronaphthalene | *46*, 291 |
| 2-Nitronaphthalene | *46*, 303 |
| 3-Nitroperylene | *46*, 313 |
| 2-Nitropropane | *29*, 331 (1982) |
| | *Suppl. 7*, 67 (1987) |
| 1-Nitropyrene | *33*, 209 (1984) |
| | *Suppl. 7*, 67 (1987) |
| | *46*, 321 |
| 2-Nitropyrene | *46*, 359 |
| 4-Nitropyrene | *46*, 367 |
| *N*-Nitrosatable drugs | *24*, 297 (1980) (*corr. 42*, 260) |
| *N*-Nitrosatable pesticides | *30*, 359 (1983) |
| *N'*-Nitrosoanabasine | *37*, 225 (1985) |
| | *Suppl. 7*, 67 (1987) |
| *N'*-Nitrosoanatabine | *37*, 233 (1985) |
| | *Suppl. 7*, 67 (1987) |
| *N*-Nitrosodi-*n*-butylamine | *4*, 197 (1974) |
| | *17*, 51 (1978) |
| | *Suppl. 7*, 67 (1987) |
| *N*-Nitrosodiethanolamine | *17*, 77 (1978) |
| | *Suppl. 7*, 67 (1987) |
| *N*-Nitrosodiethylamine | *1*, 107 (1972) (*corr. 42*, 251) |
| | *17*, 83 (1978) (*corr. 42*, 257) |
| | *Suppl. 7*, 67 (1987) |
| *N*-Nitrosodimethylamine | *1*, 95 (1972) |
| | *17*, 125 (1978) (*corr. 42*, 257) |
| | *Suppl. 7*, 67 (1987) |

| | |
|---|---|
| N-Nitrosodiphenylamine | 27, 213 (1982) |
| | Suppl. 7, 67 (1987) |
| para-Nitrosodiphenylamine | 27, 227 (1982) (corr. 42, 261) |
| | Suppl. 7, 68 (1987) |
| N-Nitrosodi-n-propylamine | 17, 177 (1978) |
| | Suppl. 7, 68 (1987) |
| N-Nitroso-N-ethylurea (see N-Ethyl-N-nitrosourea) | |
| N-Nitrosofolic acid | 17, 217 (1978) |
| | Suppl. 7, 68 (1987) |
| N-Nitrosoguvacine | 37, 263 (1985) |
| | Suppl. 7, 68 (1987) |
| N-Nitrosoguvacoline | 37, 263 (1985) |
| | Suppl. 7, 68 (1987) |
| N-Nitrosohydroxyproline | 17, 304 (1978) |
| | Suppl. 7, 68 (1987) |
| 3-(N-Nitrosomethylamino)propionaldehyde | 37, 263 (1985) |
| | Suppl. 7, 68 (1987) |
| 3-(N-Nitrosomethylamino)propionitrile | 37, 263 (1985) |
| | Suppl. 7, 68 (1987) |
| 4-(N-Nitrosomethylamino)-4-(3-pyridyl)-1-butanal | 37, 205 (1985) |
| | Suppl. 7, 68 (1987) |
| 4-(N-Nitrosomethylamino)-1-(3-pyridyl)-1-butanone | 37, 209 (1985) |
| | Suppl. 7, 68 (1987) |
| N-Nitrosomethylethylamine | 17, 221 (1978) |
| | Suppl. 7, 68 (1987) |
| N-Nitroso-N-methylurea (see N-Methyl-N-nitrosourea) | |
| N-Nitroso-N-methylurethane (see N-Methyl-N-nitrosourethane) | |
| N-Nitrosomethylvinylamine | 17, 257 (1978) |
| | Suppl. 7, 68 (1987) |
| N-Nitrosomorpholine | 17, 263 (1978) |
| | Suppl. 7, 68 (1987) |
| N'-Nitrosonornicotine | 17, 281 (1978) |
| | 37, 241 (1985) |
| | Suppl. 7, 68 (1987) |
| N-Nitrosopiperidine | 17, 287 (1978) |
| | Suppl. 7, 68 (1987) |
| N-Nitrosoproline | 17, 303 (1978) |
| | Suppl. 7, 68 (1987) |
| N-Nitrosopyrrolidine | 17, 313 (1978) |
| | Suppl. 7, 68 (1987) |
| N-Nitrososarcosine | 17, 327 (1978) |
| | Suppl. 7, 68 (1987) |
| Nitrosoureas, chloroethyl (see Chloroethyl nitrosoureas) | |
| Nitrous oxide (see Anaesthetics, volatile) | |
| Nitrovin | 31, 185 (1983) |
| | Suppl. 7, 68 (1987) |
| NNA (see 4-(N-Nitrosomethylamino)-4-(3-pyridyl)-1-butanal) | |
| NNK (see 4-(N-Nitrosomethylamino)-1-(3-pyridyl)-1-butanone) | |

| | |
|---|---|
| Nonsteroidal oestrogens (*see also* Oestrogens, progestins and combinations) | *Suppl. 7*, 272 (1987) |
| Noresthisterone (*see also* Progestins; Combined oral contraceptives) | 6, 179 (1974) 21, 461 (1979) |
| Norethynodrel (*see also* Progestins; Combined oral contraceptives) | 6, 191 (1974) 21, 461 (1979) (*corr. 42*, 259) |
| Norgestrel (*see also* Progestins; Combined oral contraceptives) | 6, 201 (1974) 21, 479 (1979) |
| Nylon 6 | 19, 120 (1979) *Suppl. 7*, 68 (1987) |

## O

| | |
|---|---|
| Ochratoxin A | 10, 191 (1976) 31, 191 (1983) (*corr. 42*, 262) *Suppl. 7*, 271 (1987) |
| Oestradiol-17β (*see also* Steroidal oestrogens) | 6, 99 (1974) 21, 279 (1979) |
| Oestradiol 3-benzoate (*see* Oestradiol-17β) | |
| Oestradiol dipropionate (*see* Oestradiol-17β) | |
| Oestradiol mustard | 9, 217 (1975) |
| Oestradiol-17β-valerate (*see* Oestradiol-17β) | |
| Oestriol (*see also* Steroidal oestrogens) | 6, 117 (1974) 21, 327 (1979) |
| Oestrogen-progestin combinations (*see* Oestrogens, progestins and combinations) | |
| Oestrogen-progestin replacement therapy (*see also* Oestrogens, progestins and combinations) | *Suppl. 7*, 308 (1987) |
| Oestrogen replacement therapy (*see also* Oestrogens, progestins and combinations) | *Suppl. 7*, 280 (1987) |
| Oestrogens (*see* Oestrogens, progestins and combinations) | |
| Oestrogens, conjugated (*see* Conjugated oestrogens) | |
| Oestrogens, nonsteroidal (*see* Nonsteroidal oestrogens) | |
| Oestrogens, progestins and combinations | 6 (1974) 21 (1979) *Suppl. 7*, 272 (1987) |
| Oestrogens, steroidal (*see* Steroidal oestrogens) | |
| Oestrone (*see also* Steroidal oestrogens) | 6, 123 (1974) 21, 343 (1979) (*corr. 42*, 259) |
| Oestrone benzoate (*see* Oestrone) | |
| Oil Orange SS | 8, 165 (1975) *Suppl. 7*, 69 (1987) |
| Oral contraceptives, combined (*see* Combined oral contraceptives) | |
| Oral contraceptives, investigational (*see* Combined oral contraceptives) | |
| Oral contraceptives, sequential (*see* Sequential oral contraceptives) | |
| Orange I | 8, 173 (1975) *Suppl. 7*, 69 (1987) |

| | |
|---|---|
| Orange G | 8, 181 (1975) |
| | *Suppl. 7*, 69 (1987) |
| Organolead compounds (*see also* Lead and lead compounds) | *Suppl. 7*, 230 (1987) |
| Oxazepam | 13, 58 (1977) |
| | *Suppl. 7*, 69 (1987) |
| Oxymetholone (*see also* Androgenic (anabolic) steroids) | 13, 131 (1977) |
| Oxyphenbutazone | 13, 185 (1977) |
| | *Suppl. 7*, 69 (1987) |

**P**

| | |
|---|---|
| Panfuran S (*see also* Dihydroxymethylfuratrizine) | 24, 77 (1980) |
| | *Suppl. 7*, 69 (1987) |
| Paper manufacture (*see* Pulp and paper manufacture) | |
| Parasorbic acid | 10, 199 (1976) (*corr. 42*, 255) |
| | *Suppl. 7*, 69 (1987) |
| Parathion | 30, 153 (1983) |
| | *Suppl. 7*, 69 (1987) |
| Patulin | 10, 205 (1976) |
| | 40, 83 (1986) |
| | *Suppl. 7*, 69 (1987) |
| Penicillic acid | 10, 211 (1976) |
| | *Suppl. 7*, 69 (1987) |
| Pentachloroethane | 41, 99 (1986) |
| | *Suppl. 7*, 69 (1987) |
| Pentachloronitrobenzene (*see* Quintozene) | |
| Pentachlorophenol (*see also* Chlorophenols; Chlorophenols, occupational exposures to) | 20, 303 (1979) |
| Perylene | 32, 411 (1983) |
| | *Suppl. 7*, 69 (1987) |
| Petasitenine | 31, 207 (1983) |
| | *Suppl. 7*, 69 (1987) |
| *Petasites japonicus* (*see* Pyrrolizidine alkaloids) | |
| Petroleum refining (occupational exposures in) | 45, 39 (1989) |
| Phenacetin | 3, 141 (1973) |
| | 24, 135 (1980) |
| | *Suppl. 7*, 310 (1987) |
| Phenanthrene | 32, 419 (1983) |
| | *Suppl. 7*, 69 (1987) |
| Phenazopyridine hydrochloride | 8, 117 (1975) |
| | 24, 163 (1980) (*corr. 42*, 260) |
| | *Suppl. 7*, 312 (1987) |
| Phenelzine sulphate | 24, 175 (1980) |
| | *Suppl. 7*, 312 (1987) |
| Phenicarbazide | 12, 177 (1976) |
| | *Suppl. 7*, 70 (1987) |
| Phenobarbital | 13, 157 (1977) |
| | *Suppl. 7*, 313 (1987) |

| | |
|---|---|
| Phenoxyacetic acid herbicides (see Chlorophenoxy herbicides) | |
| Phenoxybenzamine hydrochloride | 9, 223 (1975) |
| | 24, 185 (1980) |
| | Suppl. 7, 70 (1987) |
| Phenylbutazone | 13, 183 (1977) |
| | Suppl. 7, 316 (1987) |
| meta-Phenylenediamine | 16, 111 (1978) |
| | Suppl. 7, 70 (1987) |
| para-Phenylenediamine | 16, 125 (1978) |
| | Suppl. 7, 70 (1987) |
| N-Phenyl-2-naphthylamine | 16, 325 (1978) (corr. 42, 257) |
| | Suppl. 7, 318 (1987) |
| ortho-Phenylphenol | 30, 329 (1983) |
| | Suppl. 7, 70 (1987) |
| Phenytoin | 13, 201 (1977) |
| | Suppl. 7, 319 (1987) |
| Piperazine oestrone sulphate (see Conjugated oestrogens) | |
| Piperonyl butoxide | 30, 183 (1983) |
| | Suppl. 7, 70 (1987) |
| Pitches, coal-tar (see Coal-tar pitches) | |
| Polyacrylic acid | 19, 62 (1979) |
| | Suppl. 7, 70 (1987) |
| Polybrominated biphenyls | 18, 107 (1978) |
| | 41, 261 (1986) |
| | Suppl. 7, 321 (1987) |
| Polychlorinated biphenyls | 7, 261 (1974) |
| | 18, 43 (1978) (corr. 42, 258) |
| | Suppl. 7, 322 (1987) |
| Polychlorinated camphenes (see Toxaphene) | |
| Polychloroprene | 19, 141 (1979) |
| | Suppl. 7, 70 (1987) |
| Polyethylene | 19, 164 (1979) |
| | Suppl. 7, 70 (1987) |
| Polymethylene polyphenyl isocyanate | 19, 314 (1979) |
| | Suppl. 7, 70 (1987) |
| Polymethyl methacrylate | 19, 195 (1979) |
| | Suppl. 7, 70 (1987) |
| Polyoestradiol phosphate (see Oestradiol-17β) | |
| Polypropylene | 19, 218 (1979) |
| | Suppl. 7, 70 (1987) |
| Polystyrene | 19, 245 (1979) |
| | Suppl. 7, 70 (1987) |
| Polytetrafluoroethylene | 19, 288 (1979) |
| | Suppl. 7, 70 (1987) |
| Polyurethane foams | 19, 320 (1979) |
| | Suppl. 7, 70 (1987) |
| Polyvinyl acetate | 19, 346 (1979) |
| | Suppl. 7, 70 (1987) |

| | |
|---|---|
| Polyvinyl alcohol | *19*, 351 (1979) |
| | *Suppl. 7*, 70 (1987) |
| Polyvinyl chloride | *7*, 306 (1974) |
| | *19*, 402 (1979) |
| | *Suppl. 7*, 70 (1987) |
| Polyvinyl pyrrolidone | *19*, 463 (1979) |
| | *Suppl. 7*, 70 (1987) |
| Ponceau MX | *8*, 189 (1975) |
| | *Suppl. 7*, 70 (1987) |
| Ponceau 3R | *8*, 199 (1975) |
| | *Suppl. 7*, 70 (1987) |
| Ponceau SX | *8*, 207 (1975) |
| | *Suppl. 7*, 70 (1987) |
| Potassium arsenate (*see* Arsenic and arsenic compounds) | |
| Potassium arsenite (*see* Arsenic and arsenic compounds) | |
| Potassium bis(2-hydroxyethyl)dithiocarbamate | *12*, 183 (1976) |
| | *Suppl. 7*, 70 (1987) |
| Potassium bromate | *40*, 207 (1986) |
| | *Suppl. 7*, 70 (1987) |
| Potassium chromate (*see* Chromium and chromium compounds) | |
| Potassium dichromate (*see* Chromium and chromium compounds) | |
| Prednisone | *26*, 293 (1981) |
| | *Suppl. 7*, 326 (1987) |
| Procarbazine hydrochloride | *26*, 311 (1981) |
| | *Suppl. 7*, 327 (1987) |
| Proflavine salts | *24*, 195 (1980) |
| | *Suppl. 7*, 70 (1987) |
| Progesterone (*see also* Progestins; Combined oral contraceptives | *6*, 135 (1974) |
| | *21*, 491 (1979) (*corr. 42*, 259) |
| Progestins (*see also* Oestrogens, progestins and combinations) | *Suppl. 7*, 289 (1987) |
| Pronetalol hydrochloride | *13*, 227 (1977) (*corr. 42*, 256) |
| | *Suppl. 7*, 70 (1987) |
| 1,3-Propane sultone | *4*, 253 (1974) (*corr. 42*, 253) |
| | *Suppl. 7*, 70 (1987) |
| Propham | *12*, 189 (1976) |
| | *Suppl. 7*, 70 (1987) |
| β-Propiolactone | *4*, 259 (1974) (*corr. 42*, 253) |
| | *Suppl. 7*, 70 (1987) |
| *n*-Propyl carbamate | *12*, 201 (1976) |
| | *Suppl. 7*, 70 (1987) |
| Propylene | *19*, 213 (1979) |
| | *Suppl. 7*, 71 (1987) |
| Propylene oxide | *11*, 191 (1976) |
| | *36*, 227 (1985) (*corr. 42*, 263) |
| | *Suppl. 7*, 328 (1987) |
| Propylthiouracil | *7*, 67 (1974) |
| | *Suppl. 7*, 329 (1987) |

| | |
|---|---|
| Ptaquiloside (*see also* Bracken fern) | *40*, 55 (1986) |
| | *Suppl. 7*, 71 (1987) |
| Pulp and paper manufacture | *25*, 157 (1981) |
| | *Suppl. 7*, 385 (1987) |
| Pyrene | *32*, 431 (1983) |
| | *Suppl. 7*, 71 (1987) |
| Pyrido[3,4-*c*]psoralen | *40*, 349 (1986) |
| | *Suppl. 7*, 71 (1987) |
| Pyrimethamine | *13*, 233 (1977) |
| | *Suppl. 7*, 71 (1987) |
| Pyrrolizidine alkaloids (*see also* Hydroxysenkirkine; Isatidine; Jacobine; Lasiocarpine; Monocrotaline; Retrorsine; Riddelline; Seneciphylline; Senkirkine) | *10*, 333 (1976) |

## Q

| | |
|---|---|
| Quercetin (*see also* Bracken fern) | *31*, 213 (1983) |
| | *Suppl. 7*, 71 (1987) |
| *para*-Quinone | *15*, 255 (1977) |
| | *Suppl. 7*, 71 (1987) |
| Quintozene | *5*, 211 (1974) |
| | *Suppl. 7*, 71 (1987) |

## R

| | |
|---|---|
| Radon | *43*, 173 (1988) (*corr. 45*, 283) |
| Reserpine | *10*, 217 (1976) |
| | *24*, 211 (1980) (*corr. 42*, 260) |
| | *Suppl. 7*, 330 (1987) |
| Resorcinol | *15*, 155 (1977) |
| | *Suppl. 7*, 71 (1987) |
| Retrorsine | *10*, 303 (1976) |
| | *Suppl. 7*, 71 (1987) |
| Rhodamine B | *16*, 221 (1978) |
| | *Suppl. 7*, 71 (1987) |
| Rhodamine 6G | *16*, 233 (1978) |
| | *Suppl. 7*, 71 (1987) |
| Riddelliine | *10*, 313 (1976) |
| | *Suppl. 7*, 71 (1987) |
| Rifampicin | *24*, 243 (1980) |
| | *Suppl. 7*, 71 (1987) |
| Rockwool (*see* Man-made mineral fibres) | |
| The rubber industry | *28* (1982) (*corr. 42*, 261) |
| | *Suppl. 7*, 332 (1987) |
| Rugulosin | *40*, 99 (1986) |
| | *Suppl. 7*, 71 (1987) |

## S

| | |
|---|---|
| Saccharated iron oxide | *2*, 161 (1973) |
| | *Suppl. 7*, 71 (1987) |

Saccharin                                                         22, 111 (1980) (corr. 42, 259)
                                                                  Suppl. 7, 334 (1987)
Safrole                                                           1, 169 (1972)
                                                                  10, 231 (1976)
                                                                  Suppl. 7, 71 (1987)
The sawmill industry (including logging) (see The lumber and
    sawmill industry (including logging))
Scarlet Red                                                       8, 217 (1975)
                                                                  Suppl. 7, 71 (1987)
Selenium and selenium compounds                                   9, 245 (1975) (corr. 42, 255)
                                                                  Suppl. 7, 71 (1987)
Selenium dioxide (see Selenium and selenium compounds)
Selenium oxide (see Selenium and selenium compounds)
Semicarbazide hydrochloride                                       12, 209 (1976) (corr. 42, 256)
                                                                  Suppl. 7, 71 (1987)
Senecio jacobaea L. (see Pyrrolizidine alkaloids)
Senecio longilobus (see Pyrrolizidine alkaloids)
Seneciphylline                                                    10, 319, 335 (1976)
                                                                  Suppl. 7, 71 (1987)
Senkirkine                                                        10, 327 (1976)
                                                                  31, 231 (1983)
                                                                  Suppl. 7, 71 (1987)
Sepiolite                                                         42, 175 (1987)
                                                                  Suppl. 7, 71 (1987)
Sequential oral contraceptives (see also Oestrogens, progestins   Suppl. 7, 296 (1987)
    and combinations)
Shale-oils                                                        35, 161 (1985)
                                                                  Suppl. 7, 339 (1987)
Shikimic acid (see also Bracken fern)                             40, 55 (1986)
                                                                  Suppl. 7, 71 (1987)
Shoe manufacture and repair (see Boot and shoe manufacture
    and repair)
Silica (see also Amorphous silica; Crystalline silica)            42, 39 (1987)
Slagwool (see Man-made mineral fibres)
Sodium arsenate (see Arsenic and arsenic compounds)
Sodium arsenite (see Arsenic and arsenic compounds)
Sodium cacodylate (see Arsenic and arsenic compounds)
Sodium chromate (see Chromium and chromium compounds)
Sodium cyclamate (see Cyclamates)
Sodium dichromate (see Chromium and chromium compounds)
Sodium diethyldithiocarbamate                                     12, 217 (1976)
                                                                  Suppl. 7, 71 (1987)
Sodium equilin sulphate (see Conjugated oestrogens)
Sodium fluoride (see Fluorides)
Sodium monofluorophosphate (see Fluorides)
Sodium oestrone sulphate (see Conjugated oestrogens)
Sodium ortho-phenylphenate (see also ortho-Phenylphenol)          30, 329 (1983)
                                                                  Suppl. 7, 392 (1987)

Sodium saccharin (*see* Saccharin)
Sodium selenate (*see* Selenium and selenium compounds)
Sodium selenite (*see* Selenium and selenium compounds)
Sodium silicofluoride (*see* Fluorides)
Soots — *3*, 22 (1973); *35*, 219 (1985); *Suppl. 7*, 343 (1987)
Spironolactone — *24*, 259 (1980); *Suppl. 7*, 344 (1987)
Stannous fluoride (*see* Fluorides)
Steel founding (*see* Iron and steel founding)
Sterigmatocystin — *1*, 175 (1972); *10*, 245 (1976); *Suppl. 7*, 72 (1987)
Steroidal oestrogens (*see also* Oestrogens, progestins and combinations) — *Suppl. 7*, 280 (1987)
Streptozotocin — *4*, 221 (1974); *17*, 337 (1978); *Suppl. 7*, 72 (1987)
Strobane® (*see* Terpene polychlorinates)
Strontium chromate (*see* Chromium and chromium compounds)
Styrene — *19*, 231 (1979) (*corr. 42*, 258); *Suppl. 7*, 345 (1987)
Styrene-acrylonitrile copolymers — *19*, 97 (1979); *Suppl. 7*, 72 (1987)
Styrene-butadiene copolymers — *19*, 252 (1979); *Suppl. 7*, 72 (1987)
Styrene oxide — *11*, 201 (1976); *19*, 275 (1979); *36*, 245 (1985); *Suppl. 7*, 72 (1987)
Succinic anhydride — *15*, 265 (1977); *Suppl. 7*, 72 (1987)
Sudan I — *8*, 225 (1975); *Suppl. 7*, 72 (1987)
Sudan II — *8*, 233 (1975); *Suppl. 7*, 72 (1987)
Sudan III — *8*, 241 (1975); *Suppl. 7*, 72 (1987)
Sudan Brown RR — *8*, 249 (1975); *Suppl. 7*, 72 (1987)
Sudan Red 7B — *8*, 253 (1975); *Suppl. 7*, 72 (1987)
Sulfafurazole — *24*, 275 (1980); *Suppl. 7*, 347 (1987)
Sulfallate — *30*, 283 (1983); *Suppl. 7*, 72 (1987)

Sulfamethoxazole                                              24, 285 (1980)
                                                              Suppl. 7, 348 (1987)

Sulphisoxazole (see Sulfafurazole)
Sulphur mustard (see Mustard gas)
Sunset Yellow FCF                                             8, 257 (1975)
                                                              Suppl. 7, 72 (1987)
Symphytine                                                    31, 239 (1983)
                                                              Suppl. 7, 72 (1987)


T

2,4,5-T (see also Chlorophenoxy herbicides; Chlorophenoxy     15, 273 (1977)
    herbicides, occupational exposures to)
Talc                                                          42, 185 (1987)
                                                              Suppl. 7, 349 (1987)
Tannic acid                                                   10, 253 (1976) (corr. 42, 255)
                                                              Suppl. 7, 72 (1987)
Tannins (see also Tannic acid)                                10, 254 (1976)
                                                              Suppl. 7, 72 (1987)
TCDD (see 2,3,7,8-Tetrachlorodibenzo-para-dioxin)
TDE (see DDT)
Terpene polychlorinates                                       5, 219 (1974)
                                                              Suppl. 7, 72 (1987)
Testosterone (see also Androgenic (anabolic) steroids)        6, 209 (1974)
                                                              21, 519 (1979)

Testosterone oenanthate (see Testosterone)
Testosterone propionate (see Testosterone)
2,2',5,5'-Tetrachlorobenzidine                                27, 141 (1982)
                                                              Suppl. 7, 72 (1987)
2,3,7,8-Tetrachlorodibenzo-para-dioxin                        15, 41 (1977)
                                                              Suppl. 7, 350 (1987)
1,1,1,2-Tetrachloroethane                                     41, 87 (1986)
                                                              Suppl. 7, 72 (1987)
1,1,2,2-Tetrachloroethane                                     20, 477 (1979)
                                                              Suppl. 7, 354 (1987)
Tetrachloroethylene                                           20, 491 (1979)
                                                              Suppl. 7, 355 (1987)
2,3,4,6-Tetrachlorophenol (see Chlorophenols; Chlorophenols,
    occupational exposure to)
Tetrachlorvinphos                                             30, 197 (1983)
                                                              Suppl. 7, 72 (1987)
Tetraethyllead (see Lead and lead compounds)
Tetrafluoroethylene                                           19, 285 (1979)
                                                              Suppl. 7, 72 (1987)
Tetramethyllead (see Lead and lead compounds)
Thioacetamide                                                 7, 77 (1974)
                                                              Suppl. 7, 72 (1987)

| | |
|---|---|
| 4,4'-Thiodianiline | *16*, 343 (1978) |
| | *27*, 147 (1982) |
| | *Suppl. 7*, 72 (1987) |
| Thiotepa (*see* Tris(1-aziridinyl)phosphine sulphide) | |
| Thiouracil | *7*, 85 (1974) |
| | *Suppl. 7*, 72 (1987) |
| Thiourea | *7*, 95 (1974) |
| | *Suppl. 7*, 72 (1987) |
| Thiram | *12*, 225 (1976) |
| | *Suppl. 7*, 72 (1987) |
| Tobacco habits other than smoking (*see* Tobacco products, smokeless) | |
| Tobacco products, smokeless | *37* (1985) (*corr. 42*, 263) |
| | *Suppl. 7*, 357 (1987) |
| Tobacco smoke | *38* (1986) (*corr. 42*, 263) |
| | *Suppl. 7*, 357 (1987) |
| Tobacco smoking (*see* Tobacco smoke) | |
| *ortho*-Tolidine (*see* 3,3'-Dimethylbenzidine) | |
| 2,4-Toluene diisocyanate (*see also* Toluene diisocyanates) | *19*, 303 (1979) |
| | *39*, 287 (1986) |
| 2,6-Toluene diisocyanate (*see also* Toluene diisocyanates) | *19*, 303 (1979) |
| | *39*, 289 (1986) |
| Toluene diisocyanates | *39*, 287 (1986) (*corr. 42*, 264) |
| | *Suppl. 7*, 72 (1987) |
| Toluenes, α-chlorinated (*see* α-Chlorinated toluenes) | |
| *ortho*-Toluenesulphonamide (*see* Saccharin) | |
| *ortho*-Toluidine | *16*, 349 (1978) |
| | *27*, 155 (1982) |
| | *Suppl. 7*, 362 (1987) |
| Toxaphene | *20*, 327 (1979) |
| | *Suppl. 7*, 72 (1987) |
| Tremolite (*see* Asbestos) | |
| Treosulphan | *26*, 341 (1981) |
| | *Suppl. 7*, 363 (1987) |
| Triaziquone (see Tris(aziridinyl)-*para*-benzoquinone)) | |
| Trichlorfon | *30*, 207 (1983) |
| | *Suppl. 7*, 73 (1987) |
| 1,1,1-Trichloroethane | *20*, 515 (1979) |
| | *Suppl. 7*, 73 (1987) |
| 1,1,2-Trichloroethane | *20*, 533 (1979) |
| | *Suppl. 7*, 73 (1987) |
| Trichloroethylene | *11*, 263 (1976) |
| | *20*, 545 (1979) |
| | *Suppl. 7*, 364 (1987) |
| 2,4,5-Trichlorophenol (*see also* Chlorophenols; Chlorophenols, occupational exposure to) | *20*, 349 (1979) |

2,4,6-Trichlorophenol (*see also* Chlorophenols; Chlorophenols, occupational exposures to)    *20*, 349 (1979)

(2,4,5-Trichlorophenoxy)acetic acid (*see* 2,4,5-T)

Trichlorotriethylamine hydrochloride    *9*, 229 (1975)
*Suppl. 7*, 73 (1987)

$T_2$-Trichothecene    *31*, 265 (1983)
*Suppl. 7*, 73 (1987)

Triethylene glycol diglycidyl ether    *11*, 209 (1976)
*Suppl. 7*, 73 (1987)

4,4',6-Trimethylangelicin plus ultraviolet radiation (*see also* Angelicin and some synthetic derivatives)    *Suppl. 7*, 57 (1987)

2,4,5-Trimethylaniline    *27*, 177 (1982)
*Suppl. 7*, 73 (1987)

2,4,6-Trimethylaniline    *27*, 178 (1982)
*Suppl. 7*, 73 (1987)

4,5',8-Trimethylpsoralen    *40*, 357 (1986)
*Suppl. 7*, 366 (1987)

Triphenylene    *32*, 447 (1983)
*Suppl. 7*, 73 (1987)

Tris(aziridinyl)-*para*-benzoquinone    *9*, 67 (1975)
*Suppl. 7*, 367 (1987)

Tris(1-aziridinyl)phosphine oxide    *9*, 75 (1975)
*Suppl. 7*, 73 (1987)

Tris(1-aziridinyl)phosphine sulphide    *9*, 85 (1975)
*Suppl. 7*, 368 (1987)

2,4,6-Tris(1-aziridinyl)-*s*-triazine    *9*, 95 (1975)
*Suppl. 7*, 73 (1987)

1,2,3-Tris(chloromethoxy)propane    *15*, 301 (1977)
*Suppl. 7*, 73 (1987)

Tris(2,3-dibromopropyl) phosphate    *20*, 575 (1979)
*Suppl. 7*, 369 (1987)

Tris(2-methyl-1-aziridinyl)phosphine oxide    *9*, 107 (1975)
*Suppl. 7*, 73 (1987)

Trp-P-1    *31*, 247 (1983)
*Suppl. 7*, 73 (1987)

Trp-P-2    *31*, 255 (1983)
*Suppl. 7*, 73 (1987)

Trypan blue    *8*, 267 (1975)
*Suppl. 7*, 73 (1987)

*Tussilago farfara* L. (*see* Pyrrolizidine alkaloids)

# U

Ultraviolet radiation    *40*, 379 (1986)

Underground haematite mining with exposure to radon    *1*, 29 (1972)
*Suppl. 7*, 216 (1987)

Uracil mustard    *9*, 235 (1975)
*Suppl. 7*, 370 (1987)

| | |
|---|---|
| Urethane | 7, 111 (1974) |
| | *Suppl. 7*, 73 (1987) |

## V

| | |
|---|---|
| Vinblastine sulphate | *26*, 349 (1981) (*corr. 42*, 261) |
| | *Suppl. 7*, 371 (1987) |
| Vincristine sulphate | *26*, 365 (1981) |
| | *Suppl. 7*, 372 (1987) |
| Vinyl acetate | *19*, 341 (1979) |
| | *39*, 113 (1986) |
| | *Suppl. 7*, 73 (1987) |
| Vinyl bromide | *19*, 367 (1979) |
| | *39*, 133 (1986) |
| | *Suppl. 7*, 73 (1987) |
| Vinyl chloride | 7, 291 (1974) |
| | *19*, 377 (1979) (*corr. 42*, 258) |
| | *Suppl. 7*, 373 (1987) |
| Vinyl chloride-vinyl acetate copolymers | 7, 311 (1976) |
| | *19*, 412 (1979) (*corr. 42*, 258) |
| | *Suppl. 7*, 73 (1987) |
| 4-Vinylcyclohexene | *11*, 277 (1976) |
| | *39*, 181 (1986) |
| | *Suppl. 7*, 73 (1987) |
| Vinyl fluoride | *39*, 147 (1986) |
| | *Suppl. 7*, 73 (1987) |
| Vinylidene chloride | *19*, 439 (1979) |
| | *39*, 195 (1986) |
| | *Suppl. 7*, 376 (1987) |
| Vinylidene chloride-vinyl chloride copolymers | *19*, 448 (1979) (*corr. 42*, 258) |
| | *Suppl. 7*, 73 (1987) |
| Vinylidene fluoride | *39*, 227 (1986) |
| | *Suppl. 7*, 73 (1987) |
| *N*-Vinyl-2-pyrrolidone | *19*, 461 (1979) |
| | *Suppl. 7*, 73 (1987) |

## W

| | |
|---|---|
| Wollastonite | *42*, 145 (1987) |
| | *Suppl. 7*, 377 (1987) |
| Wood industries | *25* (1981) |
| | *Suppl. 7*, 378 (1987) |

## X

| | |
|---|---|
| 2,4-Xylidine | *16*, 367 (1978) |
| | *Suppl. 7*, 74 (1987) |
| 2,5-Xylidine | *16*, 377 (1978) |
| | *Suppl. 7*, 74 (1987) |

## Y

Yellow AB                                                     *8*, 279 (1975)
                                                              *Suppl. 7*, 74 (1987)
Yellow OB                                                     *8*, 287 (1975)
                                                              *Suppl. 7*, 74 (1987)

## Z

Zearalenone                                                   *31*, 279 (1983)
                                                              *Suppl. 7*, 74 (1987)
Zectran                                                       *12*, 237 (1976)
                                                              *Suppl. 7*, 74 (1987)
Zinc beryllium silicate (*see* Beryllium and beryllium compounds)
Zinc chromate (*see* Chromium and chromium compounds)
Zinc chromate hydroxide (*see* Chromium and chromium
  compounds)
Zinc potassium chromate (*see* Chromium and chromium
  compounds)
Zinc yellow (*see* Chromium and chromium compounds)
Zineb                                                         *12*, 245 (1976)
                                                              *Suppl. 7*, 74 (1987)
Ziram                                                         *12*, 259 (1976)
                                                              *Suppl. 7*, 74 (1987)